FOOD ALLERGY:
ADVERSE REACTIONS TO
FOODS AND FOOD ADDITIVES
Second Edition

Blackwell Science
Editorial Offices:
238 Main Street, Cambridge, Massachusetts 02142, USA
Osney Mead, Oxford OX2 0E1, England
25 John Street, London WC1N 2BL, England
23 Ainslie Place, Edinburgh EH3 6AJ, Scotland
54 University Street, Carlton, Victoria 3053, Australia

Other Editorial Offices:
Arnette Blackwell SA, 224, Boulevard Saint Germain, 75007 Paris, France
Blackwell Wissenschafts-Verlag GmbH Kurfürstendamm 57, 10707 Berlin, Germany
Zehetnergasse 6, A-1140 Vienna, Austria

Distributors:
USA
  Blackwell Science, Inc.
  238 Main Street
  Cambridge, Massachusetts 02142
  (Telephone orders: 800-215-1000 or 617-876-7000; Fax orders: 617-492-5263)
Canada
  Copp Clark Professional
  200 Adelaide Street, West, 3rd Floor
  Toronto, Ontario M5H 1W7
  (Telephone orders: 416-597-1616, 1-800-815-9417
  fax: 416-597-1617)
Australia
  Blackwell Science Pty., Ltd.
  54 University Street
  Carlton, Victoria 3053
  (Telephone orders: 03-9347-0300; fax orders 03-9349-3016)
Outside North America and Australia
  Blackwell Science, Ltd.
  c/o Marston Book Services, Ltd.
  P.O. Box 269
  Abingdon
  Oxon OX14 4YN
  England
(Telephone orders: 44-01235-465500; fax orders 44-01235-465555)

Acquisitions: Chris Davis
Production: Ellen Samia
Typeset, printed and bound by Maple-Vail

© 1997 by Blackwell Science, Inc.

Printed in the United States of America

97 98 99 5 4 3 2 1

Library of Congress Cataloging-in-Publication Data

Food allergy : adverse reactions to foods and food additives / [edited by] Dean D. Metcalfe, Hugh A. Sampson, Ronald A. Simon.—2nd ed.
p.   cm.
Includes bibliographical reference and index.
ISBN 0-86542-432-2 (alk. paper)
1. Food allergy. 2. Food additives—Health aspects.
I. Metcalfe, Dean D.   II. Sampson, Hugh A.   III. Simon, Ronald A.
[DNLM: 1. Food Hypersensitivity. 2. Food Hypersensitivity—
immunology. 3. Food Additives—adverse effects.   WD 310 F68567
1996]
RC596.F6543   1996
616.97′5—dc20
DNLM/DLC
for Library of Congress   96-43618
                                                                   CIP
Dr. Metcalfe's work as an editor and author was performed outside of the scope of his work as a U.S. government employee.

FOOD ALLERGY: ADVERSE REACTIONS TO FOODS AND FOOD ADDITIVES

Second Edition

Edited by

Dean D. Metcalfe, MD

Chief, Laboratory of Allergic Diseases
National Institute of Allergy and Infectious Diseases
National Institutes of Health
Bethesda, Maryland

Hugh A. Sampson, MD

Director, Pediatric Clinical Research Center
Professor of Pediatrics
Johns Hopkins University School of Medicine
Baltimore, Maryland

Ronald A. Simon, MD

Head, Division of Allergy, Asthma, and Immunology
Scripps Clinic and Research Foundation
La Jolla, California

Blackwell Science

CONTENTS

v

Part 3: Adverse Reactions to Food Additives

Part 4: Contemporary Topics in Adverse Reactions to Foods

CONTRIBUTORS

James D. Astwood, PhD
Post-doctoral Associate
Monsanto Company
St. Louis, Missouri

Fred M. Atkins, MD
National Jewish Center for Immunology and
    Respiratory Medicine
Department of Pediatrics
Denver, Colorado

Sami L. Bahna, MD
MPH Professor of Pediatrics and Medicine
University of South Florida
Co-Director, Allergy and Immunology Program
All Children's Hospital
St. Petersburg, Florida

James L. Baldwin, MD
Clinical Assistant Professor
Department of Internal Medicine
Allergy Division
University of Michigan Medical School
Ann Arbor, Michigan

Kim E. Barrett, PhD
Associate Professor of Medicine
Divisions of Allergy/Immunology and Gastroen-
    terology
University of California, San Diego
School of Medicine
San Diego, California

Carsten Bindslev-Jensen, MD, PhD, DSc
Department of Dermatology
Odense University Hospital
Odense, Denmark

Bengt Bjorksten, MD
Department of Pediatrics
University Hospital
Linkoping, Sweden

S. Allan Bock, MD
Clinical Professor
Department of Pediatrics
University of Colorado Health Sciences Center
Staff Physician
Department of Pediatrics
National Jewish Center for Immunology and
    Respiratory Medicine
Denver, Colorado

John V. Bosso, MD
Allergy and Asthma Consultants of Rockland
    and Bergin
West Nyack, New York

Jean Bousquet, MD
Clinique des Maladies Respiratoires
Centre Hospitalier Universitaire
Montpellier, France

A. Wesley Burks, MD
Associate Professor of Pediatrics
Children's Hospital
Little Rock, Arkansas

Robert K. Bush, MD
Professor of Medicine
University of Wisconsin
Madison, Wisconsin

Pascal Chañez, MD
Clinical Professor of Medicine
University of Rochester
Rochester, New York

John J. Condemi, MD
Clinical Professor of Medicine
University of Rochester
Rochester, New York

Anne Ferguson, MD, FRCP, FRCPath
Professor of Gastroenterology
University of Edinburgh
Edinburgh, United Kingdom

Roy L. Fuchs
Director of Regulatory Science
Monsanto-Ceregen
St. Louis, Missouri

David J. Hill, MD, FRACP
Department of Allergy
Royal Children's Hospital
Melbourne, Australia

Clifford S. Hosking, MD, FRACP, FRCPA
Department of Allergy
Royal Children's Hospital
Melbourne, Australia

Steffen Husby, MD, DSc
Department of Pediatrics
Arhus University Hospital
Arhus, Denmark

Donald W. Jacobsen, PhD
Department of Cell Biology/Clinical Pathology
Cleveland Clinic Foundation
Cleveland, Ohio

Celide Barnes Koerner, PhD
Johns Hopkins University School of Medicine
Baltimore, Maryland

N.-I. Max Kjellman, MD
Department of Pediatrics
University Hospital
Linkoping, Sweden

Alan M. Lake, MD
Associate Professor of Pediatrics
Johns Hopkins School of Medicine
Baltimore, Maryland

Paul B. Lavrik, PhD
Research Scientist
Regulatory Science
Monsanto-Ceregen
St. Louis, Missouri

Samuel B. Lehrer, PhD
Research Professor of Medicine
Section of Clinical Immunology and Allergy
Tulane University School of Medicine
New Orleans, Louisiana

Dean D. Metcalfe, MD
Head, Mast Cell Physiology Section
Laboratory of Clinical Investigation
National Institute of Allergy and Infectious Diseases
National Institutes of Health
Bethesda, Maryland

François-B. Michel, MD
Professor Respiratory Diseases
University Medical School
Head of Department, Respiratory Diseases
Clinique des Maladies Respiratoires
Hôpital Arnaud de Villeneuve
Montpellier, France

Kyung-Up Min, MD
Department of Internal Medicine
College of Medicine
Seoul National University
Seoul, Korea

Anne Muñoz-Furlong
Publisher of Food Allergy News
Founder of Food Allergy Network
Fairfax, Virginia

M. Stephen Murphy, MD
Senior Lecturer in Pediatrics and Child Health
The University of Birmingham
Institute of Child Health
Birmingham, United Kingdon

Julie A. Nordlee, MS
Research Analyst

Department of Food Science and Technology
University of Nebraska
Lincoln, Nebraska

Carol E. O'Neil, PhD, MPH
Department of Medicine
Section of Clinical Immunology
Tulane University School of Medicine
New Orleans, Louisiana

Claudio Ortolani, MD
Head, Department of Allergy and the "Bizzozero" Internal Medicine Division
Niguarda Hospital
Milan, Italy

Richard S. Panush, MD
Professor and Chair
Department of Medicine
St. Barnabus Medical Center
Livingston, New Jersey

Elide Anna Pastorello, MD
Associate Professor of Clinical Methodology
Department of Internal Diseases
University of Milan
Milan, Italy

Lars K. Poulsen, MSc, PhD
Associate Professor, University of Copenhagen
Head of Laboratory
Laboratory of Medical Allergology
Allergy Unit
National University Hospital
Copenhagen, Denmark

Hugh A. Sampson, MD
Professor of Pediatrics
Johns Hopkins School of Medicine
Baltimore, Maryland

Alan L. Schocket, MD, MSHA
Staff Physician
National Jewish Center for Immunology and Respiratory Medicine
Medical Director

Qual Med
Denver, Colorado

Howard J. Schwartz, MD
Clinical Professor of Medicine
Case Western Reserve University School of Medicine
Associate Physician
Department of Medicine
University Hospital
Cleveland, Ohio

John C. Selner, MD
Allergy Respiratory Institute of Colorado
Denver, Colorado

Ronald A. Simon, MD
Head, Division of Allergy and Immunology
Scripps Clinic and Research Foundation Medical Group
La Jolla, California

Laurie J. Smith, MD
Associate Professor
Medicine and Pediatrics
Uniformed Services University of the Health Sciences Center
Assistant Chief
Allergy Clinical Immunology Service
Walter Reed Army Center
Washington, District of Colombia

Herman Staudenmayer, MD
Allergy Respiratory Institute of Colorado
Denver, Colorado

Donald D. Stevenson, MD
Senior Consultant
Division of Allergy, Asthma, and Immunology
Scripps Clinic and Research Foundation
La Jolla, California

Stephan Strobel, MD, PhD, FRCP
Professor
Division of Cell and Molecular Biology
Institute of Child Health
London, United Kingdom

Steve L. Taylor, PhD
Professor and Head
Department of Food Science and Technology
University of Nebraska
Lincoln, Nebraska

Stephen A. Tilles, MD
Assistant Professor
Division of Allergy and Clinical Immunology
Oregon Health Sciences University
Portland, Oregon

T. Ray Vaughn, MD
Austin Allergy Associates
Austin, Texas

W. Allan Walker, MD
Conrad Taff Professor of Nutrition and Pediat-
   rics
Harvard Medical School
Chief, Combined Program in Pediatric Gastroen-
   terology and Nutrition
Children's Hospital
Boston, Massachusetts

John O. Warner, MD, FRCP, DCH
Professor of Child Health
University of Southampton
Child Health
Southampton General Hospital
Southampton, United Kingdom

Richard W. Weber, MD
Associate Faculty Member
National Jewish Center for Immunology and
   Respiratory Medicine
Denver, Colorado

Katharine M. Woessner
Senior Fellow
Division of Allergy, Asthma, and
Immunology
Scripps Clinic and Research Foundation
La Jolla, California

John W. Yunginger, MD
Professor of Pediatrics
Mayo Medical School
Consultant in Pediatrics and Internal Medicine
Mayo Clinic and Foundation
Rochester, Minnesota

PREFACE

*I*t is the pleasure of the editors to present the 2nd Edition of Food Allergy: Adverse Reactions to Food and Food Additives. As in the 1st Edition, we have attempted to create a book that in one volume would cover pediatric and adult adverse reactions to foods and food additives, stress efforts to place adverse reactions to foods and food additives on a sound and scientific basis, select authors to present subjects on the basis of their acknowledged expertise and reputation, and reference each contribution thoroughly. The growth in knowledge in this area since the previous edition has been gratifying, and is reflected in the increased length of this edition. Again, this book is directed toward clinicians, nutritionists, and scientists interested in food reactions, but we also hope that others interested in such reactions will find the book to be a valuable resource.

The text is divided into a review of food allergy (adverse reactions to food antigens), adverse reactions to food additives, and contemporary topics. The number of chapters addressing these areas have been increased from twenty-nine chapters in the 1st Edition to thirty-eight chapters in the 2nd Edition. Basic science begins with overview chapters on immunology of particular relevance to the gastrointestinal tract as a target organ in allergic reactions and the properties that govern reactions initiated at this site. Antigen absorption is reviewed as a unique event in gastrointestinal function. Two new chapters have been added: first, a chapter on food biotechnology and genetic engineering and issues in allergic diseases, and second, a chapter on oral tolerance, an area of significant interest to developing new strategies to treat allergic diseases.

The section on clinical adverse reactions to foods now begins with separate overview chapters on immediate reactions to foods in infants and children as well as in adults, and then presents chapters dealing with distinct clinicopathologic entities (eczema, urticaria, respiratory diseases, anaphylaxis, gluten-sensitive enteropathy, exercise and pressure-induced syndromes, and occupational reactions to food allergens). New chapters have been added addressing the oral allergy syndrome, and infantile colic and food hypersensitivity.

Adverse reactions to food additives are covered as a separate division. Chapters address specific additive sensitivities, including those to sulfites, monosodium glutamate, tartrazine, benzoates, and parabens. A new chapter has been added on adverse reactions to BHA and BHT.

The final division of the book is contemporary topics in adverse reactions to foods. This includes discussions of the pharmacologic properties of foods, the history and prevention of food allergy, diets and nutrition, neurologic reactions to foods and food additives, psychiatry and adverse reactions to foods, connective tissue and inflammatory bowel disease, and a review of unproven diagnostic and therapeutic techniques. New chapters have been added on the management of food allergy, on food toxicology, and on behavior and adverse food reactions.

Each of the chapters in this book is capable of standing alone, but when placed together present a mosaic of the ideas and research in adverse reactions to foods and food additives. Overlap is again unavoidable, but held to a minimum. Ideas of one author may sometimes differ from those of another, but in general there is remarkable consistency from chapter to chapter. We the editors thus present the 2nd

Edition of a book that we believe represents a fair, balanced, and a defensible review of adverse reactions to foods and food additives. The 2nd Edition is the end product of the coordinated effort of three editors and fifty authors from nine countries, designed to again summarize the best of the thought and research on adverse reactions to foods and food additives.

Dean D. Metcalfe
Hugh A. Sampson
Ronald A. Simon

Part One

ADVERSE REACTIONS TO FOOD ANTIGENS: BASIC SCIENCE

MUCOSAL IMMUNITY

Steffen Husby

Introduction

Mucosal membranes are daily brought into contact with innumerable food and microbial structures that are recognized by the mucosal immune system. An understanding of normal mucosal immune reactions in the gastrointestinal tract is relevant to the study of food allergy, which is broadly defined as an abnormal reaction of the immune system to dietary antigens. Furthermore, the mucosal immune system may be involved in the allergic reaction itself as one of the main target organs, in addition to the skin and the lungs.

The mucous membranes contain vital defense systems to combat microorganisms, and a unique organization has evolved in the mucosal immune system in comparison with the systemic immune system. Despite anatomical differences between the diverse mucosal surfaces of the gastrointestinal tract, the lungs, the oral cavity and the associated salivary glands, the mammary glands, and the genitourinary tract, the defense systems of these organs bear striking similarities. The concept of a common mucosal immune system was put forth almost two decades ago (1), and experimental data support the existence of a common mucosal immune system in humans (2). The term "common mucosal immune system" or "mucosal-associated lymphoid tissue (MALT)" emphasizes the trafficking of cells within the mucosal immune system, although quantitative differences and certain regional preferences do exist between the different organs.

Historically, the study of mucosal immunity began with Besredka's studies of dysentery in rabbits that were protected after oral immunization (3) and the observation that antibodies could be identified in the feces of patients with dysentery before the antibodies could be detected in their blood (4). The discovery of IgA in 1953 (Heremans) and the demonstration of secretory IgA in the early 1960s (5, 6) initiated a detailed characterization of the mucosal immune system.

The significance of the mucosal immune system for the development of food allergy was recognized in the original description of passive cutaneous anaphylaxis by Prausnitz and Küstner (7), who described Küstner's allergy to fish. The absorption of dietary antigens and the development of food allergy was further discussed in several papers at that time (8, 9). Gruskay and Cooke (10) demonstrated ovalbumin-derived antigen in the blood of children given crystalline ovalbumin by mouth. Children recovering from acute diarrhea had higher levels of ovalbumin in their blood than did controls.

This chapter will concentrate on the immune system of the gastrointestinal tract; in addition, it will describe the structure of the local immune system and the process by which it normally recognizes and handles innocuous dietary antigens, versus potentially harmful microorganisms. A wealth of information on this subject has been derived from animal experiments. Where possible, data obtained in humans with more immediate relevance to the clinical situation will be emphasized. The best-studied disorders with regard to intestinal immunology and inflammation are the inflammatory bowel diseases and the enteropathies, which will be mentioned where appropriate. Two basic areas of particular importance in food allergy—antigen uptake and oral tolerance—will be covered in greater detail in chapters 5 and 6, respectively.

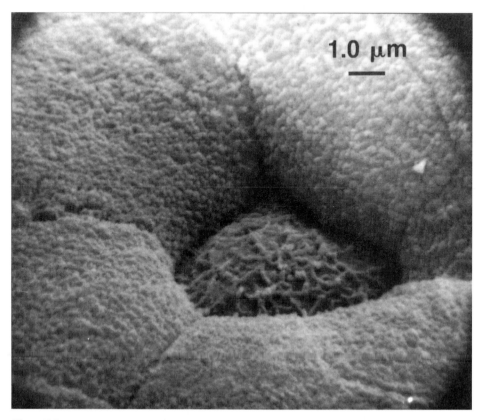

Figure 1.1

Scanning electron micrograph of the surface of a human Peyer's patch with an M cell in the center. From: Kato T, Owen RL. Structure and function of intestinal mucosal epithelium. Handbook of Mucosal Immunology. San Diego: Academic Press, 1994. Used with permission.

Anatomy of Gut-Associated Lymphoid Tissue (GALT)

The gastrointestinal tract in the human consists of a surface area of 200–300 m^2, covered with a one-cell-thick layer known as the intestinal absorptive epithelium. The epithelium of the small intestine is structured within crypts and villi. Epithelial cells, called enterocytes, divide within the crypts and pass upward to the tip of the villi, where they are shed. Although the epithelium contains predominantly epithelial cells, it also includes goblet cells, Paneth cells, and several other cell types. Lymphoid cells are also present throughout the entire length of the gastrointestinal tract; they may constitute as much as 20% of the total cell numbers.

The lymphoid cells are essentially organized in three compartments: (1) as lymphoid follicles, including the appendix and solitary nodules; (2) interspersed as single cells in the epithelium as intraepithelial lymphocytes (IELs); and (3) as single cells in the lamina propria.

The small intestine—in particular, the ileum—contains Peyer's patches, which are lymphoid follicles (Fig. 1.1) in the mucosa. Considerable differences exist among species, and approximately 100–200 patches may be found in humans. The Peyer's patch typically is separated into the follicular area or germinal center, the parafollicular area, and the dome at the gut lumen. The dome has a unique organization of follicle-associated epithelium (FAE) (11) that contains cuboidal epithelium with few goblet cells. M cells, which have microfolds instead of microvilli on their surface (12), replace the epithelial cells at the lumen.

The organization of the Peyer's patch enables it to act as a primary component of the afferent, inductive pathway of the mucosal immune system. Small clusters of lymphocytes (Fig. 1.2), which consist of mostly CD8+ T cells (13), are observed in close proximity to the basal cell surface of the M cell. In total, a vast number of B cells and T cells are observed in the patch, with sIgA-positive B cells (about 60% of the cells) predominant in the follicular area (14). Relatively few macrophages or dendritic cells are found in the patch.

The bronchi (15) and other secretory tissues harbor similar nodules, although they are not as pronounced as the organization seen in the gastrointestinal tract. During inflammation the nodules become considerably more pronounced.

Development of Mucosal Immunity

DEVELOPMENT BEFORE BIRTH

The human fetus develops a gastrointestinal tract with columnar epithelium and villi at 9 to 10 weeks of gestation (16). Lymphoid cells may be identified as IELs in the fetal gut at 11 weeks of gestation (17, 18), mostly in the form of CD8+ cells. About half of these IELs are positive for γ/δ T-cell receptors (19). Many of the cells found in the lamina propria at this time are probably macrophages.

At 14 weeks of gestation, clusters of T and B cells with accessory cells are seen (18). These clusters develop into well-defined Peyer's patches with a central B-cell zone and surrounding T cells around 19 weeks of gestation. The lamina propria contains CD3-positive T cells—most being CD4+—from 14 weeks of gestation. No B cells and plasma cells are observed in the gut lamina propria before the time of birth at 40 weeks of gestation, although they increase rapidly in number thereafter (20). In the salivary glands, immunocytes producing IgA of either the IgA1 and IgA2 subclasses may be observed before term. The majority of these plasmablasts or plasma cells express J-chains, indicating that these cells do not merely extravasate from the systemic tissues but primarily are destined for the mucosal immune system (21).

DEVELOPMENT AFTER BIRTH

The inducing components of the mucosal immune system are largely developed at the time of birth. The effector pathway, particularly of the B-cell system, is predominantly antigen-dependent and develops after birth. Intrauterine infections may well accelerate the development process in premature infants (22).

Plasmablasts and plasma cells populate the gut lamina propria after the age of 2 to 4 weeks. In the gut, IgM-producing cells dominate up to the age of one month, before being slowly replaced by IgA-immunocytes, even after the age of two years (23). Like mature infants, prematurely born infants of gestational age as young as 29 weeks express IgA and the poly-immunoglobulin receptor (pIgR) [also called secretory component (SC)] after the first 2 to 3 weeks of life, as well as expressing HLA-DR in the epithelium. This expression indicates the mucosal immune system's capacity to develop even at this age (24). Nasal and bronchial mucosa contain a larger proportion of IgG-immunocytes than that seen in the gastrointestinal tract. Furthermore, IgD-plasma cells may also be observed in these tissues—in particular, in IgA deficiency (25).

A model for immune enteropathy has been developed with the use of explants of fetal gut tissue (26). T-cell activation caused morphological changes, including villous atrophy that resembled the changes seen in coeliac disease or the patchy lesions in cow milk enteropathy. Some explants were destroyed by the T-cell activation. The cytokine IFN-γ may be responsible for part of the morphological changes observed (27).

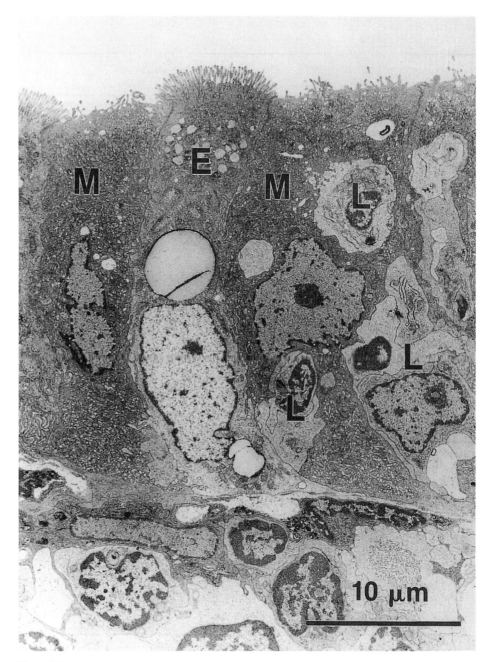

Figure 1.2

Electron micrograph of a Peyer's patch showing two M cells (M), one of which enfolds two lymphocytes (L). The enterocyte (E) has abundant microvilli, which are scarce on the M cells. From: Kato T, Owen RL. Structure and function of intestinal mucosal epithelium. Handbook of Mucosal Immunology. San Diego: Academic Press, 1994. Used with permission.

Humoral Immunity

SECRETORY IMMUNOGLOBULINS

Quantitative Aspects

IgA is the predominant immunoglobulin at mucosal surfaces (28). IgA is produced at a rate of 30–100 mg/kg/day (29), a level exceeding the production rates of all other immunoglobulins combined. This production is a consequence of the large numbers of IgA-immunocytes at the mucosal surfaces and reflects the function of IgA as a major defense mechanism against pathogens.

IgA Transport

The IgA-immunocytes in the gastrointestinal tract produce IgA mainly as dimers or larger polymers that are stabilized by a disulfide-linked polypeptide called joining- or J-chain (30). Pentameric IgM also contains J-chains. Polymeric IgA or pentameric IgM in secretions also contain secretory component (SC), which forms part of the polyimmunoglobulin (pIg) receptor. The pIg receptor is a member of the immunoglobulin superfamily (31), and the gene for human SC has been cloned (32). The pIg receptor is synthesized in secretory epithelial cells and expressed on the basolateral cell membrane, where it binds IgA or IgM to facilitate transportation of IgA across the epithelium (Fig. 1.3). The Ig–polyIg receptor complex is endocytosed into chlatrin-coated pits and, while enclosed in endosomes, is transported through the cell to be released at the luminal side. SC stays bound by disulfide- and non-covalent bonds to IgA or IgM in the lumen, whereas the rest of the pIg receptor (the cytoplasmic tail) is probably degraded. Besides mediating transport, SC probably functions to provide the immunoglobulin with an increased resistance toward proteolysis and acidity in the gastrointestinal secretions (33).

Antigen Transport

In rodents (but not in humans), pIg receptor is expressed on hepatocytes. Large concentrations of IgA were observed in rodent bile, and polymeric IgA (pIgA) or antigens complexed with pIgA were shown to be transported from the portal blood to the bile (34, 35). Furthermore, it has been shown that this transport is mediated by the pIg receptor (36). SC/pIg receptor-mediated transport of antigen–pIgA complexes has recently been suggested as a more general mechanism for disposal of antigen through epithelial membranes, particularly in the intestine. In a model system, SC-bearing epithelial cells transport IgA immune complexes from the basolateral to the apical surface where the IgA immune complexes are released (37). This mechanism may represent an important route for antigen clearance. The expression of SC on epithelial cells is regulated by cytokines such as IFN-γ (38) and in particular IL-4 (39). This regulation could be an important additional defense mechanism in inflammation in the mucosa.

IgA Isotypes

Several different isotypes of IgA have been described. In humans, IgA is observed in two subclasses, IgA1 and IgA2, with different proportions of IgA1 and IgA2 present in various body fluids (40). In serum, IgA1 accounts for approximately 85% of all IgA, most of which is monomeric. Some secretions contain larger proportions of IgA2, depending upon the site of production. In the upper respiratory and gastrointestinal tract, most plasma cells (approximately 95%) produce IgA1, whereas in the colon and rectum approximately 60% of the IgA immunocytes produce IgA2 (41).

The IgA1 and A2 subclasses differ in their heavy-chain hinge region (29). In its hinge region, IgA1 contains a heavily glycosylated 13-amino-acid stretch in which cystein residues are responsible for disulfide bonding that is lacking in IgA2. The extended hinge region may give the IgA1-Fab part greater flexibility (42).

Certain bacterial species, including *Neisseria meningitidis, Streptococcus pneumoniae,* and *Haemophilus influenzae,* have evolved proteases that cleave IgA1 at specific sites in the extended hinge region (43, 44). The IgA1-proteases in the *Haemophilus* and *Neisseria* species are serine proteases and are closely related. The proteases from pneumococci, for example, show no homology and are metalloproteases. The activity of the IgA-proteases protects the bacteria against the effector functions located on the Fc-

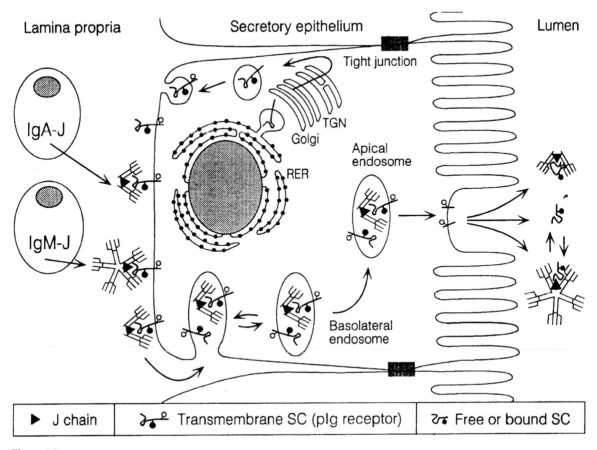

Figure 1.3

Transport of IgA and IgM and production of secretory immunoglobulins. *(left)* Production of polymeric IgA and pentameric IgM (polyIg) with J-chain by mucosal plasma cells. *(center)* Synthesis and core glycosylation of transmembrane secretory component (SC) in the rough endoplasmatic reticulum (RER). Transport through the trans-Golgi network
(TGN) and phosphorylation is followed by expression as the polymeric Ig (pIg) receptor at the basolateral plasma membrane. Endocytosis and transcytosis to apical endosomes follows. *(right)* Cleavage and release of secretory Ig with bound
SC as well as excess of free SC at the luminal surface. From Brandtzaeg P. APMIS 1995;103:1–19. Used with permission.

fragment of IgA. Furthermore, the attachment of the
IgA-Fab fragments to the bacteria may prevent further
attack by phlogistic antibodies and, therefore, increase
the invasiveness of the bacteria (45). Kilian *et al.* (46)
observed that children with an atopic disorder (and
who were frequently exposed to passive smoking) at
the age of 18 months, but not at later ages (3 and 5
years), had increased levels of IgA1-protease–producing bacteria—particularly *Streptococcus mitis*—in laryngeal swabs when compared with controls.

Immunoglobulin M

IgM-producing plasma cells are found in considerable
numbers in the gut mucosa. In contrast to IgA,
IgM has strong phlogistic properties, as it activates
complement and promotes phagocytosis. IgM found
in secretions may be regarded as a secretory immunoglobulin. It is transported by the polyIg receptor and,
in secretions, usually has bound SC, although not via
covalent bonds like IgA. In selective IgA deficiency,

IgM concentrations may be increased in secretions. Thus, IgM may partially compensate for the lack of IgA (47).

SYSTEMIC IMMUNOGLOBULINS

IgG consists of four subclasses that differ structurally in their Fc polypeptide heavy chains IgG1 through IgG4, with numbering according to their concentrations in human serum (48, 49). IgG subclasses IgG1 and IgG3 (and IgM) strongly activate the complement system (discussed below). Under normal conditions, the majority of IgG antibodies are produced systemically and extravasate into the lamina propria, where they dominate. During inflammation, the number of IgG-producing immunocytes in the mucosa increases, as does local IgG production.

The secretory immunoglobulins, which are predominantly secretory IgA, constitute a "first line of defense in the mucosa" that confers upon the mucosa the function of "immune exclusion" (50). When microorganisms penetrate the mucosa, they activate a second line of defense as part of an "immune elimination." IgG and IgM are the predominant immunoglobulin type formed in such cases, whereas IgE is the predominant form for nematode infections. Transport of IgE into the gut lumen has been reported as an IL-4–dependent function in conjunction with an experimental infection using *Trichinella spiralis* (51). Consequently, IgE may play a more important role in immune exclusion than previously recognized.

COMPLEMENT SYSTEM

The complement system is a cascade amplification defense system. Two activation pathways exist: the classical and the alternative activation pathway.

The classical pathway of the complement system is activated through C1q attachment to multiple immunoglobulin Fc portions, which further catalyze assembly of the central C3-convertase. IgM and IgG—especially IgG1 and IgG3—activate complement through the classical pathway. IgA (52), IgE (53), and the IgG4 subclass do not activate, or only very weakly activate, complement through the classical pathway.

The alternative pathway is activated by certain polysaccharides, microorganisms, cell organelles, or aggregated immunoglobulins directly through complement factor C3 with the participation of five additional proteins: factor B, factor D, factor H, factor I, and properdin (54). Both pathways act on C3, which further induces assembly of the terminal complement complex C5 through C9 and eventually lysis of the cell membrane (for a review of this topic, see 55). In the blood, a sensitive marker for complement activation is the measurement of C3dg, a C3 breakdown product (56).

Both the classical and the alternative pathways may be active in the normal mucosa as part of immune elimination, but few studies have investigated this possibility because of methodological difficulties. Activation of the complement system may be detected in the intestinal mucosa, however, and could represent an important factor in the mucosal and submucosal lesions seen in the intestines of patients with inflammatory bowel disease (57, 58).

INNATE DEFENSE FACTORS

The innate defense factors may be defined as humoral factors that are secreted onto mucosal surfaces and carry out their protective functions without the presence of specific antibodies. Although not so well appreciated, these factors are relevant components of the mucosal defense against microorganisms. Mucus is released by goblet cells of the gastrointestinal tract and covers the mucosal surfaces. It has been shown that mucus inhibits the bacterial attachment to the epithelial cell layer. The most important specific components of the mucus are lactoferrin, lysozyme, peroxidases, and high-molecular-weight glycoproteins.

Lactoferrin

Human lactoferrin is an 80 kDa glycoprotein composed of a single polypeptide chain of 691 residues. Lactoferrin binds trivalent iron, Fe^{3+}, avidly and with less affinity, Fe^{2+}. The iron binding serves as the basis for most of the biological function. Lactoferrin is found in most exocrine secretions, and in milk and blood. A relatively high content of lactoferrin in human milk may increase the bioavailability of iron, which is observed at low levels in the breast milk. Conflicting data on this point have been reported (59). Lactoferrin has documented bacteriostatic or bactericidal effects on a number of microorganisms. This effect probably depends on direct damage of the bacterial membrane by lactoferrin and on depletion of iron needed for the metabolism of the microorganism.

Lysozyme

Lysozyme is a polypeptide of 14.6 kDa that exerts its action by cleaving peptidoglycans of the bacterial cell wall (60) via activation of bacterial autolysins and aggregation of bacteria due to a cationic effect. Its activity depends heavily on the pH and ionic strength. Lysozyme is found in human saliva and milk in concentrations up to 250 μg/mL (61), which is almost 10^3 times more than the level found in cow milk.

High-Molecular-Weight Glycoproteins

High-molecular-weight glycoproteins are found in saliva and in intestinal secretions. Mucin itself is a glycoprotein that gives mucus its viscous and elastic properties. The high-molecular-weight glycoproteins exert their effect in several ways as they agglutinate bacteria and prevent the bacteria from adhering to mucosal membranes. Bacteria mainly adhere by attachment to carbohydrate receptors—for example, on epithelial cells in the colon (62). By interfering with this process, glycoproteins may act as a countermeasure for bacterial adherence.

Cellular Immune System: Inductive Sites

A number of different cell types play a role in the mucosal immune response—some as part of the inductive arm of the MALT, some as part of the effector arm, and some cells having combined function. In general, however, the division in inductive and effector sites is instructive. The participating cells are listed in Table 1.1.

EPITHELIAL CELLS

General Characteristics

The enterocytes are approximately 25 μm high and 8 μm wide. They are characterized by their abundant

Table 1.1
Organization of the Mucosal Immune
System: Cell Types Involved

Inductive Sites	Effector Sites
epithelial cells	T cells (IEL, LPL)
M cells	macrophages
T cells	plasmablasts/plasma cells
macrophages/dendritic cells	eosinophils
B cell	mast cells

microvilli, which increase their surface area enormously. The enterocytes are separated by junctional complexes that contain tight junctions. The main function of the enterocyte is the absorption of nutrients, minerals, and water. The cell membrane enzymes and carrier systems serve these purposes. Three other mechanisms play important roles in mucosal immunology: antigen transport, antigen presentation, and cytokine production.

Antigen Transport

Apart from the degradation and transfer of degraded proteins and carbohydrates, the epithelial cells transport small amounts of undegraded macromolecules. Transport may occur by receptor-mediated endocytosis, by nonselective pinocytosis, or by direct penetration of the cell membrane by certain viruses and toxins (63).

Receptor-mediated endocytosis involves the transport of maternal immunoglobulins in suckling mammals. The transport diminishes by the event of "gut closure," which in the rat takes place at 20 to 22 days of age (64). A similar transport does not occur in humans, where the placenta contains Fcγ receptors and transports IgG in utero.

Nonspecific absorption of protein has been shown to occur for smaller and larger peptides, which are absorbed and transported across the enterocyte, predominantly in endosomes. This transport has been demonstrated in adult and fetal rat tissues (65, 66). In addition, uptake has been indicated to occur intercellularly across the tight junctions after trauma (67).

In humans, uptake of intact dietary antigen has been demonstrated in IgA-deficient individuals (68). In healthy adults, intact or antibody-bound dietary protein such as ovalbumin was detected in a quantity of 0 to 20 ng/mL of serum, corresponding to a fraction of 10^{-5} of the intake (69). Larger amounts were absorbed in children. An increase was observed in children with coeliac disease when they were challenged with gluten and had villous atrophy of the small intestinal mucosa (70). Larger amounts of dietary antigen are absorbed in premature infants, with a reduction in the unspecific uptake of dietary protein observed around term (71, 72).

Antigen Presentation

Virtually all nucleated cells express class I MHC antigens. Enterocytes also have the capacity to express class II MHC antigens on their surfaces, as shown in experimental animals (73) and in humans (74). The MHC antigens are expressed on the tips of the villi, whereas SC is expressed in the crypts. The expression of MHC antigens confers upon the cell an important immunological function: antigen presentation for T cells. Enterocytes appear to process antigens only to a limited degree, however, because of limited enzymatic capacity. This situation may change during intestinal inflammation, as increased expression of HLA-DR and -DP (but not HLA-DQ) was seen in colon enterocytes from patients with inflammatory bowel disease (75).

Influence by Cytokines

After exposure to IFN-γ, cultured enterocytes showed increased permeability (76) as well as increased uptake and processing of protein (77). Interleukin-4 (IL-4) may exert a similar influence on the intestinal epithelium (78), although it is usually considered to have actions opposite to those of IFN-γ (discussed below). In addition, epithelial cells secrete cytokines such as IL-6 (79). Thus, cytokines may directly influence the function of the epithelium.

M CELLS

The surface of the Peyer's patch contains M cells, a type of cell that was discovered two decades ago. M cells replace the epithelial cells at the dome of the Peyer's patch, forming a pocket (11). The M cells (Fig. 1.2) appear to play an important role in sampling of antigen from the gut lumen and transporting both soluble and particulate antigens. In addition, microbial particles such as reovirus type 1 and 3 (80), HIV-1, and even bacteria such as *Salmonella, Yersinia enterocolitica,* and *Vibria cholera* (81) may take advantage of the M cell to gain access to the host. M cells have a low lysosome content and transport antigens from the lumen with only minor enzymatic degradation (82). Whether M cells present antigen for neighboring T cells remains controversial, as HLA antigens have not been detected on human M cells (83). Recent experiments have shown expression of MHC antigens on M cells in the rat, however, (84), so a certain level of presentation of more or less degraded antigens is a possibility. The basolateral surface of the M cell is extensively folded and surrounds the cells in the vicinity. These cells are predominantly lymphocytes, dendritic cells, and macrophages, which are thought to participate in the further degradation and presentation of antigens.

DENDRITIC CELLS AND MACROPHAGES

Peyer's patches and the lamina propria contain a heterogeneous population of large, macrophage-like cells that express class II HLA antigen. In the human colon, as much as 10% of cells in the lamina propria are phenotypically macrophages (85). To date, these cells have been studied to only a limited degree, as they are heterogenous and difficult to obtain for functional analysis. Whether the cells are macrophages or may be regarded as dendritic cells is a source of controversy. The function of these cells is partly related to antigen presentation, as they possess class II antigen, and partly to function as phagocytes (86). Under normal circumstances, however, these cells produce only small amounts of IL-1 (87) and express little of the ICAM-1 adhesion molecule (88). This condition indicates that the cells are not very active in attracting T cells for antigen presentation. Further work is needed to clarify the importance of macrophages/dendritic cells in normal and diseased mucosa.

B-CELL DEVELOPMENT

The molecular mechanisms that regulate the development of the B cells in Peyer's patches have been studied to a considerable degree (for review, see 89). The B cell goes through early antigen-dependent phases with immunoglobulin isotype switching and later undergoes antigen-independent proliferation and differentiation (Fig. 1.4). In humans, the heavy-chain immunoglobulin genes are encoded on chromosome 14 in the order of $5'\text{-}J_H\text{-}C\mu\text{-}C\delta\text{-}C\gamma3\text{-}C\gamma1$-pseudo $C\epsilon\text{-}C\alpha1$-pseudo $C\gamma\text{-}C\gamma2\text{-}C\gamma4\text{-}C\epsilon\text{-}C\alpha2\text{-}3'$ (90). The switching from IgM+, IgD+ B cells to IgA+ cells involves a series of gene rearrangements

Regulation Of Terminal Differentiation To IgA Synthesis

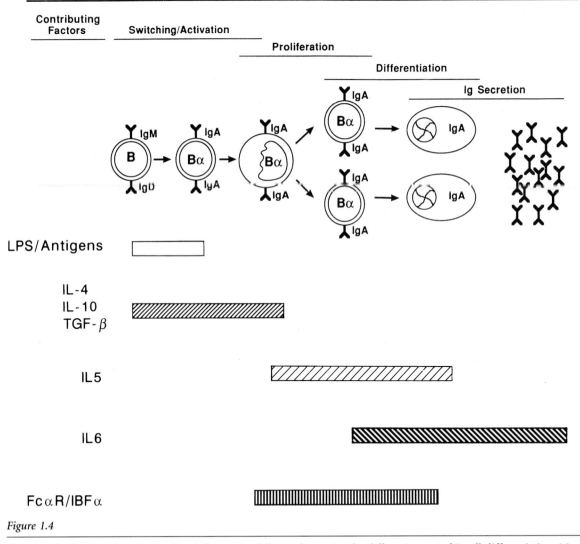

Figure 1.4

Cytokines in B-cell differentiation. The influence by different factors on the different stages of B-cell differentiation. Mature B cells switch to IgA+ cells influenced by several cytokines (IL-4, IL-10, and TGF-β). IL-5 promotes further proliferation and clonal expansion, and IL-6 induces B-cell differentiation into plasma cells that secrete IgA. (Modified from McGhee JR, *et al.* J Clin Immunol 1989;9: 175–199 1989.)

and joining of gene segments. The process of switching from IgM+, IgD+ to IgA+ cells is influenced by LPS and antigen, and is directed by various cytokines released by T cells. A distinct type of T cells—so-called switch T cells—may possibly be important in Peyer's patches (91). In mice, IL-4 is a potent inducer of the switch to IgG and IgE-positive cells (92), whereas interferon-γ (IFN-γ) may induce B cells to express IgG of several subclasses and suppress IgE responses (for review, see 93). Transforming growth factor β (TGF-β), together with stimulation by LPS, has been shown to initiate the switching of B cells to IgA production (94) by the induction of the germ-line Cα gene (95).

The later stages of IgA-expressing B-cell activation are aided by IL-5, which promotes activation and differentiation of IgA+ cells into plasmablasts (96, 97), and IL-6, which induces high levels of IgA secretion (98). A more definitive demonstration that IL-6 has primary importance for IgA antibody responses in the mucosa was obtained in a study of the use of transgenic mice with disruption of the gene for IL-6 (99). These mice had reduced numbers of IgA+ cells in their intestines and lungs, and exhibited diminished mucosal antibody responses following vaccination with ovalbumin or vaccinia virus. Furthermore, intranasal infection with vaccinia viruses that expressed IL-6 restored the IgA response in the lungs.

MUCOSAL T CELLS

Mucosal T cells consist of a heterogeneous population with different markers based on their final location in the mucosa. Basically, T cells migrate to Peyer's patches and then migrate further to become IELs or lamina propria lymphocytes (Fig. 1.5).

Lymphocytes are, in general, characterized on the basis of their surface markers, whose number has increased rapidly in the last 10 to 20 years (5th International Leukocyte Workshop, 1993). This greater recognition has particularly applied to T cells, also permitting an understanding of T-cell function. The CD3 molecule represents the T-cell receptor and defines the specific cell as a T cell (Fig. 1.6). The T-cell receptor is a member of the immunoglobulin

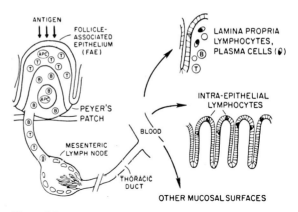

Figure 1.5

The organization of gut-associated lymphoid tissue into three major compartments: Peyer's patches, intraepithelial lymphocytes, and lamina propria lymphocytes, with indications of lymphocyte migration. Reproduced with permission from: Elson, Co. The immunology of inflammatory bowel disease. In: Inflammatory bowel disease. Philadelphia, Lea & Febiger, 1988.

superfamily with a rather limited V gene repertoire (100) that exists in the form of either α/β chains or γ/δ chains. T cells may be divided into two subpopulations based on the phenotype of the TCR α/β chain and the TCR γ/δ chain.

The presence of the CD4+ accessory molecule identifies the helper/inducer T-cell subset, while the CD8+ accessory molecule identifies the suppressor/inducer subset (Fig. 1.6). Additional subsets may be identified based on the presence of the CD45RA/45RO antigen, which differentiates between a "memory" cell subset versus a "naive" T-cell subset.

T cells with a helper-cell function and usually characterized by positive CD4+ staining may be further divided into Th1 and Th2 subsets based on their cytokine production (101). The Th1 cell response is based on the production of the cytokines IFN-γ, IL-2, and TNF-α. The Th2 cell response is associated with the production of IL-4, IL-5, IL-6, and IL-10 (Table 1.2). This distinction has been identified in experiments conducted in mice, but a similar pattern has been observed in human blood lymphocytes, particularly in relation to allergic disorders, where T cells display a Th2-like overactivity (102). The existence of separate CD4+ lymphocyte subsets on the basis of cytokine production has been disputed, how-

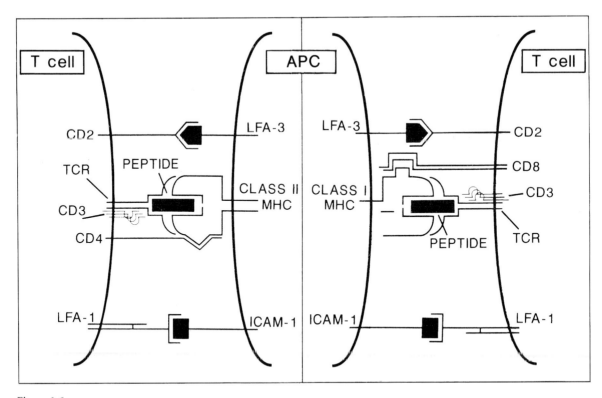

Figure 1.6

Antigen presentation, T-cell surface markers and co-stimulatory factors, and integrins/adressins involved in the interaction between T cells and antigen-presenting cells (APC).

ever, as the same T-cell clones may secrete different combinations of cytokines depending on the environment, most importantly the cells that present antigen to the T cells (103). The clinical correlate is the predominant production of Th1 or Th2 cytokines depending on the stage of disease.

Table 1.2
Cytokine Production by T Helper Cells
Separated in the Th1 and Th2 Subsets

Th1	Th2
IL-2	IL-4
IFN-γ	IL-5
lymphotoxin	IL-6
	IL-10

Cellular Immunity: Effector Sites

INTRAEPITHELIAL LYMPHOCYTES

Intraepithelial lymphocytes (IELs) are interspersed within the gastrointestinal epithelium and may constitute as much as 20% of the total cell population. IELs comprise small lymphocytes and large granular lymphocytes in varying proportions (104, 105).

The characterization of IELs with surface markers does not show a strict division of subsets as seen for peripheral blood lymphocytes; rather, IELs appear to constitute a heterogenous population of CD3-positive T cells (106, 107). In humans (108) and in experimental animals, most of these cells are CD8-positive; in contrast, "double-positive" IELs, which have markers for both CD-4 and CD-8, have been observed in considerable numbers in mice (107). Other cells, reportedly 3%–10% of the IELs, are "double-negative" T cells that do not have either CD-4 or CD-8 on their surface (109).

In mouse experiments, IELs produce cytokines such as IL-2, IL-3, and IL-6 accompanied by the proinflammatory cytokines IFN-γ, TNF-α, and TGF-β, but probably not IL-4 or IL-5 (110). On the other hand, a Th2-like pattern of cytokine production with IL-5 and IL-6 for CD4+ IELs has been reported (111).

In the mouse, gut IELs differ in T-cell receptor expression compared with that of circulating T cells, as the IELs preferentially (>90%) express γ/δ chains as compared with the α/β chains, which are expressed on the circulating T cells (112). In humans, only a few γ/δ positive T cells have been found in the small intestine (113), although the majority of T cells in the colon are γ/δ positive (108). It is conceivable that the number of human intestinal γ/δ T cells varies considerably from subject to subject, but such cells tend to become more numerous in the distal part of the gastrointestinal tract, the colon, and the rectum.

In inflammatory states such as enteropathies, these patterns of cell characteristics may change dramatically. In coeliac disease, for example, an increase in the double-negative T cells has been observed (109). In contrast, a striking increase in the proportion of γ/δ positive cells has been seen in biopsies from the small intestine (109, 114).

Apart from cytokine production, a distinct pattern of reactivity has been observed from IELs. The cells are easily activated, as indicated by increased activity of the microtubule-associated protein kinase-2 (MAP-2K) (115). They do not, however, react to proliferative signals such as pokeweed mitogen, as do peripheral blood T cells (115, 116). These results indicate a constant state of activation for the IELs. This condition could represent an adjustment of the IELs to function in a completely different milieu than that observed in the peripheral circulation.

Taken together, the function of IELs is still incompletely understood. The most important roles played by IELs are probably the removal of aged or infected epithelial cells, the influencing of the development of the epithelial cell layer, the regulation of oral hyporesponsiveness (discussed below), and the

recruitment of granulocytes for the ongoing immune defense.

LAMINA PROPRIA LYMPHOCYTES

T Cells

The lamina propria contains an abundance of T and B lymphocytes, macrophages, and dendritic cells. In contrast to intraepithelial lymphocytes, these T cells are mostly CD4-positive and of the helper/inducer subset (117). Almost equal numbers of CD45RA+ and CD45RO+ cells have been found, suggesting the presence of both "naive" and "memory" T cells (118). Other markers of the memory T-cell subset are not found on lamina propria T cells, which may well contain a specialized memory T-cell subset (119a, 119b). The lamina propria lymphocytes produce high levels of mRNA for the cytokines IL-2, IL-4, and IL-5 and of IL-2 receptors (both IL-2Rα and IL-2Rβ) (120) as compared with peripheral blood lymphocytes. This production level indicates a constant state of activation, with even higher levels observed in specimens from patients with inflammatory bowel disease (120).

B Cells

The cells of the B-cell lineage in the lamina propria are mostly plasmablasts and plasma cells, which produce immunoglobulins. Quantitatively, large numbers of these immunocytes are normally located in the lamina propria. About 10^{10} immunoglobulin-producing cells have been estimated to populate one meter of normal human small intestine (121).

Most (70%–90%) of the immunocytes produce IgA, with fewer IgM and IgG-producing cells noted. The IgA-producing cells are mostly of the IgA1 subclass and are located in the proximal part of the gastrointestinal tract. Increasing amounts of IgA2-secreting cells are seen in the distal tract, with about 60% IgA2 found in the large intestine. For IgG subclass-producing cells, the distribution in the distal gastrointestinal tract follows that of plasma cells and immunoglobulin levels in the blood with IgG1 > IgG2 > IgG3 > IgG4 (122). In the upper respiratory tract, a pattern of IgG1 > IgG3 > IgG2 is observed.

In disease states such as infection or enteropathy, the distribution of immunoglobulin-producing cells changes considerably. In inflammatory bowel disease, an increase of IgG-producing cells and an increase in IgA1-producing cells is observed (124). Specimens from patients with ulcerative colitis have increased levels of cells producing IgG1, whereas patients with Crohn's disease have high levels of IgG2-producing cells (125).

Few IgE-producing cells are normally observed in the gastrointestinal mucosa, even though their numbers may be higher in the mucosa than those observed in other lymphoid tissues (126). Most IgE-associated cells in the mucosa are mast cells (127).

MAST CELLS

Mast cells may be observed (see chapter 2) scattered throughout the gastrointestinal tissues and, more abundantly, adjacent to blood and lymphatic vessels and nerves. Mast cells are usually identified by their granules, which stain metachromatically. In rodents, two subtypes of mast cells have been described: connective-tissue mast cells and mucosal mast cells, which differ depending on their structure, mediator content, and distribution (128, 129, 130). A similar pattern is seen in humans, where mixed populations of mast cells are seen in all tissues (131).

Mast cells are important in allergic reactions, as they release a number of vasoactive substances following activation of the IgE receptors (129). The preformed mediators include histamine, serotonin, and mast-cell-specific enzymes such as chymase, tryptase, and cathepsin G, which are released from the cytoplasmic granules. In addition, newly synthesized mediators such as nitric oxide and arachidonic acid metabolites may be formed and released immediately.

It is now realized that mast cells produce a number of cytokines. Human lung and skin mast cells have been shown to produce TNF-α (132) and IL-4 (133). Mast cells are the main source of IL-4, IL-5, and IL-6 in mucosal inflammation of the nose in allergic rhinitis (134). The mast cells themselves are influenced by a number of cytokines such as IL-3, GM-CSF (135), and stem cell growth factor, the *c-kit* ligand (136, 137).

EOSINOPHILS

The eosinophil granulocyte is seen in the blood, but is predominantly found in the mucosal tissues (for review, see 137a, 137b). The eosinophil is distinguished based on its characteristic eosinophilic granules. These granules contain lysosomal hydrolases and several cationic proteins such as major basic protein, eosinophil cationic protein (ECP), and eosinophilic protein X (EPX). Furthermore, the granules are responsible for the protein that forms the Charcot-Leyden crystals in sputum and feces (138), which are a characteristic sign of eosinophil-related disease.

Eosinophils express receptors for several immunoglobulins on their surfaces, such as the low-affinity receptor for IgG and the receptor for IgA (139, 140). In addition, a low-affinity receptor for IgE is observed on eosinophils (141). IgA—in particular, secretory IgA—is a potent inducer of eosinophilic degranulation (142). Eosinophils express a number of integrins, such as LFA-1 (CD11a) and CD18, and adhesion molecules, such as L-selectin and ICAM-1, which are important for their migration to inflamed tissues (143).

Eosinophil development takes place in the bone marrow and is stimulated by three cytokines: GM-CSF, IL-3, and IL-5. In mice, the presence of IL-5 has been demonstrated to be a crucial factor, as an antibody to IL-5 inhibits the eosinophilia, without diminishing IgE-levels, induced by the helminth *Nippostrongylus brasiliensis* (144). The eosinophils themselves produce several cytokines such as IL-6 (145) and TGF-β (146).

The Integrated Mucosal Immune System

B-CELL MIGRATION

It has been shown in experimental animals that B cells committed for IgA production are primed and develop into plasma cell precursors in Peyer's patches (Fig. 1.5). The cells subsequently leave the patches via the lymphatics (145a, 145b) and usually expand in the regional lymph nodes, spreading to mucosal effector sites—primarily the lamina propria and glandular tissues (146a, 146b, 147). A study in humans found that IgA antibody-producing cells appeared in the blood seven days after the ingestion of capsules containing killed *Streptococcus mutans* and reached maximal levels 10 to 12 days after ingestion. Secretory IgA anti-*S. mutans* antibodies were detected in saliva and tear fluid two weeks after the ingestion and reached a maximum after three weeks (2). This study indicates a common mucosal immune system in humans and illustrates the timing of the human mucosal immune response, although timing may be faster with recall immune responses.

T-CELL MIGRATION

The T cells that populate the intestinal epithelium (intraepithelial lymphocytes) and the lamina propria are thought to originate from Peyer's patches or the lymphoid follicles (Fig. 1.5). Here they come in contact with antigen, are activated, and mature in the germinal centers of the follicle or Peyer's patches. IgA-committed T cells then leave the mucosa, migrate to the lymph, and then move into the blood. From the bloodstream, the cells return to the gastrointestinal tract, where they locate within the lamina propria to become lamina propria lymphocytes (LPLs) or within the intestinal epithelium to become IELs (147, 148).

Based on experiments in mice, some IELs are now believed to originate in the bone marrow and migrate directly to the epithelium (149). Studies suggest that at least two types of IELs with different migration patterns are present within the phenotypic appearance of IELs. These two types of T cells were distinguished by the presence of CD8 α/β chains and α/α chains, respectively (150). Both types were found within both the TCR α/β and γ/δ populations. The CD8 α/α population arose independently of development in the thymus and may be a subpopulation of T cells that migrates directly to the mucosa from the bone marrow. Preliminary results suggest that a similar pattern may be observed in humans, with one thymus-independent IEL-type migrating directly to the mucosa and one thymus-dependent IEL-type maturing in Peyer's patches and possibly the regional lymph nodes (151).

HOMING OF T CELLS

The organ specificity of lymphocyte migration has been associated with determinants on high endothelial venules (HEV) in the Peyer's patches (152). The molecular mechanisms of the migration pattern of the mucosal T cells—in particular, IELs—are probably complex but a major determinant is integrin/adressin interactions. Integrin molecules mediate cell–cell and cell–extracellular matrix adhesion (153), and have important functions in lymphocyte homing. The corresponding receptors for integrins are called adressins.

High endothelial venules of the lymphoid follicles and Peyer's patches contain adressins, which are recognized by lymphocyte integrins primarily identified by the corresponding monoclonal antibody MEL-14 (154) and were eventually identified as LECAM-1. The adressin ELAM-1 is the main adhesion molecule for T cells homing to the skin (155).

Recent research has identified an integrin $\alpha 4\beta 7$ that is expressed in high concentrations on IELs and on subsets of T cells, which are believed to be predominantly mucosal T cells (156, 157, 158). Furthermore, a major adressin on the HEV of Peyer's patches and in the lamina propria is the mucosal vascular adressin, MAdCAM-1. The related $\alpha E\beta 7$ integrin has been shown to mediate binding of lymphocytes to MAdCAM-1 (159). This binding is not specific, as $\alpha 4\beta 7$ and probably also $\alpha E\beta 7$ interact with multiple adhesion molecules such as VCAM-1 and fibronectin, but preferably with MAdCAM-1 (160). The $\alpha 4\beta 7$ molecule probably holds primary importance in T-cell homing to mucosal effector sites in the epithelium and the lamina propria.

STIMULATION

It is apparent that multiple factors are involved in the generation of the mucosal immune response. In summary, the antigen is encountered by the immune system, preferentially in Peyer's patches, where antigen-presenting cells such as dendritic cells/macrophages or B cells present the antigen to T cells. B cells (especially IgA+ cells) and T cells are activated and migrate from the patches to the regional lymph nodes, and then to mucosal effector sites such as the lamina propria or the epithelium itself. Different cell types such as mast cells and eosinophils may influence or augment the ensuing effector response.

The nature of the antigen(s) may have similar importance. Bacterial cell wall components such as LPS potentiate B-cell responsiveness. Certain antigenic structures, such as microbial cholera toxin (161) and the cholera toxin subunit B (CT-B), elicit strong mucosal immune responses and may act as potent adjuvants for immunization with other antigens (162, 163). The mechanism for the adjuvant effect of cholera toxin is not definitively known, but may involve stimulation of macrophage function by increased production of IL-1 and by enhancement of antigen presentation (164). An important observation for the study of allergic disorders is that, in mice, the oral administration of antigen together with cholera toxin, followed by a subsequent intraperitoneal challenge with the antigen alone, not only abrogates oral hyporesponsiveness, but also produces IgE responses and IgE-mediated anaphylaxis (165).

HYPORESPONSIVENESS

Despite the considerable numbers of IgA+ immunocytes present in the gastrointestinal tract, it has proved difficult to elicit mucosal immune responses with nonliving and nonproliferating antigens, both in humans and experimental animals (166). In addition, oral immunization may diminish the immune response from systemic immunization at a later time, in a process called oral tolerance.

The term "oral tolerance" was first coined by Chase (167), who described a reduction of cutaneous hapten sensitization in mice by prior feeding of the hapten. Oral tolerance has been convincingly demonstrated in rodents fed a variety of antigens, such as bacteria *(Streptococcus mutans)* and heterologous blood cells, or soluble protein antigens, such as ovalbumin (168, 169, 170). Species differences do exist, however; for example, the rabbit does not seem to develop oral tolerance (171). Oral tolerance has been described in both the humoral and the cellular im-

mune systems. Interestingly, antigen feeding at low doses suppresses cellular immunity, but leaves the humoral responsiveness intact (172). In addition, the induction of oral tolerance in established disease has been achieved in experimental animals with down-regulation of preexisting IgE antibodies (173), and delayed hypersensitivity has been demonstrated after oral feeding of antigen (174).

In general, immune hyporesponsiveness may occur by clonal deletion, clonal anergy, or suppression (175) (Table 1.3). In the case of oral tolerance, local and systemic suppressor T-cell circuits may be operating (176, 177, 178). The digestion and absorption of antigen by the intestine apparently produces tolerogenic forms of the antigen in the circulation (179, 180). For at least protein antigens, a major mechanism appears to be the accumulation in Peyer's patches of antigen-specific suppressor T cells, which later populate systemic lymphoid tissues such as the spleen (176). Approximately one month after feeding antigen to the animal, suppressor T cells cannot be identified, but the animal remains unresponsive to the fed antigen, suggesting the operation of mechanisms such as clonal deletion or anergy. A series of recent studies on experimental encephalomyelitis indicated immune suppression by CD8+ cells to be the main mechanism. These cells were shown to secrete TGF-β as a regulatory cytokine (181).

In humans, oral hyporesponsiveness has been studied to only a limited extent. Korenblatt *et al.* (182) studied the antibody levels to bovine serum albumin (BSA). From previous studies, they knew that antibodies to foods tended to decrease with age. They discovered that subjects without serum antibody to BSA prior to feeding with BSA were unresponsive to both oral and parenteral challenge; in contrast, subjects with a measurable antibody level tended to show increased antibody levels after challenge. In another study (183), a diminished cutaneous response to an experimental hapten was observed after antigen feeding. These results are consistent with either an-

Table 1.3
Mechanisms for the Induction of Tolerance

Central/thymus:	clonal deletion
Peripheral:	clonal anergy
	suppression

ergy or a suppressive mechanism occurring in the subjects with low antibody levels. A recent study by Husby *et al.* (184) investigated the systemic and secretory immune responses to keyhole limpet hemocyanin (KLH). The results indicated that systemic T-cell tolerance may occur concurrently with B-cell immunization.

A secretory immune response was included in the characterization of oral tolerance, but only a few studies have examined the secretory immune response directly (170). The measured levels of salivary antibodies were low in these studies, so a secretory immune response may not be an obligatory event. In humans, antibodies were detectable in salivary and intestinal secretions after the induction of systemic T-cell tolerance.

GENETIC CONTROL

The genes—in particular, those found within the MHC complex—exert a profound influence on immune responsiveness (185). The same is true for immune responses within the mucosa (186). In experimental animals, a strong genetic dependence on the immune response to orally administered cholera toxin has been observed (187). Coeliac disease, which may be considered a model for human immune enteropathy, depends heavily on the HLA-DQ antigen (188). The simultaneous presence of these haplotypes (DR2, DQA, and DQB) is associated with an increased density of γ/δ T cells in the jejunal mucosa (189) and secretory anti-gliadin antibodies (190). These results indicate a close connection between the MHC genes and T- and B-cell immune responses in the gastrointestinal mucosa.

IgE-associated immune responses have proved difficult to study in the mucosa. Human IgE responsiveness and atopy is, to a high degree, genetically dependent (191). IgE responsiveness has been suggested to relate to a locus on chromosome 11, although that finding has been disputed. Recently, a strong linkage between IgE levels and the IL-4 gene (or a gene close to the IL-4 gene) has been demonstrated (192). Given the important influence of several cytokines on mucosal immune responses, cytokine genes may well exert additional control of mucosal immune responses.

Table 1.4
Potential Immunologic Therapeutic Modalities

1. Exploitation of oral tolerance
2. Blocking of cytokine production or cytokine receptor blockade
3. Use of inhibitory cytokines (e.g., IL-10, TGF-β)
4. Blocking of integrin–adressin interactions
5. MHC–peptide toxin conjugates
6. Blocking of accessory molecules in the T-cell/antigen–presenting cell interactions

Perspectives

The mucosal immune system contains complex regulatory pathways that depend on an intact cellular immune system. The development of food allergy represents an incompletely understood disruption of these regulatory mechanisms. The mainstay of allergy treatment is the avoidance of the foods that cannot be tolerated. A number of immunologic therapies, such as regulation of cytokine release by T cells, may become feasible in inflammatory diseases in the not-too-distant future, however (Table 1.4). An increased understanding of mucosal immunity may form the basis for new therapeutic modalities for the treatment of allergic and autoimmune disorders.

REFERENCES

1. Bienenstock J, Befys AD. Mucosal immunology. Immunology 1980;41:249–270.
2. Czerkinsky C, Prince SJ, Michalek SM, Jackson S, Russell MW, Moldoveanu Z, McGhee JR, Mestecky J. IgA antibody-producing cells in peripheral blood after antigen ingestion: evidence for a common mucosal immune system in humans. Proc Natl Acad Sci USA 1987;84:2449–2453.
3. Besredka A. In: Plotz H, ed. Local Immunization. Baltimore: Williams & Wilkins, 1927,1–181.
4. Davies A. An investigation into the serological properties of dysentery stools. Lancet 1922;ii:1009–1012.
5. Hanson LÅ. Comparative immunological studies of the immune globulins of human milk and of blood serum. Int Arch Allergy 1961;18:241–249.
6. Tomasi TB, Tan EM, Solomon A, Prendergast RA. Characteristics of an immune system common to certain external secretions. J Exp Med 1965;121:101–124.
7. Prausnitz C, Küstner H. Studien bei die ueberempfindlichkeit. Centralbl f Bakt Akt Orig 1921;86:160–169.
8. György P, Moro E, Witebsky E. Eichlar-empfindlichkeit bei eczema infantum. Klin wochenschr 1930;9:1012–1017.
9. Lippard VW, Schloss OM, Johnson PA. Immune reactions induced in infants by intestinal absorption of incompletely digested cow's milk protein. Am J Dis Child 1936;51:562–574.

10. Gruskay FL, Cooke RE. Gastrointestinal absorption of unaltered protein in normal infants and in infants recovering from diarrhea. Pediatrics 1955;16:763–796.

11. Bockman DE, Cooper MD. Pinocytosis by epithelium associated with lymphoid follicles in the bursa of Fabricius, appendix and Peyer's patches. An electron microscopic study. Am J Anat 1973;136:455–478.

12. Owen RL, Jones AL. Epithelial cell specialization within human Peyer's patches: an ultrastructural study of intestinal lymphoid follicles. Gastroenterology 1974;66:189–203.

13. Bjerke K, Brandtzaeg P, Fausa O. T cell distribution is different in follicle-associated epithelium of human Peyer's patches and villous epithelium. Clin Exp Immunol 1988;74:270–275.

14. Butcher EC, Rouse RV, Coffman RL, Nottenburg CN, Hardy RR, Weissman IL. Surface phenotype of Peyer's patch germinal center cells: implications for the role of germinal centers in B cell differentiation. J Immunol 1982;129:2698–2707.

15. Bienenstock J, Johnson N. A morphologic study of rabbit bronchial lymphoid aggregates and lymphoepithelium. Lab Invest 1976;35:343–348.

16. Moxey PC, Trier JS. Specialized cell types in the human fetal small intestine. Anat Rec 1979;195:463–482.

17. Orlic D, Lev R. An electron microscopic study of intraepithelial lymphocytes in human fetal small intestine. Lab Invest 1977;37:554–561.

18. Spencer J, MacDonald TT, Finn T, Isaacson PG. The development of gut associated lymphoid tissue in the terminal ileum of fetal human intestine. Clin Exp Immunol 1986;64:536–543.

19. Spencer J, Isaacson PG, Diss TC, MacDonald TT. Expression of disulphide linked and non-disulphide linked forms of the T cell receptor gamma/delta heterodimer in human intestinal intraepithelial lymphocytes. Eur J Immunol 1989;19:1335–1338.

20. Spencer J, Dillon SB, Isaacson PG, MacDonald TT. T cell subclasses in human fetal ileum. Clin Exp Immunol 1986;65:553–558.

21. Thrane PS, Rognum TO, Brandtzaeg P. Ontogenesis of the secretory immune system and innate defence factors in human parotid glands. Clin Exp Immunol 1991;86:342–348.

22. Stoll BJ, Lee FK, Hale E, et al. Immunoglobulin secretions by the normal and the infected newborn infant. J Pediatr 1993;122:780–786.

23. Savilahti E. Immunoglobulin-containing cells in the intestinal mucosa and immunoglobulins in the intestinal juice in children. Clin Exp Immunol 1972;11:415–425.

24. Rognum TO, Thrane PS, Stoltenberg L, Vege Å, Brandtzaeg P. Development of intestinal mucosal immunity in fetal life and the first postnatal month. Ped Res 1992;32:145–149.

25. Brandtzaeg P, Gjeruldsen ST, Korsrud F, Baklien K, Berdal P, Ek J. The human secretory immune system shows striking heterogeneity with regard to involvement of J chain-positive IgD immunocytes. J Immunol 1979;122:503–510.

26. MacDonald TT, Spencer J. Evidence that activated mucosal T cells play a role in the pathogenesis of enteropathy in human small intestine. J Exp Med 1967, 1341–1349.

27. Lionetti P, Breese E, Braegger CP, Murch SH, Taylor J, MacDonald TT. T-cell activation can induce either mucosal destruction or adaptation in cultured fetal small intestine. Gastroenterology 1993;05:373–381.

28. Chodirker WB, Tomasi TB. Gamma-globulins: quantitative relationships in human serum and nonvascular fluids. Science 1963;242:1080–1081.

29. Mestecky J, McGhee JR. Immunoglobulin A (IgA): molecular and cellular interactions involved in IgA biosynthesis and immune response. Adv Immunol 1987;40:153–245.

30. Koshland ME. The coming of age of the immunoglobobulin J chain. Ann Rev Immunol 1985;3:425–453.

31. Mostov KE, Friedlander M, Blobel G. The receptor for transepithelial transport of IgA and IgM contains multiple immunoglobulin-like domains. Nature 1984;308:37–43.

32. Krajci P, Solberg R, Sandberg M, Oyen O, Jahnsen T, Brandtzaeg P. Molecular cloning of the human transmembrane secretory component (poly-Ig receptor) and its mRNA expression in human tissue. Biochem Biophys Res Commun 1991;158:783–789.

33. Bakos MA, Kurosky A, Goldblum RM. Characterization of a critical binding site for human polymeric Ig on secretory component. J Immunol 1991;147:3419–3426.

34. Jackson GFD, Lemaitre-Coelho I, Vaerman J-P, Bazin H, Beckers A. Rapid disappearance from serum of intravenously injected myeloma IgA and its secretion into bile. Eur J Immunol 1978;8:123–126.

35. Phillips JO, Russell MW, Brown TA, Mestecky J. Selective hepatobiliary transport of human polymeric IgA in mice. Mol Immunol 1984;21:907–914.

36. Orlans E, Peppard J, Fry JF, Hinton RH, Mullock BM. Secretory component as the receptor for polymeric IgA on rat hepatocytes. J Exp Med 1979;150:1577–1581.

37. Kaetzel CS, Robinson JK, Chintalacharuvu KR, Vaerman J-P, Lamm ME. The polymeric immunoglobulin receptor (secretory component) mediates transport of immune complexes across epithelial cells: a local defence function for IgA. Proc Natl Acad Sci USA 1991;88:8796–8800.

38. Sollid LM, Kvale D, Brandtzaeg P, Markussen G, Thorsby E. Interferon-gamma enhances expression of secretory component, the epithelial receptor for polymeric immunoglobulins. J Immunol 1987;138:4304–4306.

39. Phillips JO, Everson MP, Moldoveanu Z, Lue C, Mestecky J. Synergistic effect of IL-4 and IFN-γ on the expression of polymeric Ig receptor (secretory component) and IgA binding by epithelial cells. J Immunol 1990;145:1740–1744.

40. Conley ME, Delacroix DL. Intravascular and mucosal immunoglobulin A: two separate but related systems of immune defense? Ann Int Med 1987;106:892–899.

41. Kett K, Brandtzaeg P, Radl J, Haaijman JF. Different subclass distribution of IgA-producing cells in human lymphoid organs and various secretory tissues. J Immunol 1986;136:3631–3635.

42. Pumphrey RSH. Computer models of the human immunoglobulins. Binding sites and molecular interactions. Immunol Today 1986;7:206–211.

43. Mehta SK, Plaut AG, Calvanico NJ, Tomasi TB. Human immunoglobulin A: production of an Fc fragment by an enteric microbial proteolytic enzyme. J Immunol 1973;111:1274–1276.

44. Kilian M, Mestecky J, Schroenloher RE. Pathogenic species of the genus Haemophilus and Streptococcus pneumoniae produce immunoglobulin A1 protease. Infect Immun 1979;26:143–149.

45. Kilian M, Reinholdt J. A hypothetical model for the development of invasive infection due to IgA1-protease producing bacteria. In: McGhee JR, Mestecky J, 1987.

46. Kilian M, Husby S, Høst A, Halken S. Increased proportions of bacteria capable of cleaving IgA1 in the pharynx of infants with atopic disease. Ped Res 1995, in press.

47. Savilahti E. IgA deficiency in children. Immunoglobulin-con-

taining cells in the intestinal mucosa, immunoglobulins in secretions and serum IgA levels. Clin Exp Immunol 1972;13:395–406.

48. Grey HM, Kunkel HG. H chain subgroups of myeloma proteins and normal 7S γ-globulin. J Exp Med 1964;120:253–266.

49. Terry WD, Fahey JL. Subclasses of human γ2-globulin based on differences in the heavy polypeptide chains. Science 1964;146:400–401.

50. Stokes CR, Swarbrick ET, Soothill JF. Genetic differences in immune exclusion and partial tolerance to ingested antigens. Clin Exp Immunol 1983;52:678–684.

51. Ramaswamy K, Hakimi J, Bell RG. Evidence for an interleukin 4-inducible immunoglobulin E uptake and transport mechanism in the intestine. J Exp Med 1994;180:1793–1803.

52. Russell MW, Mansa B. Complement-fixing properties of human IgA antibodies: alternative pathway complement activation by plastic bound, but not specific antigen-bound IgA. Scand J Immunol 1989;30:175–183.

53. Ishizaka K. Cellular events in the IgE antibody response. Adv Immunol 1976;23:1–75.

54. Götze O, Müller-Eberhard HJ. Lysis of erythrocytes by complement in absence of antibody. J Exp Med 1970;132:898–903.

55. Mollnes TE, Lachman PJ. Regulation of complement. Scand J Immunol 1988;27:127–142.

56. Brandslund I, Siersted HC, Svehag S-E, Teisner B. Double-decker rocket immunoelectrophoresis C3 split products with C3d specificities in plasma. J Immunol Methods 1981;44:63–68.

57. Halstensen TS, Mollnes TE, Brandtzaeg P. Persistent complement activation in submucosal blood vessels of active inflammatory bowel disease: immunohistochemical evidence. Gastroenterology 1989;97:10–19.

58. Halstensen TS, Mollnes TE, Garred P, Fausa O, Brandtzaeg P. Epithelial deposition of immunoglobulin G1 and activated complement (C3b and terminal complement complex) in ulcerative colitis. Gastroenterology 1990;98:1264–1271.

59. Hurley LS, Lönnerdal B. Trace elements in human milk. In: Hanson LÅ, ed. Biology of Human Milk. New York: Raven Press, 87–88.

60. Chipman DM, Sharon N. Mechanism of lysozyme action. Lysozyme is the first enzyme for which the relation between structure and function has become clear. Science 1969;165:454–465.

61. Goldman AS, Garza C, Nichols BL. Immunologic factors in human milk during the first year of lactation. J Pediatr 1982;100:563–567.

62. Wold AE, Thorssén M, Hull S, Svanborg Edén S. Attachment of *Escheria coli* via mannose- or Galα1-4Galβ-containing receptors to human colonic epithelial cells. Infect Immun 1988;56:2531–2537.

63. Walker WA, Isselbacher KJ. Uptake and transport by the intestine. Possible role in clinical disorders. *Gastroenterology* 1974;76:531–550.

64. Rodewald R. Intestinal transport of antibodies in the newborn rat. J Cell Biol 1973;58:189–211.

65. Walker WA, Cornell R, Davenport LM, Isselbacher KJ. Macromolecular absorption. Mechanism of horseradish peroxidase uptake and transport in adult and neonatal rat intestine. J Cell Biol 1972;54:195–205.

66. Colony PC, Neutra MR. Macromolecular transport in the fetal rat intestine. Gastroenterology 1985;89:294–306.

67. Rhodes RS, Karnovsky MJ. Loss of macromolecular barrier function associated with surgical trauma to the intestine. Lab Invest 1971;25:220–229.

68. Cunningham-Rundles C, Brandeis WE, Good RA, Day NB. Bovine antigens and the formation of circulating immune complexes in selective immunoglobulin A deficiency. Proc Natl Acad Sci USA 1978;75:3387–3389.

69. Husby S, Jensenius JC, Svehag S-E. Passage of undegraded dietary antigen into the blood of healthy adults. Quantification, estimation of size distribution and relation of uptake to levels of specific antibodies. Scand J Immunol 1985;22:83–92.

70. Husby S, Foged N, Høst A, Svehag S-E. Passage of dietary protein into the blood of children with coeliac disease. Quantification and size distribution of absorbed antigen. Gut 1987;28:1062–1072.

71. Roberton DM, Paganelli R, Dinwiddie R, Levinsky RJ. Milk antigen absorption in the preterm and term neonate. Archs Dis Childh 1982;57:369–372.

72. Jacobsson I, Lindberg T, Lothe L, Axelsson I, Benediktsson B. Human α-lactalbumin as a marker of macromolecular absorption. Gut 1986;27:1029–1034.

73. Bland PW, Warren LG. Antigen presentation by epithelial cells of the rat small intestine. I. Kinetics, antigen specificity and blocking by anti-Ia antisera. Immunology 1986;58:1–7.

74. Mayer L, Shlien R. Evidence for function of Ia molecules on gut epithelial cells in man. J Exp Med 1987;166:1471–1483.

75. Mayer L, Eisenhardt D, Salomon P, Bauer W, Plous R, Piccinini L. Expression of Class II molecules on intestinal epithelial cells in humans, Differences between normal and inflammatory bowel disease. Gastroenterology 1991;100:3–12.

76. Mandera JL, Stafford J. Interferon-γ directly affects barrier function of cultured intestinal epithelial monolayers. J Clin Invest 1989;83:724–727.

77. Mayer L. Interferon-γ and class II antigen expression on enterocytes. In: Walker WA, Harmatz PR, Wershil BR, eds. Immunophysiology of the Gut. New York: Academic Press, 111–117.

78. Colgan SP, Resnick MB, Parkos CA, et al. IL-4 directly modulates function of a model human intestinal epithelium. J Immunol 1994;153:2122–2129.

79. Hedges S, Svansbor C, Svenson M. Interleukin-6 response of epithelial cell lines to bacterial stimulation in vitro. Infect Immun 1992;60:1295–1301.

80. Wolf JL, Rubin DH, Finberg R, Kauffaman RS, Sharpe AH, Trier JS, Fields BN. Intestinal M-cells: a pathway for entry of reovirus into the host. Science 1981;212:471–472.

81. Owen RL, Apple RT, Bhalla DK. Morphometric and cytochemical analysis of lysosomes in rat Peyer's patch follicle epithelium: their reduction in volume fraction and acid phosphatase content in M cells compared to adjacent enterocytes. Anat Res 1986;216:521–527.

82. Owen RL, Pierce NF, Apple RT, Cray WC. M cell transport of vibrio cholerae from the intestinal lumen into Peyer's patches: a mechanism for antigen sampling and for microbial transepithelial migration. J Infect Dis 1986;153:1108–1118.

83. Bjerke K, Brandtzaeg P. Lack of relation between expression of HLA-DR and secretory component (SC) in follicle-associated epithelium of human Peyer's patches. Clin Exp Immunol 1988;71:502–507.

84. Allen CH, Mendrick DL, Trier JS. Rat intestinal M cells contain acidic endosomal–lysosomal compartments and express class II major histocompatibility complex determinants. Gastroenterology 1993;104:698–708.

85. Bull DM, Bookman MA. Isolation and functional characterization of human intestinal mucosal lymphoid cells. J Clin Invest 1977;59:966.

86. Mahida YR, Jewell DP. Macrophage activity in inflammatory bowel disease (letter and comment). Gut 1990;31:1086–1087.

87. Mahida YR, Wu K, Jewell DP. Enhanced production of interleukin 1-β by mononuclear cells isolated from mucosa with active ulcerative colitis or Crohn's disease. Gut 1989;30:835– 838.

88. Sturgess RP, McCartney JC, Makgoba MW, Hung C-H, Haskard DO, Ciclitira PJ. Differential upregulation of intercellular adhesion molecule-1 in coeliac disease. Clin Exp Immunol 1990;82:489–492.

89. Strober W, Ehrhardt RO. Regulation of IgA B cell development. In: Ogra PL, et al. Handbook of Mucosal Immunology. San Diego: Academic Press, 1994, 159–176.

90. Flanagan JG, Rabbits TH. Arrangement of human immunoglobulin heavy chain constant region genes implies evolutionary duplication of a segment containing τ, ε and α genes. Nature (London) 1982;300:709–713.

91. Kawanishi H, Slatzman LE, Strober W. Mechanisms regulating IgA class-specific immunoglobulin production in murine gut-associated lymphoid tissues. I. T cells derived from Peyer's patches that switch sIgM B cells to sIgA B cells in vitro. J Exp Med 1983;157:433–450.

92. Coffman RL, Ohara J, Bond JW, Carty J, Zlotnick A, Paul WE. B cell stimulatory factor-1 enhances the IgE response of lipopolysaccharide-activated B cells. J Immunol 1986; 136.919 951.

93. Finkelman FD, Holmes J, Katona IM, Urban JF, et al. Lymphokine control of in vivo immunoglobulin isotype selection. Ann Rev Immunol 1990;8:303–333.

94. Coffman RL, Lebman DA, Schrader B. Transforming growth factor β specifically enhances IgA production by lipopolysaccharide-activated murine B lymphocytes. J Exp Med 1989;170:1039–1044.

95. Lebman DA, Nomura DY, Coffman RL, Lee FD. Molecular characterization of germ-line immunoglobulin α transcripts produced during transforming growth factor type β-induced isotype switching. Proc Natl Acad Sci USA 1990;87:3962–3966.

96. Murray PD, McKenzie DT, Swain SL, Kagnoff MF. Interleukin 5 and interleukin 4 produced by Peyer's patch T cells selectively enhance immunoglobulin A expression. J Immunol 139:2699–2674.

97. Beagley KW, Eldridge JH, Kiyono H, Everson MP, Koopman WJ, Honjo T, McGhee JR. Recombinant murine IL-5 induces high rate IgA synthesis in cycling IgA-positive Peyer's patch B cells. J Immunol 1988;141:2035–2042.

98. Beagley KW, Eldridge JH, Lee F, Kiyono H, Everson MP, Koopman WJ, Hirano T, Kishimoto T, McGhee JR. Interleukins and IgA synthesis: human and murine IL-6 induce high rate IgA secretion in IgA-committed B cells. J Exp Med 1989;169:2133–2148.

99. Ramsay AJ, Husband AJ, Ramshaw IA, et al. The role of interleukin-6 in mucosal IgA antibody responses in vivo. Science 1994;264:561–563.

100. Robinson MA. The human T-cell receptor beta-chain gene complex contains at least 57 variable gene segments. J Immunol 1990;146:4392–4397.

101. Mosmann TR, Coffman RL. Th1 and Th2 cells: different patterns of lymphokine secretion lead to different functional properties. Ann Rev Immunol 1989;7:145–173.

102. Romagnani S. Lymphokine production by human T cells in disease states. Ann Rev Immunol 1994;12:227–257.

103. Gajewski TF, Pinnas M, Wong T, Fitch FW. Murine Th1 and Th2 clones proliferate optimally in response to distinct antigen-presenting cell populations. J Immunol 1991; 146:1750–1758.

104. Guy-Grand D, Griscelli C, Vasalli P. The mouse gut lymphocyte, a novel type of T cell. J Exp Med 1978;148:1661–1677.

105. Davies MDJ, Parrott DMV. Preparation and purification of lymphocytes from the epithelium and lamina propria of murine small intestine. Gut 1981;22:481–488.

106. Goodman T, Lefrancois L. Intraepithelial lymphocytes. Anatomical site, not T cell receptor form, dictates phenotype and function. J Exp Med 1989;170:1569–1581.

107. Lefrancois L. Phenotypic complexity of intraepithelial lymphocytes of the small intestine. J Immunol 1991;147:1746–1751.

108. Deusch K, Luling F, Reich K, Classen M, Wagner H, Pfeffer K. A major fraction of human intraepithelial lymphocytes simultaneously expresses the γ/δ T cell receptor, the CD8 accessory molecule and preferentially uses the $V_\delta 1$ gene segment. Eur J Immunol 1991;21:1053–1059.

109. Spencer J, MacDonald TT, Diss TC, Walker-Smith JA, Ciclitira PJ, Isaacson PG. Changes in intraepithelial lymphocyte subpopulations in coeliac disease and enteropathy associated T cell lymphoma (malignant histiocytosis of the intestine). Gut 1989;30:339–346.

110. Barrett TA, Bajewski TF, Danielpour D, Chang EB, Beagley KW, Bluestone JA. Differential function of intestinal intraepithelial lymphocyte subsets. J Immunol 1992;149:1124–1130.

111. Fujihashi K, Yamamoto M, McGhee JR, Kiyuono H. αβ T cell receptor-positive intraepithelial lymphocytes with CD4+, CD8− and CD4 +, CD8+ phenotypes from orally immunized mice secrete Th2-like function for B cell responses. J Immunol 1993;51:6681–6691.

112. Bandeira A, Itohara S, Bonneville M, Burlen-Defranoux O, Mota-Santos T, Coutinho A, Tonegawa S. Extrathymic origin of intraepithelial lymphocytes bearing T-cell antigen receptor γδ. Proc Natl Acad Sci USA 1991;88:43–47.

113. Brandtzaeg P, Bosnes V, Halstensen TS, Scott H, Sollid LM, Valnes KN. T lymphocytes in human gut epithelium express preferentially the α/β antigen receptor and are often CD45/UCHL1-positive. Scand J Immunol 1989;30:123–128.

114. Halstensen TS, Scott H, Brandtzaeg P. Intraepithelial T cells of the TcRγ/δ+CD8− and Vδ1/Jδ1+ phenotypes are increased in coeliac disease. Scand J Gastroenterol 1989;30:665–672.

115. Sydora BC, Mixter PF, Holcombe HR, Eghtesady P, Williams K, Amaral MC, Nel A, Kronenberg M. Intestinal intraepithelial lymphocytes are activated and cytolytic but do not proliferate as well as other T cells in response to mitogenic signals. J Immunol 1993;150:2179–2191.

116. Mosley RL, Whetsell M, Klein JR. Proliferative capacities of murine intestinal intraepithelial lymphocytes (IEL): IEL expressing TCRαβ and TCRγδ are largely unresponsive to proliferative signals mediated via conventional stimulation of the TCR-CD3 complex. Int Immunol 1991;3:563–568.

117. Janossy G, Tidman N, Selby WS, Thomas JA, Granger S, Kung PC, Goldstein G. Human T lymphocytes of inducer

and suppressor type occupy different microenvironments. Nature 1980;288:81–84.

118. Halstensen, etal. Immunol 1990;71:460–466.

119a. James SP, Zeitz M. Human gastrointestinal mucosal T cells. In: Ogra PL, Mestecky J, Lamm ME, Strober W, McGhee JR, Bienenstock J, eds. Handbook of Mucosal Immunology. San Diego: Academic Press, 1994, 275–285.

119b. Zeitz M, Breen WC, Peffer NJ, James SP. Lymphocytes isolated from the intestinal lamina propria of normal non-human primates have increased expression of genes associated with T cell activation. Gastroenterology 1988;94:647–655.

120. Maatsura T, West GA, Yungman KR, Klein JS, Fiocchi C. Immune activation genes in inflammatory bowel disease. Gastroenterology 1993;104:448–458.

121. Brandtzaeg P, Baklien K. Immunohistochemical studies of the formation and epithelial transport of immunoglobulins in normal and diseased human intestinal mucosa. Scand J Gastroenterol 1976;11(suppl. 36):1–40.

122. Nilssen DE, Söderström R, Brandtzaeg P, Kett K, Helgeland L, Karlsson G, Söderstöm T, Hansson LÅ. Isotype distribution of mucosal IgG-producing cells in patients with various IgG-subclass deficiencies. Clin Exp Immunol 1991;83:17–24.

123. Kilian M, Mestecky J, Russell MW. Defense mechanisms involving Fc-dependent functions of immunoglobulin A and their subversion by bacterial immunoglobulin A proteases. Microbial Rev 1988;52:296–303.

124. Kett K, Brandtzaeg P. Local IgA subclass alterations in ulcerative colitis and Crohn's disease of the colon. Gut 1987;28:1013–1021.

125. Kett K, Rognum TO, Brandtzaeg P. Mucosal subclass distribution of IgG-producing cells is different in ulcerative colitis and Crohn's disease. Gastroenterology 1987;93:919–924.

126. Tada T, Ishizaka K. Distribution of γE-forming cells in lymphoid tissue of the human and monkey. J Immunol 1970;104:377–387.

127. Rognum TO, Brandtzaeg P. IgE-positive cells in human intestinal mucosa are mainly mast cells. Int Arch Allergy Appl Immunol 1989, 256–260.

128. Enerbäck L. Mucosal mast cells in rat and in man. Int Arch Allergy Appl Immunol 1987;82:249–255.

129. Galli SJ. New insights into "the riddle of the mast cells": microenvironmental regulation of mast cell development and phenotypic heterogeneity. Lab Invest 1990;62:5–33.

130. Abe T, Swieter M, Imai T, Hollander ND, Befys AD. Mast cell heterogeneity: two-dimensional gel electrophoretic analyses of rat peritoneal and intestinal mast cells. Eur J Immunol 1990;20:1941–1947.

131. Lowman MA, Rees PH, Benyon RC, Church MK. Human mast cell heterogeneity: histamine release from mast cells dispersed from skin, lung, adenoids, tonsils, and colon in response to IgE-dependent and nonimmunologic stimuli. J Allergy Clin Immunol 1988;81:590–597.

132. Walsh LJ, Trinchieri G, Waldorf HA. Human dermal mast cells contain and release tumor necrosis factor α which induces endothelial leukocyte adhesion molecule-1. Proc Natl Acad Sci USA 1991;88:4220.

133. Bradding P, Feather IH, Howarth PH, et al. Interleukin 4 is localized to and released by human mast cells. J Exp Med 1992;176:1381–1390.

134. Bradding P, Feather IH, Wilson S, et al. Immuno-locatization

of cytokines in the nasal mucosa of normal and perennial rhinitic subjects. The mast cell as a source of IL-4, II-5, and IL-6 in human allergic mucosal inflammation. J Immunol 1993;153:3853–3865.

135. Mossman TR, Bond MW, Coffman RL, Ohara J, Paul WE. T-cell and mast cell lines respond to B-cell stimulatory factor 1. Proc Natl Acad Sci USA 1986;83:5654–5658.

136. Bischoff SC, Dahinden CA. C-kit ligand: a unique potentiator of mediator release by human lung mast cells. J Exp Med 1992;175:237–243.

137a. Columbo M, Horowitz EM, Botana LM, MacGlashan DW, Bochner BS, Gillis S, Zsebo KM, Galli SJ, Lichtenstein LM. The human recombinant c-kit receptor ligand, rhSCF, induces mediator release from human cutaneous mast cells and enhances IgE-dependent mediator release from both skin mast cells and peripheral blood basophils. J Immunol 1992;149:599–608.

137b. Weller PF. The immunobiology of eosinophils. N Engl J Med 1991;324:1110–1118.

138. Weller PF, Bach D, Austen KF. Human eosinophilic lysophospholipase: the sole protein component of Charcot-Leyden crystals. J Immunol 1982;128:1346–1349.

139. Kerr MA, Mazengera RL, Stewart WW. Structure and function of immunoglobulin A receptors on phagocytic cells. Biochem Soc Trans 1990;18:215–217.

140. Monteiro RC, Kubagawa H, Cooper MD. Cellular distribution, regulation and biochemical nature of an Fcα receptor in humans. J Exp Med 1990;171:597–613.

141. Grangette C, Gruart V, Ouassi MA, et al. IgE receptor on human eosinophils (FcERII): comparison with B cell CD23 and association with an adhesion molecule. J Immunol 1989;143:3580–3588.

142. Abu-Ghazaleh RI, Fujisawa T, Mestecky J, Kyle RA, Gleich GJ. IgA-induced eosinophil degranulation. J Immunol 1989;142:2393–2400.

143. Hartnell A, Moqbell R, Walsh BM, Bradley B, Kay AB. Tc gamma and CD11/CD18 receptor expression on normal density and low density human eosinophils. Immunology 1990;69:264–270.

144. Coffman RL, Seymour BWP, Hudak S, Jackson J, Rennick D. Antibody to interleukin-5 inhibits helminth-induced eosinophilia in mice. Science 1989;245:308–310.

145a. Hamid Q, Barkans J, Meng Q, Abrams JS, Kay AB, Moqbel R. Human eosinophils synthesize and secrete interleukin-6, in vitro. Blood 1992;80:1496–1501.

145b. Reynolds JD, Pabst R. The emigration of lymphocytes from Peyer's patches in sheep. Eur J Immunol 1984;14:7–13.

146a. Wong DTW, Elovic A, Matossian K, et al. Eosinophils from patines with blood eosinophilia express transforming growth factor β1. Blood 1991;78:2702–2707.

146b. Craig SW, Cebra JJ. Peyer's patches: an enriched source of precursors for IgA-producing immunocytes in the rabbit. J Exp Med 1971;134:188–200.

147. Husband AJ, Gowans JL. The origin and antigen-dependent distribution of IgA-containing cells in the intestine. J Exp Med 1978;148:1146–1160.

148. Dunkley ML, Husband AJ. The induction and migration of antigen-specific helper cells for IgA responses in the intestine. Immunology 1986;57:379–385.

149. Poussier P, Edouard P, Lee C, Binnie M, Julius M. Thymus-independent development of T cells expressing T cell recep-

tor α/β in the intestinal epithelium: evidence for distinct circulation patterns of gut- and thymus-derived T lymphocytes. J Exp Med 1992;176:187–199.

150. Guy-Grand D, Cerf-Bensussan N, Malissen B, Malassis-Seris M, Briottet C, Vassali P. Two gut intraepithelial CD8+ lymphocyte populations with different T cell receptors: a role for the gut epithelium in T cell differentiation. J Exp Med 1991;173:471–481.

151. Deusch K, Reich K. Phenotypic features of human intestinal intraepithelial lymphocytes in health and disease. Mucosal Immunology Update 1994;2:10–15.

152. Butcher EC, Scollay RG, Weissman IL. Organ specificity of lymphocyte migration: mediation of highly selective lymphocyte interaction with organ-specific determinants on high endothelial venules. Eur J Immunol 1980;10:556–561.

153. Dustin ML, Springer TA. T-cell receptor cross-linking transiently stimulates adhesiveness through LFA-1. Nature 1989;341:619–624.

154. Gallatin WM, Weissman IL, Butcher EC. A cell-surface molecule involved in organ-specific homing of lymphocytes. Nature 1983;304:30–34.

155. Picker LJ, Kishimoto TK, Smith CW, Warnock RA, Butcher EC. ELAM-1 is an adhesion molecule for skin-homing T cells. Nature 1991;349:796–799.

156. Yuan Q, Jiang W-m, Hollander D, Leung E, Watson JD, Krissansen GW. Identity between the novel integrin β_7 subunit and an antigen found highly expressed on intraepithelial lymphocytes in the small intestine. Biochem Biophys Res Comm 1991;176:1443–1449.

157. Cepek KL, Parker CM, Madara JL, Brenner MB. Integrin $\alpha^E\beta_7$ mediates adhesion of T lymphocytes to epithelial cells. J Immunol 1993;150:3459–3470.

158. Roberts K, Kilshaw PJ. The mucosal T cell integrin $\alpha_{M290}\beta_7$ recognizes a ligand on mucosal epithelial cell lines. Eur J Immunol 1993;23:1630–1635.

159. Berlin C, Berg EL, Briskin MJ, et al. $\alpha_4\beta_7$ integrin mediates lymphocyte binding to the mucosal vascular adressin MAd-CAM-1. Cell 1993;74:185–195.

160. Andrew DP, Berlin C, Honda S, et al. Distinct but overlapping epitopes are involved in $\alpha_4\beta_7$-mediated adhesion to vascular cell adhesion molecule-1, mucosal adressin-1, fibronectin, and lymphocyte aggregation. J Immunol 1994; 153:3847–3861.

161. Pierce NF. The role of antigen form and function in the primary and secondary intestinal immune responses to cholera toxin and toxoid in the rat. J Exp Med 1978;148:1108–1118.

162. Elson CO, Ealding W. Generalized systemic and mucosal immunity in mice after mucosal stimulation with cholera toxin. J Immunol 1984;132:2736–2741.

163. Elson CO, Ealding W. Cholera toxin feeding did not induce oral tolerance in mice and abrogated oral tolerance to an unrelated protein antigen. J Immunol 1984;133:2892–2897.

164. Bromander A, Holmgren J, Lycke N. Cholera toxin stimulates IL-production and enhances antigen presentation by macrophages in vitro. J Immunol 1991;146:2908–2914.

165. Snider et al, 1994.

166. Mestecky J, McGhee JR. New strategies for oral immunization. Curr Topics Microbiol Immunol 1989;146:3.

167. Chase MS. Inhibition of experimental drug allergy by prior feeding of the sensitizing agent. Pros Soc Exp Biol Med 1946;61:257–259.

168. Hanson DGN, Vaz NM, Maia LCS, Hornbrook MM, Lynch JM, Roy CA. Inhibition of specific immune responses by feeding protein antigen. Int Arch Allergy Appl Immun 1977;55:1518–1524.

169. Kagnoff MF. Effects of antigen-feeding on intestinal and systemic immune responses II. Suppression of delayed-type hypersensitivity reactions. J Immunol 1978;120:1509–1513.

170. Challacombe SJ, Tomasi TB. Systemic tolerance and secretory immunity after oral immunization. J Exp Med 1980;152:1459–1472.

171. Peri B, Rothberg RM. Circulating antitoxin in rabbits after ingestion of diphtheria toxoid. Infect Immun 1981;32:1148–1154.

172. Mowat AMcl, Strobel S, Drummond HE, Ferguson A. Immunological responses to fed protein antigens in mice I. Reversal of oral tolerance to ovalbumin by cyclophosphamide. Immunology 1982;45:105–113.

173. Lafont S, André C, Andre F, Gillon J, Fargier M-C. Abrogation by subsequent feeding of antibody response, including IgE, in parenterally immunized mice. J Exp Med 1982;155:1573–1578.

174. Lamont AG, Bruce MG, Watret KC, Ferguson A. Suppression of an established DTH response to ovalbumin by feeding antigen after immunization. Immunol 1988;64:135–139.

175. Ramsdell F, Fowlkes BJ. Clonal deletion versus clonal anergy: the role of the thymus in inducing self-tolerance. Science 1991;248:1342–1348.

176. Mattingly JA, Waksman BH. Immunological suppression after oral administration of antigen I. Specific suppressor cells formed in rat Peyer's patches after oral administration of sheep erythrocytes and their systemic migration. J Immunol 1978;121:1878–1883.

177. Richman LK, Chiller JM, Brown WR, Hanson DG, Vaz NM. Entcrically induced immunologic tolerance I. Induction of suppressor T lymphocytes by intragastric administration of soluble protein. J Immunol 1978;121:2429–2434.

178. MacDonald TT. Immunosuppression caused by antigen feeding II. Suppressor T cells mask Peyer's patch B cell priming to orally administered antigen. Eur J Immunol 1983;13:138–142.

179. Bruce MG, Ferguson A. The influence of intestinal processing on the immunogenicity and molecular size of absorbed, circulating ovalbumin in mice. Immunology 1986;59:295–300.

180. Michael JG. The role of digestive enzymes in orally induced immune tolerance. Immunol Invest 1989;18:1049–1054.

181. Miller A, Lider O, Roberts AB, Sporn MB, Weiner HL. Suppressor T cells generated by oral tolerization to myelin basic protein suppress both in vitro and in vivo immune responses by the release of transforming growth factor beta after antigen-specific triggering. Proc Natl Acad Sci USA 1992;89:421–423.

182. Korenblatt PE, Rothberg RM, Minden P, Farr RS. Immune responses of human adults after oral and parenteral exposure to bovine serum albumin. J Allergy 1968;41:226–235.

183. Lowney ED. Suppression of contact sensitization in man by prior feeding of antigen. J Invest Dermatology 1973;61:90–93.

184. Husby S, Mestecky J, Moldoveanu Z, Holland S, Elson CO. Oral tolerance in humans. T cell but not B cell tolerance after antigen feeding. J Immunol 1994;152:4663–4670.

185. Benaceraf B. Role of MHC gene products in immune regulation. Science 1981;212:1229–1238.

186. Stokes CR, Swarbrick ET, Soothill JF. Genetic differences in immune exclusion and partial tolerance to ingested antigens. Clin Exp Immunol 1983;52:678–684.

187. Elson CO. Cholera toxin as a mucosal adjuvant: effects of H-2 major histocompatibility complex and Ips genes. Infection and Immunity 1992;60:2874–2879.

188. Sollid LM, Markussen G, Ek J, Gjerde H, Vartdal F, Thorsby E. Evidence for a primary association of celiac disease to a particular HLA-DQ α/β heterodimer. J Exp Med 1989;169:345–350.

189. Holm K, Mäki M, Savilahti E, Lipsanen V, Laippala P, Koskimies S. Interpithelial γ/δ T cell receptor lymphocytes and genetic susceptibility to coeliac disease. Lancet 1992; 339:1500–1503.

190. Arranz E, Bode J, Kingstone K, Ferguson A. Intestinal antibody pattern of coeliac disease: association with γ/δ T cell receptor expression by intraepithelial lymphocytes, and other indices of potential coeliac disease. Gut 1994;35:476–482.

191. Marsh DG, Meyers DA, Bias WB. The epidemiology and genetics of atopic allergy. N Engl J Med 1981;305:1551–1559.

192. Marsh DG, Neely JD, Breazeale DR, Ghosh B, Freidhoff LR, Ehrlich-Kautzky E, Schou C, Krishnaswamy G, Beaty TH. Linkage analysis of IL-4 and other chromosome 5q31.1 markers and total serum immunoglobulin E concentrations. Science 1994;264:1152–1158.

2

MAST CELLS, BASOPHILS, AND IMMUNOGLOBULIN E

Kim E. Barrett

The mast cell, its circulating counterpart the basophil, and immunoglobulins of the E class (IgE), which bind to these cells with extremely high affinity, are the major constituents of the immediate hypersensitivity reactions known as allergies. In the particular case of food allergy, defined as an immunologically mediated adverse reaction to a foodstuff, substantial evidence suggests that the symptoms of these reactions are often initiated when food-specific, cell-bound IgE molecules are cross-linked on the surface of gastrointestinal mast cells. This mast cell activation stimulates the release and de novo synthesis of a host of potent chemical mediators, including histamine, proteoglycans, leukotrienes, and cytokines. These substances can exert a variety of effects on the surrounding intestinal tissue. They may also, by virtue of their effects on intestinal epithelial permeability, permit passage of food antigens from the lumen of the gut into the systemic circulation, thus providing for allergic reactions in more distant organs, the recruitment of other participating cell types, and perpetuation of the response as a whole.

Given the central role for mast cells and IgE in mediating food allergies, this chapter covers what is known of the derivation, properties, and function of mast cells, with emphasis on human studies and the particular mast cell type found in the gastrointestinal tract. Also covered are studies that have increased our understanding of how the synthesis of IgE is controlled, and why, although IgE synthesis may occur in both normal and atopic individuals, IgE synthesized by the latter group may be more able to mediate various immediate hypersensitivity responses.

Mast Cells and Basophils

Mast cells and basophils are cells that are known to diverge at an early stage of their development. The tissue mast cell is derived from circulating mononuclear precursors, whereas mature basophils are circulating polymorphonuclear cells that appear to be more closely related developmentally to the eosinophil than the mast cell. Nevertheless, mast cells and basophils have many similarities of properties and function, making it logical to consider them together. For instance, they both possess high-affinity, Fc receptors for IgE, through which they can be activated to release mediators. They are both granulated cell types, with a proteoglycan granular matrix providing storage for other mediators. Many mediators, but not all, are shared by mast cells and basophils, as is the capacity to synthesize generated secondary mediators such as eicosanoids.

More important, perhaps, than the differences between mast cells and basophils is the determination, built upon by recent investigations, that mast cells themselves represent a heterogeneous population of cell types (1). This concept is particularly pertinent to the discussion of food allergy, since the mast cells of the mucosa of the gastrointestinal tract may differ quite markedly from those in connective tissue sites such as the skin. Therefore, this chapter discusses mast cell heterogeneity as it refers to the intestine, with particular emphasis on studies that have extended observations of such heterogeneity to the situation in humans.

To summarize, this section of the chapter is intended to present available information regarding the derivation, functional properties, and mediators of mast cells. Important differences between mast cells and basophils are pointed out, and information pertaining directly to intestinal mast cells, based on studies in humans where possible, is emphasized.

MAST CELL HETEROGENEITY: THE CASE OF THE MUCOSAL MAST CELL

Mast cells resident in the intestinal mucosa of rodents, and in this site and possibly others in humans, are thought to be a subpopulation with characteristic properties (1). These cells may be a distinct population, as in rodents, or may represent one extreme of a spectrum of mast cell properties in humans. In either event, it is these so-called mucosal mast cells that are likely to be the first mast cell subset responsive to substances presented by the oral route.

The concept of mast cell heterogeneity essentially originated with the studies of Enerbäck, who showed that mast cells in the mucosal layers of the rat small intestine differed from their connective tissue counterparts in terms of their staining properties, sensitivity to fixation, and responsiveness to the basic secretagogue compound 48/80 (2–4). Subsequent studies revealed that rat mucosal mast cells contained and synthesized unique mediators, and that they were functionally unresponsive to many of the activators and inhibitors of connective tissue mast cells, exemplified by rat peritoneal mast cells (5–8). Some of the major differences between rodent mucosal and connective tissue mast cells are summarized in Table 2.1.

We are beginning to gain an appreciation of the extent to which the mast cell heterogeneity identified in rodents is also manifest in humans. Cytochemical heterogeneity is apparent between human mast cell subpopulations, based both on staining characteristics and the biochemical or immunologic detection of specific mediators. Thus, recent ultrastructural studies suggest that all human mast cell subpopulations contain heparin, whereas gastrointestinal and some lung mast cells also contain appreciable amounts of a second granular proteoglycan, chondroitin sulfate E (9–13). Similarly, mast cells in the intestinal mucosa contain only the tryptic protease tryptase (T mast cells), whereas human skin mast cells contain both this protease and another enzyme of chymotryptic specificity, chymase (TC mast cells) (14).

Functional heterogeneity between mucosal and connective tissue mast cells of the rat became appreciated when methods were developed to obtain the mucosal mast cells of this species in suspension by enzymatically dispersing the intestine. When the cells so obtained were compared with the peritoneal mast cells of the same animals, significant differences were observed in their responsiveness to various agents. For example, rat peritoneal mast cells released substantial amounts of their histamine in response to basic secretagogues such as compound 48/80 and the bee venom peptide 401, and neuropeptides including vasoactive intestinal peptide (VIP), endorphins, and

Table 2.1
Comparison of Rat Connective Tissue-Type and Mucosal Mast Cells

Property	Connective Tissue-Type Mast Cells	Mucosal Mast Cells
Location	Connective tissue Serosal cavities	Intestinal mucosa Other sites?
Metacromasia and fixation	Readily demonstrated High pH, formalin	Hard to demonstrate Low pH, Carnoy's
Growth factors	SCF, others?	IL-3, IL-4
IgE-dependent activation	Yes	Yes
Effect of compound 48/80	Degranulation	Proliferation
Proteoglycan	Heparin	Chondroitin sulfate di-B
Eicosanoid	Predominantly PGD_2	LTC_4, PGD_2
Protease	RMCP I	RMCP II

Table 2.2
Functional Heterogeneity of Human Mast Cells and Basophils

Stimulus	Mast Cell Types Tested for Histamine Release			
	Intestinal Mast Cells	Lung Mast Cells	Skin Mast Cells	Basophils
Antigen	+	++	+	++
Compound 48/80	−	−	+	−
Calcium ionophores	++	++	++	++
Morphine	−	−	++	−
C5a	NR			++
F-Met peptides	−	−	−	++
Substance P	−	−	++	−

Histamine release is characterized as absent (−, <5%), moderate (+, 15%–20%), or marked (++, >20%). NR, not reported. Cell preparations were of various purities.

neurotensin, while rat mucosal mast cells were completely unresponsive to these agents (5, 15). Similarly, histamine release from rat peritoneal mast cells was inhibited by the antiallergic drugs theophylline and disodium cromoglycate (cromolyn sodium), whereas release from the mucosal cells was not (6). Several laboratories went on to examine whether such functional heterogeneity was also seen among human mast cell subsets. Initial studies in both humans and nonhuman primates compared the properties of lung and intestinal mast cells (16, 17). For these two cell types, while cytochemical heterogeneity was readily apparent, few—if any—functional differences were seen, leading some authors to conclude that functional heterogeneity, with its obvious clinical implications, was not a prominent feature of the mast cell in humans. With hindsight, the described studies probably compared the wrong two mast cell populations, however. The ability to define T and TC human mast cell subsets (14) suggests that human lung mast cells may be quite similar to human intestinal mucosal mast cells, in that the majority of mast cells in both sites are of the T phenotype. When the functional properties of human intestinal mucosal mast cells were compared with those of a TC subset, human skin mast cells, functional heterogeneity was apparent (18, 19). Human skin mast cells are responsive to many of the secretagogues that activate rat peritoneal mast cells, including compound 48/80, neuropeptides, polylysine, and morphine, while human intestinal (and lung) mast cells are not. To the author's knowledge, no secretagogues have yet been identified

that activate the latter cell type but not the former, although such T mast cell–specific agents undoubtedly exist. Functional heterogeneity of human mast cells is summarized in Table 2.2.

Current evidence thus suggests that mast cells of the human intestinal mucosa, like those of the rat, represent a specialized mast cell subtype in terms of their cytochemical and functional properties. Such mast cell heterogeneity has obvious implications for the development of antiallergic therapies targeted to the gastrointestinal tract. Mast cell heterogeneity presumably has its origins in site-specific pathways for mast cell development.

MAST CELL AND BASOPHIL ONTOGENY

Significant progress has been made in recent years in our understanding of the precursors, development, and growth factor requirements for mast cells and basophils. Much of this information has been obtained using experimental animals, particularly mice, but some general principles might be extrapolated to the situation in humans.

Mast Cells

For both mice and rats, mast cells can be propagated in cultures of a variety of starting cell sources, including bone marrow, peripheral blood, spleen, thymus, and lymph node tissues (20). Mast cells are thought to be derived, at least in rodents, from the pluripotent hemopoietic stem cell that is also able to give rise to neutrophils, macrophages, and erythrocytes (21). The differentiation of this stem cell to a mast cell pheno-type in culture is absolutely dependent on the presence of the T-cell-derived cytokine, interleukin-3 (IL-3) (22). Other cytokines may also be important in mast cell propagation. In particular, IL-4 can synergistically enhance murine mast cell growth, although it is unable to stimulate mast cell proliferation in the absence of IL-3 (22, 23). In the murine system, cytokines have also been implicated in the generation of specific mast cell subpopulations, at least in vitro. Based on the appearance of specific proteases, IL-9 and IL-10 appear to be important accessory factors driving differentiation to a mucosal-like phenotype. In contrast, the fibroblast-derived growth factor, stem cell factor (SCF, also known as *kit* ligand), supports the development of connective tissue-type mast cells (24–26).

The requirement of IL-3 for mast cell growth in vitro parallels an in vivo T-cell dependence of at least one mast cell type. Proliferation of intestinal mucosal mast cells in mice and rats has long been known to be dependent on soluble T-cell-derived factors. Neither nude mice nor severely T-cell-depleted rats exhibited the characteristic intestinal mucosal mast cell hyperplasia that accompanies nematode infection in these species (27, 28). More recent studies have specifically implicated IL-3 and IL-4 in nematode-driven intestinal mast cell hyperplasia, at least in mice (29). These animals exhibit normal numbers of mast cells in the unparasitized state, however, suggesting that other factors are also responsible for the survival of mast cells in tissues. Moreover, mast cells in connective tissue sites show no in vivo requirement for T-cell influences in their proliferation. The findings suggest that other environmental influences can stimulate or augment mast cell growth and differentiation. This hypothesis is supported by the observation that in vitro derived, IL-3-dependent murine mast cells, which display cytochemical properties reminiscent of mucosal mast cells, can be induced to change their phenotype to one more reminiscent of connective tissue mast cells by coculture with fibroblasts (30). This experiment has also provided the principal evidence for the hypothesis that the mast cell heterogeneity observed in rodents between cells in mucosal and connective tissue sites actually reflects differences in the state of maturity of these cells. It has been argued that the rodent mucosal mast cell, while exhibiting several specific biochemical markers that are not found in connective tissue (or peritoneal) cells, is an immature connective tissue cell that can be induced to differentiate further if provided with appropriate environmentally derived factors—perhaps the cytokines discussed above.

A competing hypothesis of mast cell ontogeny argues that different mast cell types in a given species arise as distinct lineages. In humans, it appears that T and TC mast cells develop by divergent pathways, or at least that TC mast cells do not develop from T mast cells, as patients with immunodeficiencies affecting T lymphocytes had profoundly depressed numbers of T mast cells in their intestinal mucosa while the number of submucosal TC mast cells was unaffected (31). Furthermore, in the mouse at least, it appears that transdifferentiation between mast cell types can occur, because the connective tissue-type peritoneal mast cells in this species were able to repopulate both mucosal and connective tissue sites of mast-cell-deficient mice (32). The transplanted cells took on the histochemical phenotype appropriate to the tissue site in which they were placed.

Despite the substantial progress made in identifying regulatory mechanisms for mast cell development in rodents, our knowledge of human mast cell ontogeny and differentiation remains quite limited. Human mast cells can be derived in vitro in the presence of SCF, whereas IL-3 and IL-4 do not appear to lead to the development of mast cells in human cultures, at least when added independently (33–35). Moreover, soluble SCF appears to be capable of generating only T mast cells, whereas coculture of precursor cells with fibroblasts, or with conditioned medium obtained from a bone marrow cell line from a patient with mastocytosis, allows the development of cells with the TC phenotype (36, 37). These findings suggest that a quantitatively or qualitatively different signal for growth may be provided by membrane-bound SCF, and/or that additional growth factors might be involved in the development of TC mast cells compared with the T mast cell population (37, 38).

We conclude that the anatomic microenvironment that a mast cell precursor encounters on establishing tissue residence has a profound effect on the subsequent phenotype of that cell. Fibroblasts, nerves, epithelial cells, endothelial cells, and others are all potential contributors to the local cytokine milieu influencing differentiation (36, 37, 39). Identification of the factors involved will facilitate our understanding of mast cell heterogeneity and may have therapeutic implications for diseases in which mast cell hyperplasia is observed.

Basophils

For the purposes of discussing ontogeny, basophils clearly merit separate consideration from mast cells. Although both basophils and mast cells may be derived from bone marrow precursors, their development appears to be regulated separately. Indeed, evidence suggests that mast cells and basophils demonstrate a reciprocal relationship in various species.

In vitro growth of basophils has been examined in most detail using tissue sources of human origin. Basophil proliferation has been obtained in cultures of fetal liver, peripheral blood, bone marrow, and umbilical cord blood, and is dependent on cytokines since cell growth is observed only in the presence of a variety of conditioned media (40–43). There is evidence that the basophil-promoting activity, which has been partially purified, is not granulocyte macrophage colony stimulating factor (GM-CSF), IL-1, IL-2, interferon-γ (IFN-γ) IFN-α, or erythroid-potentiating activity (44). Likewise, survival and/or growth of mouse basophils in vitro cannot be supported by IL-3 and SCF (45). While not specific for the basophil lineage, IL-3, IL-5, and GM-CSF do appear to direct the differentiation of peripheral blood precursors along the basophil–eosinophil pathway (46). One known growth factor that also appears to influence basophilic differentiation and proliferation is the neurotropic polypeptide nerve growth factor (NGF). This factor stimulated basophil growth in cultures of cord blood when added either alone or in combination with T-lymphocyte-conditioned medium, but its activity in promoting basophil differentiation was apparently dependent on the presence of T cells in the cord blood culture (47). Hence NGF is unlikely to

be the final cytokine that acts directly on basophil precursors, although its indirect activity in promoting their differentiation is probably important in vivo, particularly as it appears to be specific for basophilic, rather than eosinophilic, differentiation (see below).

Basophils and eosinophils are often seen in association in allergic responses, and may share several mediators and activating signals. It was, therefore, of interest to determine in what way these two cell types were related. Denburg and coworkers have demonstrated that a common basophil–eosinophil progenitor exists in human peripheral blood, and that numbers of these progenitors may be increased in atopic patients (48, 49). Differentiation of this precursor along either pathway can be stimulated by factors present in medium conditioned by leukemic T cells, and the activities for eosinophil differentiation versus basophil differentiation are partially separable (50). Transforming growth factor β may be one important factor that aids a switch from eosinophil to basophil commitment (51). Activities promoting basophil and eosinophil growth have also been identified in supernatants from nasal epithelial cells, keratinocytes, and nasal polyp mononuclear cells, and may be produced more readily using cells obtained from allergic donors (52). The findings support the hypothesis that basophils and eosinophils accumulate at sites of allergic inflammation because circulating progenitors are stimulated to proliferate and differentiate locally, under the influence of soluble hemopoietic factors derived from mucosal cell populations. Studies to date have been carried out largely with reference to the nasal mucosa, but the observation that other epithelial cell lines can also produce basophil-promoting activities suggests the findings might be extrapolated to other mucosal sites, such as the intestine.

Much remains to be elucidated about how basophil differentiation is controlled in vivo, and about its relationship to eosinophil differentiation. Clonally derived Eo-type colonies from cord blood can contain cells that are either basophilic or eosinophilic, or have mixed basophilic and eosinophilic granulation and biochemical markers. Thus, basophils and eosinophils probably differ only in the terminal events of their differentiation, which possibly explains why basophil growth and eosinophil growth appear to be reciprocally regulated (50). Depending on receptor density for basophil or eosinophil growth-promoting activities, as well as the available concentrations of these factors, a committed basophil–eosinophil progenitor will become either a basophil or an eosinophil.

MEDIATORS

The pathologic relevance of mast cells and basophils stems largely from their ability to synthesize a diverse collection of potent chemical mediators. Some of these mediators are common to basophils and all mast cell types, whereas others may be synthesized only by cell subsets. Mast cell (and basophil) mediators are commonly considered to fall into three main groups: preformed mediators that are rapidly eluted from the granule following activation; preformed mediators that remain granule-associated or elute slowly following activation; and mediators that are synthesized de novo following activation, often by the metabolism of membrane phospholipids. In addition, rapidly emerging data indicate that mast cells and basophils are important sources of the pleiotropic intercellular mediators known as cytokines. In general, these polypeptide mediators require protein synthesis for their release (53, 54). The complete catalog of substances that has been identified in mast cells and basophils is thus extensive (55). This doubtless accounts for the multiple possible consequences of allergic reactions. Some mast cell and basophil mediators are listed in Table 2.3, and selected members of this list are covered in more detail below.

Considering readily elutable granule-associated mediators, the prototype substance of this group is histamine. This biogenic amine, synthesized by the enzymatic decarboxylation of the amino acid histidine, has been identified in all mast cells and basophils so far studied. In fact, in a number of species, including humans, mast cells and basophils represent essentially the only repository of tissue histamine outside of the nervous system and that found in enteroendocrine cells. Histamine release is widely used as a marker of mast cell activation. It can be readily measured in tissue fluids such as plasma, and circulating levels of the amine are transiently increased in patients undergoing allergic reactions such as following antigen provocation. In experimen-

Table 2.3
Mast Cell and Basophil Mediators

Substances rapidly eluted from the granule under physiologic conditions
Histamine
5-Hydroxytryptamine (rodents)
Chemotactic factors
Exoglycosidases
Activators of kinin, complement and clotting systems
Vasoactive intestinal polypeptide analogues

Substances remaining granule-associated after activation
Proteoglycans
Proteinases (tryptase, chymase)
Peroxidase
Superoxide dismutase

Secondary mediators synthesized upon activation
Prostaglandins
Leukotrienes
Platelet-activating factor

Mediators whose release requires protein synthesis
IL-2, 3, 4, 5, 6
IFN-γ
TNF-α*
Endothelin-1

---

*Some TNF-α may also be stored within mast cells and rapidly released upon activation.

tal models of food allergy, challenge of animals with intraluminal antigen leads to a decrease in tissue histamine, presumably reflecting release of the amine from mast cells and loss into the lumen or circulation (56). Once released, histamine can exert a variety of effects on surrounding tissues via specific H_1, H_2, and H_3 receptors. The importance of histamine in allergic reactions is reflected in the frequent prescription of antihistamine drugs to treat some allergic disorders.

The amount of histamine present in various mast cell subsets may vary markedly. In general, basophils and mast cells in the intestinal mucosa contain smaller quantities of the amine than do mast cells in the connective tissues. In keeping with this in vivo observation, murine mast cells grown in tissue culture show increased amounts of stored histamine when cocultured with fibroblasts (30). The decreased storage of histamine in certain mast cells may reflect the fact that such cells also contain granules with a different type of proteoglycan matrix, of lower overall charge than heparin.

The presence in mast cells of amines with known

neurotransmitter properties raises the possibility that mast cells can communicate with the nervous system. There is morphological evidence for such a contention in the striking spatial association between mast cells and nerves in the intestinal mucosa of rats and humans (57, 58). Functional evidence for neuronal interactions with immediate hypersensitivity also exists (58) and is reviewed further below, but it is also of note that immunoreactive forms of neuropeptides such as VIP have been shown to occur as releasable mediators in some mast cell types (59).

Important granule-associated mast cell and basophil mediators include proteoglycans and a variety of enzymes. The particular proteoglycan class synthesized by a given mast cell (or basophil) has been suggested as a classifying feature, as have certain proteases (see above). Proteoglycans are a special class of glycoproteins and are a major granular constituent of basophils and all mast cells. The molecule consists of a protein core to which sugar side chains are covalently linked. The side chains, known as glycosaminoglycans, are of similar size and composition for a given proteoglycan, and consist of repeating disaccharide units. The nature of this disaccharide defines the class of proteoglycan as well as conferring a specific degree of negative charge density on the molecule as a whole. Mast cells may contain either heparin, a highly charged proteoglycan, or the less charged molecules chondroitin sulfate E or chondroitin sulfate di-B. These latter compounds are sometimes referred to as "oversulfated" as they have one more sulfate moiety per disaccharide unit than other chondroitin sulfates. They have one less negative charge per disaccharide than heparin, however, resulting in a significantly lower overall negative charge than the latter molecule.

In the rat, connective tissue mast cells contain heparin as their granular proteoglycan, while mast cells in mucosal sites contain chondroitin sulfates of the di-B class. In humans, all mast cell subsets appear to contain heparin (13), with intestinal mast cells (9) and some lung mast cells (10, 11) also containing chondroitin sulfate E. When the basophils of a patient with chronic myelogenous leukemia were examined, they contained mainly chondroitin-4-sulfate, as do human basophils cultured from cord blood and, interestingly, eosinophils (60).

It is to be expected that the granules of mast cells at mucosal sites would have a lower capacity than their connective tissue counterparts to store mediators such as histamine (as is true in the rat) but that the tissue availability of mediators following granule extrusion might be enhanced. Furthermore, other site-specific consequences based on proteoglycan content can be envisioned since heparin and the chondroitin sulfates have biological activity in addition to their function as a storage matrix. For example, both classes of proteoglycan can stabilize proteases, influence lymphocyte function, and inhibit certain aspects of the complement cascade, but only heparin possesses significant anticoagulant activity (11).

Mast cells and basophils are also noted for the various enzymes that they contain. One major class is the serine proteases (61). In rats, two such proteases have been identified, both of chymotryptic specificity and termed rat mast cell proteases (RMCP) I and II. These enzymes are antigenically distinct and appear to occur exclusively in different mast cell classes: RMCP I in connective tissue mast cells and RMCP II in mucosal mast cells (62). Likewise, a family of murine mast cell proteinases has been identified. These proteinases appear to be both developmentally regulated and differentially expressed in mast cell subpopulations (24–26). In humans, mast cell subsets have been classified by whether they contain a tryptic protease (tryptase) or this enzyme in association with another of chymotryptic specificity (chymase) (14). The first mast cell class, termed T, is present in the intestinal mucosa and accounts for 90% of human lung mast cells. The second mast cell class, termed TC, is predominant in the skin. Basophils contain small amounts of tryptase, and apparently no chymase (61).

Possible functions for mast cell tryptase have been studied extensively. The enzyme generates the anaphylatoxin C3a from complement component C3, inactivates high-molecular-weight kininogen, and inactivates the thrombin-induced clotting activity of fibrinogen (63). The enzymatic activity may be modulated extensively by proteoglycans such as heparin and chondroitin sulfate E (64). Tryptase is released during mast cell activation, and its persistence in the circulation relative to histamine may indicate that it will be a useful clinical marker of putative mast cell involvement in disease (65). Intriguing recent data also indicate that tryptase is mitogenic for fibroblasts and smooth muscle cells (61). Mast cell chymase is not discussed in detail here as it does not occur in intestinal mucosal mast cells. It does appear to have proinflammatory actions, being able to degrade components of the extracellular matrix (66). This activity might be important if food antigens gain access to mast cells of the submucosa, particularly in the context of existing epithelial damage.

Finally, we should consider the potent mediators that can be newly synthesized by mast cells and basophils upon activation. In the main, these mediators are generated when membrane-derived arachidonic acid is metabolized by cyclooxygenase to yield prostaglandins, and by lipoxygenase to yield hydroxyeicosatetraenoic acids (HETEs) and leukotrienes. Intestinal mast cells may also generate the potent ulcerogenic compound platelet-activating factor (67). There is some controversy about the ability of various human mast cell populations to synthesize arachidonate metabolites. A reasonable consensus would seem to be that human intestinal mast cells synthesize comparable quantities of leukotriene C_4 (LTC_4) and prostaglandin D_2 (PGD_2) (68), human lung mast cells may show some preference for PGD_2 generation (68, 69) (but may make greater absolute quantities of both mediators than intestinal cells), and skin mast cells have a marked preference for metabolism of arachidonic acid via the cyclooxygenase route to PGD_2 (19). Human basophils synthesize LTC_4 but apparently no PGD_2; this characteristic has been used to distinguish mast cell involvement and basophil involvement in late-phase reactions following nasal antigen challenge. The leukocyte chemotactic leukotriene LTB_4 is generated in sites of allergic reactions but has not been conclusively identified as a human mast cell product (70), although it is synthesized by some animal mast cells. LTB_4 synthesis is not detected in highly purified human basophil preparations (71).

The generation of eicosanoid metabolites is of particular relevance to the gastrointestinal tract. The leukotrienes are potent spasmogens and mucus secretagogues and have been implicated in the generation of intestinal inflammation (72). This latter effect may result from the promotion of inflammatory cell influx, or the activation of resident inflammatory cells, or both. PGD_2 can cause active water and electrolyte secretion in the intestine, and LTC_4 blocks active electrolyte absorption (73).

A final—and rapidly emerging—class of mast cell mediators is the cytokines. Initial studies revealed that various mast cell lines, or mast cells derived from rodents, could synthesize and release a broad array of these intercellular messengers, including IL-3, IL-4, IL-5, IL-6, TNF-α, TGF-β, and GM-CSF (53, 54). In some cases, these findings have now been extended to humans (notably for IL-4, IL-5, IL-6, and TNF-α) (74). Human basophils have also been reported to synthesize IL-4 (75). Synthesis of these polypeptides can occur either spontaneously or in response to stimuli such as specific antigen. Evidence also exists for secretory pathways that are independent of those leading to the release of other mediators such as histamine (76, 77). In addition, mast cells appear to represent an unusual source of TNF-α in that at least part of the cellular production of this cytokine is preformed and stored within the cell, and thus is available for rapid release independent of protein synthesis (78). Likewise, because mast cells synthesize other cytokines that both regulate mast cell growth (IL-3, IL-4) and control IgE synthesis (IL-4, IL-5), the possibility exists that mast cells self-regulate two key aspects of immediate hypersensitivity.

Basophils share many of the mast cell mediators described; they also contain substances that are not synthesized by any mast cell subsets. This fact apparently results from the developmental relationship between basophils and eosinophils. Basophils contain significant quantities of the eosinophil products Charcot-Leyden crystal protein (lysophospholipase) and major basic protein, while neither mediator can be detected in either human lung or skin mast cells (79). Basophils may, therefore, exhibit functional as well as antigenic similarities to eosinophils by virtue of their specific mediators.

In summary, novel mast cell and basophil mediators are identified quite routinely. The ability to obtain pure populations of human mast cells and basophils, coupled with the tools of molecular biology, has facilitated the identification of such mediators, and will also likely suggest novel roles for these cell types.

FUNCTIONAL ASPECTS OF MAST CELLS AND BASOPHILS AND CONSEQUENCES OF ACTIVATION

Stimuli for Cell Activation

The list of substances capable of inducing mediator release from mast cells and basophils is almost as long as the list of mediators themselves (Table 2.4). Mast cells and basophils may be activated in vivo by endogenous or exogenous substances, or in vitro by a variety of experimental tools such as ionophores and phorbol esters. In general, several features of the stimulus–secretion pathway induced by the various secretagogues are common to all agents. They include mobilization of intracellular calcium stores, changes in membrane potential, hydrolysis of phosphatidyl inositides, activation of guanosine 5'-triphosphate-binding proteins, and phosphorylation of cellular constituents. It is beyond the scope of this chapter to describe in detail the pathways leading to the final secretory event in mast cells and basophils; the reader is referred to a review on this topic (80). One note of caution should be introduced, however. Most of the available information regarding mast cell stimulus–secretion coupling has been obtained with mast cell

Table 2.4
Stimuli of Mast Cell and Basophil Activation

IgE-dependent stimuli of physiologic relevance
Antigen
Histamine-releasing factors
IL-3

Other endogenous stimuli
ATP
Neuropeptides
Anaphylatoxins
Substances released by physical stimuli
Bile acids
Endothelin-1

Exogenous stimuli
Drugs and drug solubilizers
Radiocontrast media
Bacterial peptides
Bacterial lectins
Bee venom peptides

Stimuli used experimentally
Anti-IgE antibodies
D_2O
Compound 48/80
Calcium ionophores

---

populations other than those from intestinal mucosal sites. Subtle differences may exist in the activation sequence between the various mast cell subsets or between mast cells and basophils.

Considering physiologic stimuli of mast cell and basophil activation, all cell populations so far examined respond to the stimulus of IgE-receptor cross-linking. In vivo, this response is mediated by specific antigens; it may also be reproduced experimentally by antibodies directed against IgE or antireceptor antibodies. Other important endogenous secretagogues may also interact with IgE. For example, many (but not all) of the histamine-releasing factors that are produced by a variety of cell types (mononuclear cells, platelets, and epithelial cells) are dependent on the presence of a certain type of IgE molecule on the cell surface for their histamine-releasing activity (81). IgE molecules capable of mediating this activity are designated IgE$^+$ and are described in more detail below. IgE$^+$ also mediates histamine release from basophils induced by IL-3 and D_2O (heavy water). The exact mechanism whereby these diverse stimuli interact with cell-fixed IgE molecules remains to be determined.

One group of endogenous mast-cell-activating agents that have received substantial recent attention comprise the neuropeptides. These secretagogues may be of particular relevance to the intestine as there is a striking morphological association of mast cells with peptidergic nerve endings in this tissue (58). At the ultrastructural level, mucosal mast cells and nerves are seen to be in intimate contact, raising the potential for communication. Various mast cell types can be activated in vitro by neuropeptides such as substance P (15). Intestinal mast cells in vivo can also be induced to release their mediators under nervous stimulation. When rats were presented with an isolated audiovisual cue, which had previously been associated with antigenic challenge following a classic conditioning protocol, plasma levels of the intestinal mast cell mediator, RMCP II, were increased (82). Similarly, some facets of intestinal anaphylaxis are largely dependent on intact enteric nervous system function (58, 83). The ability of the nervous system to control elements of the allergic response will doubtless be the subject of much ongoing investigation.

Basophils, and possibly some mast cell populations, are readily activated by anaphylatoxins, which are the split complement components C5a and C3a. Another stimulus of possible physiologic relevance is the exposure of mast cells and basophils to hyperosmolar conditions.

Mast cells have also been shown recently to release mediators in response to one of their own products, endothelin-1, implying an autocrine loop that can amplify allergic responses (84). Another class of stimuli of particular relevance to the gastrointestinal tract include the bile acids (85). The ability of these molecules to cause histamine release may relate to their actions on colonic fluid and electrolyte transport (86).

Numerous exogenous agents are known to activate mast cells and basophils. Some of these are primarily useful as experimental tools. For example, the calcium-transporting ionophore A23187 has been used extensively to probe the involvement of calcium in the secretory process. Similarly, basic agents such as compound 48/80 and the bee venom peptide 401 can cause marked histamine release from some mast cell populations (although not apparently from basophils). These basic compounds apparently interact with a cell surface receptor on mast cells, raising the possibility that an endogenous ligand exists for this site, in addition to its usefulness as an experimental mode of cell activation.

Exogenous stimuli of mast cells and basophils may also be of clinical relevance. A wide variety of drugs, contrast media, and drug-stabilizing agents have been shown to activate mast cells or basophils, or both, and mediator release may account for the adverse effects of these agents. In general, such drugs appear to have direct histamine-releasing properties that are unlikely to be mediated via specific IgE molecules, although allergic reactions to penicillin represent one important exception to this rule. Morphine and related agents are able to degranulate human skin mast cells via a specific opiate receptor. Other drugs may acquire mast-cell-activating properties after metabolic transformation into reactive species.

Finally, mast cells in situ, and particularly in the skin, can be activated by a variety of physical stimuli, including heat, cold, pressure, and vibration. Such stimuli may well produce their effects by releasing peptidergic neurotransmitters, as discussed above.

Inhibitors of Cell Activation

The clinical consequences of mast cell and basophil activation are often treated on a symptomatic basis. Thus antihistamines have had a long-standing place in the treatment of rhinitis, and leukotriene antagonists show promise as therapeutic agents for asthma. Given the multitude of mediators that are released in an immediate hypersensitivity reaction, good rationale exists for using drugs that would prevent mast cell or basophil activation rather than simply counteracting the effects of released mediators. Several drugs have been described—some only experimentally—that can inhibit mediator release from mast cells and basophils. They will be referred to here as "antiallergic" drugs. Many of these agents, however, display a high degree of species or tissue specificity.

Most antiallergic drugs have been targeted to diseases of the lung, and may or may not be active in stabilizing intestinal mucosal mast cells. For example, disodium cromoglycate (cromolyn sodium) is a highly potent inhibitor of histamine release from rat peritoneal mast cells, but is without significant effect on mucosal mast cells from this species (6) or from human intestinal specimens (16). This may account for the fact that therapeutic trials of this agent in gastrointestinal disorders that may involve mast cell activation have yielded conflicting and often disappointing results. Nedocromil, a newer cromolyn-like agent, was developed for use in pulmonary disease, but reportedly has inhibitory effects on both mucosal and connective tissue mast cells (87). Theophylline may be a broader-spectrum antiallergic drug in that it can block histamine release from rat peritoneal mast cells and from all human and primate mast cell populations tested (16, 17), though, interestingly, not from rat mucosal mast cells (6). It is also able to block histamine release from basophils. β-Adrenergic agents show a similar spectrum of activity.

A final class of antiallergic drugs that is widely used are the steroids. These agents are very effective in inhibiting late symptoms that follow bronchial antigen provocation in humans, but do not appear to block immediate hypersensitivity reactions or mast cell mediator release (88). They are, however, good inhibitors of in vitro basophil activation, provided the cells are incubated with the drugs for prolonged periods (usually overnight) before challenge (89). Evidence also suggests that, while not reducing release of histamine by mast cells, steroids might nevertheless be effective inhibitors of mast cell cytokine production (90). The efficacy of steroids in inhibiting intestinal mast cell mediator release has not yet been reported. In fact, similar to the situation for mast cell activators, to date we have no drugs available that are selective inhibitors for the intestinal mucosal mast cell class. This state of affairs presumably reflects the research bias of investigators and drug companies that has existed to date, toward therapies for asthma as their primary objective. Now that appropriate model systems (cultured cells and dispersed intestinal mast cells) exist, it may be practical to screen for agents that stabilize mucosal mast cells. Any such agents, if active in vivo, might well be important additions to the therapeutic possibilities for food allergy, and potentially for other intestinal diseases.

Consequences of Intestinal Mast Cell Activation

In light of the foregoing discussion of mast cell mediators, it is obvious that the stimulation of mast cells in the intestine has the potential to affect many surrounding cell types.

One common symptom of food allergy and other immune-related intestinal disorders is diarrhea. Diarrhea is a result of an imbalance in the normal active electrolyte-transporting properties of the intestinal epithelium (91). In health, sodium and chloride absorption predominates, but a variety of pathologic conditions can inhibit this active absorption or stimulate active chloride secretion. The resulting net active secretion of ions will promote passive net secretion of water and hence diarrhea. Mast cells might influence this process in at least three ways: direct effects of mast cell mediators on secretory epithelial cells; stimulation of synthesis of chloride secretagogues by other mucosal cell types and neurons; and alteration of the sensitivity of the epithelium to the normal neurohumoral "tone," such that levels of hormones and neurotransmitters previously below the threshold for secretory actions become effective. All three of these mechanisms have been observed in experimental models. For example, antigen challenge of sensitized intestinal tissues leads to net chloride secretion in a number of species (91). The effect is partially due to release of neurotransmitters since it can be attenuated by tetrodotoxin (83). Mast cell mediators such as histamine and adenosine can also have potent effects directly on epithelial cells, as can be demonstrated using model intestinal cell lines (73). Using this same model system, chronic exposure to mast cell mediators can render epithelial cells hyperresponsive to a number of agents, including VIP and the acetylcholine analogue carbachol (73). Mast cells may, therefore, be important determinants of fluid homeostasis in the intestine, and their modulation may be therapeutic in cases of immune-related diarrhea.

Mast cell activation in the intestine may also have inflammatory consequences. Mast cells contain and can synthesize a variety of factors that are chemotactic for eosinophils, neutrophils, and mononuclear cells (55). Furthermore, mast cell mediators—including cytokines—have been implicated in the up-regulation of adhesion molecules on endothelial cells, including E and P selectins. This action promotes leukocyte rolling, adhesion, and eventual emigration into inflammatory foci. Galli has referred to this process as part of the "mast cell–leukocyte–cytokine cascade" (92). Mast cell mediators may also be directly proinflammatory. Platelet-activating factor has been shown to be a potent ulcerogen (93), and leukotriene synthesis is associated with several models of intestinal inflammation (72).

Mast cell activation may also lead to profound effects on intestinal permeability. This effect may be related to epithelial abnormalities (94, 95). Antigen challenge of sensitized intestinal tissues can lead to villous edema and enterocyte desquamation. The increase in intestinal permeability that accompanies these epithelial changes encompasses permeability to both small molecules and macromolecular antigens; one important consequence is that bystander antigens in the gut lumen will also gain access to the systemic circulation (94). This process may provide a mechanism for multiple food allergies (96).

Finally, the ability of mast cell mediators to affect intestinal motor function is under exploration. Antigen challenge of sensitized tissue leads to selective excitation and inhibition of specific neural circuitry within the intestine. This process, in turn, results in a stereotypical pattern of altered motility, integrated with secretory changes. Clinically, this pattern likely accounts for strong muscular contractions and cramping, copious secretion, rapid intestinal transit, and diarrhea. The precise mediators responsible for these events have not yet been elucidated, and may be different in various intestinal segments and different muscle layers. Histamine, eicosanoids, and cytokines are likely important contributors to disordered motility in both acute and chronic settings, however (83).

A number of consequences of intestinal mast cell activation have been observed in parasitized animals in which a mast cell hyperplasia occurs. In this context, some responses might be considered protective. For example, mast cell mediators can cause mucus secretion, increased smooth muscle contraction and peristalsis, and increased vascular permeability (83, 95). These responses probably aid in the expulsion of parasites, but if activated inappropriately by food antigens, they may contribute to the symptoms of the food-allergic patient.

In summary, mast cells can influence many of the physiologic systems of the intestine. Knowledge in this area is likely to impact on our ability to intervene when normal intestinal function is dysregulated by allergic responses.

Immunoglobulin E

GENERAL CHARACTERISTICS

IgE is the least prevalent of the five antibody classes in terms of serum levels, which range in the normal human subject between 17 and 450 ng/mL and comprise approximately 0.002% of total serum immunoglobulin. The antibody is synthesized in monomeric form and contains a relatively high proportion of carbohydrate (approximately 12%), giving it a molecular weight of around 200,000. In addition to the circulating pool of IgE, another, possibly larger pool of IgE molecules is fixed to circulating basophils and tissue mast cells. This pool, in the absence of antibody cross-linking, which promotes receptor endocytosis, has the potential to be long-lived, as the Fc ϵ receptors for IgE on mast cells and basophils are of extremely high affinity, with affinity constants (K_a) ranging

from 10^9 to 10^{10} M^{-1}. In addition, other cell types bear low-affinity IgE receptors that are apparently unrelated to the high-affinity receptors of mast cells and basophils (97). The low-affinity receptor, present on lymphocytes, eosinophils, and macrophages, is the cellular differentiation marker CD23. Soluble forms of this antigen have also been identified. CD23 presumably does not contribute significantly to binding the cell-fixed pool of IgE because of its low affinity ($K_a = 2-6 \times 10^6$ M^{-1}), but apparently has important regulatory functions, particularly for IgE synthesis. It is beyond the scope of this chapter to discuss the structure and function of IgE receptors in detail. Readers are referred to recent reviews on this topic (97, 98).

Genomic and complementary DNAs have been cloned for the heavy chains of human, rat, and mouse IgE molecules (99). The amino acid sequences of these clones reveal a relatively high level of homology between mouse and rat ϵ chains, but much less between mouse (or rat) and human ϵ chains. There is reasonable homology in the region of human and mouse ϵ chains thought to be involved in binding to the high-affinity IgE receptor on mast cells. Doubtless this relationship accounts for the fact that human IgE can sensitize mouse mast cells for histamine release. In other regions of the chain, however, considerable sequence divergence is observed. The rate of evolution of the ϵ chain when the human sequence is compared with the mouse is higher than any other immunoglobulin chain except the δ chain. This fact raises the possibility that IgE may have somewhat different physiologic roles in humans and rodents.

In fact, the physiologic role of IgE is not well understood. It has been presumed to be an important mediator of the host defense to parasites, as high levels of both specific and polyclonal antibody are synthesized in the parasitized subject (97). IgE does, however, have a clear pathologic role in the allergic response. Some individuals, termed atopic, respond inappropriately to innocuous antigens with the synthesis of high levels of IgE, which can then sensitize mast cells and basophils for mediator release. Moreover, the IgE synthesized by atopic individuals may be functionally distinct from that found in normal subjects (100). This novel concept of a functional heterogeneity of IgE is described in more detail below.

REGULATION OF IgE SYNTHESIS

It is generally accepted that normal human peripheral lymphocytes do not spontaneously secrete IgE when placed in culture, even when measurable levels of IgG are detected. The cells can be induced to secrete IgE if provided with appropriate cytokines and cellular interactions, however. IL-4 appears to play a pivotal role in isotype switching and the induction of IgE synthesis from highly purified human B cells, but an absolute requirement also exists for an interaction with T cells of the CD4 phenotype (101). Other cytokines, although not essential for the promotion of IgE synthesis, may also play an important role (101, 102). For example, both IL-5 and IL-6, although unable to induce IgE synthesis when added singly, may enhance the effect of suboptimal doses of IL-4. Thus, the effect of these cytokines in combination with IL-4 could be termed synergistic. Another factor that interacts with the action of IL-4 is CD23 (the low-affinity IgE receptor or FcεRII) in either its soluble or membrane-bound form, which induces IgE-producing cells to become plasma cells (97). There are also a number of suppressive signals for in vitro IgE production by normal human lymphocytes (102). Interferons (IFN) of the γ and α classes, prostaglandin E_2, IL-12, and T cells of the CD8 phenotype have all been shown to inhibit IL-4-induced IgE synthesis (97, 103, 104).

Cytokines promoting IgE production are predominantly synthesized by the TH2 subset of T lymphocytes, while inhibitory signals such as IFN-γ are derived from TH1 cells (105). Recent studies suggest that TH2 cells are selectively expanded in severe allergic disease (105). Likewise, mast cells and basophils may also regulate IgE responses due to their capacity to synthesize IL-4 (74, 75).

Peripheral lymphocytes isolated from atopic patients have the ability to secrete IgE spontaneously when placed in culture, as do cells isolated from patients with the hyper-IgE syndrome (102). For the former group, this spontaneous IgE production can be further increased by IL-4 treatment, but the cytokine has little or no effect on the presumably already maximal secretion seen with cells of the latter patient group. Again, suppressive factors have been identified. The spontaneous IgE synthesis by cells from both atopic and hyper-IgE patients can be inhibited by IFN-γ and IFN-α. The spontaneous IgE synthesis of the patient lymphocytes may relate to the inherent ability of these cells to secrete cytokines. Normal peripheral blood lymphocytes secrete large quantities of interferons in culture with little IL-4. In contrast, cells from hyper-IgE patients release high levels of IL-4 with little interferon. Since IL-4 is known to down-regulate IFN-γ production, the possibility is raised that a normal feedback control for IgE production is somehow disturbed in hyper-IgE (and potentially atopic) patients. No difference is observed in IL-2 production between cells of normal and hyper-IgE patients, although the latter group release increased amounts of soluble CD23. This variation is perhaps to be expected, as IL-4 is known to induce the expression of CD23 and its release from the cell surface.

In total, results of studies in the human system, and particularly those that compare normal subjects and patients with the hyper-IgE syndrome, have emphasized the central role played by IL-4 in the induction of IgE synthesis. Furthermore, the observation that interferons suppress the response suggests that they might be used therapeutically in patients with elevated circulating IgE levels (105).

The foregoing discussion has emphasized the involvement of cytokines in the control of IgE production. The requirement for a cognate T-cell–B-cell interaction should also be stressed. Highly purified human B cells were unable to synthesize IgE when provided with only cytokines (101). The T-cell requirement could not be substituted by conditioned medium, or by placing the B cells and T cells in the same culture well but physically separating them by a membrane. Several T-cell markers and adhesion molecules appear to be important in the IgE response, as IL-4-stimulated IgE secretion in mixed T-cell–B-cell cultures could be blocked by antibodies to CD2, CD4, LFA-1, CD3, and Leu 4. Antibodies to class II antigens were also very effective in this regard, although antibodies against class I had no effect on IgE synthesis. As IL-4 increases expression of class II molecules, it may have dual effects on IgE synthesis by influencing both antibody-synthesizing and antigen-presenting cells. IgE synthesis is also regulated via cell–cell interactions mediated by a newly described molecule, CD40-ligand, which is expressed on T cells (among others) (97). This molecule binds to CD40 on IgE-producing B cells, thereby inducing them to become memory cells.

To summarize, it is apparent that the synthesis of IgE is tightly controlled, with a complex network of regulatory cytokines and cellular interactions. Some features of this network are presented in Figure 2.1. In normal individuals, IgE synthesis apparently occurs at a very low rate. Disruption of the tight control of IgE synthesis may, however, lead to allergic sensitization. In the context of the gastrointestinal tract, there is the potential for sensitization to food antigens to occur in predisposed persons at times when the permeability of the epithelial barrier is increased, such as during infancy. Subsequent exposure to the antigen could perpetuate the process, and facilitate sensitization to other substances when intestinal per-

meability was increased by local anaphylaxis. Patients with food allergy may display local IgE production, most likely from IgE-containing plasma cells in the intestinal mucosa. Such patients reportedly have high levels of fecal IgE, which can occur in the absence of high serum levels of the antibody (106). In contrast, control patients with nonintestinal allergic disease rarely had detectable fecal IgE despite elevated circulating levels. Further, an IL-4 inducible transepithelial transport system for IgE has recently been described in the rat intestine (107). This study raises the possibility that IgE might function as a secretory immunoglobulin in the mucosal immune system, particularly in the setting of parasitic disease. At present, however, it is unclear whether the regulatory scheme for IgE synthesis depicted in Figure 2.1 can be extended to the control of local IgE synthesis in the gastrointestinal tract.

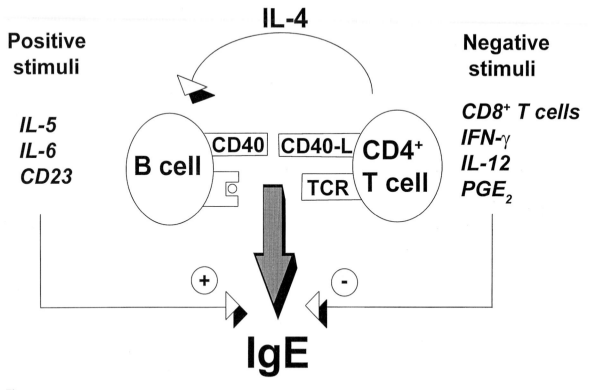

Figure 2.1

Features of the regulation of IgE synthesis in man. For explanation, see text.

FUNCTIONAL HETEROGENEITY
OF IgE MOLECULES

A number of laboratories have recently described factors derived from a variety of cell sources that can cause histamine release from human basophils. The activity of some, but not all, of these histamine-releasing factors (HRFs) is dependent on the presence of cell surface IgE; furthermore, their activity has allowed the delineation of two functional subtypes of IgE, termed IgE$^+$ and IgE$^+$ (81, 100). Only IgE$^+$ is able to sensitize basophils for HRF-induced histamine release, and IgE$^+$ synthesis occurs in atopic, but not in normal, individuals.

Normal and atopic individuals do not differ in their ability to synthesize HRFs, but they do differ in their ability to respond to such factors by virtue of the absence or presence of IgE$^+$. Lichtenstein and coworkers have hypothesized that the clinical severity of an allergic response in a given patient is related to the acquisition of IgE$^+$ (81). They believe that the presence of IgE$^+$ provides an explanation of why only a subset of patients will exhibit a late-phase response to an antigen; such responding patients have IgE$^+$, and HRFs are responsible for the delayed basophil histamine release that occurs. Since patients displaying late-phase responses to antigen (particularly asthmatic patients) tend to have more severe disease, functional IgE heterogeneity may account for the observation that patients with similar serum IgE levels and immediate skin test responsiveness may differ markedly in their clinical responsiveness on exposure to antigen. Only one human gene for IgE—and hence only one possible isotype—is known. The molecular basis of the two subtypes of IgE may, therefore, reflect some form of post-translational modification, possibly differential glycosylation.

To summarize, it appears to be possible to divide IgE molecules into two functional classes, based on their ability to support HRF-induced histamine release from human basophils. IgE$^+$, synthesized by atopic individuals, can also sensitize basophils for histamine release by heavy water (D_2O) and IL-3. The ability to synthesize IgE, and the nature of the IgE synthesized, may thus define three classes of subjects: those who do not make IgE toward a given antigen, and are not allergic; those who make IgE$^-$

to a given antigen and have positive skin tests, but relatively mild clinical symptoms; and those who are atopic and make IgE$^+$ antibodies, to a given antigen, by virtue of these antibodies their clinical response when exposed to the antigen will be more severe. Assays should soon be available that can determine which IgE type is being produced by a given patient, and such assays will obviously have substantial clinical utility.

Evidence for Involvement
of Mast Cells and Basophils
in Gastrointestinal Disease

FOOD ALLERGY

Many adverse reactions to foods can be shown to be allergic in nature; that is, they are mediated by the combination of food antigens with specific, cell-fixed IgE molecules. Thus, many food-allergic patients have positive skin test reactions to dietary antigens that correlate well with reactions to blindly administered foods (108). Skin test reactivity presumably mirrors serum food-specific IgE responses, as can be demonstrated by transferring skin test reactivity to nonallergic subjects with serum from patients (Prausnitz-Küstner test). There is also evidence that local IgE synthesis may be important when allergic disease occurs in the gastrointestinal tract. A study of children with food allergy revealed measurable fecal levels of IgE while serum levels could be either elevated or normal (106). These results were in contrast to findings for children who had extraintestinal allergic diseases, such as atopic eczema or rhinitis, in whom serum levels of IgE were elevated but fecal levels of the antibody were undetectable. Normal children also had undetectable levels of fecal IgE.

The ability of human intestinal mast cells to respond to food antigens has been studied in a variety of settings. Human jejunal biopsies were used to demonstrate IgE-dependent mast cell degranulation in vitro (109). In patients with either a colostomy or ileostomy, local passive sensitization was used to demonstrate that intestinal mast cells in vivo can respond to food antigens (110). Reimann and associates used an endoscopic technique to apply food antigens directly to the gastric mucosa in allergic patients (111). They noted local erythema and edema accompanied by histamine release in sensitive subjects. Food allergy may be linked to other allergic disorders, particularly in children. Food challenge of children with atopic dermatitis produced increases in levels of plasma histamine, presumably reflecting mast cell degranulation at intestinal and other sites (112). The ability of intestinal mast cell degranulation to alter intestinal permeability may increase the likelihood for more systemic manifestations of food allergy.

The foregoing discussion has emphasized a role for IgE-dependent hypersensitivity reactions in food allergy. There is also the possibility that mast cells are triggered by other mechanisms. IgG_4 has been implicated as an anaphylactic antibody in some animal models of food allergy. Split complement products may also be important, as complement deposition has been noted in the intestinal tissues of patients sensitive to cow's milk. Furthermore, the ability of neuropeptides to cause mast cell mediator release might provide a neural axis whereby mast cells respond to food ingestion. The ongoing definition of stimuli for mast cell activation—particularly those specific for the gastrointestinal tract—will doubtless further our understanding of mast cell involvement in adverse reaction to foods.

INFLAMMATORY BOWEL DISEASE

Some authors have argued that the inflammatory bowel diseases of ulcerative colitis and Crohn's disease result from an immunologic response to a dietary constituent. The main impetus for this line of reasoning comes from the increasing incidence of inflammatory bowel disease in developed societies and some population groups. It has been difficult to ascribe a definitive role for food-specific IgE antibodies, however, because of the conflicting data obtained from a number of studies (reviewed in 20). This issue has been revisited by a recent multicenter study of a large group of patients with Crohn's disease (113). This study suggested that an exclusion diet was significantly more effective than steroid treatment in main-

taining remission achieved initially with the use of an elemental diet. The range of foods capable of precipitating symptoms was broad, however, with several subjects reporting problems with a number of foods. Moreover, the overall rate of remission, even with the exclusion diet, was still relatively disappointing (113). Some groups have claimed an association of inflammatory bowel disease with atopy, or that patients with ulcerative colitis gave a personal or family history of atopy twice as frequently as control subjects. The observation has also been made that patients with inflammatory bowel disease have a higher incidence of positive skin tests to food antigens than control subjects, but this latter finding may reflect the decreased ability of the diseased mucosa in patients to exclude such antigens, with a consequent higher potential for systematic sensitization to occur. There is also evidence against a role for food sensitivity in the pathogenesis of inflammatory bowel disease. Some workers have failed to find an association of inflammatory bowel disease with atopy. Similarly, levels of serum IgE directed against food antigens are reportedly normal in patients with ulcerative colitis. Two reports did suggest that IgE-positive lymphocytes are increased in the intestinal mucosa of inflammatory bowel disease, although more recent studies with a highly specific monoclonal anti-IgE antibody failed to substantiate these findings.

In total, it appears unlikely that dietary antigens and immediate hypersensitivity reactions to them are of paramount importance in the pathogenesis of inflammatory bowel disease, except, perhaps, in a subset of patients. This conclusion in no way rules out a role for the mucosal mast cell. Increased mast cell numbers have been reported to occur in the lesional tissue of both ulcerative colitis and Crohn's disease, as well as in animal models of inflammatory bowel disease. Electron microscopic studies of intestinal specimens from patients with Crohn's disease have shown that the mast cells are activated and are undergoing degranulation, although the stimulus responsible for these changes is unknown (114). Conceivably, mast cells could be activated by cytokines released by other cell types migrating into the inflammatory focus. Likewise, mast cells isolated from the lesional tissue of patients with inflammatory bowel disease reportedly display a high level of spontaneous mediator release (presumably reflecting in vivo activation). The cells can also be activated by proteins obtained from intestinal epithelial cells (which have no effect on mast cells obtained from normal mucosa) or from control subjects (115, 116). The potential also exists for mast cell activation by neuropeptides or anaphylatoxins as described above. If a stimulus for mast cell activation can be identified, it may provide an important locus for therapeutic intervention in inflammatory bowel disease because mast cells have the potential to generate much of the symptomatology involved.

In summary, it currently remains unresolved to what extent, if any, mast cells and IgE participate in inflammatory bowel disease, due to a large number of conflicting studies. There is persuasive—but at present only circumstantial—evidence that mast cells and their mediators might be important in the pathogenesis of inflammatory bowel disease, if not as the initial inciting cell types, then as participants in the subsequent ongoing inflammation. Much further work is required in this area to raise this hypothesis above the level of speculation.

OTHER CONDITIONS

Activation of intestinal mast cells, either by food antigens or by other stimuli, has been proposed as a pathogenetic mechanism in several other gastrointestinal disorders. In general, the evidence for these proposals is considerably more sketchy than that linking the mast cell to inflammatory bowel disease. As we learn more about the properties of intestinal mast cells in humans, and the various ways in which they can be activated for mediator release, it is to be expected that speculation regarding mast cell involvement in various diseases can be put on a firmer footing.

Mast cells have been proposed as participants in celiac disease (117). Although the histologic picture in this condition is reminiscent of delayed rather than immediate hypersensitivity, mast cell involvement is suggested by the finding of an intestinal mast cell hyperplasia in patients. Furthermore, following treatment by gluten withdrawal from the diet, mast cell

numbers returned to normal. It is possible that the observed alterations in mast cell numbers are secondary to the mucosal damage occurring in the disease. To date, no evidence has been presented as to whether the mast cells present in the intestines of patients with celiac disease are activated.

An allergic etiology has been proposed for the unusual gastrointestinal disorder of eosinophilic gastroenteritis. This disease, characterized by eosinophilic infiltrates of the stomach and small intestine and a peripheral eosinophilia, is provoked in at least a subset of patients by the ingestion of specific foods, and some patients exhibit marked elevations in circulating IgE levels. Therapeutic benefit has been achieved by dietary manipulation or the use of corticosteroids, again supporting the possibility that immediate hypersensitivity reactions of some type are involved in the pathogenesis of the disease.

Mast cell involvement has also been proposed in both gastric and duodenal ulcer disease. Reports have suggested a role for mast cell mediators in the generation of stomach ulcers in both clinical settings (118) and experimental models. Mast cell involvement has been demonstrated in both stress and ethanol-induced ulceration of the rat stomach, and mast cell stabilizers, such as disodium cromoglycate and sulfasalazine, can reduce damage to the rat gastric epithelium (119–121). Given the emerging appreciation that the majority of peptic ulcer disease is related to infection with *Helicobacter pylori,* it is also interesting to note the preliminary reports that this microorganism may lead to activation of mucosal mast cells (122, 123). The role of mast cells in these processes most likely relates to their histamine content. Histamine is an important mediator of gastric damage, possibly because of its effects on gastric acid secretion. Stimuli for mast cell degranulation, including antigen-IgE cross-linking, have been shown to induce histamine release and increase acid secretion inappropriately (124). Furthermore, histamine has been implicated as an inhibitor of an important mucosal defensive factor, namely duodenal mucosal bicarbonate secretion (125). In summary, the balance of available evidence suggests that it is highly likely that mast cells contribute to the pathogenesis of both gastric and duodenal ulcer disease, and that these cells may

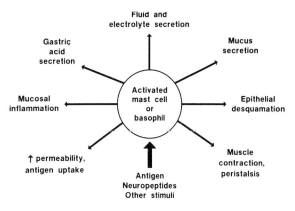

Figure 2.2

Some consequences of mast cell or basophil activation in the gastrointestinal tract.

even be primary elicitors of pathology in certain settings.

Conclusion

It has been the aim of this chapter to convey that the activation of mast cells and basophils, mediated by antigen-specific IgE molecules or by other agents, has the ability to generate a wide variety of symptoms in the gastrointestinal tract that are relevant to food allergy and other enteric diseases. Some of the consequences of intestinal mast cell activation are shown in Figure 2.2. Areas of current research emphasis, such as characterization of mucosal mast cells, identification of gut-specific, antiallergic agents, and delineation of the control of IgE synthesis, should lead to new clinical applications for the therapy of multiple allergic and inflammatory disorders.

Acknowledgments

The assistance of Julie Lessem with manuscript preparation is gratefully acknowledged. Studies from the author's laboratory have been supported by grants from the National Institutes of Health (AI24992, DK28305, DK47756). The author is a faculty member of the Biomedical Sciences Ph.D. Program, University of California, San Diego, School of Medicine.

REFERENCES

1. Barrett KE, Pearce FL. Mast cell heterogeneity. In: Foreman JC, ed. Immunopharmacology of mast cells and basophils. London: Academic Press, 1993, 29–42.
2. Enerbäck L. Mast cells in rat gastrointestinal mucosa. I. Effects of fixation. Acta Pathol Microbiol Scand 1966;66:289–302.
3. Enerbäck L. Mast cells in rat gastrointestinal mucosa. II. Dye-binding and metachromatic properties. Acta Pathol Microbiol Scand 1966;66:303–312.
4. Enerbäck L. Mast cells in rat gastrointestinal mucosa. III. Reactivity towards compound 48/80. Acta Pathol Microbiol Scand 1966;66:313–322.
5. Befus AD, Pearce FL, Gauldie J, Horsewood P, Bienenstock J. Mucosal mast cells. I. Isolation and functional characteristics of rat intestinal mast cells. J Immunol 1982;128:2475–2480.
6. Pearce FL, Befus AD, Gauldie J, Bienenstock J. Mucosal mast cells. II. Effects of anti-allergic compounds on histamine secretion by isolated intestinal mast cells. J Immunol 1982;128:2481–2486.
7. Pearce FL, Befus AD, Bienenstock J. Mucosal mast cells. III. Effect of quercetin and other flavonoids on antigen-induced histamine secretion from rat intestinal mast cells. J Allergy Clin Immunol 1984;73:819–823.
8. Stevens RL, Lee TDG, Seldin DC, Austen KF, Befus AD, Bienenstock J. Intestinal mucosal mast cells from rats infected with *Nippostrongylus brasiliensis* contain protease-resistant chondroitin sulfate di-B proteoglycans. J Immunol 1986;137:291–295.
9. Gilead L, Livni N, Eliakim R, *et al.* Human gastric mast cells are chondroitin sulphate E-containing mast cells. Immunology 1987;62:23–28.
10. Stevens RL, Fox CC, Lichtenstein LM, Austen KF. Identification of chondroitin sulfate E proteoglycans in the secretory granules of human lung mast cells. Proc Natl Acad Sci USA 1988;85:2284–2287.
11. Thompson HL, Schulman ES, Metcalfe DD. Identification of chondroitin sulfate E in human lung mast cells. J Immunol 1988;140:2708–2713.
12. Metcalfe DD, Soter NA, Wasserman SI, Austen KF. Identification of sulfated mucopolysaccharides including heparin in the lesional skin of a patient with mastocytosis. J Invest Dermatol 1980;74:210–215.
13. Craig SS, Irani AA, Metcalfe DD, Schwartz LM. Ultrastructural localization of heparin to human mast cells of the MC_T and MC_{TC} types by labelling with antithrombin III-gold. Lab Invest 1993;69:552–561.
14. Irani AA, Schechter NM, Craig SS, Deblois G, Schwartz LB. Two types of human mast cells that have distinct neutral protease compositions. Proc Natl Acad Sci USA 1986;83:4464–4468.
15. Shanahan F, Denburg JA, Fox J, Bienenstock J, Befus D. Mast cell heterogeneity: effects of neuroenteric peptides on histamine release. J Immunol 1985;135:1331–1337.
16. Fox CC, Wolf EJ, Kagey-Sobotka A, Lichtenstein LM. Comparison of human lung and intestinal mast cells. J Allergy Clin Immunol 1988;81:89–94.

17. Barrett KE, Szucs EF, Metcalfe DD. Mast cell heterogeneity in higher animals: a comparison of the properties of autologous lung and intestinal mast cells from non-human primates. J Immunol 1986;137:2001–2008.

18. Lowman MA, Rees PH, Benyon RC, Church MK. Human mast cell heterogeneity: histamine release from mast cells dispersed from skin, lung, adenoids, tonsils, and colon in response to IgE-dependent and nonimmunologic stimuli. J Allergy Clin Immunol 1988;81:590–597.

19. Lawrence ID, Warner JA, Cohan VL, Hubbard WC, Kagey-Sobotka A, Lichtenstein LM. Purification and characterization of human skin mast cells. Evidence for human mast cell heterogeneity. J Immunol 1987;139:3062–3069.

20. Barrett KE, Metcalfe DD. Mucosal mast cells and IgE. In: Jones AL, Heyworth MF, eds. Immunology of the gastrointestinal tract and liver. New York: Raven Press, 1988, 65–92.

21. Kitamura Y, Shimada M, Go S, Matsuda H, Hatanaka K, Seki H. Distribution of mast cell precursors in hemopoietic and lymphopoietic tissues of mice. J Exp Med 1979;150:482–490.

22. Schmitt E, Fassbender B, Beyreuther K, Spaeth E, Schwarzkopf R, Rüde E. Characterization of a T cell-derived lymphokine that acts synergistically with IL3 in the growth of murine mast cells and is identical with IL-4. Immunobiology 1987;174:406–419.

23. Mossman TR, Bond MW, Coffman RL, Ohara J, Paul WE. T-cell and mast cell lines respond to B-cell stimulatory factor 1. Proc Natl Acad Sci USA 1986;83:5654–5658.

24. Gurish MF, Ghildyal N, McNeil HP, Austen KF, Gillis S, Stevens RL. Differential expression of secretory granule proteases in mouse mast cells exposed to interleukin 3 and c-*kit* ligand. J Exp Med 1992;175:1003–1012.

25. Ghildyal N, Friend DS, Nicodemus CF, Austen KF, Stevens RL. Reversible expression of mouse mast cell protease 2 mRNA and protein in cultured mast cells exposed to IL-10. J Immunol 1993;151:3206–3214.

26. Eklund KK, Ghildyal N, Austen KF, Stevens RL. Induction by IL-9 and suppression by IL-3 and IL-4 of the levels of chromosome 14-derived transcripts that encode late-expressed mouse mast cell proteases. J Immunol 1993;151:4266–4273.

27. Ruitenberg EJ, Elgersma A. Absence of intestinal mast cell response in congenitally athymic mice during *Trichinella spiralis* infection. Nature 1976;264:258–260.

28. Mayrhofer G, Fisher R. Mast cells in severely T-cell depleted rats and the response to infestation with *Nippostrongylus brasiliensis*. Immunology 1979;37:145–155.

29. Madden KB, Urban Jr. JF, Ziltener HJ, Schrader JW, Finkelman FD, Katona IM. Antibodies to IL-3 and IL-4 suppress helminth-induced intestinal mastocytosis. J Immunol 1991;147:1387–1391.

30. Dayton ET, Pharr P, Ogawa M, et al. 3T3 fibroblasts induce cloned interleukin 3-dependent mouse mast cells to resemble connective tissue mast cells in granular constituency. Proc Natl Acad Sci USA 1988;85:569–572.

31. Irani AA, Buckley R, Haynes B, Schecter NM, Schwartz LB. Selective depletion of T mast cells in intestinal mucosa of patients with defective T lymphocyte function. J Allergy Clin Immunol 1987;79:179.

32. Kitamura Y, Kamakura Y, Fujita J, Nakano T. Differentiation and transdifferentiation of mast cells; a unique member of the hematopoietic cell family. Int J Cell Cloning 1987;5:108–121.

33. Mitsui H, Furitsu T, Dvorak AM, et al. Development of human mast cells from umbilical cord blood cells by recombinant human and murine c-*kit* ligand. Proc Natl Acad Sci USA 1993;90:735–739.

34. Saito H, Hatake K, Dvorak AM, et al. Selective differentiation and proliferation of hematopoietic cells induced by recombinant interleukins. Proc Natl Acad Sci USA 1988;85:2288–2292.

35. Dvorak AM, Saito H, Estrella P, Kissell S, Arai N, Ishizaka T. Ultrastructure of eosinophils and basophils stimulated to develop in human cord blood mononuclear cell cultures containing recombinant human interleukin 5 or interleukin 3. Lab Invest 1989;61:116–132.

36. Furitsu T, Saito H, Dvorak AM, et al. Development of human mast cells *in vitro*. Proc Natl Acad Sci USA 1989;86:10039–10043.

37. Li L, Macpherson JJ, Adelstein S, et al. Conditioned medium from a cell strain derived from a patient with mastocytosis induces preferential development of cells that possess high affinity IgE receptors and the granule protease phenotype of mature cutaneous mast cells. J Biol Chem 1995;270:2258–2263.

38. Miyazawa K, Williams DA, Gotoh A, Nishimaki J, Broxmeyer HE, Toyama K. Membrane-bound Steel factor induces more persistent tyrosine kinase activation and longer lifespan of c-*kit* gene-encoded protein than its soluble form. Blood 1995;85:641–649.

39. Weiss RR, Whitaker-Menezes D, Longley J, Bender J, Murphy GF. Human dermal endothelial cells express membrane-associated mast cell growth factor. J Invest Dermatol 1995;104:101–106.

40. Rimmer EF, Horton MA. *In vitro* culture of basophils from human bone marrow. Leuk Res 1986;10:1241–1248.

41. Ogawa M, Nakahata T, Leary AG, Sterk AR, Ishizaka K, Ishizaka T. Suspension culture of human mast cells/basophils from umbilical cord blood mononuclear cells. Proc Natl Acad Sci USA 1983;80:4494–4498.

42. Razin E, Cordon-Cardo C, Good RA. Growth of a pure population of mouse mast cells *in vitro* with conditioned medium derived from concanavalin A-stimulated splenocytes. Proc Natl Acad Sci USA 1981;78:2559–2561.

43. Denburg JA, Telizyn S, Richardson M, Bienenstock J. Basophil/mast cell precursors in human peripheral blood. Blood 1983;61:775–780.

44. Hutt-Taylor SR, Harnish D, Richardson M, Ishizaka T, Denburg JA. Sodium butyrate and a T lymphocyte cell line-derived differentiation factor induce basophilic differentiation of the human promyelocytic leukemia cell line HL-60. Blood 1988;71:209–215.

45. Dvorak AM, Seder RA, Paul WE, Morgan ES, Galli SJ. Effects of interleukin-3 with or without the c-*kit* ligand, stem cell factor, on the survival and cytoplasmic granule formation of mouse basophils and mast cells *in vitro*. Am J Pathol 1994;144:160–170.

46. Denburg JA, Wooley M, Leber B, Linden M, O'Byrne P. Basophil and eosinophil differentiation in allergic reactions. J Allergy Clin Immunol 1994;94:1135–1141.

47. Matsuda H, Switzer J, Coughlin MD, Bienenstock J, Denburg JA. Human basophilic cell differentiation promoted by 2.5S nerve growth factor. Int Arch Allergy Appl Immunol 1988;86:453–457.

48. Denburg JA, Telizyn S, Messner H, et al. Heterogeneity of human peripheral blood eosinophil-type colonies: evidence for a common basophil-eosinophil progenitor. Blood 1985;66:312–318.

49. Denburg JA, Otsuka H, Ohnishi M, Ruhno J, Bienenstock J, Dolovich J. Contribution of basophil/mast cell and eosinophil growth and differentiation to the allergic tissue inflammatory response. Int Arch Allergy Appl Immunol 1987;82:321–326.

50. Tanno Y, Bienenstock J, Richardson M, Lee TDG, Befus AD, Denburg JA. Reciprocal regulation of human basophil and eosinophil differentiation by separate T-cell-derived factors. Exp Hematol 1987;15:24–33.

51. Sillaber C, Geissler K, Scheurer R, et al. Type beta transforming growth factors promote interleukin-3 (IL-3)-dependent differentiation of human basophils but inhibit IL-3-dependent differentiation of human eosinophils. Blood 1992;80:634–641.

52. Ohnishi M, Ruhno J, Dolovich J, Denburg JA. Allergic rhinitis nasal mucosal conditioned medium stimulates growth and differentiation of basophil/mast cell and eosinophil progenitors from atopic blood. J Allergy Clin Immunol 1988;81:1149–1154.

53. Gordon JR, Burd P, Galli SJ. Mast cells as a source of multifunctional cytokines. Immunol Today 1990;11:458–464.

54. Plant M, Pierce JH, Watson CJ, Hanley-Hyde J, Nordan RP, Paul WE. Mast cell lines produce lymphokines in response to cross-linkage of Fc epsilon RI or to calcium ionophore. Nature 1989;339:64–67.

55. Bach MK. Mediators of anaphylaxis and inflammation. Annu Rev Microbiol 1982;36:371–414.

56. Saavedra-Delgado AM, Metcalfe DD. The gastrointestinal mast cell in food allergy. Ann Allergy 1983;51:185–189.

57. Stead RH, Tomioka M, Quinonez G, Simon GT, Felten SY, Bienenstock J. Intestinal mucosal mast cells in normal and nematode-infected rat intestine are in intimate contact with peptidergic nerves. Proc Natl Acad Sci USA 1987;84:2975–2979.

58. McKay DM, Bienenstock J. The interaction between mast cells and nerves in the gastrointestinal tract. Immunol Today 1994;15:533–538.

59. Goetzl EJ, Sreedharan SP, Turck CW. Structurally distinctive vasoactive intestinal peptides from rat basophilic leukemia cells. J Biol Chem 1988;263:9083–9086.

60. Stracke ML, Metcalfe DD. Glycosaminoglycans and proteoglycans in inflammatory cells. In: Reed CE, ed. Proceedings of the XII international congress of allergology and clinical immunology. St. Louis: CV Mosby, 1986, 267–274.

61. Caughey GH. Serine proteinases of mast cell and leukocyte granules. A league of their own. Am J Respir Crit Care Med 1994;150:S138–S142.

62. Gibson S, Miller HRP. Mast cell subsets in the rat distinguished histochemically by their content of serine proteases. Immunology 1986;58:101–104.

63. Schwartz LB. Tryptase from human pulmonary mast cells. In: Kay AB, Austen KF, Lichtenstein LM, eds. Asthma: physiology, immunopharmacology and treatment. Third international symposium. London: Academic Press, 1984, 19–37.

64. Alter SC, Metcalfe DD, Bradford TR, Schwartz LB. Regulation of human mast cell tryptase. Effects of enzyme concentration, ionic strength and the structure and negative charge density of polysaccharides. Biochem J 1987;248:821–827.

65. Schwartz LB, Metcalfe DD, Miller JS, Earl H, Sullivan T. Tryptase levels as an indicator of mast cell activation in systemic anaphylaxis and mastocytosis. N Engl J Med 1987;316:1622–1626.

66. Briggaman RA, Schecker NM, Fraki JE, Lazarus GS. Degradation of the epidermal–dermal junction by proteolytic enzymes from human skin and human polymorphonuclear leukocytes. J Exp Med 1984;160:1027–1042.

67. Hogaboam CM, Wallace JL. Intestinal PAF synthesis: the role of the mast cell. J Lipid Mediators Cell Signalling 1994;10:103–105.

68. Fox CC, Kagey-Sobotka A, Schleimer RP, Peters SP, MacGlashan DW, Lichtenstein LM. Mediator release from human basophils and mast cells from lung and intestinal mucosa. Int Arch Allergy Appl Immunol 1985;77:130–136.

69. Leung KPB, Flint KC, Hudspith BN, et al. Some further properties of human pulmonary mast cells recovered by bronchoalveolar lavage and enzymic dispersion of lung tissue. Agents Actions 1987;20:213–215.

70. MacGlashan DW, Schleimer RP, Peters SP, et al. Comparative studies of human basophils and mast cells. Fed Proc 1983;42:2504–2509.

71. Warner JA, Freeland HS, MacGlashan DW, Lichtenstein LM, Peters SP. Purified human basophils do not generate LTB$_4$. Biochem Pharmacol 1987;36:3195–3199.

72. Wallace JL, MacNaughton WK, Morris GP, Beck PL. Inhibition of leukotriene synthesis markedly accelerates healing in a rat model of inflammatory bowel disease. Gastroenterology 1989;96:29–36.

73. Barrett KE. Immune-related intestinal secretion. III. Acute and chronic effects of mast cell mediators on chloride secretion by a human colonic epithelial cell line. J Immunol 1991;147:959–964.

74. Bradding P, Roberts JA, Britten KM, et al. Interleukin-4, -5, and -6 and tumor necrosis factor-α in normal and asthmatic airways: evidence for the human mast cell as a source of these cytokines. Am J Respir Cell Mol Biol 1994;10:471–480.

75. MacGlashan Jr. D, White JM, Huang S-K, Ono SJ, Schroeder JT, Lichtenstein LM. Secretion of IL-4 from human basophils. The relationship between IL-4 mRNA and protein in resting and stimulated basophils. J Immunol 1994;152:3006–3016.

76. Schroeder JT, MacGlashan Jr. DW, Kagey-Sobotka A, White JM, Lichtenstein LM. IgE-dependent IL-4 secretion by human basophils. The relationship between cytokine production and histamine release in mixed leukocyte cultures. J Immunol 1994;153:1808–1817.

77. Leal-Berumen I, Conlon P, Marshall JS. IL-6 production by rat peritoneal mast cells is not necessarily preceded by histamine release and can be induced by bacterial lipopolysaccharide. J Immunol 1994;152:5468–5476.

78. Gordon JR, Galli SJ. Mast cells as a source of both preformed and immunologically-inducible TNF-α/cachectin. Nature 1990;346:274–276.

79. Lieferman KM, Gleich GJ, Kephart GM, et al. Differences between basophils and mast cells: failure to detect Charcot-Leyden crystal protein (lysophospholipase) and eosinophil granule major basic protein in human mast cells. J Immunol 1986;136:852–855.

80. Beaven MA, Metzger H. Signal transduction by Fc receptors: the FcϵRI case. Immunol Today 1993;14:222–226.

81. Lichtenstein LM. Histamine releasing factors and IgE heterogeneity. J Allergy Clin Immunol 1988;81:814–820.

82. MacQueen G, Marshall J, Perdue M, Siegel S, Bienenstock J. Pavlovian conditioning of rat mucosal mast cells to secrete rat mast cell protease II. Science 1989;243:83–85.

83. Cooke HJ. Neuroimmune signalling in regulation of intestinal ion transport. Am J Physiol 1994;266:G167–G178.

84. Egger D, Geuenich S, Denzlinger C, et al. IL-4 renders mast

cells functionally responsive to endothelin. J Immunol 1995;154.1830–1837.

85. Quist RG, Ton-Nu H-T, Lillienau J, Hofmann AF, Barrett KE. Activation of mast cells by bile acids. Gastroenterol 1991;101:446–456.

86. Gelbmann CM, Schteingart CD, Thompson SM, Hofmann AF, Barrett KE. Mast cells and histamine contribute to bile-acid stimulated secretion in the mouse colon. J Clin Invest, 1995; 9S:2831–2839.

87. Eady RP, Greenwood B, Jackson DM, Orr TSC, Wells E. The effect of nedocromil sodium and sodium cromoglycate in the *Ascaris*-sensitive monkey. Brt J Pharmacol 1985;85:323–325.

88. Pipkorn U, Proud D, Lichtenstein LM, *et al.* Effect of short-term systemic glucocorticoid treatment on human nasal release after antigen challenge. J Clin Invest 1987;80:957–961.

89. Schleimer RP, MacGlashan DW, Gillespie E, Lichtenstein LM. Inhibition of basophil histamine release by anti-inflammatory steroids. J Immunol 1982;129:1632–1636.

90. Wershil BK, Furuta GT, Lavigne JA, Choudhury AR, Wang Z-S, Galli SJ. Dexamethasone or cyclosporine A suppress mast cell–leukocyte cytokine cascades. Multiple mechanisms of inhibition of IgE- and mast cell-dependent cutaneous inflammation in the mouse. J Immunol 1995;154:1391–1398.

91. Barrett KE, Dharmsathaphorn K. Secretion and absorption: small intestine and colon. In: Yamada T, ed. Textbook of gastroenterology. Philadelphia: J.B. Lippincott Company, 1991, 265–294.

92. Galli SJ. New concepts about the mast cell. N Engl J Med 1993;328:257–265.

93. Wallace JL, Whittle BJR. Profile of gastrointestinal damage induced by platelet-activating factor. Prostaglandins 1986;32:137–141.

94. Turner MW, Boulton P, Shields JG, *et al.* Intestinal hypersensitivity reactions in the rat. I. Uptake of intact protein, permeability to sugars and their correlation with mucosal mast cell activation. Immunology 1988;63:119–124.

95. Perdue MH, McKay DM. Integrative immunophysiology in the intestinal mucosa. Am J Physiol 1994;267:G151–G165.

96. Sanderson IR, Walker WA. Uptake and transport of macromolecules by the intestine: possible role in clinical disorders (an update). Gastroenterol 1993;104:622–639.

97. Sutton BJ, Gould HJ. The human IgE network. Nature 1993;366:421–428.

98. Ravetch JV, Kinet J-P. Fc receptors. Ann Rev Immunol 1991;9:457–492.

99. Liu F-T. Gene expression and structure of immunoglobulin epsilon chains. CRC Crit Rev Immunol 1986;6:47–69.

100. MacDonald SM, Lichtenstein LM. Histamine releasing factors and heterogeneity of IgE. Springer Sem Immunopathol 1990;12:415–428.

101. Vercelli D, Jabara HH, Arai K, Geha RS. Induction of human IgE synthesis requires interleukin 4 and T/B cell interactions involving the T cell receptor/CD3 complex and MHC class II antigens. J Exp Med 1989;169:1295–1307.

102. Romagnani S, Del Prete G, Maggi E, *et al.* Role of interleukins in induction and regulation of human IgE synthesis. Clin Immunol Immunopathol 1989;50:513–523.

103. Renz H, Lack G, Saloga J, *et al.* Inhibition of IgE production and normalization of airways responsiveness by sensitized CD8 T cells in a mouse model of allergen-induced sensitization. J Immunol 1994;152:351–360.

104. Kiniwa M, Gately M, Gubler U, Chizzonite R, Fargeas C, Delespesse G. Recombinant interleukin-12 suppresses the synthesis of immunoglobulin E by interleukin-4 stimulated human lymphocytes. J Clin Invest 1992;90:262–266.

105. Leung DYM. Mechanisms controlling the human immunoglobulin E response: new directions in the therapy of allergic diseases. Ped Res 1993;33(suppl):S56–S62.

106. Kolmannskog S, Haneberg B. Immunoglobulin E in feces from children with allergy. Evidence of local production of IgE in the gut. Int Arch Allergy Appl Immunol 1985;76:133–137.

107. Ramaswamy K, Hakimi J, Bell RG. Evidence for an interleukin 4-inducible immunoglobulin E uptake and transport mechanisms in the intestine. J Exp Med 1994;180:1793–1803.

108. Atkins FM, Steinberg SS, Metcalfe DD. Evaluation of immediate adverse reactions to foods in adult patients. I. Correlation of demographic, laboratory, and prick skin test data with response to controlled oral food challenge. J Allergy Clin Immunol 1985;75:348–355.

109. Selbekk BH, Aas K, Myron J. *In vitro* sensitization and mast cell degranulation in human jejunal mucosa. Scand J Gastroenterol 1978;13:87–92.

110. Gray I, Harten M, Walzer M. Studies in mucous membrane hypersensitiveness: allergic reaction in passively sensitized mucous membranes of ileum and colon in humans. Ann Intern Med 1940;13:2050–2056.

111. Reimann H-J, Ring J, Ultsch B, *et al.* Release of gastric histamine in patients with urticaria and food allergy. Agents Actions 1982;12:111–113.

112. Sampson HA, Jolie PL. Increased plasma histamine concentrations after food challenges in children with atopic dermatitis. N Engl J Med 1984;311:372–376.

113. Riordan AM, Hunter JO, Cowan RE, *et al.* Treatment of active Crohn's disease by exclusion diet: East Anglian multicentre controlled trial. Lancet 1993;342:1131–1134.

114. Dvorak AM, Monahan RA, Osage JE, Dickersin GR. Crohn's disease: transmission electron microscopic studies. II. Immunologic inflammatory response. Alterations of mast cells, basophils, eosinophils, and the microvasculature. Hum Pathol 1980;11:606–619.

115. Fox CC, Lazenby AJ, Moore WC, Yardley JH, Bayless TM, Lichtenstein LM. Enhancement of human intestinal mast cell mediator release in active ulcerative colitis. Gastroenterol 1990;99:119–124.

116. Fox CC, Lichtenstein LM, Roche JK. Intestinal mast cell responses in idiopathic inflammatory bowel disease. Histamine release from human intestinal mast cells in response to gut epithelial proteins. Dig Dis Sci 1993;38:1105–1112.

117. Strobel S, Busuttil A, Ferguson A. Human intestinal mucosal mast cells. Expanded population in untreated coeliac disease. Gut 1983;24:222–227.

118. Andre C, Moulinier B, Andre F, Daniere S. Evidence for anaphylactic reactions in peptic ulcer and varioliform gastritis. Ann Allergy 1983;51:325–328.

119. Ogle CW, Cho CH. Effects of sulphasalazine on stress ulceration and mast cell degranulation in rat stomachs. Eur J Pharmacol 1985;112:285–286.

120. Beck PL, Morris GP, Wallace JL. Reduction of ethanol-induced gastric damage by sodium cromoglycate and FPL-52694. Role of leukotrienes, prostaglandins and mast cells in the protective mechanism. Can J Physiol Pharmacol 1989;67:287–293.

121. Rioux KP, Wallace JL. Mast cell activation augments gastric

mucosal injury through a leukotriene-dependent mechanism. Am J Physiol 1994;266:G863–G869.

122. Queiroz DM, Mendes EN, Rocha GA, *et al.* Histamine content of the oxyntic mucosa from duodenal ulcer patients. Effect of *Helicobacter pylori* eradication. Am J Gastroenterol 1993;881:1228–1232.

123. Kurose I, Granger DN, Evans Jr. DJ, *et al. Helicobacter pylori*-induced microvascular protein leakage in rats: role of neutro-phils, mast cells and platelets. Gastroenterol 1994;107:70–79.

124. Catto-Smith AG, Patrick MK, Scott RB, Davison JS, Gall DG. The gastric response to mucosal IgE-mediated reactions. Am J Physiol 1989;257:G704–G708.

125. Hogan DL, Yao B, Barrett KE, Isenberg J. Histamine inhibits prostaglandin E_2-stimulated rabbit duodenal bicarbonate secretion via H_2-receptors and enteric nerves. Gastroenterol, 1995; 108:1676–1682.

3

FOOD ANTIGENS

John W. Yunginger

*F*ood antigens are derived from animal or vegetable sources and, in most cases, consist of proteins or glycoproteins. This chapter discusses the food antigens that have commonly been implicated in producing IgE-mediated reactions in humans. Foods may contain naturally occurring pharmacologically active ingredients or may acquire additives or contaminants during processing; adverse reactions related to these materials are discussed elsewhere in this book.

Historically, adverse reactions to foods were initially described anecdotally, with reports concerning deliberate food challenge feedings subsequently appearing to document food-induced reactions in sensitive persons. Advances in laboratory technology during the past two decades have permitted in vitro study of food antigens; nevertheless, relatively few food antigens have been isolated, purified to homogeneity, and characterized in detail.

Fish

Fish hypersensitivity is commonly seen in countries where fish consumption is high. Codfish allergens have been investigated in the greatest detail. Compared with other meats for human consumption, codfish muscle contains relatively more water (81.2%), less protein (17.6%), and markedly less lipid (0.3%) (1).

BIOCHEMISTRY

All animal muscle tissue contains contractile proteins, sarcoplasmic proteins, and connective tissue proteins (1). Contractile proteins comprise the majority of muscle protein and are soluble in salt solutions of high ionic strength. Sarcoplasmic proteins, on the other hand, are soluble in water or in dilute salt solutions (1). Except for a portion of collagen that is soluble in neutral salt solution, the connective tissue proteins are insoluble at physiologic pH.

ALLERGENS

The most extensively characterized food allergen is Gad c 1 (allergen M), a parvalbumin from codfish (*Gadus callarias* L.). Parvalbumins control the flow of Ca^{++} into and out of the cell and are found only in the muscles of fish and amphibians.

Allergen M was purified by ion-exchange chromatography, gel filtration, and isoelectric focusing (2, 3). Gad c 1 contains 113 amino acid residues and one glucose molecule. It has a molecular mass of 12,328 daltons and an isoelectric point of 4.75 (4). A high degree of amino acid sequence homology is observed between Gad c 1 from cod and the corresponding parvalbumins of other fish species. The tertiary configuration of the molecule has also been established as a single polypeptide chain having three domains (AB, CD, and EF) (5). The CD and EF domains each bind one calcium ion. Synthetic peptides corresponding to residues 13–32 (domain AB), 49–64 (domain CD), and 88–103 (domain EF) have been prepared and shown to bind specific IgE from the sera of cod-sensitive individuals. Rocket line immunoelectrophoresis shows that the Gad c 1 hexadecapeptide 49–64 cross-reacts with birch pollen allergen (6). Gad c 1 is remarkably heat-stable and remains resistant to partial proteolysis; its allergenicity is decreased by polymerization or by acetylation of the Tyr-30 residue (7). The latter chemical modifications cannot be exploited commercially to reduce the allergenicity of cod, however.

Crossed radioimmunoelectrophoresis (CRIE) reveals a number of codfish allergens that are distinct from Gad c 1 (8, 9), but these materials have not yet been well characterized. For example, an allergenic protein with molecular mass of 63 kD has been isolated from codfish surimi (10), a Japanese food product prepared from minced, thoroughly washed fish meat that lacks most soluble sarcoplasmic proteins but contains myofibrillar proteins (11).

Persons allergic to fresh tuna or fresh salmon may be able to tolerate ingestion of canned tuna or canned salmon (12). The prolonged cooking undergone by these products may denature the allergenic components.

Crustaceans

The crustacean family, which is part of the order Decadoda, includes shrimp, prawns, crabs, lobsters, and crayfish (crawfish). A listing of edible crustaceans has been published previously (13).

SHRIMP

Several groups of investigators have shown that tropomyosins represent the major allergens in shrimp. Shanti et al. (14) purified a 34 kD heat-stable allergen from boiled aqueous extracts of fresh unshelled Indian prawns (Penaeus indicus); this allergen was shown to be identical to tropomyosin purified from the same shrimp. Two IgE-binding epitopes were demonstrated (residues 50–66 and 153–161). IgE binding to shrimp tropomyosin could be inhibited as much as 95% by the addition of tropomyosins from different crustaceans (lobster, prawn, and crab) and as much as 80% by the addition of tropomyosin from Drosophila, another arthropod. Daul et al. (15) isolated a similar 36 kD acidic glycoprotein (Pen a 1; pI 5.2, 2.9% carbohydrate) from the brown shrimp, Penaeus aztecus; Pen a 1 demonstrated 60% to 87% homology with muscle protein tropomyosins from various sources. In addition, Witteman et al. (16) demonstrated that a monoclonal antibody raised to Dermatophagoides pteronyssinus house dust mite cross-reacted with tropomyosin from yet another shrimp, Cragnon cragnon. Finally, Leung et al. (17) cloned, expressed, and sequenced a 34 kD heat-stable

shrimp allergen (Met e 1) from Metapenaeus ensis that proved highly homologous to multiple isoforms of tropomyosin.

Using traditional protein separation techniques, Nagpal et al. (18) isolated another allergen from cooked Indian prawns (Peneaus indicus) that was subsequently identified as tRNA.

CRAWFISH AND LOBSTER

Halmepuro et al. (19) used crossed immunoelectrophoresis (CIE) and CRIE to study antigens and allergens from crawfish (Procambarus clarkii) and spiny lobster (Panulirus argus). Using sera from several crustacean-sensitive persons, IgE antibodies were noted to multiple shared crawfish and lobster allergens. Some of these allergens may be cross-reacting tropomyosins.

Cow's Milk

In much of the world, milk from cattle (Bos taurus) accounts for nearly all of the milk produced for human consumption. Approximately 50% of all U.S. milk production is sold as fluid milk or related products, while another 25% is processed into cheese (20).

CHEMISTRY

Cow's milk contains approximately 86.6% water, 4.1% fat, 3.6% protein, 5.0% lactose, and 0.7% ash (20). Milk allergens consist of proteins, and the characteristics of the major milk proteins are given in Table 3.1. The α-, β, and κ-caseins, β-lactoglobulins, and α-lactalbumin are the major gene products of the mammary gland; the γ-casein and proteose-peptones result from post-translational proteolysis (20). The caseins are found with calcium phosphate in hydrated spherical micelles. At the pH level found in milk (6.6–6.7), β-lactoglobulin exists as a dimer. Milk also contains trace amounts of bovine albumin and immunoglobulins (derived from bovine serum), lactoferrin, lactoperoxidase, alkaline phosphatase, and catalase (21). The heat stabilities of milk proteins vary widely, with serum proteins and β-casein being

Table 3.1
Characteristics of the Major Milk Proteins

Protein	Concentration (g/L)	Percentage of Total Protein	Molecular Weight (D)
Caseins:	24–28		
α_s-caseins	15–19		23,612–25,228
α_{s1}	12–15	34	
α_{s2}	3–4	8	
β-caseins	9–11	25	23,980
κ-caseins	3–4	9	19,005
γ-caseins	1 2	4	11,557–20,520
Whey proteins:	5 7		
β-lactoglobulin	2–4	9	18,263
α-lactalbumin	1.0–1.5	4	14,174
proteose-peptones	0.6–1.8	4	
blood proteins:			
albumin	0.1–0.4	1	67,000
immunoglobulins	0.6–1.0	2	160,000–200,000

Modified from (20).

the most labile, and β-lactoglobulin and α-lactalbumin being the most stable.

ALLERGENS

The allergenicities of individual milk proteins have been studied via skin tests, immunoassays, and oral challenge feedings. Although casein produced the highest rate of skin test reactivity (68%) in children with milk allergy (22), β-lactoglobulin produced the highest rate (66%) of positive oral challenges (23). Most children reacted to more than one milk protein. Skin test reactivity to cow milk proteins is closely correlated with the results obtained from immunoassays for milk-protein-specific IgE antibodies, although such immunoassays are less sensitive, particularly to casein and bovine albumin (24).

Most milk-allergic individuals are sensitized to more than one milk protein (21). Some allergic individuals have IgE antibodies directed only to proteolytic digests of milk proteins, however (25).

The antigenic determinants of milk proteins appear to be continuous rather than conformational. Ball *et al.* (26) synthesized hexapeptides and dodecapeptides of β-lactoglobulin, which were used to screen sera from 14 milk-sensitive individuals for IgE antibodies. One of these peptides (peptide 4, TDYKKYLLFCME; residues 97–108) significantly inhibited the binding of all sera in an IgE anti-β-

lactoglobulin radioimmunoassay, suggesting that this peptide contains a major continuous IgE binding epitope. Similar observations were made by Kohno *et al.* (27), who found that serum IgE antibodies from 11 milk-sensitive children could bind equally well to native α-casein and to urea-denatured, acid-treated, alkaline-treated, or heat-denatured α-casein.

Eggs

Infertile eggs from chickens *(Gallus domesticus)* are used widely for human consumption. The average egg weighs 58 g and contains 8%–11% shell, 56%–61% albumen (white), and 27%–32% yolk (28). The albumen, in turn, is composed mainly of water (87%–89%) and protein (9%–11%), while the yolk contains 50% water, 32%–35% lipid, and 16% protein (28).

CHEMISTRY

The characteristics of major egg proteins have been summarized by Powrie and Nakai (28) and are listed in Table 3.2. The major protein in the egg albumen is ovalbumin, a phosphoglycoprotein. Purified ovalbumin has three components (A_1, A_2, and A_3) that differ only in terms of their phosphate contents. Conalbumin (ovotransferrin) is a glycoprotein that binds metallic ions. Ovomucoid is highly glycosylated

Table 3.2
Characteristics of the Major Egg Proteins

Protein	Percentage of Total Protein	Molecular Weight (D)	pI
Albumen			
Ovalbumin	54	44,500	4.5
Conalbumin (ovotransferrin)	12	76,000	6.1
Ovomucoid	11	28,000	4.1
Ovomucin	3.5	$5.5–8.3 \times 10^6$	4.5–5.0
Lysozyme	3.4	14,300	10.7
Yolk			
Granule:			
Lipovitellin	70	400,000	
Phosvitin	16	160,000–190,000	
Low-density lipoprotein	12	—	
Plasma:			
Low-density lipoprotein	64	$3–10 \times 10^6$	
Livetin	14	45,000–150,000	

Modified from (28).

(20%–25%) and contains three separate domains, each cross-linked by three disulfide bonds. Ovomucin contains 30% carbohydrate and contributes to the gelatinous nature of egg albumen. The primary structure of lysozyme, the most basic albumen protein, has been reported. Egg albumen contains numerous trace proteins, including catalase, ovoflavoprotein, ficin inhibitor, ovoglycoprotein, G_2 and G_3 globulins, ovomacroglobulin, ribonuclease, ovoinhibitor, and avidin.

Egg yolk contains several types of particles (yolk spheres, granules, myelin figures, and low-density lipoproteins) that are dispersed uniformly in a protein (livetin) solution (28). Yolk may be separated by ultracentrifugation into granule and plasma fractions; the granule fraction contains 60% proteins and 35% lipids, while the plasma fraction contains 80% lipid and 18% protein. The high-density lipoprotein fraction of yolk granules—the lipovitellin—can be separated into α- and β-lipovitellins by electrophoresis; both exist as dimers with molecular mass of 400 kD. Phosvitin, which contains 10% phosphorus, can be separated into α- and β-phosvitin by gel filtration; this protein is the principal iron carrier in the yolk. In addition, low-density lipoproteins are present in both the granule and plasma fractions of egg yolk. Livetins are derived from the blood of the hen and can be separated into α-, β-, and γ-fractions by electrophoresis.

ALLERGENS

In most published studies of egg allergy, the egg albumen has proved more allergenic than the egg yolk. In studies based on skin test (29–31), immunoassay (31, 32), immunoblotting (33), and CRIE (32, 34, 35), the major allergens have been identified as ovalbumin (Gal d 1), ovomucoid (Gal d 3), and conalbumin (ovotransferrin, Gal d 2). Recent studies employing highly purified egg white proteins have, however, shown ovomucoid to be the major egg white allergen in egg-sensitive children with atopic dermatitis (31). IgE antibodies can also be directed to egg yolk proteins (33), and cross-reactivity may exist between egg yolk and egg albumen proteins, and between eggs of various birds (36). Ovomucoid, in particular, is quite heat-stable (28). Individuals sensitive to this component may react to foods containing cooked eggs as well as to raw eggs. As with most other foods, the pattern of reactivity to egg proteins varies considerably from one person to another (34). Individuals who experience both inhalant allergy to birds and allergic reactions after ingestion of eggs have IgE antibodies directed to α-livetin (chicken serum albumin), which is a component of both feathers and egg yolk (37).

Elsayed *et al.* have investigated the allergenicity of ovalbumin in some detail. The NH_2-terminal decapeptide of ovalbumin (38) and peptide 323–339 (39) were synthesized, and both proved capable of partially inhibiting binding of IgE antibodies to solid-phase ovalbumin in inhibition immunoassays. Epitope mapping of region 11–70 of ovalbumin showed a wide distribution of allergenicity over region 33–70 (40). Japanese investigators have established an ovalbumin-specific human CD4+ T-cell line capable of secreting high levels of IL-5 following stimulation with intact ovalbumin or ovalbumin peptide 323–339 (41).

Legumes

Legumes are dicotyledonous seed plants that include peanuts, soybeans, peas, lentils, and beans. Collectively, legumes account for only 6% of the world's food crops, but constitute 19% of the world's food protein (42). Approximately 80% of legume seed nitrogen is contained in two types of storage globulins: legumin and vicilin. Selected properties of these globulins are shown in Table 3.3 (43).

PEANUTS

The principal varieties of peanuts (Arachis hypogaea) grown in the United States are Virginia, Spanish, and

Runner. The Virginia variety produces a uniformly long kernel grown primarily for shelled, whole-kernel use. The Spanish variety produces a shorter, rounded kernel. The Runner variety produces kernels of variable length that are typically used for peanut oil or peanut butter.

Chemistry

Peanut kernels contain 45%–50% oil, 25%–30% protein, 5%–12% carbohydrate, 5% moisture, 3% fiber, and 2.5% ash (44). The peanut skin (testa) contains 49% carbohydrate and 19% fiber (45), along with tannins and pigments; these materials produce undesirable colors in peanut products unless they are removed during the initial processing (46).

Peanut proteins were originally classified as albumins (water-soluble) or globulins (saline-soluble). The globulins, in turn, were subdivided into arachin and conarachin fractions (the legumin and the vicilin storage proteins of the peanut, respectively) based on their differing precipitability in ammonium sulfate (47). The compositions of arachin and conarachin are not easily defined because of their ability to undergo reversible association and dissociation in solution under different conditions of temperature, pH, and ionic strength.

Native arachin in the seed has a molecular mass of at least 600 kD (44), but readily dissociates into arachin, with a dimer molecular mass of 330 kD, and a monomer with molecular mass of 170 kD (48, 49). Arachin has two polymorphic forms: A and B (50). Arachin A contains alpha, beta, gamma, and delta peptide chains, while arachin B lacks the alpha chain. Using electrophoresis in polyacrylamide gels containing sodium dodecylsulfate (SDS-PAGE), arachin may be dissociated into a variable number of subunits ranging from 71 kD to 10 kD in molecular mass (51).

Conarachin can be separated by ultracentrifugation into 7.8S and 12.6S components, with calculated molecular masses of 142 and 295 kD, respectively (52). The latter component is designated as conarachin II, or α-conarachin. Using SDS-PAGE, conarachin II can be dissociated into multiple subunits having molecular masses ranging from 62 to 18 kD (53).

The albumin fraction of peanuts contains agglutinins, lectin-reactive glycoproteins, protease inhibi-

Table 3.3
Comparison of Selected Characteristics of the Two Major Legume Seed Storage Globulins—Legumins and Vicilins

Characteristics	Legumins	Vicilins
Sedimentation coefficient	11S	7S
Molecular weight range	300–400 kD	150–250 kD
Solubility in salt solution	less soluble	more soluble
Temperature of coagulation	higher, more stable	lower, less stable
Structure	hexamers, composed of bicatenar monomers having one acidic and one basic subunit	subunits frequently noncovalently associated in trimers or hexamers
Carbohydrate	0	+
Disulfide bonds	+	0

Modified from Pernollet & Mosse (43).

tors, α-amylase inhibitors, and phospholipases (reviewed in Yunginger *et al.* [54]).

Allergens

Peanut allergens are relatively heat-stable and are thus present in both raw and roasted peanuts (55). In a study of various commercial peanut-containing foods, only hydrolyzed peanut protein and peanut oil did not show allergenic activity in inhibition immunoassays (56). The lack of allergenicity of high-temperature processed peanut oil has also been demonstrated by double-blind cross-over feeding tests in peanut-sensitive persons (57). Cold-pressed peanut oils may contain peanut allergen, however (58).

Using immunoassays, Australian investigators have examined the allergenicities of α-arachin, conarachin I, the concanavalin A–reactive glycoprotein, peanut agglutinin, and peanut phospholipase D (59). All test sera contained IgE antibodies to α-arachin and conarachin I, but fewer sera proved reactive to peanut agglutinin and phospholipase D. The allergenicity of the concanavalin A–reactive glycoprotein was confirmed in subsequent skin test experiments (60). The concanavalin A–reactive glycoprotein has a monomeric molecular mass of 65 kD, a pI of 4.6, and a carbohydrate content of 2.4%. It is allergenically stable at temperatures as high as 100°C and over the pH range 2.8–10.0. Removal of the carbohydrate group slightly decreases, but does not eliminate, the allergenicity of the molecule (60).

Using ion-exchange chromatography to fractionate extracts of Runner peanuts, Burks *et al.* have isolated Ara h 1 (61), an allergenic glycoprotein with molecular mass of 63.5 kD and a pI of 4.55, and Ara h 2 (62), a protein with molecular mass of 17 kD and a mean pI of 5.2. Although the physicochemical characteristics of Ara h 1 closely resemble those of the concanavalin A–reactive glycoprotein allergen described by the Australian group, Ara h 1 does not bind concanavalin A. Burks *et al.* have also confirmed the allergenicity of peanut agglutinin (63).

SOYBEANS

The major food crop of the legume family is the soybean *(Glycine max)* (42). Its oil is intended mainly for human consumption, while most soybean protein meal is used for animal feed.

Chemistry

Soybeans contain 32% to 42% protein; the proteins may be separated into globulin (80%–90%) and whey (10%–15%) fractions by precipitation of the globulin fraction at pH 4.5.

The globulins may be separated into 2S, 7S, 11S, and 15S fractions by ultracentrifugation (64). The 2S fraction contains 20% of extractable protein and includes heat-stable components having molecular masses of 18.2 and 32.6 kD, as well as trypsin inhibitor and cytochrome c activity (65). The 7S fraction contains 35% of the extractable protein and consists mainly of β-conglycinin (the soybean vicilin storage protein), β-amylase, lipoxygenase, and a lectin (66). A glycoprotein, β-conglycinin has a molecular mass of 180 kD (67). It is a trimer composed of three major subunits (alpha', alpha, and beta) that have molecular masses of 76, 72, and 53 kD, respectively (68). The 11S fraction also contains 35% of extractable protein and consists almost entirely of glycinin, the soybean legumin globulin. Glycinin, which has a molecular mass ranging from 320 to 360 kD, is composed of six subunits; each subunit consists, in turn, of one acidic and one basic polypeptide chain linked covalently. These chains have molecular masses ranging from 10 to 45 kD (69, 70). The 15S fraction accounts for 10% of extractable protein and contains mainly aggregated glycinin (71).

The whey fraction contains several biologically active substances, including a hemagglutinin, a trypsin inhibitor, and a urease (65).

Allergens

Many soybean fractions contain allergens. Using immunoassay procedures, Japanese investigators have identified cross-reacting allergens in the 2S, 7S, and 11S soybean globulin fractions (65). Immunoblotting studies using sera from soy-sensitive persons with atopic dermatitis have shown that IgE antibodies were directed preferentially to a 7S globulin with a molecular mass of 30 kD (72). Burks *et al.* (73) have demonstrated IgE antibodies directed to 7S and 11S soybean globulins by both ELISA and immunoblotting procedures. Moroz and Yung (74) reported a soybean-sensitive patient who reacted to purified Kunitz soybean trypsin inhibitor in both a skin test and via an immunoassay; the allergenicity of soybean trypsin inhibitor has been confirmed by Burks *et al.* (63). Ingestion of soybean oil does not pose risks to soybean-sensitive individuals (75).

Using serum from a patient with inhalant sensitivity to soybean flour, Bush *et al.* (76) demonstrated by SDS-PAGE immunoblots the existence of IgE antibodies to multiple soybean flour components having apparent molecular masses between 14 and 54 kD. Indeed, soybean lecithin has been reported as one cause of baker's asthma (77). Epidemics of asthma caused by inhalation of soybean dust have been traced to two soybean-hull-derived proteins, Gly m 1A (7.5 kD, pI 6.8) and Gly m 1B (7.0 kD, pI 6.1–6.2) (78).

Cereal Grains

Cereal grains include wheat, maize (corn), rice, barley, sorghum, oats, millet, and rye. These grains collectively account for 72% of the world's food protein (42). Cereal grain proteins include the water-soluble albumins, the saline-soluble globulins, the 70% aqueous ethanol-soluble prolamins, and the acid- or alkali-soluble glutelins (43).

WHEAT

Wheat grains contain a small proximal germ and a large distal endosperm, in which starch and protein are stored. The endosperm is surrounded by an aleurone layer and an outer protective bran layer; together, these two layers contain most of the wheat grain's fiber and minerals. The endosperm contains 100% of the starch, 72% of the protein, and 50% of the lipid within the grain (79).

Chemistry

The prolamin protein of wheat is gliadin, and the glutelin protein is glutenin. Gliadin is composed of two sets of polypeptides—one about 30 kD in molecular mass (α-, β-, or γ-gliadins) and another about 60 kD in molecular mass (ω-gliadin) (43). When a lump of flour–water dough is kneaded in a stream of running water, the starch and water-soluble proteins wash away, leaving behind a rubbery mixture of gliadin and glutenin called gluten.

Allergens

Blands *et al.* (80) used CIE and CRIE to study wheat flour antigens and allergens. Forty different antigens were noted, half of which cross-reacted with rye flour extract. Using sera from 13 allergic bakers, 18 allergenic components were identified, including three major allergens. Subsequently, Australian investigators (81, 82) used immunoassays to demonstrate that sera from asthmatic bakers contained IgE antibodies to several wheat proteins, including the albumin, wheat germ agglutinin, a concanavalin A-purified glycoprotein, and a trypsin inhibitor. Furthermore, when wheat flour was treated with 1% potassium hydroxide to facilitate extraction of the globulin, gliadin, and gluten, IgE antibodies could be demonstrated to these components (83). French investigators have documented sensitization to *Aspergillus orizae*-derived α-amylase added to wheat flour to enhance carbohydrate fermentation by yeast (84).

More recently, Spanish investigators have used serum from individuals having baker's asthma to identify a 15 kD salt-soluble allergen in wheat flour (85) and a corresponding 14.5 kD allergen in barley flour (86). These allergens, which are glycosylated monomeric subunits of cereal α-amylase/trypsin inhibitors (87), produce positive skin prick test results in more than 80% of individuals with baker's asthma (88). The allergenicity of α-amylase inhibitor subunits has been confirmed by other investigators as well (89).

BARLEY AND RYE

The prolamins of barley *(Hordeum vulgare)* are called hordeins, while those of rye *(Secale cereale)* are known as secalins (43). In addition to the prolamin components listed previously for wheat, cereal flours also contain α-amylase (α-1,4-glucan 4-glucanohydrolase) and β-amylase (α-1,4-glucan maltohydrolase). Using immunoassay and immunoblotting techniques, Sandiford and colleagues (90) demonstrated the presence of serum IgE antibodies to purified barley α-amylase (54 kD) and barley β-amylase (64 kD) in 29 of 30 persons with baker's asthma. Garcia-Casado *et al.* (91) have isolated homodimeric 25 kD proteins from both rye and barley. The amino acid sequences of these proteins were closely homologous to other cereal α-amylase/trypsin inhibitor proteins, but neither demonstrated inhibitory activities for α-amylase or trypsin. The monomeric 13.5 kD protein from rye, designated as Sec c 1, produced positive skin tests in 70% of rye-sensitive persons tested.

RICE

Rice *(Oryza sativa)* forms the staple diet of one-half of the world's population (42). Nevertheless, relatively little information has been published on allergy to rice.

Chemistry

In contrast to wheat, barley, and rye, rice storage proteins consist of 8% prolamins and 80% glutelins. Each storage protein is found in a separate protein body in the rice endosperm (92).

Allergens

Shibasaki *et al.* (93) separated defatted rice flour into glutelin and globulin components; the latter components were further fractionated by gel filtration. In immunoassays using sera from rice-sensitive patients, IgE antibodies were demonstrated to both the glutelin and globulin fractions. Subsequently, other investigators (94) isolated a 16 kD saline-soluble rice protein that bound serum IgE antibodies from rice-sensitive individuals. This binding could be inhibited by preincubation of sera with not only rice extract, but also extracts of wheat, corn, Japanese millet *(Panicum crus-galli* L. var. *frumentaceum Trin.)*, and Italian millet *(Setaria italica* Beauv. var. *germanica schrad.)*, suggesting that this protein is responsible for the cross-allergenicity among cereal grains (95). Indeed, when cloned and sequenced, this protein showed 40% homology with wheat α-amylase inhibitor and 20% homology with barley trypsin inhibitor (96).

Other Foods

COTTONSEED

Cotton *(Gossypium* spp.) has been cultivated for centuries as a source of textile fiber. In addition, the cottonseed is utilized as a source of edible oil and protein for humans and animals.

Chemistry

Cottonseed meal constitutes 60% of the harvested fiber-free seed (97). The cotyledons contain the major deposits of storage oil and protein. Cottonseed contains three major classes of proteins (2S, 5S, and 9S) in nearly equal amounts (97). The 2S proteins are albumins (water-soluble) and represent the source of the major cottonseed allergen, CS-1A (vide infra) (98). The higher-molecular-weight proteins comprise globulin storage proteins, with subfractions of acalin A and acalin B (99). The molecular masses of these components range from 22 kD for the 2S fraction, to 130 kD and 240–300 kD for acalin A and acalin B, respectively (99).

The widespread use of cottonseed in human foods has been hindered by the presence in the seed of pigment glands containing gossypol, a yellow polyphenolic compound that is toxic to humans when it is ingested in its unbound form (100). Raw cottonseed kernels may contain from 0.6% to 2.0% free gossypol; the FDA limit for free gossypol in human food products and ingredients is 450 ppm (100). Genetic engineering, which has resulted in varieties of cottonseed that are virtually free of pigment glands, has spurred renewed interest in cottonseed-containing products meant for the human diet (101).

Allergens

The isolation and partial characterization of cottonseed allergens was performed by Spies *et al.* in a series of reports from 1939 to 1960 (reviewed in [102]). Several allergenic fractions were isolated from cottonseed meal by a variety of techniques (reviewed in [102]). The principal heat-stable proteinaceous fraction, designated as CS-1A, could be further purified to a fraction designated as CS-13 Endo. The latter material contained 17.8% nitrogen and 7.7%

carbohydrate, and was unaffected by pepsin digestion (103). Unfortunately, no further characterization of this allergenic fraction has been undertaken via more modern laboratory techniques.

TOMATO

The tomato *(Lycopersicon esculentum)* is a member of the Solanaceae (nightshade) family. Tomato allergens have been isolated from red, ripe tomatoes by sequential homogenization, dialysis, ammonium sulfate precipitation, and ion-exchange chromatography (104, 105). The most allergenic fraction (fraction G) contained 8% nitrogen and 21% hexoses and accounted for only 0.15% of extractable solids. The allergen content of unripe tomatoes was lower than that of ripe tomatoes.

SESAME SEED

Sesame *(Sesamum indicum)* is an East Indian herb of the Pedaliaceae family whose seeds are commonly used in baked goods or halvah candy. Malish *et al.* (106) utilized density-gradient ultra-centrifugation to fractionate sesame seed extract. Using immunoassay, they noted allergenic activity in multiple components with molecular masses ranging from less than 8 to 84 kD.

CABBAGE

Cabbage *(Brassica oleracea capitata)* is a member of the Brassicaceae (mustard) family. Blaiss *et al.* (107) fractionated cabbage extract by gel filtration and obtained five peaks of UV-absorbing material at 280 nm. Using inhibition immunoassay, several allergenic components were identified with apparent molecular masses between 20 and 67 kD.

MUSTARD

Spanish investigators have isolated, sequenced (108), cloned, and expressed (109) Sin a 1, the major allergen of yellow mustard seed *(Sinapis alba L.)*. This basic 14 kD protein consists of two disulfide-linked polypeptide chains of 39 and 88 amino acids and is derived from the 1.7S storage protein of the seed. A closely related allergenic protein, Bra j 1, has been isolated from oriental mustard seeds *(Brassica juncea)* (110). This protein is also a 2S albumin with two polypeptide chains and multiple isoforms with molecular mass between 16.0 and 16.4 kD. The amino acid sequences of Sin a 1 and Bra j 1 are closely related, and IgE antibodies from mustard-sensitive persons recognize a heavy-chain epitope common to both allergens (111).

Phylogeny of Animal and Vegetable Foods

Allergy reference textbooks often contain phylogenetic tables of animal (Table 3.4) and vegetable (Table 3.5) foods (112). Food-sensitive persons are often advised to avoid eating other closely-related foods. Such advice is conservative and perhaps warranted in cases where individuals exhibit anaphylactic reactivity to certain foods. In clinical practice, patients often report cross-reactivity among various fish and among various crustaceans, with less cross-reactivity noted within vegetable food groups. From a practical point of view, food-allergic patients should be educated about food groupings and advised to use caution when first eating other members of the same food group.

Cross-Allergenicity Among Foods and Pollens

Some allergic individuals exhibit cross-reactivity between pollen allergens and vegetable allergens. These cross-reactions have been described between melon, banana, and ragweed pollen (113); celery and mugwort pollen (114); potato and grass pollen (115); and apple, cherry, pear, peach, and birch pollen (116). In addition, some individuals sensitized to natural rubber latex also react to certain foods, including banana, avocado, kiwi, apricot, grape, passionfruit, and pineapple (117–119). Many of these cross-reactions are caused by pathogenesis-related proteins and profilins.

Table 3.4
Classification of Foods from Animal Sources.

Molluscs	Crustaceans	Fish	
Abalone	Crab	Sturgeon	Halibut
Mussel	Crayfish	Hake	Catfish
Oyster	Lobster	Anchovy	Sole
Scallop	Shrimp	Sardine	Pike
Clam		Herring	Founder
Squid	*Reptiles*	Haddock	Drum
	Turtle	Bass	Mullet
Amphibians		Trout	Weakfish
Frog	*Birds*	Salmon	Mackerel
	Chicken	Whitefish	Tuna
Mammals	Duck	Scrod	Pompano
Beef	Goose	Shad	Bluefish
Pork	Turkey	Eel	Snapper
Goat	Guinea hen	Carp	Sunfish
Mutton	Squab	Codfish	Swordfish
Venison	Pheasant		
Horsemeat	Partridge		
Rabbit	Grouse		
Squirrel			

Reprinted with permission from Metcalfe DD. The diagnosis of food allergy: theory and practice. In: Spector SL, ed. Provocative challenge procedures: background and methodology. Mt. Kisco, New York: Futura Publishing Co., 1989.

Table 3.5
Classification of Foods from Plant Sources

Grain family	Ginger family	Buckwheat family	Mulberry family
Wheat	Ginger	Buckwheat	Mulberry
Graham flour	Turmeric	Rhubarb	Fig
Gluten flour	Cardamon		Hop
Bran		*Potato family*	Breadfruit
Wheat germ	*Pine family*	Potato	
Rye	Juniper	Tomato	*Maple family*
Barley		Eggplant	Maple syrup
Malt	*Orchid family*		
Corn	Vanilla	*Gooseberry family*	*Palm family*
Oats		Gooseberry	Coconut
Rice	*Madder family*	Current	Date
Wild rice	Coffee		Sago
Sorghum		*Honeysuckle family*	
Cane	*Tea family*	Elderberry	*Pomegranate family*
	Tea		Pomegranate
Mustard family		*Citrus family*	
Mustard	*Pedalium family*	Orange	*Ebony family*
Cabbage	Sesame seed	Grapefruit	Persimmon
Cauliflower		Lemon	
Broccoli	*Mallow family*	Lime	*Rose family*
Brussels sprouts	Okra	Tangerine	Raspberry
Turnip	Cottonseed	Kumquat	Blackberry
Rutabaga			Loganberry
Kale	*Spurge family*	*Pineapple family*	Boysenberry
Collard	Tapioca	Pineapple	Dewberry
Celery cabbage			Strawberry
Kohlrabi	*Arrowroot family*	*Papaw family*	
Radish	Arrowroot	Papaya	*Banana family*
Horseradish			Banana
Watercress	*Arum family*	*Birch family*	Plantain
	Taro	Filbert	
		Hazelnut	

Table 3.5
(Continued)

Grape family	*Plum family*	*Parsley family*	Licorice
Grape	Plum	Parsley	Acacia
Raisin	Prune	Parsnip	Senna
	Cherry	Carrot	
Myrtle family	Peach	Celery	*Morning glory family*
Allspice	Apricot	Celeriac	Sweet potato
Cloves	Nectarine	Caraway	Yam
Paprika	Almond	Anise	
Guava		Dill	*Sunflower family*
	Laurel family	Coriander	Jerusalem artichoke
Mint family	Avocado	Fennel	Sunflower seed
Mint	Cinnamon		
Peppermint	Bay leaf	*Heath family*	*Pepper family*
Spearmint		Cranberry	Black pepper
Thyme	*Olive family*	Blueberry	
Sage	Green olive		*Nutmeg family*
Marjoram	Ripe olive	*Legythis family*	Nutmeg
Savory	Red pepper	Brazil nut	
	Green pepper		*Walnut family*
Gourd family	Bell pepper	*Composite family*	English walnut
Pumpkin	Chili	Leaf lettuce	Black walnut
Squash	Tabasco	Head lettuce	Butternut
Cucumber	Pimento	Endive	Hickory nut
Cantaloupe		Escarole	Pecan
Muskmelon	*Lily family*	Artichoke	
Honeydew melon	Asparagus	Dandelion	*Cashew family*
Persian melon	Onion	Oyster plant	Cashew
Casaba	Garlic	Chicory	Pistachio
Watermelon	Leek		Mango
	Chive	*Legume family*	
Apple family	Aloe	Navy bean	*Beech family*
Apple		Kidney bean	Beechnut
Pear	*Goosefoot family*	Lima bean	Chestnut
Quince	Beet	String bean	
	Spinach	Soybean	*Fungi family*
Poppy family	Swiss chard	Lentil	Mushroom
Poppy seed		Black-eyed pea	Yeast
		Pea	
		Peanut	*Sterculia family*
			Cocoa
			Chocolate

Reprinted with permission from Metcalfe DD. The diagnosis of food allergy: theory and practice. In: Spector SL, ed. Provocative challenge procedures: background and methodology. Mt. Kisco, New York: Futura Publishing Co., 1989.

PATHOGENESIS-RELATED (PR) PROTEINS

PR proteins are disease-resistance gene products that are widely distributed in plants. They are usually produced in response to plant injury by microbes, but may also be induced by chemicals, osmotic stress, or air pollution (120). The major allergens of several tree pollens, including birch (Bet v 1), alder (Aln g 1), hornbeam (Car a 1), and hazel (Cor a 1) show 50% to 70% structural homology with PR proteins (121). For example, recombinant Bet v 1 produced positive skin test responses in persons allergic to birch pollen and apples, cherries, or hazelnuts (122). Moreover, an allergen homologous to Bet v 1 could be detected in apple, pear, and celery using a Bet v 1-specific monoclonal antibody (123).

PROFILINS

Profilins are actin-binding proteins found in all eukaryotic cells (121). Plant profilins are highly homologous (121) and are thought to play an important role in plant cell growth and in pollen germination.

One of the purified birch pollen allergens, Bet v 2, is a profilin (124) and cross-reacts with celery profilin (125). Subsequently, profilins have been identified in a variety of other foods (onion, avocado, carrot, tomato, orange, cucumber, peach, cherry, pear, strawberry, nectarine, potato, peanut, almond, pea, parsley, kiwi, walnut, apple, corn, soy, and spinach) (126) and wheat (127), as well as in timothy grass and mugwort pollens (128), and natural rubber latex (129).

Acknowledgments

The author acknowledges the secretarial assistance of Ms. Marian Bortolon and Ms. JoAnn Lower.

REFERENCES

1. Hultin HO. Characteristics of muscle tissue. In: Fennema OR, ed. Food chemistry, 2nd ed. New York: Marcel Dekker, 1985, 725–789.
2. Aas K, Jebsen JW. Studies of hypersensitivity to fish. Partial purification and crystallization of a major allergenic component of cod. Int Arch Allergy Appl Immunol 1967;32:1–20.
3. Elsayed S, Aas K. Isolation of purified allergens (cod) by isoelectric focusing. Int Arch Allergy Appl Immunol 1971;40:428–438.
4. Elsayed S, Bennich H. The primary structure of allergen M from cod. Scand J Immunol 1975;4:203–208.
5. Elsayed S, Apold J. Immunochemical analysis of cod fish allergen M: locations of the immunoglobulin binding sites as demonstrated by the native and synthetic peptides. Allergy 1983;38:449–459.
6. Elsayed S, Apold J, Holen E, Vik H, Florvaag E, Dybendal T. The structural requirements of epitopes with IgE binding capacity demonstrated by three major allergens from fish, egg, and tree pollen. Scand J Clin Lab Invest 1991;204S:17–31.
7. Apold J, Elsayed S. The effect of amino acid modification and polymerization on the immunochemical reactivity of cod allergen M. Molec Immunol 1979;16:559–564.
8. Aukrust L, Apold J, Elsayed S, Aas K. Crossed immunoelectrophoretic and crossed radioimmunoelectrophoretic studies employing a model allergen from codfish. Int Arch Allergy Appl Immunol 1978;57:253–262.
9. Aukrust L, Grimmer O, Aas K. Demonstration of distinct allergens by means of immunological methods. Comparison of crossed radioimmunoelectrophoresis, radioallergosorbent test, and in vivo passive transfer test. Int Arch Allergy Appl Immunol 1978;57:183–192.
10. Mata E, Favier C, Moneret-Vautrin DA, Nicholas JP, Han Ching L, Gueant JL. Surimi and native codfish contain a common allergen identified as a 63-kDa protein. Allergy 1994;49:442–447.
11. Lee CM. Surimi manufacturing and fabrication of surimi-based products. Food Technol 1986;3:115–124.
12. Bernhisel-Broadbent J, Strause D, Sampson HA. Fish hypersensitivity. II. Clinical relevance of altered fish allergenicity caused by various preparation methods. J Allergy Clin Immunol 1992;90:622–629.
13. Lemanske RF, Taylor SL. Standardized extracts, foods. Clin Rev Allergy 1987;5:23–36.
14. Shanti KN, Martin BM, Nagpal S, Metcalfe DD, Rao PV. Identification of tropomyosin as the major shrimp allergen and characterization of its IgE-binding epitopes. J Immunol 1993;151:5354–5363.
15. Daul CB, Slattery M, Reese G, Lehrer SB. Identification of the major brown shrimp allergen as the muscle protein tropomyosin. Int Arch Allergy Immunol 1994;105:49–55.
16. Witteman AM, Akkerdaas JH, van Leeuwen J, van der Zee JS, Aalberse RC. Identification of a cross-reactive allergen (presumably tropomyosin) in shrimp, mite, and insects. Int Arch Allergy Immunol 1994;105:56–61.
17. Leung PS, Chu KH, Chow WK, Ansari A, Bandea CI, Kwan HS, Nagy SM, Gershwin ME. Cloning, expression, and primary structure of *Metapenaeus ensis* tropomyosin, the major heat-stable shrimp allergen. J Allergy Clin Immunol 1994;94:882–890.
18. Nagpal S, Metcalfe DD, Subba Rao PV. Identification of a shrimp-derived allergen as tRNA. J Immunol 1987;138:4169–4174.
19. Halmepuro L, Salvaggio JE, Lehrer SB. Crawfish and lobster allergens: identification and structural similarities with other crustacea. Int Arch Allergy Appl Immunol 1987;84:165–172.
20. Swaisgood HE. Characteristics of edible fluids of animal origin: milk. In: Fennema OR, ed. Food chemistry, 2nd ed. New York: Marcel Dekker, 1985, 791–827.
21. Baldo BA. Milk allergies. Aust J Dairy Technol 1984;39:120–128.
22. Goldman AS, Sellars WA, Halpern SR, Anderson DW, Furlow TE, Johnson CH. Milk allergy. II. Skin testing of allergic and normal children with purified milk proteins. Pediatrics 1963;32:572–579.
23. Goldman AS, Anderson DW, Sellars WA, Halpern SR, Saperstein S, Knicker WT, Halpern SR. Milk allergy I. Oral challenge with milk and isolated milk proteins in allergic children. Pediatrics 1963;32:425–443.
24. Vanto T, Smogorzewska EM, Viander M, Kalimo K, Koivikko A. Leukocyte migration inhibition test in children with cow milk allergy. Allergy 1987;42:612–618.
25. Haddad ZH, Kalra V, Verma S. IgE antibodies to peptic and peptic-tryptic digests of betalactoglobulin: significance in food hypersensitivity. Ann Allergy 1979;42:368–371.
26. Ball G, Shelton MJ, Walsh BJ, Hill DJ, Hosking CS, Howden ME. A major continuous allergenic epitope of bovine beta-lactoglobulin recognized by human IgE binding. Clin Exp Allergy 1994;24:758–764.
27. Kohno Y, Honma K, Saito K, Shimojo N, Tsunoo H, Kaminogawa S, Niimi H. Preferential recognition of primary protein structures of alpha-casein by IgG and IgE antibodies of patients with milk allergy. Ann Allergy 1994;73:419–422.
28. Powrie WD, Nakai S. Characteristics of edible fluids of animal origin: eggs. In: Fennema OR, ed. Food chemistry, 2nd ed. New York: Marcel Dekker, 1985, 829–855.
29. Bleumink E, Young E. Studies on the atopic allergen in hen's

egg. I. Identification of the skin reactive fraction in egg white. Int Arch Allergy Appl Immunol 1969;35:1–19.

30. Bleumink E, Young E. Studies on the atopic allergen in hen's egg. II. Further characterization of the skin-reactive fraction in egg-white; immuno-electrophoretic studies. Int Arch Allergy Appl Immunol 1971;40:72–88.

31. Bernhisel-Broadbent J, Dintzis HM, Dintzis RZ, Sampson HA. Allergenicity and antigenicity of chicken egg ovomucoid (*Gal d* III) compared with ovalbumin (*Gal d* I) in children with egg allergy and in mice. J Allergy Clin Immunol 1994;93:1047–1059.

32. Hoffman DR. Immunochemical identification of the allergens in egg white. J Allergy Clin Immunol 1983;71:481–486.

33. Anet J, Back JF, Baker RS, Barnett D, Burley RW, Howden MEH. Allergens in the white and yolk of hen's egg. A study of IgE binding by egg proteins. Int Arch Allergy Appl Immunol 1985;77:364–371.

34. Langeland T. A clinical and immunological study of allergy to hen's egg white. III. Allergens in hen's egg white studied by crossed radioimmunoelectrophoresis (CRIE). Allergy 1982;37:521–530.

35. Langeland T, Harbitz O. A clinical and immunological study of allergy to hen's egg white. V. Purification and identification of a major allergen (antigen 22) in hen's egg white. Allergy 1983;38:131–139.

36. Langeland T. A clinical and immunological study of allergy to hen's egg white. VI. Occurrence of proteins cross-reacting with allergens in hen's egg white as studied in egg white from turkey, duck, goose, seagull, and in hen egg yolk, and hen and chicken sera and flesh. Allergy 1983;38:399–412.

37. Szépfalusi Z, Ebner C, Pandjaitan R, Orlicek F, Scheiner O, Boltz-Nitulescu G, Kraft D, Ebner H. Egg yolk alpha-livetin (chicken serum albumin) is a cross-reactive allergen in the bird-egg syndrome. J Allergy Clin Immunol 1994;93:932–942.

38. Elsayed S, Holen E, Haugstad MB. Antigenic and allergenic determinants of ovalbumin. II. The reactivity of the NH_2 terminal decapeptide. Scand J Immunol 1988;27:587–591.

39. Johnsen G, Elsayed S. Antigenic and allergenic determinants of ovalbumin. III. MHC Ia-binding peptide (OA 323-339) interacts with human and rabbit specific antibodies. Mol Immunol 1990;27:821–827.

40. Elsayed S, Stavseng L. Epitope mapping of region 11-70 of ovalbumin (*Gal d* I) using five synthetic peptides. Int Arch Allergy Immunol 1994;104:65–71.

41. Shimojo N, Katsuki T, Coligan JE, Nishimura Y, Sasazuki T, Tsunoo H, Sakamaki T, Kohno Y, Niimi H. Identification of the disease-related T cell epitope of ovalbumin and epitope-targeted T cell inactivation in egg allergy. Int Arch Allergy Immunol 1994;105:155–161.

42. Payne PI. Breeding for protein quantity and protein quality in seed crops. In: Daussant J, Mosse J, Vaughan J, eds. Seed proteins. London: Academic Press, 1983, 223–253.

43. Pernollet J-C, Mosse J. Structure and location of legume and cereal seed storage proteins. In: Daussant J, Mosse J, Vaughan J, eds. Seed proteins. London: Academic Press, 1983, 155–191.

44. Arthur Jr. JC. Peanut protein isolation, composition, and properties. Adv Protein Chem 1953;8:393–414.

45. Lusas EW. Food uses of peanut protein. J Am Oil Chem Soc 1979;56:425–430.

46. Natarajan KR. Peanut protein ingredients: preparation, properties, and food uses. Adv Food Res 1980;26:215–273.

47. Johns CO, Jones DB. The proteins of the peanut, *Arachis hypogaea.* I. The globulins arachin and conarachin. J Biol Chem 1916;28:77–87.

48. Johnson P. The proteins of the ground-nut (*Arachis hypogaea*). I. The isolation and properties of the proteins. Trans Faraday Soc 1946;42:28–36.

49. Johnson P, Shooter EM. The globulins of the ground nut (*Arachis hypogaea*). I. Investigation of arachin as a dissociation system. Biochim Biophys Acta 1950;5:361–375.

50. Tombs MP. An electrophoretic investigation of groundnut proteins: the structure of arachins A and B. Biochem J 1965;96:119–133.

51. Shetty KJ, Rao MSN. Studies on groundnut proteins. III. Physicochemical properties of arachin prepared by different methods. Anal Biochem 1974;62:108–120.

52. Dechary JM, Talluto KF, Evans WJ, Carney WB, Altschul AM. Alpha-conarachin. Nature 1961;190:1125–1126.

53. Shetty KJ, Rao MSN. Studies on groundnut proteins: part VII—physico-chemical properties of conarachin II. Indian J Biochem Biophys 1977;14:31–34.

54. Yuninger JW, Jones RT. A review of peanut chemistry. Implications for the standardization of peanut extracts. In: Schaeffer M, Sisk C, Brede HD, eds. Regulatory control and standardization of allergenic extracts. Stuttgart: Gustav Fischer Verlag, 1987, 251–254.

55. Gillespie DN, Nakajima S, Gleich GJ. Detection of allergy to nuts by the radioallergosorbent test. J Allergy Clin Immunol 1976;57:302–309.

56. Nordlee JA, Taylor SL, Jones RT, Yuninger JW. Allergenicity of various peanut products as determined by RAST inhibition. J Allergy Clin Immunol 1981;68:376–382.

57. Taylor SL, Busse WW, Sachs MI, Parker JL, Yuninger JW. Peanut oil is not allergenic to peanut-sensitive individuals. J Allergy Clin Immunol 1981;68:372–375.

58. Hoffman DR, Collins-Williams C. Cold-pressed peanut oils may contain peanut allergen. J Allergy Clin Immunol 1994;93:801–802.

59. Barnett D, Baldo BA, Howden MEH. Multiplicity of allergens in peanuts. J Allergy Clin Immunol 1983;72:61–68.

60. Barnett D, Howden MEH. Partial characterization of an allergenic glycoprotein from peanut (*Arachis hypogaea* L.). Biochim Biophys Acta 1986;882:97–105.

61. Burks AW, Williams LW, Helm RM, Connaughton C, Cockrell G, O'Brien T. Identification of a major peanut allergen, *Ara h* I, in patients with atopic dermatitis and positive peanut challenges. J Allergy Clin Immunol 1991;88:172–179.

62. Burks AW, Williams LW, Connaughton C, Cockrell G, O'Brien TJ, Helm RM. Identification and characterization of a second major peanut allergen, *Ara h* II, with use of the sera of patients with atopic dermatitis and positive peanut challenge. J Allergy Clin Immunol 1992;90:962–969.

63. Burks AW, Cockrell G, Connaughton C, Guin J, Allen W, Helm RM. Identification of peanut agglutinin and soybean trypsin inhibitor as minor legume allergens. Int Arch Allergy Immunol 1994;105:143–149.

64. Naismith WEF. Ultracentrifuge studies on soya bean protein. Biochim Biophys Acta 1955;16:203–210.

65. Shibasaki M, Suzuki S, Tajima S, Nemoto H, Kuroume T. Allergenicity of major component proteins of soybeans. Int Arch Allergy Appl Immunol 1980;61:441–448.

66. Murphy PA. Structural characteristics of soybean glycinin and

beta-conglycinin. In: Shibles RA, ed. World soybean research conference III proceedings. Boulder, CO: Westview Press, 1985, 143–151.

67. Koshiyama I, Fukushima D. Identification of the 7S globulin with beta-conglycinin in soybean seeds. Phytochem 1976;15:157–160.

68. Shattuck-Eidens DN, Beachy RN. Degradation of beta-conglycinin in early stages of soybean embryogenesis. Plant Physiol 1985;78:895–898.

69. Brooks JR, Morr CV. Current aspects of soy protein fractionation and nomenclature. J Am Oil Chem Soc 1985;62:1347–1354.

70. Moreira MA, Hermodson MA, Larkins BA, Nielsen NC. Comparison of the primary structure of the acidic polypeptides of glycinin. Arch Biochem Biophys 1981;210:633–642.

71. Nielsen NC. Structure of soy proteins. In: Altschul AM, Wilcke HL, eds. New protein foods, vol. 5. Orlando: Academic Press, 1985, 27–64.

72. Ogawa T, Bando N, Tsuji H, Okajima H, Nishikawa K, Sasaoka K. Investigation of the IgE-binding proteins in soybeans by immunoblotting with the sera of the soybean-sensitive patients with atopic dermatitis. J Nutr Sci Vitamin 1991;37:555–565.

73. Burks AW, Brooks JR, Sampson HA. Allergenicity of major component proteins of soybean determined by enzyme-linked immunosorbent assay (ELISA) and immunoblotting in children with atopic dermatitis and positive soy challenges. J Allergy Clin Immunol 1988;81:1135–1142.

74. Moroz LA, Yang WH. Kunitz soybean trypsin-inhibitor: a specific allergen in food anaphylaxis. N Engl J Med 1980;302:1126–1128.

75. Bush RK, Taylor SL, Nordlee JA, Busse WW. Soybean oil is not allergenic to soybean-sensitive individuals. J Allergy Clin Immunol 1985;76:242–245.

76. Bush RK, Schroeckenstein D, Meier-Davis S, Balmes J, Rempel D. Soybean flour asthma: detection of allergens by immunoblotting. J Allergy Clin Immunol 1988;82:251–255.

77. Lavaud F, Perdu D, Prevost A, Vallerand H, Cossart C, Passemard F. Baker's asthma related to soybean lecithin exposure. Allergy 1994;49:159–162.

78. Gonzalez R, Polo F, Zaperto L, Caravaca F, Carreira J. Purification and characterization of major inhalant allergens from soybean hulls. Clin Exp Allergy 1992;22:748–755.

79. Baldo BA, Sutton R, Wrigley CW. Grass allergens, with particular reference to cereals. Progr Allergy 1982;30:1–66.

80. Blands J, Diamant B, Kallos P, Kallos-Deffner L, Løwenstein H. Flour allergy in bakers. I. Identification of allergenic fractions in flour and comparison of diagnostic methods. Int Arch Allergy Appl Immunol 1976;52:392–406.

81. Baldo BA, Wrigley CW. IgE antibodies to wheat flour components. Studies with sera from subjects with bakers' asthma or coeliac condition. Clin Allergy 1978;8:109–124.

82. Sutton R, Skerritt JH, Baldo BA, Wrigley CW. The diversity of allergens involved in bakers' asthma. Clin Allergy 1984;14:93–107.

83. Walsh BJ, Wrigley CW, Musk AW, Baldo BA. A comparison of the binding of IgE in the sera of patients with bakers' asthma to soluble and insoluble wheat-grain proteins. J Allergy Clin Immunol 1985;76:23–28.

84. Kanny G, Moneret-Vautrin D-A. Alpha amylase contained in bread can induce food allergy. J Allergy Clin Immunol 1995;95:132–133.

85. Gómez L, Martin E, Hernández D, Sánchez-Monge R, Barber D, del Pozo V, de Andrés B, Armentia A, Lahoz C, Salcedo G, Palomino P. Members of the alpha-amylase inhibitors family from wheat endosperm are major allergens associated with baker's asthma. FEBS Letters 1990;261:85–88.

86. Barber D, Sánchez-Monge R, Gómez L, Carpizo J, Armentia A, Lopez-Otin C, Juan F, Salcedo G. A barley flour inhibitor of insect alpha-amylase is a major allergen associated with baker's asthma disease. FEBS Letters 1989;248:119–122.

87. Sánchez-Monge R, Gómez L, Barber D, Lopez-Otin C, Armentia A, Salcedo G. Wheat and barley allergens associated with baker's asthma. Glycosylated subunits of the alpha-amylase-inhibitor family have enhanced IgE-binding capacity. Biochem J 1992;281:401–405.

88. Armentia A, Sánchez-Monge R, Gómez L, Barber D, Salcedo G. In vivo allergenic activities of eleven purified members of a major allergen family from wheat and barley flour. Clin Exp Allergy 1993;23:410–415.

89. Franken J, Stephan U, Meyer HE, Konig W. Identification of alpha-amylase inhibitor as a major allergen of wheat flour. Int Arch Allergy Immunol 1994;104:171–174.

90. Sandiford CP, Tee RD, Taylor AJ. The role of cereal and fungal amylases in cereal flour hypersensitivity. Clin Exp Allergy 1994;24:549–557.

91. Garcia-Casado G, Armentia A, Sánchez-Monge R, Sanchez LM, Lopez-Otin C, Salcedo G. A major baker's asthma allergen from rye flour is considerably more active than its barley counterpart. FEBS Letters 1995;364:36–40.

92. Tanaka K, Sugimoto T, Ogawa M, Kasai Z. Isolation and characterization of two types of protein bodies in the rice endosperm. Agric Biol Chem 1980;44:1633–1639.

93. Shibasaki M, Suzuki S, Nemoto H, Kuroume T. Allergenicity and lymphocyte-stimulating property of rice protein. J Allergy Clin Immunol 1979;64:259–265.

94. Matsuda T, Sugiyama M, Nakamura R, Torii S. Purification and properties of an allergenic protein in rice grain. Agric Biol Chem 1988;52:1465–1470.

95. Urisu A, Yamada K, Masuda S, Komada H, Wada E, Kondo Y, Horiba F, Tsuruta M, Yasaki T, Yamada M, Torii S, Nakamura R. 16-kilodalton rice protein is one of the major allergens in rice grain extract and responsible for the cross-allergenicity between cereal grains in the Poaceae family. Int Arch Allergy Appl Immunol 1991;96:244–252.

96. Izumi H, Adachi T, Fujii N, Matsuda T, Nakamura R, Tanaka K, Urisu A, Kurosawa Y. Nucleotide sequence of a cDNA clone encoding a major allergenic protein in rice seeds. Homology of the deduced amino acid sequence with members of α-amylase/trypsin inhibitor family. FEBS Letters 1992;302:213–216.

97. Ory RL, Sekul AA. Allergens in oilseeds. In: Daussant J, Mosse J, Vaughan J, eds. Seed proteins. London: Academic Press, 1983, 83–99.

98. Youle RJ, Huang AHC. Albumin storage protein and allergens in cottonseeds. J Agric Food Chem 1979;27:500–503.

99. Lusas EW, Jividen GM. Characteristics and uses of glandless cottonseed food protein ingredients. J Am Oil Chem Soc 1987;64:973–986.

100. Lusas EW, Jividen GM. Glandless cottonseed: a review of the first 25 years of processing and utilization research. J Am Oil Chem Soc 1987;64:839–854.

101. Clark SP, Baker GW, Matlock SW, Mulsow D. Cottonseed flour production: economic evaluation. J Am Oil Chem Soc 1978;55:690–694.

102. Berrens L. The chemistry of atopic allergens. In: Kallos P, Hasek M, Inderbitzin TM, Miescher PA, Waksman BH, eds. Monogr Allergy, vol. 7. Basel: S. Karger, 1971, 1–298.

103. Spies JR, Chambers DC, Coulson EJ, Bernton HS, Stevens H. The chemistry of allergens. XII. Protolysis of the cottonseed allergen. J Allergy 1953;24:483–491.

104. Bleumink E, Berrens L, Young E. Studies on the atopic allergen in ripe tomato fruits. I. Isolation and identification of the allergen. Int Arch Allergy Appl Immunol 1966;30:132–145.

105. Bleumink E, Berrens L, Young E. Studies on the atopic allergen in ripe tomato fruits. II. Further chemical characterization of the purified allergen. Int Arch Allergy Appl Immunol 1967;31:25–37.

106. Malish D, Glovsky MM, Hoffman DR, Ghekiere L, Hawkins JM. Anaphylaxis after sesame seed ingestion. J Allergy Clin Immunol 1981;67:35–38.

107. Blaiss MS, McCants ML, Lehrer SB. Anaphylaxis to cabbage: detection of allergens. Ann Allergy 1987;58:248–250.

108. Menéndez-Arias L, Moneo I, Dominguez J, Rodríguez R. Primary structure of the major allergen of yellow mustard (*Sinapis alba* L.) seed, *Sin a* I. Eur J Biochem 1988;177:159–166.

109. González de la Peña MA, Villalba M, García-López JL, Rodríguez R. Cloning and expression of the major allergen from yellow mustard seeds, *Sin a* I. Biochem Biophys Res Comm 1993;190:648–653.

110. González de la Peña MA, Menéndez-Arias L, Monsalve RI, Rodríguez R. Isolation and characterization of a major allergen from oriental mustard seeds, *Bra j* I. Int Arch Allergy Appl Immunol 1991;96:263–270.

111. Monsalve RI, González de la Peña MA, Menéndez-Arias L, Lopez-Otin C, Villalba M, Rodríguez R. Characterization of a new oriental mustard (*Brassica juncea*) allergen, *Bra j* IE: detection of an allergenic epitope. Biochem J 1993;293:625–632.

112. Sheldon JM, Lovell RG, Mathews KP. A manual of clinical allergy, 2nd ed. Philadelphia: W.B. Saunders, 1967, 1–550.

113. Anderson LB Jr, Dreyfuss EM, Logan J, Johnstone DE, Glaser J. Melon and banana sensitivity coincident with ragweed pollinosis. J Allergy 1970;45:310–319.

114. Pauli G, Bessot JC, Dietemann-Molard A, Braun PA, Thierry R. Celery sensitivity: clinical and immunological correlations with pollen allergy. Clin Allergy 1985;15:273–279.

115. Aalberse RC, Koshte V, Clemens JGJ. Immunoglobulin E antibodies that cross react with vegetable foods, pollen, and Hymenoptera venom. J Allergy Clin Immunol 1981;68:356–364.

116. Lahti A, Bjorksten F, Hannuksela M. Allergy to birch pollen and apple, and cross-reactivity of the allergens studied with the RAST. Allergy 1980;35:297–300.

117. Rodriguez M, Vega F, Garcia MT, Panizo C, Laffond E, Montalvo A, Cuevas M. Hypersensitivity to latex, chestnut, and banana. Ann Allergy 1993;70:31–34.

118. Fernandez de Corres L, Moneo I, Munoz D, Bernola G, Fernandez E, Audicana M, Urrutia I. Sensitization from chestnuts and bananas in patients with urticaria and anaphylaxis from contact with latex. Ann Allergy 1993;70:35–39.

119. Lavaud F, Prevost A, Cossart C, Guerin L, Bernard J, Kochman S. Allergy to latex, avocado pear, and banana: evidence for a 30 kD antigen in immunoblotting. J Allergy Clin Immunol 1995;95:557–564.

120. Stinzi A, Heitz T, Prasad V, Wiedemann-Merdinoglu S, Kauffmann S, Geoffroy P, Legrand M, Fritig B. Plant "pathogenesis related" proteins and their role in defense against pathogens. Biochimie 1993;75:687–706.

121. Scheiner O. Recombinant allergens: biological, immunological, and practical aspects. Int Arch Allergy Immunol 1992;98:93–96.

122. Pauli G, Oster JP, Deviller P, Bessot JC, Heiss S, Ferreira F, Kraft D, Valenta R. Skin testing with recombinant birch allergens rBet V1 and rBet V2: Diagnostic value for birch pollen and associated allergies. J Allergy Clin Immunol 1995;95:318 (abst).

123. Ebner C, Hirschwehr R, Bauer L, Breiteneder H, Valenta R, Ebner H, Kraft D, Scheiner O. Identification of allergens in fruits and vegetables: IgE cross-reactivities with the important birch pollen allergens Bet v 1 and Bet v 2 (birch profilin). J Allergy Clin Immunol 1995;95:962–969.

124. Valenta R, Duchene M, Pettenburger K, Silaber C, Valent P, Bettelheim P, Breitenbach M, Rumpold H, Kraft D, Scheiner O. Identification of profilin as a novel pollen allergen; IgE autoreactivity in sensitized individuals. Science 1991;253:557–560.

125. Vallier P, Dechamp C, Valenta R, Vial O, Deviller P. Purification and characterization of an allergen from celery immunochemically related to an allergen present in several other plant species. Identification as a profilin. Clin Exp Allergy 1992;22:774–782.

126. Van Ree R, Voitenko V, Van Leeuwen WA, Aalberse RC. Profilin is a cross-reactive allergen in pollen and vegetable foods. Int Arch Allergy Immunol 1992;98:97–104.

127. Rihs HP, Rozynek P, May-Taube K, Welticke B, Baur X. Polymerase chain reaction based cDNA cloning of wheat profilin: a potential plant allergen. Int Arch Allergy Immunol 1994;105:190–194.

128. Valenta R, Duchene M, Ebner C, Valent P, Sillaber C, Deviller P, Ferreira F, Tejkl M, Edelman H, Kraft D, Scheiner O. Profilins constitute a novel family of functional plant pan-allergens. J Exp Med 1992;175:377–385.

129. Vallier P, Balland S, Harf R, Valenta R, Deviller P. Identification of profilin as an IgE-binding component in latex from Hevea brasiliensis—clinical implications. Clin Exp Allergy 1995;25:332–339.

FOOD BIOTECHNOLOGY AND GENETIC ENGINEERING

James D. Astwood
Roy L. Fuchs
Paul B. Lavrik

Introduction

Food biotechnology and genetic engineering should have little practical consequence for the occurrence, frequency, and natural history of food allergy if simple precautions are observed. This chapter outlines the critical technological aspects of agricultural biotechnology. Genetic engineering offers several advantages over other technologies, including the precision with which modifications are made and the predictability of their consequences. Essential aspects of health safety assessment for products derived from this technology will be discussed, and the accepted strategy for addressing any potential impact on food allergy will be detailed. No single, predictive assay appears to assess the allergenic potential of specific proteins introduced into food crops (1). Using in vivo and in vitro immunological assays and comparing the amino acid sequence and important physicochemical and biological properties of proteins introduced via biotechnology with the sequence and properties of known allergens provide a sound scientific basis for an allergenicity assessment, however. The physicochemical characteristics of common food allergens have been described in this book and elsewhere (2–4): allergens tend to be stable to proteolysis, may be glycosylated, tend to be abundant, and tend to be resistant to heat (cooking or processing). Thus, these factors could possibly be used to discriminate between potentially harmful allergens and safe proteins entering the food supply.

Plant Biotechnology

The origins of modern agriculture are unknown, but cultivation of many crops has clearly been ongoing in Europe for at least 6000 years (and probably much longer in western and central Asia), where at least three species of barley, five species of wheat, several species of millets, and flax were grown contemporaneously in the area that constitutes present-day Switzerland (5). The need to increase food production in the face of ever-expanding populations has long been understood. In 1942, Karl Klages, Professor of Agronomy at the University of Idaho, estimated that if the world's population reached 5.2 billion, all of the planet's then-available arable land would need to be in production (13 billion acres) (6). Klages could not know that six years and only five miles away Orville Vogel, working at Washington State University, would introduce high-yielding semi-dwarf wheats developed in Japan that would precipitate the so-called green revolution of the 1950s and 1960s (7). The world's population now exceeds 5.2 billion people, who are sustained on far less than 13 billion acres of arable land. Indeed, it is anticipated that the world's population could reach 11.6 billion before leveling off in 2150 (8).

Modern agriculture has brought many disciplines to bear on the challenge of developing improved and higher-yielding food crop varieties: agronomy, botany, physiology, statistics, breeding and genetics, entomology, weed science, biochemistry, and, most recently, biotechnology. It is critical that agricultural advances continue for the foreseeable future. At the same time, it is imperative to manage agricultural resources appropriately so as to prevent or ameliorate the negative effects of increasing population (9).

Biotechnology is best conceived as a flavor of plant breeding. Plant breeding is itself defined as an activity that seeks to improve the heredity of plants (7). Of course, biotechnology also affords more than a simple increase in agricultural productivity—opportunities to develop more sustainable production practices (10), safer and healthier foods (11, 12), biopharmaceuticals (13), and bio-industrial commodities (14) are now being realized (15–17).

Direct and stable gene transfer into plants was first reported in 1984 (18, 19). Since then, at least 88 different plant species and many economically important crops have been genetically engineered (20) (Table 4.1), usually via *Agrobacterium* (21, 22a) or particle gun technologies (22b). The variety of traits being introduced into crops is impressive, and includes insect protection, delayed ripening, virus resistance, modified starch, herbicide tolerance, modified oils, disease resistance, and male sterility. Most traits introduced into crops result from the expression of one or more new proteins. These proteins are typically expressed at low levels and usually represent a minor percentage of the total plant protein. Several genetically engineered plant products have been commercialized to date, and many others will arrive in the marketplace in the near future (Table 4.2) (15).

None of the first-generation plant biotechnology products has resulted in direct productivity enhancements (e.g., higher yield). Instead, these products confer protection from pests, herbicides, pathogens, or other environmental insults, thereby indirectly enhancing crop productivity under these adverse conditions. For example, genetically engineered resistance to Colorado potato beetle can provide dramatic indirect yield benefits for NewLeaf[1] potatoes (23). Other

[1] New Leaf is a trademark of Monsanto Company, St. Louis, Mo.

Table 4.1
Plants That Have Been Modified Using Genetic Engineering Techniques

Alfalfa	Flax	Petunia
Allocasuarina verticillata	Foxglove	Plum
Anagallis arvensis	Geranium	Poplar
Apple	Grape	Poppy
Apricot	Horseradish	Potato
Arabidopsis thaliana	Kiwi	Raspberry
Asparagus	Lettuce	Rice
Aspen	Lemon	Rose
Atropa belladonna	Licorice	Rye
Barley	Lily	Snap dragon
Black currant	Lotus	*Solanum dulcamara*
Brassica carinata	Maize	*Solanum muricatum*
Brassica juncea	*Medicago trunculata*	Sorghum
Broccoli	Morning glory	Soybean
Brown sarson	Muskmelon	Spruce
Buckwheat	*Nicotiana bigelovii*	Strawberry
Cabbage	*Nicotiana clevlandii*	*Stylosanthes humilis*
Canola	*Nicotiana glauca*	Sugarbeet
Carnation	*Nicotiana hesperis*	Sugar cane
Carrot	*Nicotiana plumbaginifolia*	Sunflower
Cauliflower	*Nicotiana rustica*	Sweet potato
Celery	Nightshade	Tobacco
Chicory	Oats	Tomato
Chrysanthemum	Oilseed rape	Tulip
Cotton	*Onobrychis viciifolia*	Walnut
Cranberry	Orange	Wheat
Cucumber orchid	Orchardgrass	White clover
Eggplant	Papaya	Yam
European larch	Pea	
Fennel	Peach	

Table 4.2
Transgenic Plants in or Nearing the Marketplace

Genetic Trait	Crop	Primary Introduced Gene	Company
Delayed ripening fruit	Tomato	antisense PG	Calgene
	Tomato	ACC deaminase	Monsanto
	Tomato	antisense PG	Zeneca
	Tomato	antisense ACC synthase	DNA Plant Technology
Insect resistance	Potato	*cryIIIA*	Monsanto
	Cotton	*cryIA(c)*	Monsanto
	Corn	*cryIA(b)*	Monsanto Virgale Ciba-Geigy/
	Corn	*cryIA(b)*	Mycogen/Northrup King
Virus resistance	Squash	Viral coat proteins	Asgrow Seed
	Tobacco	Viral coat protein	China
Herbicide tolerance	Cotton	BXN nitrilase	Calgene
	Cotton	CP4 EPSPS	Monsanto
	Soybean	CP4 EPSPS	Monsanto
	Flax	Acetolactate synthase	University of Saskatchewan
	Corn	Basta tolerance	AgroEvo
	Canola	Basta tolerance	AgroEvo
	Canola	CP4 EPSPS/GOX	Monsanto
Male sterility	Canola	Barnase/Barstar	Plant Genetic Systems
Starch quality	Potato	antisense GB-SS	AVEBE
Oil quality modification	Canola	Thioesterase	Calgene

ACC = 1-amino-1cyclopropane-carboxylic acid.
BXN = Bromoxonyl.
CP4 EPSPS = 5-enolpyruvylshikimate-3-phosphate synthase from *Agrobacterium* sp. strain CP4.
GOX = Glyphosate oxidoreductase.
GB-SS = Granule bound starch synthase.
PG = Polygalacturonase.

approaches improve handling and taste characteristics, which in turn improves market distribution and reduces waste (e.g., FlavrSavr[2] tomato) (24). By using insect-protected crops developed through genetic engineering, the farmer no longer needs to apply expensive and environmentally unfavorable chemical pesticides. Crops that resist disease [e.g., virus-resistant squash (25, 26)], are adaptable to new crop rotation production practices [e.g., sulfonylurea-tolerant flax (10)], or are amenable to new production practices [e.g., Roundup[3]-tolerant crops (27)] also improve production efficiency.

Below we describe the development of the Colorado beetle-protected NewLeaf potato to illustrate the application of agricultural biotechnology. We then briefly summarize the food safety assessment of this product to illustrate the approaches used to ensure the safety of foods derived from genetically engi-

neered food crops. One of the key components of safety assessment is the evaluation of any allergenic concerns raised by the introduction of new proteins into the food supply. This chapter describes in detail an accepted approach to assess the allergenic potential of foods derived from any genetically engineered plant, with an in-depth examination of the allergenic potential assessment for the two proteins introduced into the NewLeaf potato.

NewLeaf Potato—A Case Study

Potato (*Solanum tuberosum* L.) ranks fourth in world production of major crops after wheat, maize, and rice (28). In the United States, potatoes represent $2.3 billion in farm gate receipts (29). Colorado potato beetle (*Leptinotarsa decemlineata*) can significantly lower yield unless expensive insecticides are used, and is considered to be the most damaging

[2]FlavrSavr is a trademark of Calgene Inc., Davis, CA.
[3]Roundup is a registered trademark of Monsanto Company, St. Louis, Mo.

potato pest (30–32). Without the use of pesticides, Colorado potato beetle (CPB) is capable of defoliating the potato plant, reducing yield by as much as 85%, and effectively excluding potato production in some geographies (33, 34). Even the use of insecticides can prove ineffective against this pest (35). To obviate the need for pesticide application, a gene *(cryIIIA)* encoding a parasporal crystal protein from *Bacillus thuringiensis* (a soil-borne bacterium), which effectively controls coleropteran pests, has been genetically engineered into potato to confer host plant protection against damage by CPB (23).

Many *cry* genes encoding insecticidal crystal proteins are found in *Bacillus,* all having different spectrums of insecticidal activity (36). To be effective against the target insect, the CryIIIA protein must be ingested where it binds to specific midgut receptors. At that location the CryIIIA protein inserts into the membrane of the midgut epithelial cells of the insect to create an ion channel that ultimately leads to cell lysis and mortality (37, 38). The specificity of Cry proteins is determined by membrane receptors present only in target insects (39). These receptors are not present in nontarget insects or on mammalian cells (39, 40), thereby defining the strict specificity and explaining the exquisite and long-established safety of the Cry proteins (36, 41, 42).

To genetically engineer the *cryIIIA* gene into plants, transformation of the *cryIIIA* gene was performed using well-established *Agrobacterium tumafaciens* transformation techniques (Fig. 4.1) (43). Using a binary vector system, genetically engineered potato plants were developed that express CryIIIA protein and the neomycin phosphotransferase (NPTII) selectable marker, which confers kanamycin resistance (Fig. 4.2A) (23). Selectable markers are required during plant regeneration. One interesting feature of the *cryIIIA* and *nptII* genes is both are prokaryotic genes. The *nptII* gene was originally isolated from the Tn5 transposon (44), and has subsequently been employed as a selectable marker in a large number of genetically engineered plants (45, 46). To obtain expression of these genes in plants, which are eukaryotes, special eukaryotic-compatible promoters from the cauliflower mosaic virus 35S RNA gene (47) were engineered into the vector to drive the expression of these genes (see Fig. 4.2A). The nucleotide sequence of the *cryIIIA* gene was also modified (without changing the amino acid sequence) to further optimize expression of the CryIIIA protein in plant cells (48).

BENEFITS OF NEWLEAF POTATOES

The resulting NewLeaf potatoes have proved very resistant to damage caused by CPB (Figs. 4.2B and 4C). Host plant resistance to CPB provides significant benefits beyond the direct economic advantage available to growers. By reducing reliance on chemical insecticides, overall exposure of farm workers and the environment to agrichemicals is reduced. A wide range of chemical agents have been used to control CPB, including carbamates, pyrethroids, and organo-

Figure 4.1

Agrobacterium-mediated plant transformation using a binary vector. To genetically engineer a desired trait into plants, a system based on the plant tumor-inducing (Ti) plasmids of *Agrobacterium tumafaciens* may be used. *Agrobacterium* has the remarkable ability to transfer, insert, and express a specific segment of DNA in the plant genome (21, 22). The gene conferring the desired trait is first subcloned (#1) into the TDNA (transfer-DNA) of a nonvirulent "disarmed" Ti plasmid vector using standard recombinant DNA techniques. The TDNA region is flanked by borders (B) that define the excision/insertion points of the TDNA on the Ti plasmid (188). The disarmed vector plasmid harbors origins of replication for propagation in both *E. coli* and *Agrobacterium* and selectable makers for bacterial (Spec) and plant cells (Kan). It is transformed (#2) into an *Agrobacterium* strain that already contains a second, nonvirulent "helper" plasmid (H). During *Agrobacterium* infection (#3) of the target plant cells, the virulence genes (189) and genes responsible for mobilization of the TDNA contained on the helper vector (H) allow transfer (#4) and ultimate integration of the TDNA region of the vector plasmid (#5), which includes the desired trait and the plant selectable marker (Kan). After plant tissue culture and appropriate selection with kanamycin (#6), mature transgenic plants are obtained.

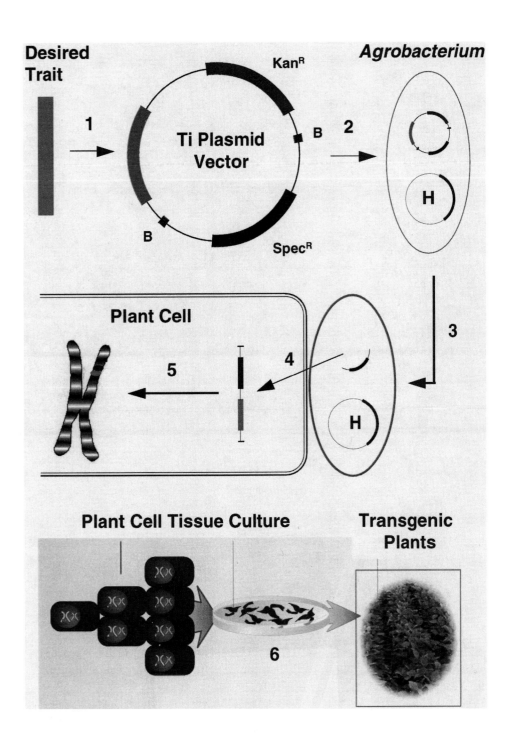

Desired Trait

Ti Plasmid Vector

Kan^R

B

B

Spec^R

1

2

Agrobacterium

H

3

Plant Cell

5

4

H

Plant Cell Tissue Culture

Transgenic Plants

6

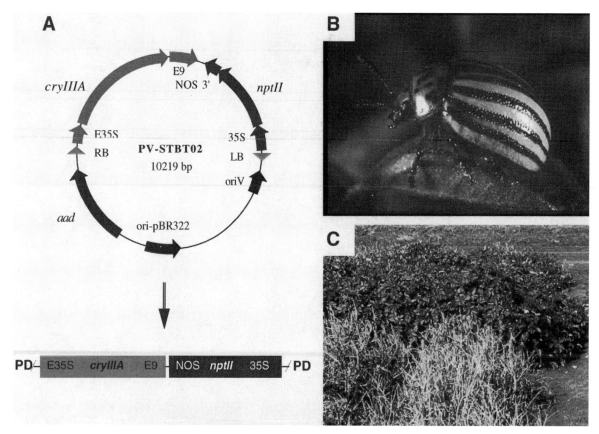

Figure 4.2

Genetic engineering of NewLeaf potatoes. (A) *Agrobacterium* Ti plasmid vector PV-STBT02 was used to transform Russet Burbank potatoes. The Ti plasmid and the genes carried by the TDNA integrated into the potato genome are illustrated. The *aad* gene encodes selectable marker conferring spectinomycin/streptomycin resistance expressed only in bacterial cells. The *nptII* gene uses the 35S promoter (35S) and a transcription terminator (NOS 3') to express neomycin phospho-transferase (kanamycin resistance) in plant cells. The *cryIIIA* gene uses the enhanced 35S promoter (E35S) and a transcription terminator sequence (E9) to express CryIIIA protein in potato cells. *Ori-pBR322* and *oriV* are *E. coli* and *Agrobacterium* origins of replication, respectively. PD marks the site of TDNA integration into potato DNA. (B) Colorado potato beetle *(Leptinotarsa decemlineata)* foraging on a potato leaf. (C) Russet Burbank (foreground) and NewLeaf (background) potato plants infested with Colorado potato beetle. NewLeaf potatoes are unaffected by the pest.

phosphates (32, 49). Both carbamates and organophosphates are toxic via dermal and oral routes of exposure. In farm use, the application of these compounds necessarily requires special work practices that, while effective, do not eliminate the potential for accidental exposure. Shipping, storage, mixing, loading, spraying, and disposal processes can all lead to mishap when handling these chemicals (50). By replacing their use with NewLeaf potatoes, agricul-

tural practices are made considerably safer for humans, animals, and the environment.

NewLeaf potatoes provide obvious benefits for the environment. Potatoes are grown in coarse soils that rely on heavy irrigation or rainfall to ensure good growing conditions and plant performance. In the past, potato fields have often represented a significant source of agrichemical pollution, especially by field run-off that may eventually enter the groundwater supply (51, 52). NewLeaf potatoes do not pose a similar risk because they reduce or eliminate use of chemical pesticides. In addition, the specificity of the CryIIIA protein enables the preservation and multiplication of beneficial insect populations. Broad-spectrum insecticides have a destructive impact on beneficial arthropod populations and can lead to a resurgence of secondary pests (53), whereas the use of NewLeaf potatoes can significantly increase the populations of natural enemies of pests like aphids (54). This enhanced control of other potato pests can lead to even further reductions in chemical pesticide use.

SAFETY ASSESSMENT OF NEWLEAF POTATOES

Safety of the CryIIIA Protein

The Cry or *Bacillus thuringiensis* proteins have a long history of safe use—spanning more than 30 years—as the active ingredients in microbial formulations (36, 41). The CryIIIA protein expressed in NewLeaf potato tubers is, in fact, identical to one of the proteins contained in commercial microbial formulations used since 1988 (29). These proteins have comparable insecticidal activities and insect specificities, with both showing stringent selectivity for CPB. In addition, both proteins share similar molecular weights and show similar immuno-reactivities. These data were used to establish that the CryIIIA protein produced in potato tubers of the NewLeaf is equivalent to the CryIIIA protein in commercial microbial products (29). Therefore, the extensive safety database developed for commercial microbial products corroborated the safety of this protein as expressed in potato tubers.

Because NewLeaf was one of the first genetically engineered products introduced into commerce, many of the studies performed with microbial products were repeated for CryIIIA and NPTII to provide additional safety assurance. The limited expression of CryIIIA in NewLeaf potato tubers ruled out the isolation of large quantities of the plant-expressed protein. Therefore, gram quantities of purified CryIIIA protein were obtained by expressing this protein in *Escherichia coli*, and safety studies were then performed with the *E. coli*-expressed protein. Minor quantities

of CryIIIA protein were purified from the potato tuber; this protein was shown to be chemically and functionally equivalent to the CryIIIA protein produced in *E. coli* (29). This equivalence assessment relied on a series of commonly used analytical assays, including establishing comparable insecticidal activities, molecular weights, immuno-reactivities, N-terminal amino acid sequences, and lack of post-translation modification.

An acute gavage study was conducted in mice with the *E. coli*-derived CryIIIA protein that confirmed its safety (29). Acute gavage studies were considered most appropriate as proteins known to be toxic act via acute mechanisms (55–57). Following EPA guidelines, a dose was used that was equivalent to more than a 2.5 million-fold safety factor, based on the average consumption of potato and the level of the CryIIIA protein present in the tuber. No adverse effects were observed in terms of food consumption, weight gain, mortality, or gross necropsy. Purified protein was also used in an in vitro digestion experiment (59) that demonstrated that the CryIIIA protein has an extremely short half-life under simulated gastric conditions (30). These studies confirmed the safety of the CryIIIA protein for human consumption.

Safety of the NPTII Protein

The second protein introduced into NewLeaf potatoes comprised the selectable marker NPTII. The NPTII protein has also been shown to present no food safety concern, as it is ubiquitous in bacteria normally contained within the human gastrointestinal tract (45, 59–62). The description and safety assessment of the NPTII protein has been discussed in detail in an FDA "processing aid food additive approval" of this protein for use in genetically engineered tomato, cotton, and canola products (63). The Environmental Protection Agency (EPA) also issued an "exemption from the requirement of a tolerance" for NPTII for use as a selectable marker, when accompanying a pesticidal trait (such as the CryIIIA protein) (64). No adverse effects were observed in the acute gavage study, which involved a greater than a 5 million-fold safety factor compared with projected consumption (61). The NPTII protein was rapidly degraded under simulated digestive conditions (61). Both studies con-

Table 4.3
Summary of Composition of NewLeaf and Russet Burbank Potatoes

| Component | NewLeaf | | Russet Burbank (66) | | Published (67) |
	Mean	Range	Mean	Range	Range
Solids (% tuber fresh weight)	19.6	18.0–21.0	20.0	19.6–20.5	16.8–24.5 [2]
Carbohydrate (g/100 g tuber)	16.0	15.4–16.5	16.0	15.7–16.4	13–17 [3]
Protein (g/100 g tuber)	2.1	2.1–2.2	2.1	2.0–2.1	1.4–2.9 [3]
Vitamin C (mg/100 g tuber)	11.4	8.7–13.6	11.6	11.0–12.3	10.3–22.0 [2]
Vitamin B_6 (μg/100 g tuber)	97.2	75.4–119	97.2	89.2–105	140–280 [3]
Folic acid (μg/100 g tuber)	6.7	5.7–7.7	7.0	5.2–8.7	4.0–20 [3]
Potassium (mg/100 g tuber)	420	388–453	416	393–438	340–600 [3]
Glycoalkaloids (mg/100 g tuber)	3.8	2.7–5.8	3.1	2.7–3.5	3.1–16.1 [2]

Values for NewLeaf and Russet Burbank are the means of tubers obtained from seven CPB-protected or parental Russet Burbank control lines grown at two field locations. At each field location, plots for each CPB-protected line were replicated six times.

firmed the mammalian safety of this protein. A report from a workshop sponsored by the World Health Organization (WHO) also supported the safety of the NPTII protein as used in genetically modified plants (46).

Wholesomeness of NewLeaf Potatoes

Potato has long been valued as an excellent source of staple starch and contributes mainly to the carbohydrate calories in the diet. Some vitamins (e.g., vitamin C and vitamin B_6) and potassium also add to potato tubers' nutritional value. Tubers from NewLeaf potato were compared with tubers from Russet Burbank potato, which was the parental variety from which NewLeaf potato was derived, and is also the dominant commercial variety in today's marketplace. Additional components were measured, with 23 variables included, as summarized in Table 4.3. The levels of these components were comparable in NewLeaf and the Russet Burbank control and were well within the ranges reported previously for Russet Burbank (29). These data established that NewLeaf potatoes are as nutritious and wholesome as traditional varieties. In addition to establishing that NewLeaf potatoes are

compositionally and nutritionally equivalent to Russet Burbank potatoes and that the CryIIIA and NPTII proteins lack any toxicological concerns, studies also showed that these potatoes pose no significant allergenic concerns for human consumption. The remainder of this chapter focuses on describing the scientific basis for an allergenicity assessment of the food products resulting from plant biotechnology.

Assessment Strategy for Food Allergy

Plant tissues can express as many as 100,000 discrete proteins. Yet, despite this large variety, allergy to food proteins is uncommon—affecting perhaps 5% of infants and as many as 2% of adults (65–67). Nevertheless, a growing body of evidence suggests that allergic disorders are increasing in prevalence and severity (68). This trend may be due to increased exposure to allergens and early-life exposure to adjuvants such as air pollution (69, 70). Interestingly, only a small number of foods or food groups (peanuts, soybeans, tree nuts, milk, eggs, fish, crustacea, molluscs, and wheat) account for more than 90% of food allergies (4). The majority of allergy sufferers exhibit immunoglobulin E (IgE)-mediated immediate hypersensitivity (71, 72). An individual's genetics also plays an important role in defining individual propensity to allergy, although recent attempts to define an "atopy" gene have met with mixed success (73). Atopic responses may be associated with mutations in the β subunit of the high-affinity IgE receptor (74) or other regions of chromosome 11q (75). Serum IgE levels and bronchial hyperreactivity have also been linked to chromosome 5 (76, 77). A full understanding of the underlying genetics of allergy, a healthier environment, vigilance to minimizing accidental and unnecessary exposure to allergens, and (as described later in this chapter) the possibility of decreasing or eliminating allergen exposure could reverse the upward trend in allergy occurrence.

Preventing the accidental transfer of allergens into the food supply is a significant component in the safety assessment of foods derived from biotechnology products (78–81). Indeed, accidental exposure to food allergens can have unfortunate consequences (82, 83). Therefore, a sound science-based approach has been developed to ensure that potential concerns are adequately addressed before foods derived from genetically engineered food crops reach the market.

Clearly, not all plant biotechnology products are destined to enter the food supply. In some cases, only a specific fraction of an agricultural commodity (e.g., oil) may be consumed. Fractions that are devoid of protein are unlikely to pose any allergy concerns. For oils such as soybean, sunflower, or peanut, protein contamination is known to be rare (84), and these commodities appear to be safely consumed even by individuals allergic to soybean (85), sunflower (86), or peanut (87) when the oil is processed appropriately. Before genetically engineered forms of these products may be marketed, however, it should be confirmed that the oil commodities actually contain no protein, especially the introduced protein. A similar approach should be used for other commodities such as starch (e.g., pea, potato, or corn) or sugar (e.g., sugarcane or sugarbeet).

When proteins introduced into crops developed through genetic engineering will definitely enter the food supply, the assessment of allergenic potential should focus on the source from which the gene was obtained, amino acid sequence comparisons to known allergens, and physicochemical and biological comparisons of the introduced protein with allergens. Previous consumption information and potential changes in the endogenous allergens of the host plant (if present) should also be addressed. The totality of these assessments provides appropriate assurance that foods derived from genetically modified plants do not introduce allergenic concerns beyond those present in the current food supply.

ANALYZING THE SOURCES OF INTRODUCED GENES

The source of the introduced gene is the first variable to consider in the allergy assessment. If a gene transferred into a food crop is obtained from a source known to be allergenic, data should be generated to prove that the gene does not encode an allergen. The U.S. Food and Drug Administration (FDA) recognizes this need and realizes that such risks to consumers can be avoided (64). The use of labels that clearly indicate the presence of ingredients that may cause harmful effects, such as allergies, gives consumers the opportunity to avoid these foods or food ingredients. For example, to assist people who suffer from coeliac disease, the FDA has determined that products containing gluten should be identified as to the source—i.e., wheat versus corn gluten (wheat gluten cannot be safely consumed by these patients, unlike corn gluten). In the case of food allergy, voluntary labeling already occurs for certain snackfoods that do not ordinarily contain peanuts, but that may come into contact with peanuts during preparation. This type of labeling provides protection for peanut allergy sufferers and helps prevent accidental and unwanted exposure. The FDA has also stated that, if known allergens are genetically engineered into food crops, the resulting foods must be labeled to appropriately inform consumers, with the label disclosing the source of the introduced genes (63, 64). Moreover, proteins derived from known allergenic sources should be treated as allergens until demonstrated otherwise. The methodology to assess whether the transferred protein is allergenic is described below.

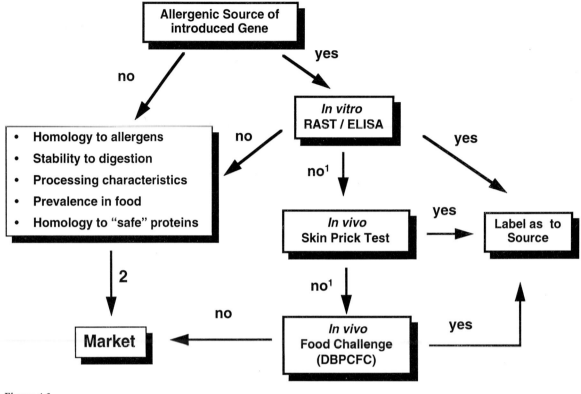

Figure 4.3

Assessment strategy for food developed through genetic engineering.
[1] Proceed to in vivo tests for genes that are obtained from common food allergy sources (peanuts, soybeans, tree nuts, milk, eggs, fish, crustacea, molluscs, and wheat).
[2] When considering further research or characteristics because one or more of the properties of the introduced protein is shared with food allergens, a consultation with a relevant regulatory agency is advised.

ALLERGENIC SOURCES OF GENES

The assessment of potential allergen transfer employs a decision tree approach (Fig. 4.3) in which each subsequent level of evaluation represents a greater degree of certainty that the source protein is *not* an allergen. The first level in the decision tree (Fig. 4.3, right side) for introduced genes from allergenic sources employs in vitro assays such as radioallergo-sorbent tests (RAST) (88, 89), enzyme-linked immunosorbent assays (ELISA) (90), or immunoblotting assays to detect the presence of allergens in the genetically modified plant or the purified gene product. These assays should use IgE fractions of serum from individuals who are actively sensitive (allergic) to the food from which the transferred gene was derived. Serum donors should meet clinically relevant criteria, which includes a convincing history (91) or positive responses in double-blind, placebo-controlled food challenges (DBPCFC) (88, 92). Data from one or more of these in vitro assays provide strong evidence of whether an allergen has been transferred. A clear positive result from the in vitro tests would require that any food including the transferred gene be labeled as containing a gene from that source.

If no differential response is observed during in vitro testing, then the protein should be assessed as though it was obtained from a nonallergenic source (Fig. 4.3, left side). For genes derived from commonly allergenic food sources such as those listed earlier (i.e., the foods responsible for 90% of food allergies), further experiments may be required to prove that the introduced protein does not encode an allergen. In vivo skin prick testing may be required for the proteins that test negative during in vitro testing and that are obtained from one of these commonly allergenic foods. Foods including proteins that test positive would also require labeling. Those proteins testing negative could then be assessed by DBPCFCs (88). Positive reactions in DBPCFCs would also mandate labeling.

The DBPCFC would involve testing with sensitive and nonsensitive patients under controlled clinical conditions. Patients who are known to be allergic to proteins from the source would be tested directly for hypersensitivity to food containing the protein encoded by the gene from the allergenic source. Food from the parental variety would be used as a negative control. The ethical considerations for this type of assessment would include, but not be limited to, factors such as likelihood of inducing anaphylactic shock in test subjects, potential value to test subjects, availability of appropriate safety precautions, and approval of local institutional review boards. If sensitive patients underwent a reaction in these tests, food derived from crops containing the protein would require labeling.

If no adverse reactions were observed in this decision-tree testing, it would be concluded that the gene obtained from the allergenic source did not encode one of the endogenous allergens. In such a case, the product would be marketed without labeling.

Brazil Nut 2S Albumin—A Case Study

One example illustrating the effectiveness of this decision-tree testing approach involves the discovery that a Brazil nut 2S albumin protein that had been engineered into soybean (93) and canola (94) encoded a major allergen of Brazil nut. The Brazil nut 2S albumin protein (a seed-specific protein) contains 18.8% of the essential amino acid methionine (95) and was initially perceived as an ideal candidate gene for enhancement of nutritional seed quality (96). Brazil nut is known to cause adverse reactions (97, 98), however, and would be described as an allergenic source of a gene. When genetically engineered into plants, the Brazil nut 2S albumin accumulation represented a significant fraction of total canola (94) and

soybean (93) seed protein. Subsequent RAST and immunoblot assays established that sera from eight of nine Brazil nut-allergic patients reacted to genetically modified soybeans containing the Brazil nut gene (99, 100). If marketed, this product must be labeled as containing a protein from Brazil nut so as to alert individuals allergic to Brazil nut. The incidence of Brazil nut allergy is currently quite small (98), presumably because few people are exposed to Brazil nuts. If the Brazil nut allergen were widely dispersed in a commodity such as soybeans, the incidence of Brazil nut allergy would likely increase. Therefore, it seems imprudent to market a product with this allergen unless significant modifications were made to the gene and resulting protein to eliminate allergenicity. At present, it is not obvious which molecular modifications would adequately resolve this problem. This example demonstrates the value and effectiveness of using in vitro assays to identify and prevent the accidental transfer of known allergens by genetic engineering.

In cases where suitable immunological reagents are not available for in vitro or in vivo testing, then the introduced protein should be assessed in the same manner as proteins from nonallergenic sources.

NONALLERGENIC SOURCES OF GENES

Two approaches may be taken to address the allergenicity of a protein prospectively. First, when a candidate gene is being considered for transfer into a plant, the gene is typically well characterized—that is, the DNA and amino acid sequences are known. As a starting point, a search for amino acid sequence homology of the introduced protein with known allergens should be performed for all genes, including those from allergenic sources.

Second, an analysis of the physicochemical properties of the introduced protein should be conducted. A key prerequisite for food protein allergenicity appears to be stability to the proteolytic and acid conditions of the human digestive system. The high concentrations of allergens in foods that cause allergy and the stability of allergens when faced with processing into specific food products are additional important factors contributing to the allergenicity of a protein. For example, soybean and peanut allergens retain their allergenic potential after the processing used in the preparation of food products such as peanut butter (4).

Amino Acid Sequence Comparisons to Known Allergens

The amino acid sequences of many allergens, including food allergens, have been reported (101), and the list continues to expand. Although many important T-cell, B-cell, and IgE binding epitopes of allergens have been mapped (102–115), the distinction between allergenic and nonallergenic epitopes remains unclear (116). The optimal peptide length for binding lies between 8 and 12 amino acids (117). T-cell epitopes of allergenic proteins and peptide fragments appear to be at least eight amino acids in length (117). In addition, exact conservation of epitope sequences is observed in homologous allergens of disparate species (110, 118, 119). Indeed, conservative substitutions introduced by site-directed mutagenesis can reduce epitope efficacy (120). The situation is more complex and less well defined for conformational epitopes (121), which means that sequence-based comparisons should be used only as indicators of potential linear epitopes.

While the molecular and structural requirements of allergenic epitopes have proved difficult to define, an immunologically relevant sequence comparison test for similarity between the amino acid sequence of the introduced protein and known allergens has been proposed. Under the test, a significant sequence similarity requires a match of at least eight contiguous identical amino acids (1). In the absence of specific epitope information, this test provides a conservative estimate of whether a theoretical possibility exists that the introduced protein shares an epitope with a known allergen.

The lack of any significant amino acid sequence homology leads to the conclusion that the introduced gene does not encode a known allergen or an evolutionarily related (homologous) protein; in addition, it can be concluded that the introduced gene does not encode an immunologically relevant epitope, as defined by the allergen database. In contrast, if significant amino acid sequence similarity is observed, the transferred protein may potentially be either an allergen or related to an allergen. The in vitro assays

described above for genes from allergenic sources should be used to determine whether the transferred protein conveys any immunologically significant cross-reactivity. In addition, the physicochemical properties of the transferred protein should be compared with those of known allergens as described below.

An important feature of the amino acid sequence analysis is retrieval of relevant allergen sequences from public domain databases such as GenBank, EMBL, PIR, and SwissProt. Two considerations should be taken into account: retrieval of as many relevant sequences as possible, and elimination of irrelevant and duplicated sequences.

The best approach is to retrieve the amino acid sequence data using appropriate keywords. For example, using "allergen" as a key word retrieves approximately 300 entries. More than 155 of these entries represent duplicates (the databases tend to accumulate repeated sequences submitted by independent laboratories or partial sequences that are subsequently resubmitted as full sequences) and irrelevant sequences, however.

On the other hand, using the keyword "allergen" retrieves IgE receptor genes like FcεR1α. This gene is important to allergy, but is not an allergen. When the list of 145 sequence entries retrieved by the keyword "allergen" was examined, many allergens were found to be overlooked. This problem is not uncommon, as even recent compendia of allergen sequences may contain as few as one food allergen sequence (122), when dozens of unique sequences actually exist. This problem may arise out of the fact that many food allergens were characterized at both the DNA and protein levels long before it became apparent that they encoded allergens. For example, all of the cow's milk proteins that have been subsequently characterized to be allergens were initially cloned and sequenced in the early 1980s (123) and cannot be retrieved with the keyword "allergen." Therefore, it is necessary to use supplemental searches using guidance from the scientific literature regarding the identity of additional food and other allergens (124).

A compendium of allergen sequences should also contain sequences of nonfood allergens. The presence of considerable cross-reactivity between food and pollen or other allergens is well established (125–

Table 4.4
Keywords Used to Assemble Allergen Sequences

Keywords	Number of Sequences		
	Retrieved	Eliminated	Final
Allergen	300	155	145
Arachis lectin	2	1	1
Bertholletia albumin	3	2	1
Bos taurus lactoglobulin	7	6	1
Bos taurus albumin	29	24	5
Gallus albumin	21	18	3
Gallus lysozyme	5	4	1
Gallus lipovitellin	1	0	1
Gallus apovitellenin	1	0	1
Glycine max lectin	1	0	1
Glycine max trypsin inhibitor	3	0	3
Mus urinary	22	16	6
Ovomucoid	1	0	1
Papaya papain	1	0	1
Rattus 2u globulin	9	8	1
Soybean glycinin	24	15	9
Triticum gliadin	33	11	22
Triticum agglutinin	3	0	3
Allergen*	209	196	13
Total	675	456	219

*These entries were retrieved from the DNA database (GenBank/EMBL).

135). It would be undesirable to express a known pollen or mite allergen in a food in any case. Table 4.4 provides an example of the keywords that can be used to assemble a valid allergen sequence database. Table 4.5 provides an example of a comprehensive list of available amino acid sequences for known allergens.

To compare the amino acid sequences of allergens present in public domain genetic databases with sequences of introduced proteins, the FASTA (136, 137) or a similar computer program should be used. If the test criteria described earlier are applied, no homology and no immunologically relevant sequence similarity should be observed with allergens. Only then can it be concluded that the genes introduced into these foods do not encode known allergens or their homologues and that none of the introduced proteins shares a linear epitope with a known allergen.

Stability to Digestion

The ability of food allergens to reach and cross the mucosal membrane of the intestine is a likely prereq-

uisite to allergenicity (138). Clearly, a protein that is stable to the proteolytic and acidic conditions of the digestive tract has an increased probability of reaching the intestinal mucosa. Intact proteins are known to be capable of crossing the mucosal membrane of the gut and entering the circulatory system (139). Many allergens exhibit proteolytic stability (2–4, 138, 140–142), although the majority have not been tested directly. Thus, physicochemical properties that favor digestive stability can serve as important indicators of allergenic potential (1).

Recently, simulated gastric (143) and intestinal (144) models of mammalian digestion described in the U.S. Pharmacopeia have been used to systematically compare the relative stability of a number of common food allergens with common safe food proteins and with proteins engineered into plants (1, 145). These digestion models have been used to investigate the digestibility of plant proteins (146, 147), animal proteins (148), and food additives (149). A similar model has also been used to examine the stability of milk allergens (150–153). The data presented in Table 4.6 show that common food allergens are, without exception, stable to digestion in this gastric model. In cases where the food allergen is less stable (i.e., not stable for 60 minutes), the fragments generated remain stable for a substantial period of time. In contrast, common plant proteins are rapidly digested in the gastric model, disappearing by the first time point (Table 4.6).

Proteins that have been expressed in genetically modified plants have also been tested for stability with this model (1, 29, 61, 154). In contrast to food allergens, all nine proteins that were expressed in plants rapidly degraded under the test conditions (Table 4.7). The time required to degrade these proteins varied between less than 10 seconds and 30 seconds in simulated gastric fluid. Allergens remained stable for at least 2 minutes (and the major allergens were stable for at least 60 minutes) in simulated gastric fluids. Interestingly, those allergens with low stability in simulated gastric fluids tended to exhibit at least some stability in simulated intestinal fluids (145). Many allergens remained stable for 24 hours in simulated intestinal fluids. Rapid degradation of the proteins expressed in genetically engineered plants greatly minimizes the likelihood that these proteins

Table 4.5
Allergen and Gliadin Sequences Retrieved from the Genetic Databases
(GenEMBL/GenPept ver. 86, Swissprot ver. 30, PIR ver. 41)

Species	Common Name	Allergen	Synonym/Function	Accession
Food (plants)				
Arachis hypogea	peanuts	*Ara h* 1	clone P41b	L34402
			clone 5A1	L33402
			clone P17	L38853
		peanut lectin	agglutinin	S14765
Bertholletia excelsa	Brazil nut	methionine-rich	2S albumin (BE2S1 gene)	X54490
Brassica juncea	leaf mustard	*Bra j* IE-L	2S albumin large chain	S35592
		Bra j IE-S	2S albumin small chain	S35591
Carica papaya	papaya	papain		M15203
Glycine max	soybean	glycinin	A1aBx subunit	X02985
			A2B1a subunit	Y00398
			A3B4 subunit	M10962
			A5A4B3 subunit	X02626
			G1 subunit	X15121
			G2 subunit	X15122
			G3 subunit	X15123
		β-conglycinin	α-subunit	X17698
			CG4 subunit	S44893
		soy lectin	soy agglutinin	K00821
		Kunitz trypsin-inhibitor	KTi-s sub-type	X80039
			KTi-a sub-type	X64447
			KTi-b sub-type	X64448
Hordeum vulgare	barley	14.5 kD	α-amylase/trypsin inhibitor	S26197
		14.5 kD	"	P32360
Malus domestica	apple	*Mal d* 1	profilin homologue	X83672
Oryza sativa	rice	RAP	rice allergenic protein	X66257
		RAG1	rice allergen 1	D11433
		RAG2	rice allergen 2	D11434
		RAG5	rice allergen 3	D11430
		RAG14	rice allergen 14	D11432
		RAG17	rice allergen 17	D11431
Phaseolus vulgaris	kidney bean	PR-1	pathogenesis related prot. 1	S11929
		PR-2	pathogenesis related prot. 2	S11930
Sinapis alba	white mustard	*Sin a* 1.1	2S albumin/amylase inhibitor	S54101
		Sin a 1.2	"	PC1247
Triticum aestivum	bread wheat	gluten	α-gliadin	U08287
		"	"	K02068
		"	α/β-gliadin	X02538
		"	"	X02539
		"	"	X02540
Triticum aestivum	bread wheat	gluten	α/β-gliadin	K03074
		"	"	K03075
		"	α/β-gliadin class I	K03076
		"	α/β-gliadin class A-I	M11074
		"	α/β-gliadin class A-II	M10092
		"	α/β-gliadin class A-III	M11076
		"	α/β-gliadin class A-IV	M11075
		"	α/β-gliadin class A-V	M11073
		"	α/β-gliadin class MM1	X17361
		"	"	X00627
		"	γ-gliadin	M36999
		"	"	M16064
		"	γ-gliadin class B	M13713
		"	γ-gliadin class B-I	M11077

Table 4.5
(Continued)

Species	Common Name	Allergen	Synonym/Function	Accession
Triticum aestivum (con't)		gluten	γ-gliadin class B-I	M11336
		"	γ-gliadin class BIII	M11335
		WGA	wheat germ agglutinin A	M25536
		WGA	wheat germ agglutinin D	M25537
Triticum durum	pasta wheat	WGA	wheat germ agglutinin	J02961
Triticum turgidum	poulard wheat	16K allergen	α-amylase inhibitor	S19296
Triticum uratu		gluten	α/β-gliadin	M16496
Food (animal)				
Bos taurus	cow	BSA	serum albumin	M73993
		β-lactoglobulin	milk globulin (whey)	X14712
		α-lactalbumin	milk albumin (whey)	J05147
		Casein	type α-S1	M33123
			type α-S1	M38641
			type α-S2	M16644
			type β	M15132
			type κ	M36641
Gadus callarias	cod fish	*Gad c* 1	β-parvalbumin, allergen M	A94236
Gallus domesticus	chicken	*Gal d* 1	ovomucoid	M10639
		Gal d 2	ovalbumin Y gene	J00922
"		"	ovalbumin	M34352
		Gal d 3	conalbumin (ovotransferrin)	Y00407
		Gal d 4	lysozyme	J00885
		"	iso-lysozyme	X61001
		Vitellogenin II	lipovitellin/phosvitin	A92941
		Apovitellenin I	low density lipoprotein II	A91484
Metapenaeus ensis	shrimp	*Met e* 1	tropomyosin	U08008
Pollen				
Agrostis alba	bent grass	*Agr a* 1	group I	E37396
Alnus glutinosa	alder tree	*Aln g* 1	*Bet v* 1 homologue	S50892
Ambrosia artemisiifloia	ragweed (short)	*Amb a* 1.1	antigen E	A39099
		Amb a 1.2	"	B39099
		Amb a 1.3	"	C39099
		Amb a 1.4	"	D53240
		Amb a 2	antigen K	E53240
		Amb a 3	Ra3	P00304
		Amb a 5	Ra5	A03371
Ambrosia trifida	ragweed (tall)	*Amb t* 5	Ra5 homologue	S39336
		Amb t 5	"	A23859
Ambrosia psilostachya	weed	*Amb p* 5 (A2)	"	L24465
		Amb p 5 (A3)	"	L24466
		Amb p 5 (B1)	"	L24467
		Amb p 5 (B2)	"	L24468
		Amb p 5 (B3)	"	L24469
Anthoxanthum odoratum	sweet vernal grass	*Ant o* I	group I	G37396
Artemisia vulgaris	mugwort	*Art v* 2	glycoprotein allergen	A38624
Betula verrucosa	birch tree	*Bet v* 1	pathogenesis related (PR)	S05376
		Bet v 1N	*Bet v* 1 isoform	X82028
		Bet v 2	profilin	B45786
		Bet v 3		X79267
Carpinus betulus	hornbeam tree	*Car b* 1	*Bet v* 1 homologue	C53288
Castanea sativa	European chestnut	*Cas s* 1	"	PC2001
Corylus avellana	hazel tree	*Cor a* 1–5	"	S30053
		Cor a 1–6	"	S30054
		Cor a 1–11	"	S30055
		Cor a 1–16	"	S30056
Cryptomeria japonica	Japanese cedar	*Cry j* 1-A		D26544

Table 4.5
(Continued)

Species	Common Name	Allergen	Synonym/Function	Accession
Cryptomeria japonica (con't)		*Cry j* 1-B		D26545
		Cry j 2		D29772
Cynodon dactylon	Bermuda grass	*Cyn d* 1		A61226
Dactylis glomerata	orchard grass	*Dac g* 2		S45354
		Dac g 3		A60359
Festuca elator	reed fescue	*Fes e* 1-A		C37396
		Fes e 2-B		D37396
Glycine max	soybean	*Gly m* cim1	cytokinin-inducible protein	U03860
Holocus lanatus	meadow velvet	*Hol l* 1	30K allergen	Z27084
Hordeum vulgare	barley	*Hor v* 9	group IX	U06640
Lolium perenne	ryegrass	*Lol p* 1	group I	M57476
		Lol p 1	"	M57474
		Lol p 1b	"	M59163
		Lol p 2-A	group II	A34291
		Lol p 2	"	A48595
		Lol p 3	group III	A33422
		Lol p 4	group IV	A60737
		Lol p 9	group IX	L13083
		Lol p 30K	30K group V allergen	S38290
		Lol p 34K	34K group V allergen	S38289
		Lol p 50K	50K allergen	S38288
Lycopersicon esculatum	tomato	LAT52	*Ole e* 1 homologue	P13447
Olea europea	olive tree	*Ole e* 1		S36872
Parietaria judaica	parietaria	*Par j* 1		X77414
Parietaria officinalis	parietaria	*Par o* 1		A53252
Phleum pratense	timothy grass	*Phl p* 1	group I	X78813
		Phl p 1	"	Z27090
		Phl p 2	group II	X75925
		Phl p 5a	group V, group IX	X70942
		Phl p 5b	group V	Z27083
		Phl p 6		Z27082
		Phl p 32K	group V-like	S38294
		Phl p 38K	group V-like	S38293
		Phl p 11	group XI/profilin	P35079
Poa pratensis	Kentucky blue-grass	*Poa p* 1	group I	F37396
		"	"	A60372
		Poa p 9 (KBG31)	group IX	M38342
		Poa p 9 (KBG41)	"	M38343
		Poa p 9 (KBG60)	"	M38344
Quercus alba	oak tree	*Que a* 1	*Bet v* 1 homologue	D53288
Secale cereale	cultivated rye	*Sec c* 30K	30K group Vallergen	S38292
Triticum aestivum	bread wheat	*Tri a* 2.1	profilin	S72384
		Tri a 2.2	"	S72374
		Tri a 2.3	"	S72375
Zea mays	maize	*Zea m* 1	*Lol p* I homologue	JC1524
		clone c13	*Ole e* I homologue	P33050
Mites				
Euroglyphus maynei	house mite	*Eur m* 1	group I, thiol protease	S21864
Dermatophagoides farinae	house mite	*Der f* 1	thiol protease	X65196
		Der f 2.1	antigen 2	D10447
		Der f 2.1	"	A61241
		Der f 2.2	"	D10448
		Der f 2.2	"	B61241

Table 4.5
(Continued)

Species	Common Name	Allergen	Synonym/Function	Accession
Dermatophagoides farinae (con't)		*Der f 2.3*	antigen 2	D10449
		Der f 2.3	"	PS0417
Dermatophagoides microceras	house mite	*Der m 1*	thiol-protease	B27634
Dermatophagoides pteronyssinus	house mite	*Der p 1*	antigen P₁	U11695
		Der p 1	"	JQ0337
		Der p 2		A60381
		Der p 3	trypsin	U11719
		Der p 4	amylase	A61242
		Der p 5	14K allergen	S06734
		Der p 7		X17699
Lepidoglyphus destructor	feces mite	*Lep d 1*		X81399
Insect Venoms				
Apis mellifera	honeybee	*Api m 1*	phospholipase A2	P00630
		Api m 3	melittin	P01501
Dolichovespula arenaria	yellow hornet	*Dol a 5*	antigen 5	M98859
Dolichovespula maculata	whiteface hornet	*Dol m 1.02*	phospholipase A1	A44563
		Dol m 2	hyaluronidase	L34548
		Dol m 5	antigen 5 clone f5	J03602
		Dol m 5	antigen 5 clone f10	J03601
Myrmecia pilosula	bulldog ant	*Myr p 1*		X70256
Polestes annularis	wasp	*Pol a 5*	antigen 5	M98857
Polestes exclamans	paper wasp	*Pol e 5*	"	P35759
Polestes fascatus	paper wasp	*Pol f 5*	"	F44522
Solenopsis invicta	red fire ant	*Sol i 2*	phospholipase	A37330
		Sol i 3		B37330
		Sol i 4		C37330
Solenopsis richteri	black fire ant	*Sol r 2*	phospholipase	E60727
		Sol r 3		D60727
Vespa crabro	European hornet	*Ves c 5.0001*	antigen 5	G44522
		Ves c 5.0002	"	H44522
Vespula flavopilosa	yellow jacket	*Ves f 5*	"	B44522
Vespula germanica	german yellowjacket	*Ves g 5*	"	A44522
Vespula maculifrons	eastern yellowjacket	*Ves m 1*	phospholipase A1	A44564
		Ves m 5	antigen 5	M35760
Vespula pensylvanica	western yellowjacket	*Ves p 5*	"	C44522
Vespula squamosa	southern yellowjacket	*Ves s 5*	"	D44522
Vespula vidua	yellowjacket	*Ves vi 5*	"	E44522
Vespula vulgaris	yellow jacket	*Ves v 5*	"	M98858
Parasitic Nematodes				
Loa loa	filarial worm	LL20	15 kDa ladder protein	U03103
Segmented Worms				
Ascaris lumbricoides	common roundworm	*Asc l 1*	aba-1	B37188
Ascaris suum	earth worm	*Asc s 1*	"	A37188
		Asc s 1	"	L03211
Animals				
Felis domesticus	cat dander	*Fel d 1.1*	antigen 4	M74952
		Fel d 1.2	"	M74953
		Fel d 1.3	"	M77341
Mus masculus	mouse urine	*Mus m 1*	major urinary protein (MUP)	M27608
			MUP I	M16355
			MUP II	M16356
			MUP III	M16359
			MUP IV	M16358
			MUP V	M16360

Table 4.5
(Continued)

Species	Common Name	Allergen	Synonym/Function	Accession
Rattus norvegicus	rat urine	*Rat n* 1	hepatic α-2u globulin	J00737
Fungi (spores)				
Alternaria alternata		*Alt a* 2	aldehyde dehydrogenase	X78227
		Alt a 6	ribosomal protein	X78222
		Alt a 7		X78225
Aspergillus fumigatus		*Asp f* 1	mitogillin toxin/ribonuclease	M83781
		Asp f 1-A		S39330
Cladosporium herberum		*Cla h* 2	enolase	X78226
		Cla h 3	aldehyde dehydrogenase	X78228
		Cla h 4	ribosomal P2	X78223
		Cla h 5		X78224
			Total number of sequences = 219	

will survive the digestive tract and be absorbed—thereby eliciting an allergic response. The human digestive system provides a highly effective mechanism to remove these proteins before they can reach the intestinal mucosa. The simulated gastric model, therefore, provides a valuable tool to assess concerns about the allergenic potential of proteins introduced into food crops.

Prevalence in Food and Sequence Similarity to Food Proteins

Many food allergens are present as major protein components in a specific food, typically ranging between 1% and 80% of total protein (155) (Table 4.6). In contrast, the introduced proteins listed in Table 4.7 are expressed in plants at levels ranging from less than 0.001% to 0.03% of the raw product on a fresh-weight basis or from less than 0.01% to 0.4% of the protein content (27, 29, 61, 156).

The low levels of these proteins, combined with the digestive lability of these proteins relative to that for known food allergens, suggest a very low probability that any of these proteins will reach the intestinal mucosa during consumption. Thus, consumption of foods containing these proteins is not likely to sensitize an allergic individual.

The final component used in the assessment of the allergenic potential of a newly expressed protein is the amino acid sequence similarity to nonallergenic food proteins. The presence of biologically homologous proteins in food—especially a food with similar levels and types of consumption—further decreases concerns of potential allergenicity (27).

MOLECULAR GENETIC EFFECTS ON THE HOST PLANT

If the host plant being genetically engineered is known to contain specific endogenous allergens, and sera are available from allergy patients, the food derived from the new plant variety should be analyzed to ensure that the composition and level of endogenous allergens were not altered during the genetic engineering process. Although no precedent exists that suggests that the genetic engineering process itself could change either the composition or level of endogenous proteins, a direct assessment to confirm this expectation is prudent for genetically engineered food products. Of course, if the plant has no history of causing allergy or a limited history that precludes the availability of sera, this assessment cannot be performed.

Immunoblotting or ELISA methods could be implemented for this assessment. Although ELISA provides a quantitative assessment of the total allergenic protein composition, the immunoblotting approach provides more detailed information on the composition of specific endogenous allergens and is, therefore, the preferred method (157). Using this immunoblot approach with IgE from soybean-sensitive and normal individuals, Burks and Fuchs (157) showed no qualitative or quantitative differences

Table 4.6
Summary of Allergen and Protein Stability in a Gastric Model

Protein	% Total Protein	Stability (min)	
		Whole Protein	Fragments
Egg White Allergens[a]			
Ovalbumin (*Gal d* 2)	54	60	—
Ovomucoid (*Gal d* 1)	11	8	—
Conalbumin (*Gal d* 3)	12	0	15
Milk Allergens[a]			
β-lactoglobulin	9	60	—
Casein	80	2	15
BSA	1	0.5	15
α-lactalbumin	4	0.5	2
Soybean Allergens			
β-Conglycinin (β subunit) (179)	18.5[b]	60	—
Kunitz trypsin inhibitor (180)	2–4	60	—
Soy lectin (181)	1–2	15	—
β-Conglycinin (α subunit) (179)	18.5[b]	2	60
Glycinin (179)	51	0.5	15
Gly m Bd 30K (182)	2–3	0	8
Peanut Allergens			
Ara h II (183)	6[c]	60	—
Peanut lectin (184)	1.3	8	—
Mustard Allergens			
Sin a I (185)	20	60	—
Bra j IE (731)	20	60	—
Common Plant Proteins			
Rubisco LSU (spinach leaf) (186)	25[b]	0 (<15 sec)	—
Rubisco SSU (spinach leaf) (186)	25[b]	0 (<15 sec)	—
Lipoxygenase (soybean seed) (187)	<1	0 (<15 sec)	—
Glycolate reductase (spinach leaf)[d]	<1	0.25	—
PEP carboxylase (corn kernel)[d]	<1	0 (<15 sec)	—
Acid phosphatase (potato tuber)[d]	<1	0 (<15 sec)	—
Sucrose synthetase (wheat kernel)[d]	<1	0 (<15 sec)	—
β-amylase (barley kernel)[d]	<1	0 (<15 sec)	—

[a] See chapter 3.
[b] Represents total amount of protein for combined subunits.
[c] Reported as % crude extract.
[d] Values estimated from the literature.

in the endogenous allergens in glyphosate-tolerant (RoundupReady[4]) soybeans compared with the parental soybean variety or with soybeans from commercial varieties. The assessment of the endogenous allergens in RoundupReady soybeans represented the first application of this approach and confirmed that the genetic engineering process caused no changes in the composition or levels of endogenous allergens.

[4] RoundupReady is a trademark of Monsanto Company, St. Louis, Mo.

SUMMARY OF ALLERGY ASSESSMENT FOR GENETICALLY ENGINEERED PLANTS

The approach described above provides substantial detail and justification for the combination of factors that should be addressed when assessing potential allergy concerns for food developed through genetic engineering. It is important to remember that no single property or assay can predict allergenicity. If a protein lacks all of the important characteristics of an

Table 4.7
Digestion by a Gastric Model of Proteins Introduced into Plants

Protein	% Total Protein	Stability (min)	
		Whole Protein	Fragments
CryIIIA	<0.01	0 (<30 sec)	—
CryIA(c)	<0.01	0.5	—
CryIA(b)	<0.01	0.5	—
CP4 EPSP synthase (CP4)	<0.1	0 (<15 sec)	—
Glyphosate oxidoreductase (GOX)	<0.01	0 (<15 sec)	—
ACC deaminase (ACCd)	0.4	0 (<15 sec)	—
β-D-glucuronidase (GUS)	0.01	0 (<15 sec)	—
NPTII	<0.01	0 (<10 sec)	—
PAT	n.d.	0	—

allergenic protein, however, no further information should be necessary prior to introduction of the new plant variety. For proteins that share one or more characteristics of allergenic proteins, a synthesis of all of the information discussed above should be considered when deciding whether to pursue further research or characterization. In the end, a more balanced approach (illustrated in Fig. 4.3) will ensure that foods derived from genetically engineered plants are safe. For example, none of the proteins introduced into crops listed in Table 4.7 shares the major characteristics of food allergens discussed in this strategy.

Allergy Assessment of CryIIIA and NPTII—A Case Study

No reports in the literature have suggested that the source of the *cryIIIA* or *nptII* genes causes allergy. The *cryIIIA* gene was isolated from *Bacillus thuringiensis* spp. *tenebrionis* (23, 48). This bacterium has never been reported to cause allergy (158). In fact, the CryIIIA protein in NewLeaf potatoes is identical to one of the proteins contained in commercial microbial formulations that have been used since 1988 (29, 158). As part of the registration of microbial formulations, EPA requires that manufacturers of these products report any adverse reactions, including allergy (or possible allergy). The EPA has stated that, since the introduction of microbial formulations con-

taining Cry proteins in 1961, no reports of allergy have occurred (159). Likewise, the gene for NPTII was obtained from bacterial sources that have no history of allergy (60). Thus, both CryIIIA and NPTII are considered to be derived from sources having no prior history of allergenicity. In addition, no immunologically significant sequence similarity and no overall amino acid homology exists between these proteins and allergen sequences listed in Table 4.5 (29, 158).

The other physicochemical characteristics (Fig. 4.3, left side) of CryIIIA and NPTII have been assessed and compared with those of food allergens as well. Both the CryIIIA and the NPTII proteins appear to be extremely labile under the simulated digestive conditions described above (Table 4.7) (29, 61). Processing of the product carries little relevance in this case because tubers are marketed without processing. The CryIIIA and NPTII proteins are denatured and inactivated upon processing, with the majority of the respective denatured proteins remaining (Lavrik, unpublished). Neither CryIIIA nor NPTII is prevalent in potato tubers, representing less than 0.01% of total protein (Table 4.7). As both CryIIIA and NPTII are assumed to have entered the food supply prior to the advent of biotechnology, a history of safe consumption has been established.

These analyses are summarized in Table 4.8. Taken together, the results led to the conclusion that NewLeaf potatoes developed via the introduction and expression of the genes encoding CryIIIA and NPTII poses no increased risk of food allergy.

Table 4.8
Characteristics of CryIIIA and NPTII
versus Food Allergens

Characteristic	Allergens	CryIIIA	NPTII
Homology to allergens	Yes	No	No
Stable to digestion	Yes	No	No
Stable to processing	Yes	n/a	n/a
Prevalent to food	Yes	No	No
Homology to "safe" proteins	No	Yes*	Yes*

n/a = not applicable.
* Safe as defined by experience in the food supply.

Removing Allergens from Foods

Genetic engineering also provides a unique opportunity to reduce the levels of specific allergens in the food supply. By introducing genes in the antisense orientation (the opposite orientation required to produce a protein), the levels of protein produced by the "sense" orientation can be dramatically reduced. This technique is used to produce the delayed-softening FlavrSavr tomato. Inhibiting the production of a polygalacturonase enzyme that normally causes softening in tomato, extended the shelf life of FlavrSavr tomato (160).

The antisense approach has been used to significantly reduce the primary allergen in rice as well. Matsuda *et al.* (161) cloned the gene encoding the 16 kDa allergenic protein from rice grain, and then introduced the gene encoding this protein in the antisense orientation into rice. The levels of the 16 kDa protein were significantly reduced in rice grain from 312 μg per seed to 60 μg per seed (162), as shown in Figure 4.4. Additional studies are under way to achieve greater reductions in this allergenic protein.

The antisense approach or more sophisticated technologies like homologous recombination and gene replacement (163) could be used in other food crops such as peanuts and soybeans to selectively reduce the levels of specific allergens. The presence of multiple allergens and multigene families makes this undertaking more complex, however. Care must be taken not to change the nutritional value of these foods when attempting to manipulate or down-regulate allergen levels.

Animal Models for Predicting Allergenicity

While animal models provide important information for understanding the mechanisms of allergenicity, these models have not been validated for assessing the allergenic potential of specific proteins in naive subjects. Examples of animal models include mouse models to evaluate IgE responses to recombinant allergens (164), an IgE-mediated rodent model (165, 166), a guinea pig model of anaphylaxis (167, 168), dog models to study asthma and food allergy (165, 169, 170), and mouse models to study possible immunotherapeutic peptide epitopes (109) and other immunoprophylactic strategies (171). In all cases, the models have been used to study only the biological or molecular mechanisms of the immunopathogenesis of established allergic responses. Variable responses from animal to animal, species to species, and within the same animal suggest that it will be extremely difficult to establish an animal model with adequate power to predict hypersensitivity reactions to foods derived from genetically modified plants.

In fact, when animal models were used in one instance to predict allergenicity, they failed to detect the presence of a potent allergen. In the Brazil nut allergen example discussed earlier, passive cutaneous anaphylaxis in mice was used as a testing criteria (172). This study reached the erroneous conclusion that the Brazil nut 2S albumin gene was a strong candidate for genetic engineering into crop plants to enhance nutritional quality of derived foods. Thus, it is important that a robust animal model be developed and validated before it can be implemented in an allergy assessment program.

Other Factors to Consider in Allergy Assessment

Other factors can influence the appropriate assessment of potential food allergy as well. Unfortunately, these factors are difficult to accommodate in current systematic assessments, although some aspects of the presented strategy can at least partially address these issues. For example, in the case of oral allergy syn-

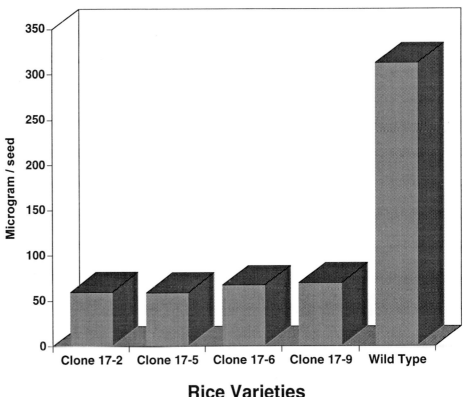

Figure 4.4

Suppression of 16 kDa rice allergen using antisense technology. Rice allergen levels were quantified by ELISA for each genetically engineered rice variety (clones 17-2, 17-5, 17-6, and 17-9) and were compared with wild-type rice seeds. By permission from Matsuda T, Nakase M, Adachi T, *et al.* Allergenic proteins in rice: strategies for reduction and evaluation. Presented at the Symposium of Food Allergies and Intolerances, Bonn, Germany, May 10–13, 1995.

drome (OAS), it is not clear that allergens responsible for this condition share physicochemical properties with common food allergens as they elicit a response in the buccal cavity immediately upon contact and may not need to be ingested. In cases where specific allergens implicated in OAS have been cloned (and for which amino acid sequences are available), however, it should be possible to perform the sequence comparisons described above. In addition, serum from OAS patients could conceivably be used in a similar fashion as has been proposed for in vitro and in vivo tests (see Fig. 4.3).

In the case of coeliac disease, the assessment strategy discussed above may not have specific relevance, although certain similar precautions should be observed. For example, genetic engineering of wheat gliadins (see Table 4.5) into a crop other than wheat would require appropriate labeling. Specific diagnostic tests—either in vitro or in vivo—have not yet been proposed or tested, however. It will be interesting to learn whether stability to digestion represents an important physicochemical parameter for offending gliadins.

Finally, the importance of cross-reactive allergens

found in pollen, fungi, insects, and other sources should not be underestimated. Wherever possible, efforts should be made to ensure that these ostensibly nonfood allergens do not proliferate in the food supply.

International Consensus— A Common Strategy

The development of national and international regulations, guidelines, and policies to assess the safety of food products derived from genetically engineered plants has led to broad discussions and a general consensus on the types of information that are appropriate to assess the potential allergenicity of such foods.

In the United States, FDA provided guidance for allergenicity assessment in its 1992 Food Policy (64). EPA also provided guidance in its draft guidelines for Pesticidal Plants (158). In addition, FDA, EPA, and the United States Department of Agriculture (USDA) co-sponsored a symposium in April 1994 that focused on assessing the allergenic potential of foods derived from genetically engineered plants (173).

Recent workshops sponsored by the Organization for Economic Cooperation and Development (OECD) (174) and the World Health Organization (WHO) (175) provided international guidance on allergenicity assessment. The most extensive effort to provide a comprehensive background on allergenicity and proposed criteria to assess allergenic concerns related to foods derived from genetically engineered plants was the result of an effort co-sponsored by the Allergy and Immunology Institute of the International Life Science Institute (ILSI) and the International Food Biotechnology Council (IFBC) (176).

Gaining international consensus on allergy assessment is critical because many genetically engineered plant products are commodity products (e.g., corn, soybean, wheat) grown and traded globally. A consensus approach provides producers, regulators, and consumers with the assurance that the risk of allergy to these products is appropriately addressed prior to their marketing, and that a consistent assessment approach is used around the world.

Conclusions and Future Considerations

The approaches recommended in this chapter are consistent with the guidance from the groups mentioned above. Using these approaches, the new plant varieties generated by genetic engineering should be introduced into the marketplace with the same confidence with which new plant varieties developed by traditional breeding have been introduced for centuries. We anticipate that new opportunities to enhance nutritional qualities and actually reduce the risk of allergy will become realized through the use of food biotechnology and genetic engineering. It will remain important to adopt new discoveries and techniques as part of an evolving strategy to assess potential allergy concerns for food developed through genetic engineering.

Acknowledgments

The authors thank Joel Ream, Terry Stone, Glen Rogan, and others who have critically reviewed and provided valuable suggestions for this chapter.

REFERENCES

1. Fuchs RL, Astwood JD. Allergenicity assessment of foods derived from genetically modified plants. Food Tech 1996; in press.
2. Metcalfe DD. Food Allergens. Clin Rev Allergy 1985;3:331–349.
3. Taylor SL, Lemanske RF, Bush RK, Busse WW. Food allergens: structure and immunologic properties. Ann Allergy 1987;59:93–99.
4. Taylor SL. Chemistry and detection of food allergens. Food Tech 1992;46:146–152.
5. Dettwiller A. Aryan agriculture. J Hered 1914;5:473–481.
6. Klages KHW. Ecological crop geography. New York: Macmillan, 1942, 1.
7. Poehlman JM. Breeding field crops, 2nd ed. Westport: AVI Publishing Inc., 1979, 1.
8. Sadik N. The state of world population 1992. New York: United Nations Population Fund, 1992.
9. Pingali P. Institutional and environmental constraints to agricultural intensification. In: McNicoll G, Cain M, eds. Rural development and population: Institutions and policy. New York: Oxford University Press, 1990.
10. McHughen A, Holm FA. Transgenic flax with environmentally

and agronomically sustainable attributes. Transgenic Research 1995;4:3–11.

11. Falco SC, Guida T, Locke M, et al. Transgenic canola and soybean seeds with increased lysine. Bio/Technology 1995;13:577–582.

12. Beauregard M, Dupont C, Teather RM, Hefford MA. Design, expression, and initial characterization of MB1, a de novo protein enriched in essential amino acids. Bio/Technology 1995;13:974–981.

13. Ma JK-C, Hein MB. Immunotherapeutic potential of antibodies produced in plants. Trends Biotechnol 1995;13:522–527.

14. Poirier Y, Nawrath C, Somerville C. Production of polyhydroxyalkanoates, a family of biodegradable plastics and elastomers, in bacteria and plants. Bio/Technology 1995;13:142–150.

15. Goy PA, Duesing JH. From pots to plots: Genetically modified plants on trial. Bio/Technology 1995;13:454–458.

16. Peacock WJ. Genetic engineering of crop plants will enhance the quality and diversity of foods. Food Australia 1994;46:379–381.

17. Van Montagu M, Goldberg RB. Plant biotechnology. Current Biology 1995;6:143–144.

18. Horsch RB, Fraley RT, Rogers SG, Sanders PR, Lloyd A, Hoffmann N. Inheritance of functional foreign genes in plants. Science 1984;223:496–498.

19. De Block M, Herrera-Estrella L, Van Montagu M, Schell J, Zambryski P. Expression of foreign genes in regenerated plants and their progeny. EMBO J 1984;3:1681–1689.

20. Fiske HJ, Dandekar AM. The introduction and expression of transgenes in plants. Sci Hort 1993;55:5–36.

21. Van Larebeke N, Engler G, Holsters M, et al. Large plasmid in Agrobacterium tumafaciens is essential for crown gall inducing activity. Nature 1974;252:169.

22. Zambryski PC. Chronicles from the Agrobacterium-plant cell DNA transfer story. Annu Rev Plant Physiol Plant Mol Biol 1992;43:465–490.

23. Perlak FJ, Stone TB, Muskopf YM, et al. Genetically improved potatoes—protection from damage by Colorado potato beetles. Plant Mol Biol 1993;22:313–321.

24. Redenbaugh K, Berner T, Emlay D, et al. Regulatory issues for commercialization of tomatoes with an antisense polygalacturonase gene. In Vitro Cell Dev Biol 1993;29P:17–26.

25. Tricoli DM, Carney KJ, Russell PF, et al. Field evaluation of transgenic squash containing single or multiple virus coat protein gene constructs for resistance to cucumber mosaic virus, watermelon mosaic virus 2, and zucchini yellow mosaic virus. Bio/Technology 1995;13:1458–1465.

26. Fuchs M, Gonsales D. Resistance of transgenic hybrid squash ZW-20 expressing the coat protein genes of zucchini yellow mosaic virus and watermelon mosaic virus 2 to mixed infections by both potyviruses. Bio/Technology 1995;13:1466–1473.

27. Padgette SR, Re DB, Barry GF, et al. New weed control opportunities: Development of soybeans with a Roundup Ready gene. In: Duke SO, ed. Herbicide-resistant crops. Agricultural, environmental, economic, regulatory, and technical aspects. CRC Lewis Publishers, 1996, 53–84.

28. Ross H. Potato breeding—problems and perspectives. Adv Plant Breeding 1986;13:1–132.

29. Lavrik PB, Bartnicki DE, Feldman J, et al. Safety assessment of potatoes resistant to Colorado potato beetle. In: Engel K-

H, Takeoka GR, Teranishi R, eds. ACS Symposium Series 605. Genetically modified foods. Safety issues. Washington: American Chemical Society, 1995, 148–158.

30. Krieg A, Huger AM, Langenbruch GA, Schnetter W. Bacillus thuringiensis var tenebrionis, a new pathotype effective against Coleoptera. Z Angew Ent 1983;96:500–508.

31. Shields EJ, Wyman JA. Effect of defoliation at specific growth stages on potato yields. J Econ Entomol 1984;77:1194–1199.

32. Casagrande RA. The Colorado potato beetle: 125 years of mismanagement. Bull Entomol Soc 1987;33:142–150.

33. Hare JD. Impact of defoliation by Colorado potato beetle on potato yields. J Econ Entomol 1980;73:369–373.

34. Ferro DN, Morzuch BJ, Margolies D. Crop loss assessment of the Colorado potato beetle (Coleoptera:Chrysomelidae) on potatoes in western Massachusetts. J Econ Entomol 1983;76:349–356.

35. Ferro DN, Boiteau G. Management of major insect pests of potato. In: Rowe RC, ed. Potato health management. St. Paul: American Phytopathology Society Press, 1992, 103–115.

36. Höfte H, Whitely HR. Insecticidal crystal proteins of Bacillus thuringiensis. Microbiol Rev 1989;53:242–255.

37. Van Rie J, Jansens S, Hofte H, Degheele D, Van Mellaert H. Receptors on the brush border membrane of the insect midgut as determinants of the specificity of Bacillus thuringiensis deltatoxins. Appl Environ Microbiol 1990;56:1378–1385.

38. Slaney AC, Robbins HL, English L. Mode of action of Bacillus thuringiensis toxin CryIIIA: An analysis of toxicity in Leptinotarsa decemlineata (Say) and Diabrotica undicimpunctata Hawardi Barber. Insect Biochem Molec Biol 1992;22:9–18.

39. Hofmann C, Vanderbruggen HV, Hofte H, Van Rie J, Jansens S, Van Mellaert H. Specificity of B. thuringiensis delta-endotoxins is correlated with the presence of high affinity binding sites in the brush border membrane of target insect midguts. Proc Natl Acad Sci USA 1988;85:7844–7848.

40. Sacchi VF, Parenti P, Hanozet GM, Giordana B, Luthy P, Wolfersberger MG. Bacillus thuringiensis toxin inhibits K^+-gradient-dependent amino acid transport across the brush border membrane of Pieris brassicae midgut cells. FEBS Letters 1986;204:213–218.

41. U.S. Environmental Protection Agency (EPA). Guidance for the reregistration of pesticide products containing Bacillus thuringiensis as the active ingredient. EPA Office of Pesticidal Programs. NTIS:PB 89-164198, 1989.

42. Aronson AI, Beckman W, Dunn P. Bacillus thuringiensis and related insect pathogens. Microbiol Rev 1986;50:1–24.

43. Newell CA, Rozman R, Hinchee MA, et al. Agrobacterium-mediated transformation of Solanum tuberosum L. cv. 'Russet Burbank.' Pl Cell Rep 1991;10:30–34.

44. Beck E, Ludwig G, Auerswald E, Riess B, Schaller H. Nucleotide sequence and exact localization of the neomycin phosphotransferase gene from transposon Tn5. Gene 1982;9:327–336.

45. Fuchs RL, Heeren RA, Gustafson ME, et al. Purification and characterization of microbially expressed neomycin phosphotransferase II (NPTII) protein and its equivalence to the plant expressed protein. Bio/Technology 1993;11:1537–1542.

46. World Health Organization (WHO). Health aspects of marker genes in genetically modified plants. Geneva: World Health Organization Food Safety Unit, 1993.

47. Odell JT, Nagy F, Chua N-H. Identification of DNA sequences required for activity of the cauliflower mosaic virus 35S promoter. Nature 1985;313:810–812.

48. Perlak FJ, Fuchs RL, Dean DA, McPherson SL, Fischhoff DA. Modification of the coding sequence enhances plant expression of insect cotton protein genes. Proc Natl Acad Sci USA 1991;88:3324–3328.

49. Tette J, Heinmiller M. Potato. In: A strategic long-range plan for the New York integrated pest management program. Geneva: New York IPM Program, 1992, 263–281.

50. Hock WK. Pesticide use: the need for proper protection, application and disposal. In: Ragsdale NN, Kuhr RJ, eds. Pesticides: minimizing the risks. New York: American Chemical Society, 1986.

51. Zaki MH, Moran D, Harris D. Pesticide in groundwater: The aldicarb story in Suffolk County, New York. Am J Public Health 1982;72:1391–1395.

52. Rothschild ER, Mauser RJ, Anderson MP. Investigation of aldicarb in groundwater in selected areas of the central sand plain of Wisconsin. Groundwater 1982;20:432–445.

53. Van den Bosch RE, Schliner EI, Dietrick EJ, Hall JC, Puttler B. Studies on succession, distribution and phenology of imported parasites of *Therioaphis trifolii,* in southern California. Ecology 1964;45:602–621.

54. Reed GL, Puls KA, Berry RE, Jenson AS, Feldman J. Effect of Colorado potato beetle suppression (Transgenic resistance) on seasonal abundance of parasites and preditors. Entomology Society of America 1992 (abs).

55. Pariza MW, Foster EM. Determining the safety of enzymes used in food processing. J Food Protect 1983;46:453–468.

56. Jones DD, Maryanski JH. Safety considerations in the evaluation of transgenic plants for human foods. In: Levin MA, Strauss HS, eds. Risk assessment in genetic engineering. New York: McGraw-Hill, 1991, 64–82.

57. Sjoblad R, McClintock JT, Engler R. Toxicological considerations for protein components of biological pesticide products. Reg Toxicol Pharmacol 1992;15:3–9.

58. Anonymous. Simulated gastric fluid, TS. In: Board of Trustees, ed. The United States Pharmacopeia XXII, The National Formulary XVII. Rockville: United States Pharmacopeial Convention Inc., 1990, 1788.

59. Flavell RB, Dart E, Fuchs RL, Fraley RT. Selectable marker genes: safe for plants? Bio/Technology 1992;10:141–144.

60. Nap J-P, Bijvoet J, Stiekema WJ. Biosafety of kanamycin-resistant transgenic plants. Transgenic Research 1992;1:239–249.

61. Fuchs RL, Ream JE, Hammond BG, Naylor MW, Leimgruber RM, Berberich SA. Safety assessment of the neomycin phosphotransferase II (NPTII) protein. Bio/Technology 1993;11:1543–1547.

62. Kok EJ, Noteborn HPJM, Kuiper HA. Food safety assessment of marker genes in transgenic crops. Trends Food Sci Technol 1994;5:294–298.

63. U.S. Food and Drug Administration (FDA), Department of Health and Human Services. Secondary direct food additives permitted in food for human consumption; food additives permitted in feed and drinking water of animals; Aminoglycoside 3′—Phosphotransferase II. Fed Regist 1994;59:26700–26711.

64. U.S. Food and Drug Administration (FDA), Department of Health and Human Services. Statement of policy: foods derived from new plant varieties. Fed Regist 1992;57:22984–23005.

65. Sampson HA. Food hypersensitivity: manifestations, diagnosis, and natural history. Food Tech 1992;46:141–144.

66. Young E, Stoneham MD, Petruckevitch A. A population study of food intolerance. Lancet 1994;343:1127–1130.

67. Jansen JJN, Kardinaal AFM, Huijbers G, Vlieg-Boerstra BJ, Martens BPM, Ockhuizen T. Prevalence of food allergy and intolerance in the adult Dutch population. J Allergy Clin Immunol 1994;93:446–456.

68. Ninan TK, Russel G. Respiratory symptoms and atopy in Aberdeen schoolchildren: evidence from two surveys 25 years apart. Brit Med J 1992;304:873–875.

69. Burr ML. Epidemiology of clinical allergy. Monogr Allergy 1993;31:1–8.

70. Bjorksten B. Risk factors in early childhood for the development of atopic diseases. Allergy 1994;49:400–407.

71. Metcalfe DD. The nature and mechanisms of food allergies and related diseases. Food Tech 1992;46:136–144.

72. Taylor SL. Food allergies. Food Tech 1985;49:116–119.

73. Panhuysen CIM, Meyers DA, Postma DS, Bleecker ER. The genetics of asthma and atopy. Allergy 1995;50:863–869.

74. Shirakawa T, Li A, Dubowitz M, *et al.* Association between atopy and variants of the β subunit of the high-affinity immunoglobulin E receptor. Nature Genet 1994;7:125–130.

75. Moffatt MF, Sharp PA, Faux JA, Young RP, Cookson WOCM, Hopkin JM. Factors confounding genetic linkage between atopy and chromosome 11q. Clin Exp Allergy 1992;22:1046–1051.

76. Xu J, Levitt RC, Panhuysen CMI, *et al.* Evidence for two unlinked loci regulating total serum IgE levels. Am J Hum Genet 1995;57:425–430.

77. Postma DS, Bleecker ER, Amelung PJ, *et al.* Genetic susceptibility to asthma: bronchial hyperresponsiveness co-inherited with a major gene for atopy. N Engl J Med 1995;333:894–900.

78. Flamm EL. Plant biotechnology: food safety and environmental issues. In: Arntzen CJ, ed. Encyclopedia of agricultural science. San Diego: Academic Press, 1994, 213–223.

79. Berkowitz DB, Kryspin-Sorensen I. Transgenic fish: Safe to eat? Bio/Technology 1994;12:247–252.

80. Barefoot SF, Beachy RN, Lilburn MS. Labeling of food-plant biotechnology products. In: CAST Number 4. Ames: Council for Agricultural Science and Technology, 1994, 1–8.

81. Miller H. Labeling of "biotech foods" is no free lunch. Bio/Technology 1995;13:1510.

82. Jones RT, Squillace DL, Yunginger JW. Anaphylaxis in a milk-allergic child after ingestion of milk-contaminated kosher-pareve-labeled "dairy-free" desert. Ann Allergy 1992;68:223–227.

83. Gern JE, Yang E, Evrard HM, Sampson HA. Allergic reactions to milk-contaminated "nondairy" products. N Engl J Med 1991;324:976–979.

84. Tattrie NH, Yaguchi M. Protein content of various processed edible oils. Can Inst Food Sci Technol J 1973;6:289–290.

85. Bush RK, Taylor SL, Nordlee JA, Busse WW. Soybean oil is not allergic to soybean sensitive individuals. J Allergy Clin Immunol 1984;73:176.

86. Halsey AB, Martin ME, Ruff ME, Jacobs FO, Jacobs RL. Sunflower oil is not allergic to sunflower seed-sensitive patients. J Allergy Clin Immunol 1986;78:408–410.

87. Taylor SL, Busse WW, Sachs MI, Parker JL, Yunginger JW. Peanut oil is not allergenic to peanut-sensitive individuals. J Allergy Clin Immunol 1981;68:372–375.

88. Sampson HA, Albergo R. Comparison of results of skin tests, RAST, and double-blind, placebo-controlled food challenges

in children with atopic dermatitis. J Allergy Clin Immunol 1984;74:26–33.

89. Yunginger JW, Adolphson CR. Standardization of allergens. In: Washington: American Society of Microbiology, 1992, 678–684.

90. Burks AW, Brooks JR, Sampson HA. Allergenicity of major component proteins of soybean determined by enzyme-linked immunosorbent assay (ELISA) and immunoblotting in children with atopic dermatitis and positive soy challenges. J Allergy Clin Immunol 1988;81:1135–1142.

91. Sampson HA, Scanion SM. Natural history of food hypersensitivity in children with atopic dermatitis. J Pediatr 1989;115:23–27.

92. Bock SA, Sampson HA, Atkins FM, et al. Double-blind, placebo-controlled food challenges (DBPCFC) as an office procedure. J Allergy Clin Immunol 1988;82:986–997.

93. Townsend JJ, Thomas LA, Kullisek ES, Daywalt MJ, Winter KRK, Altenbach SB. Improving the quality of seed proteins in soybean. In: Proceedings of the fourth biennial conference of molecular biology of soybean. Ames: Iowa State University, 1992, 4.

94. Altenbach SB, Kuo C-C, Staraci LC, et al. Accumulation of a Brazil nut albumin in seeds of transgenic canola results in enhanced levels of seed protein methionine. Plant Mol Biol 1992;18:235–245.

95. Ampe C, Van Damme J, de Castro LAB, Sampaio MJAM, Van Montagu M, Vandekerckhove J. The amino-acid sequence of the 2S sulphur-rich proteins from seeds of Brazil nut (Bertholletia excelsa H.B.K.). Eur J Biochem 1986;159:597–604.

96. Shewry PR, Napier JA, Tatham AS. Seed storage proteins: structures and biosynthesis. Plant Cell 1995;7:945–956.

97. Gillespie DN, Nakajima S, Gleich GJ. Detection of allergy to nuts by the radioallergosorbent test. J Allergy Clin Immunol 1976;57:302–309.

98. Arshad SH, Malmberg E, Krapf K, Hide DW. Clinical and immunological characteristics of Brazil nut allergy. Clin Exp Allergy 1991;21:373–376.

99. Nordlee JA, Taylor SL, Townsend JA, Thomas LA. High methionine Brazil nut protein binds human IgE. J Allergy Clin Immunol 1992;93:209 (abs).

100. Nordlee JA, Taylor SL, Townsend JA, Thomas LA, Townsend R. Investigations of the allergenicity of Brazil nut 2S seed storage protein in transgenic soybean. In: Anonymous, ed. OECD Workshop on food safety evaluation, Oxford England, 12–15 September 1994. Paris: OECD Environmental Health and Safety Unit, 1995, 121–125.

101. King TP, Hoffman D, Lowenstein H, Marsh DG, Platts-Mills TAE, Thomas W. Allergen nomenclature. Int Arch Allergy Immunol 1994;105:224–233.

102. Elsayed S, Apold J. Immunochemical analysis of cod fish allergen M: locations of the immunoglobulin binding sites as demonstrated by native and synthetic peptides. Allergy 1983;38:449–459.

103. Johnsen G, Elsayed S. Antigenic and allergenic determinants of ovalbumin-III. MHC Ia-binding peptide (OA 323-339) interacts with human and rabbit specific antibodies. Mol Immunol 1990;27:821–827.

104. Menendez-Arias L, Dominguez J, Moneo I, Rodriguez R. Epitope mapping of the major allergen from yellow mustard seeds, Sin a I. Mol Immunol 1990;27:143–150.

105. Elsayed S, Apold J, Holen E, Vik H, Florvaag E, Dybendal T. The structural requirements of epitopes with IgE binding capacity demonstrated by three major allergens from fish, egg and tree pollen. Scand J Clin Lab Invest 1991;51:17–31.

106. Greene WK, Cyster JG, Chua KY, O'Brien RM, Thomas WR. IgE and IgG binding of allergen peptides expressed from fragments of cDNA encoding the major house dust mite allergen Der p I. Journal of Immunology 1991;147:3768.

107. Zhang L, Olsen E, Kisil FT, Hill RD, Sehon AH, Mohapatra SS. Mapping of antibody binding epitopes of a recombinant Poa p IX allergen. Mol Immunol 1992;29:1383–1389.

108. Aki T, Ono K, Paik S-Y, et al. Cloning and characterization of a cDNA coding for a new allergen from the house dust mite, Dermatophagoides farinae. Int Arch Allergy Immunol 1994;103:236–239.

109. Hoyne GF, Callow MG, Kuo M-C, Thomas WR. Inhibition of T-cell responses by feeding peptide containing major and cryptic epitopes: studies with the Der p I allergen. Immunology 1994;83:190–195.

110. Mohapatra SS, Mohapatra S, Yang M, et al. Molecular basis of cross-reactivity among allergen-specific human T-cells: T-cell receptor Vα gene usage and epitope structure. Immunology 1994;81:15–20.

111. Shimojo N, Katsuki T, Coligan JE, et al. Identification of the disease-related T cell epitope of ovalbumin and epitope-targeted T cell inactivation in egg allergy. Int Arch Allergy Appl Immunol 1994;105:155–161.

112. Suphioglu C, Singh MB, Knox RB. Peptide mapping analysis of group I allergens of grass pollens. Int Arch Allergy Immunol 1993;102:144–151.

113. Bufe A, Becker WM, Schramm G, Petersen A, Mamat U, Schlaak M. Major allergen Phi p Va (timothy grass) bears at least two different IgE-reactive epitopes. J Allergy Clin Immunol 1994;94:173–181.

114. Van Milligen FJ, van't Hof W, van den Berg M, Aalberse RC. IgE epitopes on the cat (Felis domesticus) major allergen Fel d I: a study with overlapping synthetic peptides. J Allergy Clin Immunol 1994;93:34–43.

115. Van Ree R, van Leeuwen WA, van den Berg M, Weller HH, Aalberse RC. IgE and IgG cross-reactivity among Lol p I and Lol p II/II. Identification of the C-termini of Lol p I, II and III as cross-reactive structures. Allergy 1994;49:254–261.

116. O'Hehir RE, Garman RD, Greenstein JL, Lamb JR. The specificity and regulation of T-cell responsiveness to allergens. Annu Rev Immunol 1991;9:67–95.

117. Rothbard JB, Gefter ML. Interactions between immunogenic peptides and MHC proteins. Ann Rev Immunol 1991;9:527–565.

118. Singh MB, Hough T, Theerakulpisut P, et al. Isolation of CDNA encoding a newly identified major allergenic protein of rye-grass pollen: intracellular targeting to the amyloplast. Proc Natl Acad Sci USA 1991;88:1384–1388.

119. Astwood JD, Mohapatra SS, Ni H, Hill RD. Pollen allergen homologues in barley and other crop species. Clin Exp Allergy 1995;25:66–72.

120. Smith AM, Chapman MD. Reduction of IgE antibody binding to rDER P 2 variants generated by site-directed mutagenesis. In: Sehon AC, Kraft D, eds. International symposium on molecular biology of allergens and the atopic immune response, Quebec, Feb 18–22. New York: Plenum Publishing, 1996, in press.

121. Seiberler S, Scheiner O, Kraft D, Lonsdale D, Valenta R.

Characterization of a birch pollen allergen, *Bet v* III, representing a novel class of Ca^{2+} binding proteins; specific expression in mature pollen and dependence of patients IgE binding on protein bound Ca^{2+}. EMBO J 1994;13:3481–3486.

122. Scheiner O, Kraft D. Basic and practical aspects of recombinant allergens. Allergy 1995;50:384–391.

123. Bawden WS, Passey RJ, MacKinlay AG. The genes encoding the major milk-specific proteins and their use in transgenic studies and protein engineering. Biotech Gen Eng Rev 1994;12:89–137.

124. Astwood JD, Hill RD. Molecular biology of male gamete development in plants—an overview. In: Mohapatra SS, Knox RB, eds. Pollen biotechnology: Gene expression and allergen characterization. New York: Chapman & Hall, 1996, 1–37.

125. Lahti A, Bjorksten F, Hannuksela M. Allergy to pollen and apple, and cross reactivity of the allergens studied with RAST. Allergy 1980;35:297.

126. Aalberse RC, Koshte V, Clemens JGJ. Immunoglobulin E antibodies that cross-react with vegetable foods, pollen, and hymenoptera venom. J Allergy Clin Immunol 1981;68:356–364.

127. Calkhoven PG, Aalbers M, Koshte VL, Pos O, Oei HD, Aalberse RC. Cross-reactivity among birch pollen, vegetables and fruits as detected by IgE antibodies is due to at least three distinct cross-reactive structures. Allergy 1987;42:382–390.

128. De Martino M, November E, Cozza G, De Marco A, Bonazza P, Vierucci A. Sensitivity to tomato and peanut allergens in children monosensitised to grass pollen. Allergy 1988;43:206–213.

129. Subiza J, Subiza JL, Hinojosa M, et al. Anaphylactic reaction after the ingestion of chamomile tea: a study of cross-reactivity with other composite pollens. J Allergy Clin Immunol 1989;84:353–358.

130. Valenta R, Breiteneder H, Pattenburger K, et al. Homology of the major birch-pollen allergen, *Bet v* I, with the major pollen allergens of alder, hazel, and hornbeam at the nucleic acid level as determined by cross-hybridization. J Allergy Clin Immunol 1991;87:677–682.

131. Van Ree R, Voitenko V, van Leeuwen WA, Aalberse RC. Profilin is a cross-reactive allergen in pollen and vegetable foods. Int Arch Allergy Immunol 1992;98:97–104.

132. Bircher AJ, Van Melle G, Haller E, Curty B, Frei PC. IgE to food allergens are highly prevalent in patients allergic to pollens, with and without symptoms of food allergy. Clin Exp Allergy 1994;24:367–374.

133. Vocks E, Borga A, Szliska C, Seifert HU, Burrow G, Borelli S. Common allergenic structures in hazelnut, rye grain, sesame seeds, kiwi, and poppy seeds. Allergy 1993;48:168–172.

134. Schoning B, Vieths S, Petersen A, Baltes W. Identification and characterization of allergens related to *Bet v* I, the major birch pollen allergen, in apple, cherry, celery and carrot by two-dimensional immunoblotting and N-terminal microsequencing. J Sci Food Agric 1995;67:431–440.

135. Crespo JF, Pascual C, Helm R, et al. Cross-reactivity of IgE-binding components between boiled Atlantic shrimp and German cockroach. Allergy 1995;50:918–924.

136. Pearson W, Lipman D. Improved tools for biological sequence comparison. Proc Natl Acad Sci USA 1988;85:2444–2448.

137. Pearson W. Rapid and sensitive sequence comparison with FASTP and FASTA. In: Doolittle RF, ed. Methods in Enzymology, vol. 183. Molecular evolution: computer analysis of protein and nucleic acid sequences. San Diego: Academic Press, 1990, 63–98.

138. Onaderra M, Monslave RI, Mancheno JM, et al. Food mustard allergen interaction with phospholipid vesicles. Eur J Biochem 1994;225:609–615.

139. Gardner MLG. Gastrointestinal absorption of intact proteins. Ann Rev Nutr 1988;8:329–350.

140. King TP, Norman PS, Lichtenstein LM. Isolation and characterization of allergens from ragweed pollen, IV. Biochemistry 1967;6:1992–2000.

141. Kortekangas-Savolainen O, Savolainen J, Einarsson R. Gastrointestinal stability of baker's yeast allergens: an in vitro study. Clin Exp Allergy 1993;23:587–590.

142. Taylor SL. Immunologic and allergic properties of cow's milk proteins in humans. J Food Protect 1986;49:239–250.

143. Anonymous. Simulated Gastric Fluid, TS. In: Board of Trustees, ed. The United States Pharmacopeia 23, The National Formulary 18. Rockville: United States Pharmacopeial Convention, 1995, 2053.

144. Anonymous. Simulated Intestinal Fluid, TS. In: The Board of Trustees, ed. The United States Pharmacopeia 23, The National Formulary 28. Rockville: United States Pharmacopeial Convention, 1995, 2053.

145. Astwood JD, Fuchs RL. Allergenicity of foods derived from transgenic plants. In: Wuthrich B, ed. Monographs in allergy: 6th international symposium on immunological and clinical problems in food allergy, Lugano, September 24–26, 1995. Basil: Karger, 1996, in press.

146. Marquez UML, Lajolo FM. Composition and digestibility of albumin, globulins, and glutelins from *Phaseolus vulgaris*. J Agric Food Chem 1981;29:1068–1074.

147. Nielsen SS. Degradation of bean proteins by endogenous and exogenous proteases—a review. Cereal Chem 1988;65:435–442.

148. Zikakis JP, Rzucidlo SR, Biasotto NO. Persistence of bovine milk xanthine oxidase activity after gastric digestion in vivo and in vitro. J Dairy Sci 1977;60:533–541.

149. Tilch C, Elias PS. Investigation of the mutagenicity of ethylphenylglycidate. Mutation Res 1984;138:1–8.

150. Haddad ZH, Kalra V, Verma S. IgE antibodies to peptic and peptic-tryptic digests of betalactoglobulin: significance in food hypersensitivity. Ann Allergy 1979;42:368–371.

151. Schwartz HR, Nerurkar LS, Spies JR, Scanlon RT, Bellanti JA. Milk hypersensitivity: RAST studies using new antigens generated by pepsin hydrolysis of beta-lactoglobulin. Ann Allergy 1980;45:242–245.

152. Asselin J, Amiot J, Gauthier SF, Mourad W, Hebert J. Immunogenicity and allergenicity of whey protein hydrolysates. J Food Sci 1988;53:1208–1211.

153. Asselin J, Hebert J, Amiot J. Effects of in vitro proteolysis on the allergenicity of major whey proteins. J Food Sci 1989;54:1037–1039.

154. Fuchs RL, Rogan GJ, Keck PJ, Love SL, Lavrik PB. Safety evaluation of Colorado potato beetle-protected potatoes. In: Application of the principles of substantial equivalence to the safety evaluation of foods or food components from plants derived by modern biotechnology. World Health Organization, Food Safety Unit, 1995, 63–78.

155. Yuninger JW. Classical food allergens. Allergy Proceedings 1990;11:7–9.

156. Reed AJ, Magin KM, Anderson JS, et al. Delayed ripening tomato plants expressing the enzyme 1-aminocyclopropane-

1-carboxylic acid deaminase: I. Molecular characteristics. J Agric Food Chem 1996, in press.

157. Burks AW, Fuchs RL. Assessment of the endogenous allergens in glyphosate-tolerant and commercial soybean varieties. J Allergy Clin Immunol 1996;96:1008–1010.

158. U.S. Environmental Protection Agency (EPA). Neomycin phosphotransferase II; Tolerance exemption. Fed Regist 1994;59:49351–49353.

159. U.S. Environmental Protection Agency (EPA). Plant pesticide *Bacillus thuringiensis* CryIIIA delta endotoxin and the genetic material necessary for its production; tolerance exemption. Fed Regist 1995;60:21725–21728.

160. Sheehy RE, Kramer M, Hiatt WR. Reduction of polygalacturonase in tomato fruit by antisense RNA. Proc Natl Acad Sci USA 1988;85:8805–8809.

161. Matsuda T, Alvarez AM, Tada Y, Adachi T, Nakamura R. Gene engineering for hypo-allergenic rice: repression of allergenic protein synthesis in seeds of transgenic rice plants by antisense RNA. In: Anonymous, ed. Proceedings of the international workshop on life science in production and food—consumption of agricultural products—October 24–28. Japan. 1993.

162. Matsuda T, Nakase M, Adachi T, Nakamura R. Allergenic proteins in rice: strategies for reduction and evaluation. In: Anonymous, ed. Food allergies and intolerances. Bonn: DFG Senate commission on the evaluation of food safety, 1995.

163. Morton R, Hooykaas PJJ. Gene replacement. Mol Breed 1995;1:123–132.

164. Zhang L, Sehon AH, Mohapatra SS. Induction of IgE antibodies in mice with recombinant grass pollen allergens. Immunology 1992;76:158–163.

165. Andre F, Andre C, Colin L, Cavagna S. IgE in stools as indicator of food sensitization. Allergy 1995;50:328–333.

166. Perove MH, Gall DG. Transport abnormalities during intestinal anaphylaxis in the rat: effect of antiallergic agents. J Allergy Clin Immunol 1985;76:498–503.

167. Granti B, Marioni L, Rubaltelli FF. Evaluation in guinea pigs of the allergenic capacity of two infant formulae based on hydrolyzed milk proteins. Biol Neonate 1985;48:122–124.

168. Pahud J-J, Monti JC, Jost R. Allergenicity of whey protein: its modification by tryptic in vitro hydrolysis of the protein. J Pediatr Gastroenterol Nutr 1985;4:408–413.

169. Becker AB. A canine model of allergy and airway hyperresponsiveness. In: Sehon AC, Kraft D, eds. Molecular biology of allergens and the atopic immune response. New York: Plenum Publishing, 1996, in press.

170. Frick OL, Ermel RW, Buchanan BB. Food allergy in atopic dogs. In: Sehon AC, Kraft D, eds. Molecular biology of allergens and the atopic immune response. New York: Plenum Publishing, 1996, in press.

171. Holt PG. Immunoprophylaxis of atopy: light at the end of the tunnel? Immunology Today 1994;15:484–489.

172. Melo VMM, Xavier-Filho J, Lima MS, Prouvost-Danon A. Allergenicity and tolerance to proteins from Brazil nut (*Bertholletia excelsa* HBK). Food Agric Immunol 1994;6:185–195.

173. Anonymous. Conference on scientific issues related to potential allergenicity in transgenic food crops, April 18–19, 1994. Annapolis: FDA, EPA, USDA Docket 94N-0053, 1994, 1.

174. Organization for Economic and Cooperative Development (OECD), Environmental Health and Safety Division. Workshop on food safety evaluations. Paris, 1995.

175. WHO. Application of the principles of substantial equivalence to the safety evaluation of foods or food components from plants derived by modern biotechnology. Geneva: World Health Organization, Food Safety Unit, 1995, 1–80.

176. Metcalfe DD. Assessment of the allergenic potential of foods derived from genetically engineered crop plants. In: Fuchs RL, Fordham J, Metcalfe DD, *et al.* eds. Allergenicity of foods produced by genetic modification. Washington: International Food Biotechnology Council/ILSI Allergy and Immunology Institute, 1996, in press.

177. Pavek J. Western regional variety trial report, 1980–1992, WRCC-27. Moscow: University of Idaho, 1992.

178. Scherz H, Senser F. Food composition and nutrition tables 1989/90. In: Muchen GB, ed. Food composition and nutrition tables. Stuttgart: Deutsche Forshunganstalt fur Lebensmittelchemie, 1989, 542–544.

179. Murphy PA, Resurreccion AP. Varietal and environmental differences in soybean glycinin and β-conglycinin content. J Agric Food Chem 1984;32:911–915.

180. Charpentier BA, Lemmel DE. A rapid automated procedure for the determination of trypsin inhibitor activity in soy products and common foodstuffs. J Agric Food Chem 1984;32:908–911.

181. Goldberg RB, Hoschek G, Vodkin LO. An insertion sequence blocks the expression of a soybean lectin gene. Cell 1983;33:465–475.

182. Kalinski A, Weisemann JM, Matthews BF, Herman EM. Molecular cloning of a protein associated with soybean seed oil bodies that is similar to thiol proteases of the papain family. J Biol Chem 1990;265:13843–13848.

183. Burks AW, Williams LW, Connaughton C, Cockrell G, O'Brien TJ, Helm RM. Identification and characterization of a second major peanut allergen, *Ara h* II, with use of sera of patients with atopic dermatitis and positive peanut challenge. J Allergy Clin Immunol 1992;90:962–969.

184. Lotan R, Skutelsky E, Danon D, Sharon N. The purification, composition, and specificity of the anti-T lectin from peanut (*Arachis hypogaea*). J Biol Chem 1975;250:8518–8523.

185. Crouch ML, Sussex IM. Development and storage-protein synthesis in *Brassica napus* L. embryos in vivo and in vitro. Planta 1981;153:64–74.

186. Ellis RJ. The most abundant protein in the world. Trend Biochem 1979;4:241–244.

187. Siedow JN. Plant lipoxygenase: structure and function. Ann Rev Plant Physiol Plant Mol Biol 1991;42:145–188.

188. Wang K, Herrera-Estrella L, Van Montagu M, Zambryski P. Right 25-bp terminus of the nopaline T-DNA is essential for and determines direction of DNA transfer from *Agrobacterium* to the plant genome. Cell 1984;38:455–462.

189. Klee HJ, White FF, Iyer VN, Gordon MP, Nester EW. Mutational analysis of the virulence region of an *Agrobacterium tumafaciens* Ti plasmid. J Bacteriol 1983;153:878–883.

ANTIGEN ABSORPTION

Stephen Murphy
W. Allan Walker

The primary functions of the gastrointestinal tract are to permit the absorption of nutritionally important dietary components and to assist in the maintenance of homeostasis in the internal milieu. A wide range of specific absorptive mechanisms exists to facilitate the efficient uptake of essential luminal constituents. Because of these absorptive adaptations, the surface of the digestive tract lacks the protective properties possessed by the epidermis. The gut is exposed to an enormous variety of potentially noxious elements, including microorganisms, toxins, and foreign antigens, and consequently it possesses a range of protective adaptations. Within the gut, non-immunologic and immunologic processes act both independently and in concert to provide an effective "mucosal barrier."

For many years, it was believed that macromolecules were not absorbed in biologically significant quantities; this assumption arose because no transport mechanisms for such molecules had been identified and in any event it was thought that digestion ensured their degradation (1). A great deal of clinical and experimental evidence now indicates that such molecules penetrate the intestinal mucosa in quantities sufficient to evoke important immune responses. Immunologic reactions to dietary antigens are common, but the nature and intensity of these responses vary and in most instances no pathologic consequences ensue (2).

Absorption of Dietary Antigen

The uptake of macromolecules has been studied in most detail in animals that absorb biologically important quantities of immunoglobulin during the neonatal period (3). In certain mammalian species, relatively large quantities of protein are transported across the intestinal epithelium in the perinatal period. Ruminants derive very little passive immunity from transplacental passage of maternal antibody, but rely instead on the postpartum enteric absorption of maternal IgG antibodies that are present in high concentrations in the colostrum of these species (3). Rodents are passively immunized by transplacental transfer of antibody and by receptor-mediated intestinal uptake of milk IgG during the first 18 to 21 days of life (4).

In the human infant, gastrointestinal maturation is relatively more advanced at birth and the capacity for uptake of colostral proteins is less than that seen in other mammals. Passive immunity, therefore, depends on the transplacental passage of IgG; very little immunoglobulin is absorbed by the gut (5). Studies do indicate, however, that increased quantities of macromolecules penetrate the intestinal epithelium even in the human neonate. Following ingestion of bovine serum albumin (BSA), detectable levels may be present in the serum of premature infants, unlike in older children given equivalent quantities of the protein (6). Serum from infants more often contains antibody to food antigens in the first three months of life than in later infancy, again suggesting that proteins are more readily absorbed at that time (7). Morphologic studies on both monkey and human fetal intestine (8, 9) have produced evidence that the epithelial cells of the immature gut take up significant quantities of antigen. In one study, human α-lactalbumin, which is the predominant whey protein of human milk (molecular weight 14,000), was used as a marker of macromolecular absorption; in breast-fed infants, the serum concentration was highest in preterm infants and decreased progressively with increasing maturity in term infants (10). Enhanced uptake of macromolecules may be an important factor in creating a predisposition to a number of gastrointestinal disorders that characteristically occur in early life, such as necrotizing enterocolitis and food-sensitive enteropathies.

A smaller capacity for macromolecular absorption remains even in the fully mature gastrointestinal tract. In vitro studies have demonstrated the uptake of macromolecules by mature intestinal epithelial cells (11). Injection of insulin into isolated loops of adult rat small intestine induces hypoglycemia, indicating intact absorption (12). Clear evidence exists that adult human subjects also absorb antigen; both antigen and specific antibodies can be detected in the serum of individuals fed egg albumin, and 15% to 30% of normal adults develop an antibody response following ingestion of cow's milk (13, 14).

MECHANISMS OF ANTIGEN UPTAKE

A number of pathways may permit or facilitate the uptake of macromolecules. The relative importance of these mechanisms is uncertain and may vary depending on the specific antigen and on the state of gut maturity.

Enterocyte Transcellular Uptake

The lamina propria is separated from the intestinal lumen by a single layer of epithelial cells connected by relatively impermeable tight junctions. This physical barrier is not totally impervious to macromolecules, however. In the small intestine of fetal (8, 9), neonatal (15), and adult (11, 16) mammals, the enterocyte has been shown to have a capacity to take up macromolecules by endocytosis (Fig. 5.1). Molecules within the lumen contact and interact with the surface of the microvillus membrane of the cell (adsorption). The apical membrane then invaginates to form a pit whose cytoplasmic surface is coated with clathrin, a protein that plays an important role in budding and fusion of membrane vesicles and that promotes the endocytosis of luminal receptors (17). Membrane-bound cytoplasmic vesicles (phagosomes) containing the macromolecules are surrounded by a clathrin lattice and then formed (11, 18). This process is energy-dependent, being suppressed by inhibitors of glycolysis and oxidative phosphorylation (19). The phagosomes may fuse with lysosomes, and antigen digestion may occur within these large vacuoles. Small quantities of undigested or partially digested antigen may then undergo exocytosis at the basolateral cell membrane and thus enter the interstitial space.

Direct morphological and physiological evidence indicates that nonspecific transport of macromolecules across the intestinal epithelium can occur. Studies in the rat have demonstrated transcellular passage of horseradish peroxidase (HRP), a marker molecule that can be detected histochemically via light or electron microscopy. When HRP was injected into ligated segments of rat intestine, it could be detected on the surface of the enterocyte, within membrane-bound cytoplasmic structures, in the intercellular spaces between enterocytes, and in the lamina propria (11). When HRP was infused into the intestine, uptake into the cells and into the intercellular spaces and lamina propria again occurred. In addition, significant amounts of HRP were transmitted to the intestinal lymphatics and portal bloodstream (20). Uptake of various macromolecules—including HRP and BSA—proceeds more efficiently in the young animal, and diminishes with age and maturation (21–23).

Uptake of macromolecules may also occur along pathways that depend on specific surface receptors. In many mammals, IgG present in milk can be absorbed intact through a process mediated by an Fc receptor similar to that facilitating transplacental passage of maternal antibody to the fetus (25). Binding of IgG to the receptor is promoted by the acid pH of the gut lumen, followed by invagination and endocytosis. Because the cytoplasmic vesicles formed are acidic, the complexes remain intact during transport through the cell. Following exocytosis at the basolateral membrane, the receptor releases its antibody in the non-acid environment of the interstitial compartment (Fig. 5.1) (4, 25, 26).

The physiological significance of the intact uptake of other macromolecules is less clear, however. Epidermal growth factor (EGF) has emerged as a regulatory peptide that almost certainly influences the regulation of growth, regeneration, and repair in the gastrointestinal tract (27). It is present in high

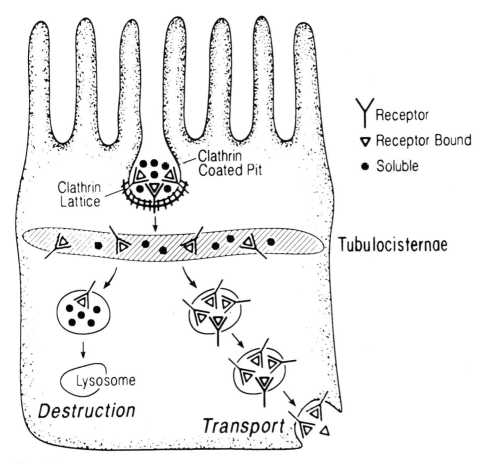

Figure 5.1

Endocytosis of macromolecules by the enterocyte. The plasma membrane between the microvilli invaginates to form vesicles. Clathrin, a protein that forms a membrane lattice, controls the curvature of the membrane. Macromolecules can enter the vesicle bound to the surrounding membrane by their own receptors or by nonspecific attraction; they can also enter free in solution. After entry, the macromolecules move to the tubulocisternae, where they are sorted and pass either to vesicles that travel toward the lysosome or to vesicles that traverse the cell to the basolateral pole. (From Figure 1 in Sanderson IR, Walker WA. Gastroenterology 1993;104:622–639.)

concentration relative to plasma in various gastrointestinal secretions, including saliva, gastric juice, and bile, as well as in milk. Not surprisingly, this finding has led to the suggestion that EGF may act directly on the mucosa from the gut lumen. The EGF receptor may be expressed primarily on the basolateral membrane, however, which suggests that EGF would have to cross the intestinal epithelium to bind with it (28, 29). Similarly, speculation has grown about the intact uptake of other regulatory peptides. Thus, nerve growth factor found in saliva and human milk is theorized to cross the intestinal epithelium (30).

Microfold (M) Cell Uptake

Peyer's patches consist of organized collections of lymphoid follicles in the small intestine. These

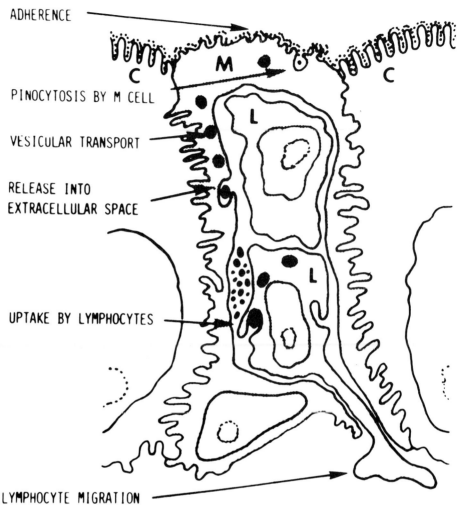

Figure 5.2

M cell after adherence and endocytosis. Macromolecules need to travel only a short distance from the apical surface to the basal pole, where they are released close to immune cells that have migrated into a "pocket" at the basal surface of the M cells. (From Owen RL. Gastroenterology 1977;72:440–451.)

lymphoid aggregates extend through the mucosa and into the submucosa, being most abundant in the distal ileum. Peyer's patches are thought to act as sampling sites for intestinal antigens; as such, they play an essential role in the initiation and expression of mucosal immunity (31) (Fig. 5.2). Primed precursor lymphocytes pass to the blood via the lymphatic system and may then migrate to other components

of the gut-associated lymphoid tissue (GALT), including the lamina propria and the intraepithelial lymphoid cell populations (IEL) (31, 32).

The epithelium overlying Peyer's patches consists of specialized cells known as microfold (or M) cells (33, 34). The luminal surface of each M cell lacks the well-developed microvilli and glycocalyx that are characteristic of the enterocyte, instead possessing irregular surface convolutions, or microfolds, that contain numerous vesicles. The M cell also differs from the enterocyte in that it is deficient in lysosomes and does not secrete IgA. M cells represent an important physiological pathway for the uptake of macromolecules from the gut lumen. They utilize the processes of endocytosis, transcellular trafficking, and exocytosis of antigens into the interstitium of the lymphoid follicle (35). Molecules that adhere to the cell surface are transported more efficiently, however. Thus, cationized BSA is absorbed much more efficiently than the unmodified protein because it adheres more readily to the luminal surface of the M cell (36). Moreover, uptake of the marker molecule ferritin is enhanced if it is first complexed with hydroxyapatite, a process that generates increased IgA production in response to this antigen (37). In addition to such nonspecific adherence, receptor-mediated binding to the surface of the M cell may possibly occur. As a result, certain infectious agents such as reovirus bind selectively to the M cell (38). The mechanisms involved in antigen uptake may also vary. Poliovirus is taken up in clathrin-coated vesicles (39). In contrast, the vesicles implicated in reovirus uptake do not appear to contain clathrin (38).

Paracellular Uptake

In recent years, it has become apparent that, in addition to water and electrolytes, large solutes can sometimes cross the gut epithelium through the paracellular route (40). The intercellular tight junction normally prevents the passage of macromolecules such as HRP. Sodium-coupled glucose transport can alter the barrier properties of the tight junctions, however, allowing peptides up to 11 amino acids in length to be absorbed between adjacent cells (41). The biological significance of this phenomenon is not clear, but peptides of this size are known to act as potent immunogens.

Closure

In most species, intestinal maturation results in a progressive diminution of dietary antigen uptake. This decrease in macromolecular penetration is referred to as "closure." It is seen most typically in the ruminant mammalian species in which bulk intestinal

absorption of intact proteins occurs during the early days of life, followed by a sudden and pronounced decrease in uptake (3, 42). In the neonatal rat, the receptor-mediated process of IgG uptake ceases abruptly about 21 days after birth (4), the result of a reduction in expression of the enterocyte Fc receptor gene (43).

Roberton *et al.* failed to detect bovine β-lactoglobulin in the serum of milk-fed term human neonates, and they concluded that gut closure was complete at birth (44). Unlike the ruminant species, however, it appears that closure in the human infant is a more subtle process. As discussed previously, various studies have shown increased antigen uptake in early infancy and a gradual reduction thereafter (7, 10). Jakobsson *et al.* found, for example, that the rise in serum concentration of human α-lactalbumin that could be detected in infants after a milk feed diminished progressively during the first eight weeks of life (10). These changes presumably reflect a progressive maturation of certain components of the "mucosal barrier."

The Mucosal Barrier

Intestinal absorption of macromolecules is limited by a variety of factors (45). These factors include various gastrointestinal secretions, the propulsive activity of the gut, the properties of the mucosal epithelium, and the mucosal immune system. Evidence suggests that the liver may act as a second line of protection against foreign antigens that do succeed in penetrating the mucosal barrier.

NONIMMUNOLOGIC COMPONENTS OF THE MUCOSAL BARRIER

Macromolecular Digestion

It has been recognized for many years that, in patients with lactase deficiency states, lactosuria is often demonstrable due to increased absorption of unhydrolyzed disaccharide (46). Much evidence exists that uptake of antigens may be similarly increased in the absence of normal luminal proteolytic activity. Increased levels of antibodies to BSA (a common food antigen) have been reported in adults with gastric achlorhydria (47). Increased uptake of BSA was demonstrated in rats that were fed this marker molecule in combination with bicarbonate so as to neutralize gastric acid (48). These observations suggest that, in the presence of adequate acid secretion, hydrolysis may limit the amount of intact protein available for absorption.

The proteolytic enzymes secreted by the exocrine pancreas also reduce intestinal uptake of intact protein. The results of various studies support this important role for luminal proteases. Thus, a patient with diabetes mellitus and pancreatic exocrine deficiency following pancreatectomy may respond to enteral administration of insulin with a fall in blood glucose, while no such response appears in a similarly treated subject with normal pancreatic function (49). Intragastric administration of lysine vasopressin and the trypsin inhibitor aprotinin was reported to result in an antidiuretic response in rats, while administration without aprotinin had no such effect (50).

In vitro studies have demonstrated that mucosal antigen uptake may be reduced in previously immunized animals compared with controls; it has also been shown that antigen–antibody complexes on the surface of the intestine are more rapidly degraded by local proteases (51). Studies were, therefore, carried out to determine the possible role of pancreatic enzymes in the degradation of antigen–antibody complexes on the surface of the small intestine (52). The breakdown of ^{125}I-labeled BSA in isolated intestinal sacs prepared from rats subjected to pancreatic duct ligation was significantly decreased in BSA-immunized animals. Moreover, if these duct-ligated animals were fed pancreatic enzyme prior to removal of the small intestine, digestion of ^{125}I-BSA in the gut sacs was enhanced. These findings led to the suggestion that pancreatic enzymes adsorbed to the mucosal surface contributed to the proteolysis of antigen–antibody complexes at this site.

In infants, gastric acid secretion is reduced in the first four weeks of life, especially in the premature infant (53). A slight reduction in pancreatic protease secretion has been noted in the full-term infant at birth (54). Immaturity of digestive processes may partially explain the enhanced antigen uptake that occurs in early infancy.

Mucus Secretion

Mucus provides a viscous coating on the mucosal surface of the gut and is believed to constitute an important component of the mucosal barrier (55). The organic constituents of this secretion consist mainly of mucin glycoproteins. These glycoproteins, in turn, consist of a protein core with carbohydrate side chains that constitute as much as 80% of the total molecular weight (56). The side chains, which consist of 2 to 22 monosaccharide units, are each linked to the protein core by an N-acetylgalactosamine. Mucin glycoproteins are a heterogenous group of substances that vary greatly, particularly with regard to the exact composition of their carbohydrate side chains. They are synthesized in the endoplasmic reticulum of mucosal goblet cells and, after packaging in the Golgi apparatus, they are secreted from the cell apex. Mucus acts as a lubricant and as a protective barrier against physical and chemical injury (55). In the presence of irritants, mucus secretion increases, with the thickness of the protective coat growing (56, 57, 58).

Evidence suggests that the protective properties of the mucus layer derive not only from its viscous nature, but also from its capacity to inhibit antigen and microorganism attachment to the microvillus membrane (56) (Fig. 5.3). Adherence of microorganisms to specific carbohydrate binding sites on the membrane appears to be essential to their pathogenicity (59). Lectin binding studies have shown that similar attachment to mucin glycoproteins occurs (60). The carbohydrate moieties of these glycoproteins provide specific binding sites for both macromolecules and microorganisms, and may competitively inhibit their attachment to membrane receptors.

Differences exist in the physical properties and chemical composition of mucin in the adult and neonatal small intestine. For example, mucin from the small intestine of the newborn rat differs from that of the adult in its buoyant density in CsCl and its mobility on SDS-PAGE (60). In the newborn rat, the mucin glycoproteins have a reduced carbohydrate content and a relatively low proportion of fucose and N-acetylgalactosamine residues (56, 60). The relevance of these observations to the functional proper-

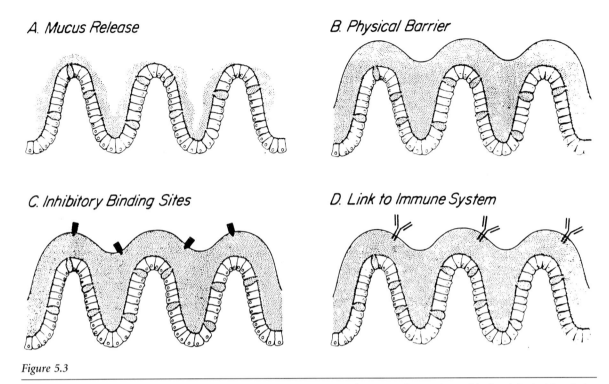

A. Mucus Release

B. Physical Barrier

C. Inhibitory Binding Sites

D. Link to Immune System

Figure 5.3

Four proposed mechanisms for mucus protection: rate and quantity of mucus release; viscous blanket (physical barrier); competitive binding sites; and link to the intestinal immune system. (From Snyder JD, Walker WA. Int Arch Allergy Appl Immunol 1981;82:351.)

ties of mucin in the immature animal is not yet clear. Evidence suggests that mucin from the neonatal rat intestine may bind cholera toxin more effectively than mucin from the adult rat (61).

Motility

Intestinal peristaltic activity likely plays an important role in limiting antigen, toxin, and microbial adherence to the microvillus membrane. In the postprandial state, persistent but irregular contractile activity in the intestine facilitates the mixing of luminal contents. The fasting state is characterized by periodic "migrating myoelectric complexes" (MMC). These complexes are associated with coordinated waves of contractile activity that migrate down the small intestine at intervals of about 90 to 120 minutes (62, 63). These waves are associated with the aboral propulsion of luminal contents (64), which may be important in

the control of bacterial overgrowth (62). The MMC has been termed the "housekeeper" of the gastrointestinal tract, with its regular propulsive waves being envisaged as clearing food residue from the small intestine following a period of digestion and absorption (65). Macromolecular and bacterial diffusion through the mucus coat and subsequent adherence to the microvillus membrane may, therefore, decline as the result of the gut's motor activity.

Studies of the ontogeny of motor activity in the preterm infant have been performed by simultaneously observing changes in intraluminal pressure at several sites along the small intestine using a multilumen perfused tube manometric apparatus (66). These studies demonstrated that motor activity is poorly developed prior to 30 weeks' gestation, but that greater pressures are generated and the contractions are propagated distally with increasing frequency as post-conceptual age grows. With advancing maturity comes a developmental progression from random to highly organized motor activity, similar to the pattern seen in older individuals. These changes presumably reflect maturation of myogenic, neural, and humoral elements in the gut during infancy. It is noteworthy that gastrointestinal motility is reduced in ill infants exposed to stresses such as hypoxia or septicemia. Immature or disordered motility patterns in the gut may, therefore, represent an important factor in increased antigen uptake.

The Intestinal Epithelium

The microvillus membrane of the enterocyte is relatively impermeable to the passage of macromolecules. In comparison with the basolateral membrane, it has distinctive physical and chemical characteristics. It is wider and has a higher protein, glycolipid, and cholesterol content (67, 68). The glycocalyx—a glycoprotein layer secreted by the enterocyte—adheres firmly to the outer surface of the microvilli and therefore forms an integral part of the cell membrane. In addition to the range of digestive enzymes included in the enterocyte, its surface membrane incorporates various specific carbohydrate moieties, as discussed earlier, which facilitate the adherence of certain microorganisms and macromolecules (59). Intact proteins that successfully penetrate the microvillus membrane by the process of endocytosis may undergo degradation by lysosomal enzymes as previously described.

The structure and composition of the microvillus membrane undergoes a number of changes during postnatal development that may influence its barrier properties. With maturation its protein/lipid ratio increases and the fluidity of the membrane decreases (69). Developmental differences also appear to exist in the binding of macromolecules and microorganisms to the membrane glycoproteins. Studies have demonstrated striking changes in the accessibility, distribution, and composition of their carbohydrate binding sites during maturation (69, 70). Maturation of the membrane, as indicated by increased structural organization and enhanced binding of lectins, may be induced by prenatal exposure to cortisone, supporting the suggestion that endogenous glucocorticoids may play an important role in mediating maturation of the mucosal barrier (71).

IMMUNOLOGIC COMPONENTS OF THE MUCOSAL BARRIER

In spite of the many nonimmunologic mechanisms restricting the uptake of macromolecules, some penetration of the mucosal epithelium occurs. As a result, the underlying tissues are exposed to significant quantities of antigen.

Antigen–GALT Interactions

Following antigenic stimulation, lymphocytes within Peyer's patches are activated and migrate via the lymphatics to the mesenteric lymph nodes. They are then transported via the lymphatic system to the systemic circulation. These activated cells home to various sites of mucosa-associated lymphoid tissue, with an especially high selectivity for the GALT. This process distributes specifically sensitized lymphoid cells throughout the lamina propria, as well as to the IEL compartment. These specifically sensitized cells are, therefore, located at sites that could facilitate their interaction with absorbed antigen. The GALT usually respond to foreign antigens in a manner that reduces their potentially harmful effects. Moreover, antigen-specific immunological responses may assist in limiting antigen uptake. The enteral administration of an antigenic substance may lead to various immunological responses. Most frequently, a state of "oral tolerance" is induced, but a local secretory IgA antibody response may also occur; only rarely does the process lead to a state of systemic immune sensitization (72).

Oral tolerance refers to the phenomenon whereby enteric exposure to an antigen induces a state of specific immunological unresponsiveness (72) (see also chapters 1 and 6). This condition has been noted in a wide range of animal species. Oral tolerance is most easily induced by soluble antigens, while administration of live allogeneic cells or virus tends to evoke both local and systemic immune responses. IgE and delayed-type hypersensitivity may be effectively tolerized by feeding of protein antigens, but these types of immune responses are most often considered important in food intolerance (72).

The unique ability of the M cell to transport macromolecules facilitates the role of Peyer's patches as sampling sites for luminal antigens. Although studies using HRP have demonstrated efficient uptake of this marker protein by M cells (as described earlier), exposure of the mucosa to higher concentrations of HRP has resulted in significant uptake by the enterocyte. Despite the avidity with which the M cell transports antigen, its total absorptive surface is small compared with that of the mucosal surface as a whole. The relative importance of these two uptake pathways may ultimately depend on the quantity of luminal antigen.

The Enterocyte as an Antigen-presenting Cell

Although Peyer's patches are clearly involved in the regulation of immune responses, several factors suggest that the villus enterocyte may also play a role in modulating the immune response to luminal antigens (73). Enterocytes are involved in the assembly and transport of secretory IgA and IgM (discussed below). They may also have the capacity to influence T-cell responses. Stimulation of helper T cells by foreign antigens depends on specialized antigen-presenting cells (APCs), including macrophages, B cells, and dendritic cells. Such APCs can endocytose and partially digest foreign proteins. Resultant peptide fragments are then bound to specialized glycoproteins—the major histocompatibility complex (MHC) class II molecules. These peptide–glycoprotein complexes are then transported to the cell surface, where they become available for presentation to the T-cell receptor. Enterocytes possess lysosomal enzymes capable of digesting proteins, and studies have shown MHC class II expression within intracellular organelles and on enterocytes' basolateral membranes. The cells of the IEL compartment are located between the basolateral surfaces of epithelial cells above the basal lamina.

These findings support the concept of antigen uptake by the enterocyte at its luminal surface, interaction of peptide products and class II MHC molecules within cytosolic organelles, and transport of the complex to the basolateral membrane where presentation to T cells of the IEL compartment might occur. These T cells are predominantly of the suppressor phenotype, and they may play an immunoregulatory role by suppressing the systemic immune response to antigens (74–76). In vitro studies have shown that rat and human enterocytes can, indeed, present soluble protein antigens to specifically primed T cells (75–

77). Surprisingly, class II-restricted presentation of antigen by enterocytes in these in vitro systems (which was expected to induce CD4+ helper T cells) activated CD8+ suppressor/cytotoxic T cells. This finding creates interest in view of the predominantly suppressor phenotype of the IEL T cells.

Secretory Immunoglobulin A (sIgA)

As much as 90% of B cells and plasma cells in the lamina propria have been shown by immunofluorescence techniques to stain positively for IgA antibody (31). The plasma cells of the lamina propria secrete IgA in a dimeric form, with the monomers being joined by a polypeptide J-chain. This dimer is then transported across the intestinal epithelial cell in association with a glycoprotein receptor found on the basolateral membrane that is known as secretory component (SC) or polyimmunoglobulin receptor. IgA is released from the epithelial cell via exocytosis and enters the gut lumen, where it maintains its association with SC. This complex (sIgA) is resistant to degradation by pancreatic proteases.

It is postulated that sIgA may play a role in limiting the uptake of antigens through the formation of immune complexes. In patients with selective IgA deficiency, high titers of antibodies directed against milk and other food antigens have been described (78, 79). In some of these IgA-deficient subjects, immune complexes containing casein and BSA can be detected in the circulation shortly after milk ingestion (80). In addition, associations have been reported between selective IgA deficiency and both coeliac disease and various allergic disorders (81). Evidence suggests that both oral and parenteral immunization with specific antigens may reduce their intestinal uptake (82, 83). Local antibodies can inhibit the absorption of soluble protein antigens by decreasing their adherence to intestinal epithelial cells. A similar effect has been demonstrated in studies in which IgA and soluble antigen were infused into the small intestine (84).

Although IgA is the predominant immunoglobulin found in intestinal secretions, other immunoglobulin classes may also play a significant role in regulating antigen uptake. Some patients with sIgA deficiency suffer from recurrent infections involving mucosal surfaces, and allergic disorders are also common; nevertheless, most such individuals remain asymptomatic (81). In some cases of sIgA deficiency, SC-linked IgM has been detected in saliva (81, 85). The salivary glands may contain large numbers of IgM-positive (rather than IgA-positive) plasma cells (86).

The GALT is not fully developed at birth (87, 88). Rather, a deficiency of immunoglobulin-containing cells is noted in the gut of newborn infants up to the age of 12 days (87). IgA is the last of the immunoglobulin classes to develop, and mucosal concentrations do not reach adult levels for several months (43, 89). This relative sIgA deficiency may contribute to the increased permeability to foreign proteins in early life.

Other Immunoglobulin Classes

Other antibody isotypes may also play an important role in controlling antigen uptake. Maternal IgG, which is acquired by transplacental uptake, may limit the absorption of enteric antigens in infant rabbits (90). It is unclear whether IgG acts by restricting uptake of specific antigens at the mucosal surface or by facilitating antigen clearance through the formation of immune complexes (91). In contrast, some experimental evidence suggests that IgG antibodies to luminal antigens may produce the opposite effect, causing increased penetration of the mucosal barrier (92).

In addition, IgE may influence the development of the mucosal barrier, as it has been shown that anaphylaxis induces goblet secretion of mucus (57). In rodents, dietary antigens enhance mucus secretion if the animal has been previously sensitized by oral immunization (93). Mucin secretion also increases following instillation of soluble immune complexes, which may facilitate their clearance from the gut lumen (94).

HEPATIC DEFENSES

The liver is an important site of phagocytosis, with 30% of its mass being composed of reticuloendothelial cells (95). Hepatic macrophages have been shown to reduce the immunogenicity of antigens, while splenic or lymph node macrophages enhance it (96). In studies in which rats with hepatic cirrhosis received injections of radio-labeled antigen, hepatic uptake was reduced, splenic uptake was increased, and enhanced antibody production occurred (97). Both the humoral and cellular responses to antigens injected into the portal circulation were shown to differ from the response to the same antigen injected into the inferior vena cava (98). Animals subjected to portacaval shunt procedures often develop hyperglobulinemia (99). The hepatic sinusoidal phagocytes have been demonstrated to possess the capacity to clear immune complexes from both the systemic and portal blood (100).

The liver also has the capacity to transport polymeric IgA from the serum into the bile (101–103). This transport system may aid in removing absorbed circulating antigen by returning it to the intestine as an IgA–antigen complex (91). IgA is poorly opsonic, and does not fix complement (85). Elimination of potentially harmful antigen may, therefore, be achieved by IgA immune complex formation, thereby preventing the initiation of immune-mediated inflammatory reactions and their associated tissue damage. Substantial evidence indicates that the liver may act as a second line of defense against the potentially injurious effects of absorbed dietary antigens.

THE INFLUENCE OF BREAST MILK

Dietary antigens, including wheat and various bovine milk proteins, have been identified in human milk (104, 105). Several studies have indicated that maternal dietary proteins transferred to breast milk may be responsible for infant colitis (105, 106). During the period in early life when potentially excessive uptake of antigen may occur, colostrum may provide important passive protection at the mucosal surface (Fig. 5.4). Human colostrum contains predominantly sIgA, which may assist in immune exclusion (107). It may limit contact between ingested antigen and the intestinal mucosa by binding to it in the gut lumen. As discussed previously, factors in milk such as EGF may also facilitate maturation of the mucosal surface (108, 109). Studies from the authors' laboratory have demonstrated decreased uptake of antigen from the gut of infant rabbits fed on breast milk compared with bottle-fed animals at one week of age (110). This finding may reflect accelerated maturation of

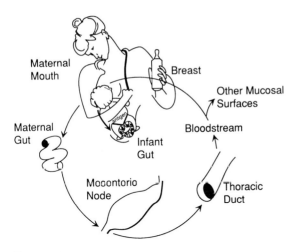

Figure 5.4

Dietary antigen entering the maternal gut reaches lymphoid follicles through specialized transport cells (M cells). This antigen commits the lymphoblasts to specific IgA production, and these then migrate via mesenteric nodes and thoracic duct into the systemic circulation. During the periods of proper hormonal stimulation, such cells populate the breast and secrete serum IgA, which then is ingested by and functions in the infant. T cells, B cells, and macrophages also are extruded into the breast milk and are immunologically active. (Reprinted, with permission, from Kleinman RE, Walker WA. The enteromammary immune system: an important new concept in breast milk host defense. Dig Dis Sci 1979;24:876.)

the mucosal barrier under the influence of breast milk and may serve to restrict systemic exposure to antigens.

Antigen Absorption in Disease States

Regulated intestinal absorption of foreign antigens is necessary for the development and maintenance of the normal protective immune responses. The intestinal barrier is incompletely developed in premature infants, which may contribute to the high incidence of necrotizing enterocolitis in this group. Corticosteroids are known to accelerate intestinal maturation, and a rat model of necrotizing enterocolitis has provided evidence that prenatal administration of cortisone can reduce intestinal uptake of ovalbumin, bacterial translocation, and mortality (111). Antigen

uptake is facilitated by adherence to enterocytes, and this process appears to occur more readily with immature cells (112). In many enteropathies, including viral gastroenteritis, enterocytes are replaced by immature crypt cells. Antigen absorption apparently increases in patients with various intestinal disorders, and the effects of intestinal pathology on paracellular uptake merits further investigation (113). Such mechanisms may underlie the development of allergic gastroenteropathies following episodes of infective gastroenteritis (113).

In recent years, interest has focused on the importance of the phenomenon known as "translocation" whereby bacteria and bacterial endotoxins may cross the intestinal barrier and enter the lymphatics and the circulation in seriously ill patients (114, 115). This process represents a major failure of the intestinal mucosal barrier and may lead to sepsis and multiorgan failure.

Conclusion

Small, but biologically significant quantities of antigen are normally absorbed intact from the intestinal lumen, although only a minority of individuals suffer untoward consequences from this contact. A complex interaction of factors, collectively constituting the "mucosal barrier," limits and regulates antigen uptake and modulates their effects. In infancy, increased quantities of foreign antigens penetrate the relatively immature barrier. This penetration is probably important in the predisposition to disorders such as necrotizing enterocolitis and food-sensitive enteropathies in early life. Breast milk appears to possess factors that protect the individual during this period of increased vulnerability.

REFERENCES

1. Sanderson IR, Walker WA. Uptake and transport of macromolecules by the intestine: possible role in clinical disorders (an update). Gastroenterology 1993;104:622–639.
2. Bahna SL. Pathogenesis of milk hypersensitivity. Immunology Today 1985;6:153–154.
3. Morris IG. Gamma globulin absorption in the newborn. In: Code CF, ed. Handbook of physiology. Alimentary canal, vol. 2. Washington, DC: American Physiological Society, 1968.
4. Borthistle BK, Kubo RT, Brown WR, Gray HM. Studies on

receptors for IgG on epithelial cells of the rat intestine. J Immunol 1977;119:471–476.

5. Leissring JC, Anderson JW, Smith DW. Uptake of antibodies by the intestine of the newborn infant. Am J Dis Child 1962;103:160–165.

6. Rothberg RM. Immunoglobulin and specific antibody synthesis during the first weeks of life in premature infants. J Pediatr 1969;75:391–399.

7. Eastham EJ, Lichauco T, Grady MI, Walker WA. Antigenicity of infant formulas: role of immature intestine in protein permeability. J Pediatr 1978;93:561–564.

8. Lev R, Orlic D. Uptake of proteins in swallowed amniotic fluid by monkey fetal intestine in utero. Gastroenterology 1973;65:60–68.

9. Moxey PC, Trier JS. Structural features of the mucosa of human fetal small intestine. Gastroenterology 1975;68:1002–1009.

10. Jakobsson I, Lindberg T, Lothe L, Axelsson I, Benediktsson B. Human α-lactalbumin as a marker of macromolecular absorption. Gut 1986;27:1029–1034.

11. Cornell R, Walker WA, Isselbacher KJ. Small intestinal absorption of horseradish peroxidase. A cytochemical study. Lab Invest 1971;25:42–48.

12. Danforth E, Moore RD. Intestinal absorption of insulin in the rat. Endocrinology 1959;65:118–126.

13. Wilson SJ, Walzer M. Absorption of undigested proteins in human beings. Am J Dis Child 1935;50:49–57.

14. Korenblat RE, Rothberg RM, Minden P. Immune responses of human adults after oral and parenteral exposure to bovine serum albumin. J Allergy 1968;41:226–235.

15. Clark SL. The ingestion of proteins and colloidal materials by columnar absorptive cells of the small intestine in suckling rats and mice. J Biophys Biochem Cytol 1959;5:41–50.

16. Casley-Smith JR. The passage of ferritin into jejunal epithelial cells. Experentia 1967;23:370–371.

17. North RJ. Endocytosis. Semin Hematol 1970;7:161–171.

18. Brodsky FM. Living with clathrin: its role in intracellular membrane traffic. Science 1984;242:1396–1402.

19. Lecce JG. In Vitro absorption of δ-globulin, by neonatal intestinal epithelium of the pig. J Physiol 1966; 184: 594–604

20. Warshaw AL, Walker WA, Cornell R, Isselbacher KJ. Small intestinal permeability to macromolecules: transmission of horseradish peroxidase into mesenteric lymph and portal blood. Lab Invest 1971;25:675–684.

21. Bamford DR. Studies in vitro of the passage of serum proteins across the intestinal wall of young rats. Proc R Soc Lond (Biol) 1966;166:30–45.

22. Udall JN, Pang K, Fritze L, Kleinman R, Walker WA. Development of gastrointestinal mucosal barrier. I. The effect of age on intestinal permeability to macromolecules. Pediatr Res 1981;15:241–244.

23. Teichberg S, Isolauri E, Wapnir RA, Roberts B, Lifschitz F. Development of the neonatal rat small intestinal barrier to nonspecific macromolecular absorption: effect of early weaning to artificial diets. Pediatr Res 1990;28:31–37.

24. Sedmak DD, Davis DH, Singh U, van de Winkel JG. Expression of IgG Fc receptor antigens in placenta and on endothelial cells in humans. An immunohistochemical study. Am J Pathol 1991;138:175–181.

25. Jones EA, Waldmann TA. The mechanism of intestinal uptake and transcellular transport of IgG in the newborn rat. J Clin Invest 1972;51:2916–2927.

26. Abrahamson DR, Rodewald R. Evidence for sorting of endocytic vesicle contents during the receptor-mediated transport of IgG across the newborn rat membrane. J Cell Biol 1981;91:270–280.

27. Marti U, Burwen SJ, Jones AL. Biological effects of epidermal growth factor, with emphasis on the gastrointestinal tract and liver: an update. Hepatology 1989;9:126–138.

28. Carpenter G. Epidermal growth factor is a major growth-promoting agent in human milk. Science 1980, 198–199.

29. Memard D, Potheir P. Radioautographic localization of epidermal growth factor receptors in human fetal gut. Gastroenterology 1991;1:640–649.

30. Siminoski K, Gonella P, Bernake J, Owen L, Neutra M, Murphy RA. Uptake and transepithelial transport of nerve growth factor in suckling rat ileum. J Cell Biol 1986;103:1979–1990.

31. Kagnoff MF. Immunology of the digestive system. In: Johnson LR, ed. Physiology of the gastrointestinal tract, 2nd ed. New York: Raven Press, 1987, 1699–1728.

32. Nagata H, Miyairi M, Seikizuka E, Morishita T, Tatemichi M, Miura S, Tsuchiya M. In vivo visualization of lymphatic microvessels and lymphocyte migration through rat Peyer's patches. Gastroenterology 1994;106:1548–1553.

33. Owen RL, Jones AL. Epithelial cell specialisation within human Peyer's patches: an ultrastructural study of intestinal lymphoid follicles. Gastroenterology 1974;66:189–203.

34. Owen RL, Nemiac P. Antigen processing structures of the mammalian intestinal tract: an SEM study of lymphoepithelial organs. In: Becker RP, Johari O, eds. Scanning electron microscopy/1978/II. AMF O'Hare, Ill.: Scanning Electron Microscopy, 1978, 367–378.

35. Owen RL. Sequential uptake of horseradish peroxidase by lymphoid follicle epithelium of Peyer's patches in the normal unobstructed mouse intestine: an ultrastructural study. Gastroenterology 1977;72:440–451.

36. Sanderson IR, Walker WA. Uptake and transport of macromolecules by the intestine: possible role in clinical disorders (an update). Gastroenterology 1993;104:622–639.

37. Amerongen MH, Weltzin RW, Mack JA, Winner LS, Michetti P, Apter FM, Kraehenbuhl JP, Neutra MR. M-cell mediated antigen transport and monoclonal IgA antibodies for mucosal immune protection. Ann Res NY Acad Sci 1992;664:18–26.

38. Wolf JL, Rubin DH, Finberg R, Kauffman S, Sharpe AH, Trier JS, Fields BN. Intestinal M cells: a pathway for entry of reovirus into the host. Science 1981;212:471–472.

39. Scinski P, Rowinski J, Wasrchol JB, Jarcabek Z, Gut W, Szczygie B, Bielecki K, Koch G. Poliovirus type 1 enters the human host through intestinal M cells. Gastroenterology 1990;98:56–58.

40. Madara JL. Pathobiology of the intestinal epithelial barrier. Am J Pathol 1990;137:1273–1281.

41. Atisook K, Madara JL. An oligopeptide permeates intestinal tight junctions at glucose-elicited dilatations. Implications for oligopeptide absorption. Gastroenterology 1991;100:719–724.

42. Kraehenbuhl JP, Campiche MA. Early stages of intestinal absorption of specific antibodies in the newborn. An ultrastructural, cytochemical, and immunological study in the pig, rat and rabbit. J Cell Biol 1969;42:345–360.

43. Simister N, Mostov KE. An Fc receptor structurally related to MHC class 1 antigens. Nature 1989;333:184–187.

44. Roberton DM, Paganelli R, Dinwiddie R, Levinsky RJ. Milk

antigen absorption in the preterm and term neonate. Arch Dis Child 1982;57:369–372.

45. Van Elburg RM, Uil JJ, de Monchy JG, Heymans HS. Intestinal permeability in pediatric gastroenterology. Scand J Gastroenterol 1992;194(suppl):19–24.

46. Gryboski JD, Thayer WR, Gabrielson IW, Spiro HM. Disacchariduria in gastrointestinal disease. Gastroenterol 1963;45: 633–637.

47. Kraft SC, Rothberg RM, Knauer CM, Svoboda AC, Monroe LS, Farr RS. Gastric acid output and circulating anti-bovine serum albumin in adults. Clin Exp Immunol 1967;2:231–236.

48. Bloch KJ, Bloch KB, Sterns M, Walker WA. Intestinal uptake of macromolecules. VI. Uptake of protein antigen in vivo in normal rats and rats infected with *Nippostrongylus brasiliensis* or subjected to mild systemic anaphylaxis. Gastroenterology 1979;77:1039–1044.

49. Crane CW, Lunt GR. Absorption of insulin from the human small intestine. Diabetes 1968;17:625–627.

50. Saffron M, Franco-Saenz R, Kong A, Papabadjopoulos D, Szoka F. A model for the study of oral administration of peptide hormones. Can J Bioch 1979;57:548–555.

51. Walker WA, Wu M, Isselbacher KJ, Bloch KJ. Intestinal uptake of macromolecules. III. Studies on the mechanism by which immunization interferes with antigen uptake. J Immunol 1975;115:854–861.

52. Walker WA, Wu M, Isselbacher KF, Bloch KJ. Intestinal uptake of macromolecules. IV. The effect of duct ligation on the breakdown of antigen and antigen–antibody complexes on the intestinal surface. Gastroenterology 1975;69:1223–1229.

53. Hyman PE, Clarke DD, Everett SL, Sonne B, Stewart D, Harada T, Walsh JH, Taylor IL. Gastric acid secretory function in preterm infants. J Pediatr 1985;106:467–471.

54. Lebenthal E, Lee PC. Development of functional response in human exocrine pancreas. Pediatrics 1980;66:556–560.

55. Allen A. Structure and function of gastrointestinal mucus. In: Johnson LR, ed. Physiology of the gastrointestinal tract. New York: Raven Press, 1981, 617–639.

56. Snyder JS, Walker WA. Structure and function of intestinal mucin: developmental aspects. Int Arch Allergy Appl Immunol 1987;82:351–356.

57. Lake AM, Bloch KJ, Sinclair KJ, Walker WA. Anaphylactic release of intestinal goblet cell mucus. Immunol 1980;39:173–178.

58. Miller HRP. Intestinal parasites. In: Chadwick VS, Philips SF, eds. Gastroenterology, vol. 2. Small intestine. London: Butterworth Scientific, 1982, 162–173.

59. Freter R. Mechanisms of association of bacteria with mucosal surfaces. In: Elliott K, O'Connor M, Whelan J, eds. Adhesion and microorganism pathogenicity. CIBA Foundation Symposium. London: Pitman Medical, 1981, 36–47.

60. Shub MD, Pang KY, Swann DA, Walker WA. Age-related changes in chemical composition and physical properties of mucus glycoproteins from rat small intestine. Biochem J 1983;215:405–411.

61. Snyder JD, Podolsky DK, Walker WA. The role of mucus in intestinal host defense: developmental differences in composition and binding to cholera toxin. Pediatr Res 1986;20:249.

62. Vantrappen G, Janssens J, Hellemans J, Ghoos Y. The interdigestive motor complex in normal subjects and patients with bacterial over-growth of the small intestine. J Clin Invest 1977;59:1158–1166.

63. Kerlin P, Phillips S. Variability of motility of the ileum and jejunum in healthy humans. Gastroenterology 1982;82:694–700.

64. Schemann M, Ehrlein H-J. Mechanical characteristics of phase II and phase III of the interdigestive migrating motor complex in dogs. Gastroenterology 1986;91:117–123.

65. Kerlin P, Zinsmeister A, Philips S. Relationship of motility to flow of contents in the human small intestine. Gastroenterology 1982;82:701–706.

66. Bisset WM, Watt JB, Rivers RPA, Milla PJ. The ontogeny of small intestinal motor activity. Pediatr Res 1986;20:692.

67. Douglas AP, Kerley R, Isselbacher KJ. Preparation and characterization of the lateral and basal plasma membranes of rat intestinal epithelial cell. Biochem J 1972;128:1329–1338.

68. Glickman RM, Bouhours JF. Characterization and distribution and biosynthesis of the major ganglioside of rat intestinal mucosa. Biochim Biophys Acta 1976;424:17–25.

69. Pang KY, Bresson JL, Walker WA. Development of the gastrointestinal mucosal barrier. Evidence for structural differences in microvillus membranes from newborn and adult rabbits. Biochim Biophys Acta 1983;727:201–208.

70. Pang KY, Walker WA. Differential effect of *Ulex europeus* (UEA) on microvillus membrane MVM from immature and immature rats. J Cell Biol 1982;95:270A.

71. Pang KY, Newman AP, Udall JN, Walker WA. Development of the gastrointestinal mucosal barrier. VII. In utero maturation of microvillus surface by cortisone. Am J Physiol 1985;249:G85–G91.

72. Mowat AMI. The regulation of immune responses to dietary protein antigens. Immunology Today 1987;8:93–98.

73. Bland P. MHC class II expression by the gut epithelium. Immunology Today 1988;9:174–178.

74. Bland PW, Warren LG. Antigen presentation by epithelial cells of the rat small intestine. I. Kinetics, antigen specificity and blocking by anti-Ia antisera. Immunology 1986;58:1–7.

75. Bland PW, Warren LG. Antigen presentation by epithelial cells of the rat small intestine. II. Selective induction of suppressor T cells. Immunology 1986;56:9–14.

76. Dobbins WO. Human intestinal intraepithelial lymphocytes. Gut 1986;27:972–985.

77. Meyer L, Schlien B. Evidence for function of Ia molecules on gut epithelial cells in man. J Exp Med 1987;166:1471–1483.

78. Huntley CC, Robbins JB, Lyerly AD, Buckley RH. Characterization of precipitating antibodies to ruminant serum and milk proteins in humans with selective IgA deficiency. New Engl J Med 1971;284:7–10.

79. Cunningham-Rundles C, Brandeis WE, Good RA, Day NK. Milk precipitins, circulating immune complexes and IgA deficiency. Proc Natl Acad Sci 1978;75:3387–3389.

80. Cunningham-Rundles C, Brandeis WE, Good RA, Day NK. Bovine antigens and the formation of circulating immune complexes in selective immunoglobulin A deficiency. J Clin Invest 1979;64:272–279.

81. Morgan G, Levinsky RJ. Clinical significance of IgA deficiency. Arch Dis Child 1988;63:579–581.

82. Walker WA, Isselbacher KJ, Bloch KJ. Intestinal uptake of macromolecules: effect of oral immunization. Science 1972;177:608–610.

83. Walker WA, Isselbacher KJ, Bloch KJ. Intestinal uptake of macromolecules. II. Effect of parenteral immunization. J Immunol 1973;111:221–226.

84. Andre C, Lambert R, Bazin H, Heremans JF. Interference of

oral immunization with the intestinal absorption of heterologous albumin. Eur J Immunol 1974;4:701–704.

85. Mestecky J, Russell MW, Jackson S, Brown TA. The human IgA system: a reassessment. Clin Immunol Immunopath 1986;40:105–114.

86. Brandtzaeg P. Human secretory immunoglobulin M. An immunochemical and immunohistochemical study. Immunology 1975;29:559–570.

87. Perkkiö M, Savilahti E. Time of appearance of immunoglobulin containing cells in the mucosa of the neonatal intestine. Pediatr Res 1980;14:953–955.

88. Cummins AG, Steele TW, LaBrooy JT, Shearman DJC. Maturation of the rat small intestine at weaning: changes in epithelial cell kinetics, bacterial flora, and mucosal immune activity. Gut 1988;29:1672–1679.

89. Ogra PL, Yamanaka T, Kaul TN, Fishaut JM. Development of mucosal immunity during the perinatal period. In: Lebenthal E, ed. Textbook of gastroenterology and nutrition in infancy, vol. I. New York: Raven Press, 1981, 211–218.

90. Kleinman RE, Harmatz PR, Jacobson LA, Udall JN, Bloch KJ, Walker WA. Passive transplacental immunization: influence on the detection of enteric antigen in the systemic circulation. Ped Res 1983;17:449–451.

91. Kleinman RE, Walker WA. Antigen processing and uptake from the intestinal tract. Clin Rev Allergy 1984;2:25–37.

92. Brandtzaeg P, Tolo K. Mucosal penetrability enhanced by serum-derived antibodies. Nature 1977;266:262–263.

93. Lake AM, Bloch KJ, Neutra MR, Walker WA. Intestinal goblet cell mucus release. II. In vivo stimulation by antigen in the immunized rat. J Immunol 1979;122:834–837.

94. Walker WA, Wu M, Bloch KJ. Stimulation by immune complexes of mucus release from goblet cells of the rat small intestine. Science 1977;197:370.

95. Popper H, Schaffner F. Progress in liver disease. New York: Grune & Stratton, 1972.

96. Inchley CJ. The activity of mouse Kupffer cells following intravenous injections of T4 bacteriophage. Clin Exp Immunol 1969;5:173–187.

97. Thomas HC, Singer CRJ, Tilney NL, Folch H, MacSween RNM. The immune response in cirrhotic rats: antigen distribution, humoral immunity, cell mediated immunity and splenic suppressor cell activity. Clin Exp Immunol 1976;26:574–582.

98. Triger DR, Cunamon MH, Wright R. Studies on hepatic uptake of antigen I. Comparison of inferior vena cava and portal vein routes of immunization. Immunology 1973;25:941–950.

99. Benjamin IS, Ryan CJ, McLay ALC, Horne CHW, Blumgart LH. The effects of portacaval shunting and portacaval trans-

position on serum IgG levels in the rat. Gastroenterology 1976;70:661–664.

100. Thomas HC, Vaez-Zadeh F. A homeostatic mechanism for the removal of antigen from the portal circulation. Immunology 1974;26:375–382.

101. Orland E, Peppard J, Reynolds J, Hall J. Rapid active transport of immunoglobulin A from blood to bile. J Exp Med 1978;147:588–592.

102. Jackson GDF, Lemaitre-Coelho I, Vaerman JP, Bazin H, Beckers A. Rapid disappearance from serum of intravenously injected rat myeloma IgA and its secretion into bile. Eur J Immunol 1978;8:123–126.

103. Harmatz PR, Kleinman RE, Bunnel BW, Bloch KJ, Walker WA. Hepatobiliary clearance of IgA immune complexes formed in the circulation. Hepatology 1982;2:328–333.

104. Kulangara AC. Dietary antigens in breast milk. Lancet 1978;2:575.

105. Jakobsson I, Lindberg T. Cow's milk as a cause of infantile colic in breast-fed infants. Lancet 1978;2:437–439.

106. Lake AM, Whitington PF, Hamilton SR. Dietary protein-induced colitis in breast-fed infants. J Pediatr 1982;101:906–910.

107. Hanson LÅ, Ahlstedt S, Andersson B, Carlsson B, Fällström SP, Mellander L, Porras O, Söderström T, Edén CS. Protective factors in milk and the development of the immune system. Pediatrics 1985;75(suppl):172–176.

108. Weaver LT, Walker WA. Epidermal growth factor and the developing human gut. Gastroenterology 1988;94:845–847.

109. Gaull GE, Wright CE, Isaacs CE. Significance of growth modulators in human milk. Pediatrics 1985;75(suppl):142–145.

110. Udall JN, Colony P, Fritze L, Pang K, Trier JS, Walker WA. Development of gastrointestinal mucosal barrier. II. The effect of natural versus artificial feeding on intestinal permeability to macromolecules. Pediatr Res 1981;15:245–249.

111. Israel EJ, Schiffrin EJ, Carter EA, Freiberg E, Walker WA. Prevention of necrotizing enterocolitis in the rat with prenatal cortisone. Gastroenterology 1990;99:1333–1338.

112. Stern M, Pang KY, Walker WA. Food proteins and gut mucosal barrier. II. Differential interaction of cow's milk proteins with the mucous coat and the surface membrane of adult and immature rat jejunum. Pediatr Res 1984;18:1252–1257.

113. Walker-Smith JA. Cow's milk intolerance as a cause of post-enteritis diarrhea. J Pediatr Gastroenterol Nutr 1982; 1:1636.

114. Saadia R, Schein M, MacFarlane C, Boffard KD. Gut barrier function and the surgeon. Br J Surg 1990;77:487–492.

115. Van Camp JM, Tomaselli V, Coran AG. Bacterial translocation in the neonate. Curr Opin Pediatr 1994;6:327–333.

6

ORAL TOLERANCE: IMMUNE RESPONSES TO FOOD ANTIGENS

Stephan Strobel

Introduction

The concept of immunologically mediated tolerance to food antigens (oral tolerance) through mucosal antigen exposure either via breast milk or through normal nutrition has been the subject of scientific debate since the late 19th century. A possible role of the oral route in suppressing adverse clinical effects was reported in 1829 by R. Dakin (1), who questioned the efficacy of the practice of preventing painful skin rashes from poison-ivy contact by prior chewing of the leaves of the plants:

> "Some good meaning, mystical, marvellous physicians, or favoured ladies with knowledge inherent, say the bane will prove the best antidote, and hence *advise the forbidden leaves to be eaten,* both as a preventive and cure to the external disease.
> I have known the experiment tried . . ."

In contrast, in 1911, H. G. Wells (author and scientist) and T. Osborne reported the prevention of systemic anaphylaxis in guinea pigs that had been previously fed with hen's egg or other proteins (2, 3). Suppression of contact sensitivity in guinea pigs by prior feeding of the sensitizing agent was reported in 1946 by Chase (4). The ease of systemic immunological suppression via the oral route became known as the Chase–Sulzberger phenomenon, in acknowledgment of an earlier report by Sulzberger (5). These pioneering observations, well before the onset of "modern immunology," were extended in the late 1970s and early 1980s. In the 1990s, oral tolerance has again attracted the interest of immunologists because it represents a central immunological principle and because it may potentially play a role in the treatment of autoimmune disorders (6–9) and food allergic diseases, which frequently have their onset in the neonatal period and early childhood (10–13).

"Oral tolerance" is often used to describe a clinical situation that is synonymous with the immunological definition of "peripheral tolerance"—i.e., that which is acquired by mature lymphocytes in the peripheral tissues (GALT)—as opposed to "central tolerance"—a tolerance that is acquired by immature lymphocytes during thymic development. "Oral tolerance" can be defined as an antigen-specific, systemic immunological hyporesponsiveness after prior oral (mucosal) administration of the antigen. Lifelong clinical and immunological tolerance to most complex mixtures of antigens (e.g., bacteria, viruses) is the rule. Clearly, however, a sizable number of individuals suffer from food-induced clinical symptoms and allergic diseases (14–20). In operational terms, food-induced allergic diseases represent a breakdown or failure of oral tolerance, either during induction or during maintenance (Fig. 6.1).

Basic Effects of Oral Tolerance on Immunity

SYSTEMIC IMMUNITY

Oral exposure to dietary (and other) antigens has two major effects on the immune system. These responses can be simplified and summarized as leading to: (1) induction of systemic immunological hyporesponsiveness (tolerance); (2) sensitization and priming; and (3) local production of secretory IgA

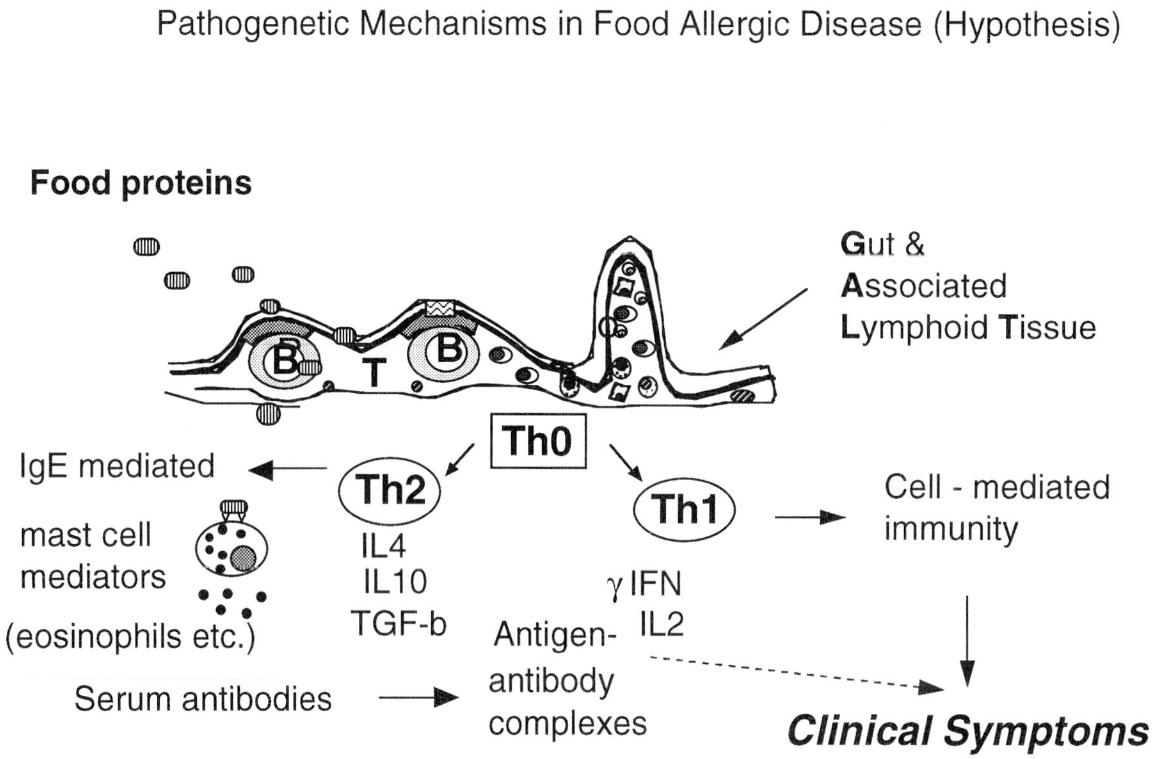

Pathogenetic Mechanisms in Food Allergic Disease (Hypothesis)

Food proteins

Figure 6.1

Hypothetical mechanisms and events in food allergic diseases. Food proteins reach the gut-associated tissue (GALT) after luminal and intracellular digestion and processing. In a normal situation, this process would lead to clinical tolerance. Under the conditions that affect the normal inductive process (biparental history of atopy, intercurrent inflammatory reactions in the gut interfering with the normal antigen presenting pathway with and without an increased uptake of antigen, etc.), the immune response can be polarized. Originating from a common precursor T lymphocyte, CD4 positive Th cells can be functionally divided on the basis of their cytokine secretion pattern after activation. Th1 effector cells predominantly secrete IFN-γ and IL-2 mediation delayed hypersensitivity responses. Th2 lymphocytes predominantly secrete IL-4, IL-5, and IL-10; thus, they are not only involved in regulating IgE production but also may down-regulate Th1 lymphocyte responses. Th0 cells lack a particular specialization and are able to secrete cytokines of either cell type (Th1 or Th2). Th1 immunity is more likely to induce cell-mediated damage to the mucosa. Th2 responses preferentially lead to IgE-mediated immunity, which could in turn affect the intestinal physiology (see Fig. 6.12a).

responses, although their mucosal induction after a feed appears to vary (21–24) (Fig. 6.2).

Little doubt exists that systemic suppression of specific immune responses arises in humans. For ethical reasons, most reports in humans are circumstantial (25, 26) except for a study in volunteers using keyhole limpet haemocyanin (27). A great deal of the in-depth scientific research work has, however, been performed in laboratory rodents with a limited range of food- and other T-cell-dependent antigens (e.g.,

milk and egg proteins, sheep erythrocytes, and organ-specific antigens) (7, 28, 29).

Most aspects of the systemic immune response of naive animals can be tolerized by single or multiple feeds. Single feeds have suppressed IgM, IgG, and IgE antibody responses (22, 30, 31) as well as cell-mediated immune responses (32–36), contact sensitivity (31, 37–39), and possibly cytotoxic responses (40). The effects on cytokine production (41–45) are variable and depend on the context in which they are

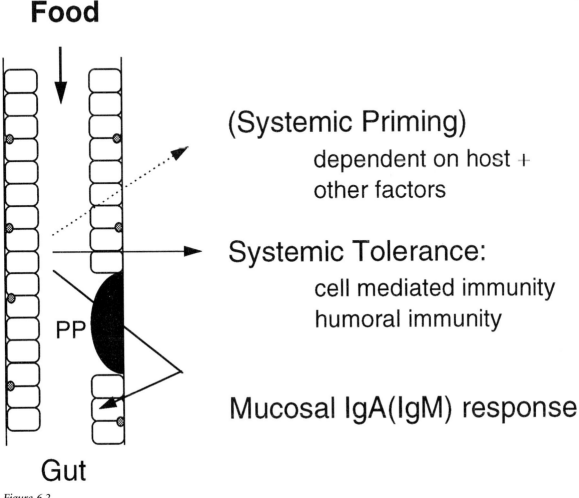

Food

(Systemic Priming)
dependent on host +
other factors

Systemic Tolerance:
cell mediated immunity
humoral immunity

PP

Mucosal IgA(IgM) response

Gut

Figure 6.2

Basic principle of immunoregulation in the gut after oral protein administration. Food enters the intestinal tract, and three major immune responses can occur. Systemic tolerance for cellular and humoral immunity is most commonly induced. The mucosal sIgA response is variable and related to the antigens encountered. Under certain conditions that depend on the host and other factors (see below), systemic priming is encountered that may affect all limbs of the immune response.

analyzed. Such antibody responses to soluble antigens are typically more difficult to suppress than cell-mediated immunity, although IgE responses appear to be exceptions to this general rule. Given that IgE and cell-mediated immunity are frequently implicated as a pathogenetic principle in food-sensitive diseases, it is interesting to note that these responses are more easily suppressed for a longer period of time with smaller amounts of antigen, either ingested (46) or administered via an aerosol (47, 48).

MUCOSAL IMMUNITY

The extent of the local mucosal immune response after oral antigen encounter is unclear. Some reports suggest that suppression of systemic immunity is accompanied by local secretory IgA production (22) or induction of Peyer's patch T lymphocytes that suppress IgG production and help IgA production in vitro (49). Other investigators have reported that the intestinal IgA antibody production is reduced by oral administration of antigens (50). These findings are also compatible with the apparent lack of food-related secretory IgA antibodies in normal individuals and could indicate that mucosal IgA production is regulated in a way similar to that of systemic immunity. Undisputed differences have been noted between secretory IgA responses and systemic immunity, however, that are not directly related to tolerance.

Mechanisms Implicated in Oral Tolerance Induction

As an oversimplification, three basic immunologic mechanisms can account for the phenomenon of oral tolerance, either singularly or in any combination. These factors are: (1) antigen-driven suppression (51–56); (2) clonal anergy (9, 31, 57, 58); and (3) clonal deletion. As yet, no comprehensive studies have addressed the existence of orally induced, peripheral, antigen-specific deletion of cells that have escaped thymic deletion. Most studies reporting clonal deletion as a mechanism of tolerance are related to intravenous injection of soluble antigen or cells during the neonatal period (59–63).

A primary factor in determining the immunological outcome after an oral antigen feed is the dose of the antigen fed. "High doses" (approximately 0.5 or more mg/g body weight in mice) of antigen induce unresponsiveness of Th1 function and probably of Th2-associated functions (44, 58, 64). The degree of clonal anergy and suppression may represent direct passage of small undegraded amounts of antigen into the circulation. It may also be dependent on filtration, processing, or both, by the intestinal epithelium. A possible involvement of enterocytes in this process cannot be ruled out. "Low doses" (less than 0.1 mg/g body weight in mice) are more likely to generate antigen-specific suppressor (regulatory) cells. On subsequent recognition of antigen, the cells secrete suppressive cytokine (e.g., TGF-β). Under these conditions, TGF-β, a multifunctional substance, may then suppress local immunity to nonspecific antigens. This form of "bystander suppression" represents an important concept in the treatment of autoimmune diseases via the oral route (58, 65).

Oral (mucosal) antigen encounter preferentially induces Th2 type responses (T lymphocytes secreting IL-4, IL-5, or IL-10) in the gut (43, 44, 47, 66). Th2 type responses in vivo (like secretion of IL-4 for IgE production), however, seem to be suppressed also (44, 67), highlighting the complex regulatory network that operates after oral antigen encounter. "Very low doses" (less than 0.005 mg/g body weight in mice) given orally have been shown to prime the animal for subsequent systemic and local immune responses (28).

Transfer of Tolerance

Several studies have demonstrated that suppression may be transferred with spleen cells after administration of a range of different antigens in the rodent system (68–70). The existence of two components of oral tolerance—suppression and anergy—was suggested in 1982 (32). Induction of "low dose" tolerance could be prevented by elimination of cyclophosphamide-sensitive cells prior to an antigen feed, whereas "high dose" tolerance was not affected (32, 51).

Adoptive transfer studies have shown that oral tolerance (in this case, suppression) is not transferable with spleen cells of already tolerant (for more than 4–6 weeks) animals. This absence of transferable tolerance in phenotypically tolerant mice provides circumstantial evidence of clonal anergy. No firm evidence currently exists for an antigen-specific, post-thymic, clonal *deletion* or the induction of an apoptotic process in vivo. The ability to "rescue" anergic cells in in vitro culture systems with IL-2 from the anergic state (58, 71) supports this statement, as lymphocytes—once deleted—could not have been "rescued" from a silent state. Obviously, suppression and clonal anergy are not mutually exclusive, and both may co-exist in an individual.

Time to Induction of Oral Tolerance and Duration

Systemic induction of tolerance is achieved soon after a single feed of antigen (7, 29, 72). Significant suppression of immunity to OVA has been demonstrated 2 days after a feed (31, 49, 54) and is well established within 5 to 7 days (7, 28, 73, 74), an observation that is reflected in most experimental protocols. The inductive process of tolerance is dependent on the antigen and the species tested, and may require repeated administration, as seen with heterologous antigens such as sheep red blood cells (SRBC). Before oral tolerance is established, animals may go through a short-lived phase of sensitization (75). Similar observations have been made for tolerance induction via an aerosol (76, 77). Some evidence also suggests that a similar process, at least for IgE antibodies, exists in humans (78).

Duration of Tolerance

Duration of tolerance after oral administration of antigens has not been systematically studied. The gastrointestinal flora likely affects the extent of suppression and its duration. Tolerance to ovalbumin in axenic mice of the C3H/HeJ type was shorter-lived than suppression observed in conventionally reared littermates (79, 80). In conventionally reared rodents, suppression of DTH has been demonstrated for as long as 17 months after a single feed (81), whereas suppression of antibody responses was lost after 3 to 6 months. These findings support the general observation that CMI responses are more easily suppressed than antibody responses.

Factors Influencing the Induction of Oral Tolerance

GENETIC BACKGROUND

The influence of genetic background as one of the most important denominators for the development of an atopic disease or reaction is generally accepted but difficult to quantify. The risk of developing allergic reactions increases in infants with atopic family members. Indeed, several studies using chromosomal analysis have suggested a potential linkage between IgE responses, atopic disease, and chromosomal markers such as 5q and 11q (82–85). An association between HLA class II molecules and immune responses to specific antigens has also been described in humans (86, 87).

In high and low responder states with regard to IgE responses shown in rodents, differences of immune responses can be linked to MHC class differences and to specific antigens (88–92). Kinetics of antigen absorption, elimination, and response to oral immunization in mice may also be linked to a particular MHC type (93, 94). It remains unresolved whether genetic differences in antigen clearance from the circulation and handling are actually correlated with the capacity to induce in vivo oral tolerance.

REGULATORY FACTORS FOR THE INDUCTION AND MAINTENANCE OF ORAL TOLERANCE

Nature of the Antigen

Tolerance can probably be induced to all thymus-dependent soluble antigens, a feature that has hampered the successful development of oral vaccines unless mucosal adjuvants are used (95, 96). Cholera toxin acts as an adjuvant and primarily stimulates the local IgA response. The nontoxic subunit has also been employed as a powerful mucosal immunization agent (97). Surprisingly, the same group has shown that conjugating soluble and particulate antigens to the recombinantly produced cholera toxin B (CTB) subunit induces profound mucosal and systemic tolerance (95) (Fig. 6.3). Minimal contamination of the purified CTB preparation with the A subunit may account for these diametrically different responses. Further in vitro studies (98) have demonstrated marked suppressive effects of CT and its CTB subunit and have concluded that one of the mechanisms of CT's mucosal effects in vivo is the inhibition of certain mucosal T-cell functions and alteration of

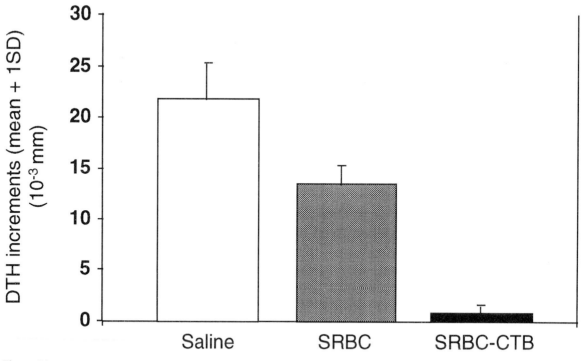

Figure 6.3

Oral tolerization by a CTB-SRBC conjugate in systemically immunized mice. Mice after systemic immunization to sheep red blood cells (SRBC) were fed SRBC, saline, or a CTB-SRBC conjugate. Delayed hypersensitivity was assessed 7 days after immunization by a footpad challenge test. Only the CTB-SRBC conjugate significantly re-tolerized the mice (compared with saline and SRBC). The kinetics and dose requirements remain unclear.

the regulatory T-cell environment in gut-associated lymphoid tissue.

Replicating organisms such as viruses and bacteria are more likely to induce active and often protective immunity. A striking example of this capability is the successful oral vaccine against the polio virus.

Tolerance induction with thymus-independent antigens is generally impossible without a thymus-dependent carrier. Even in the context of a thymus-dependent carrier, however, tolerance is directed against the carrier—not against the thymus-independent antigen. When mice were fed killed *Escherichia coli* antigen, tolerance developed against the T-dependent K antigen, while no active immunity was induced against the T-independent O antigen (99).

Particulate antigens may be preferentially taken up by the M cells of Peyer's patches and thus pro-

cessed in a more efficient way (100). There is, however, no simple relationship between solubility, processing, site of presentation to the GALT, and subsequent immunity.

Antigen Uptake

Minor amounts of protein antigens reach the circulation in an undegraded state. Circulating immunoreactive antigen levels vary considerably and are most likely linked to the analytical methods. Levels of the administered dose varying from 10^{-2} to 10^{-6} (one to several hours after administration) have been reported in both rodents (13, 101–103) and humans (104–106). Achlorhydria has been found to increase macromolecular absorption of bovine serum albumin (BSA) in adults (107, 108) without reported evidence of an increased risk of developing food allergic symptoms. In an animal model of intestinal anaphylaxis, neutralization of gastric pH delayed digestion, thereby increasing macromolecular absorption (109, 110). Administration of the protease inhibitor aprotinin reportedly reduces suppression associated with increased circulating levels of antigen (ovalbumin) (111). These observations have not been confirmed by others, however, and remain controversial (Strobel, unpublished observation).

Investigations into macromolecular (protein) uptake and the permeability of sugar molecules in premature and term infants have shown that increased permeability is correlated with reduced gestational age. This level returns to "normal" (postnatal) levels at about the 36th or 38th gestational week (105, 112, 113).

Mucosal Barrier Function

The role of the mucosal barrier in antigen handling has been extensively investigated (114, 115). Altered (increased) binding patterns of antigens to (epithelial) microvillus membrane preparations have been demonstrated in neonatal rats (116). Maturational changes of the phospholipid composition of microvillus membranes and changes in the intestinal mucus may nonspecifically alter antigen absorption (114, 115). The effects of these changes on induction of oral tolerance have not been formally studied.

Clinical Implications

A study in eczematous children without gastrointestinal symptoms has identified a subgroup of children with atopy under six years of age that exhibit an increased lactulose/rhamnose urinary excretion ratio, possibly indicating an overall increased gastrointestinal permeability (117 and Isolaury E, 1995 personal communication). It is unresolved whether the increased permeability indicates an atopic state (a primary phenomenon) or is secondarily caused by the disease process through constant low-grade intestinal antigen challenge to which the patient may be reacting in a subclinical way. A similar mechanism likely operates in children and adults with coeliac disease who have marked mucosal abnormalities without overt clinical symptoms while being on a diet that contains amounts of gluten sufficient to trigger the disease process (118–120).

Role of Digestive Flora

Evidence obtained from experiments in germ-free and conventionally reared rodents has shown that the intestinal colonization can affect the outcome of the host's immune responses after oral antigen encounter. Early experiments demonstrated that germ-free animals may have a defective immune system (121) and may not be tolerizable against SRBC. After such mice were given lipopolysaccharides (LPS) from gram-negative bacteria, tolerance could be induced (122). Further studies by several investigators using soluble OVA have shown, however, that tolerance is also induced in germ-free and LPS-unresponsive C3H/ HeJ animals (79). These results highlight the major differences in the induction of unresponsiveness noted after administration of particulate (SRBC) and soluble (OVA) antigens.

Role of the Enterocyte in Antigen Presentation

Ultrastructural studies (123) on rat and human enterocytes have identified MHC class II molecules that are found within the cytoplasm and associated with the endocytic pathway. Although antigen uptake by enterocytes is insignificant (123), it is fascinating to speculate that minor amounts of OVA-derived, processed (tolerogenic) peptides, in association with class II or I, could alternatively be presented by "traditional" APC or by T cells. Clonal anergy or memory could be induced by antigen presentation to T cells that do not express the B7 family of molecules like conventional antigen-presenting cells, and that fail to provide a second costimulatory signal via the CD28, CTLA4, or other as-yet-unidentified molecules (124–126). This finding may explain why, despite long-term tolerance for cell-mediated immunity, no antigen-specific or -responsive T lymphocytes (suppressors) could be demonstrated in longer-term tolerant mice (49, 127) (Fig. 6.4).

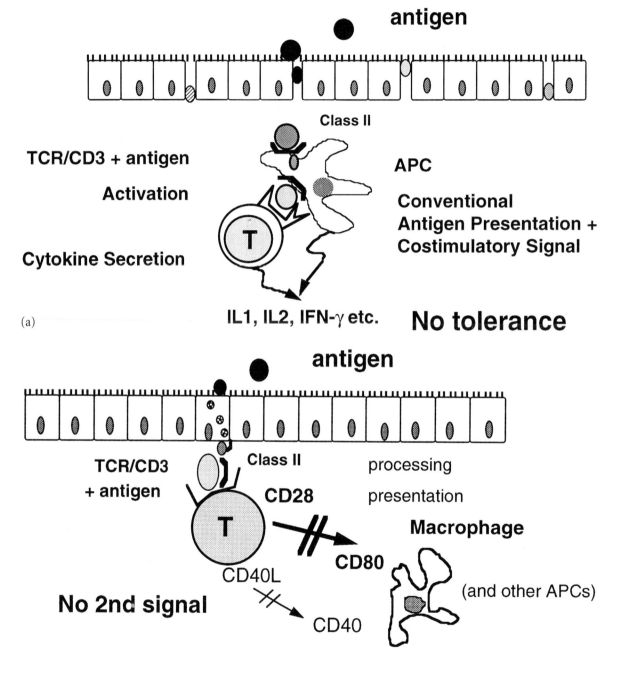

Generally, antigen is presented to CD4 (helper) T lymphocytes in association with class II molecules. In vitro, several scientists (128, 129) using rat enterocytes and enterocytes isolated from human colonic biopsies (130, 131) have demonstrated a preferential presentation to CD8+ suppressor T lymphocytes that did not express the surface marker for cytotoxicity. Most human intraepithelial lymphocytes (IEL) that are CD8+ also express CD7, supporting the idea that these cells may indeed be activated (132, 133).

It is also unresolved—although unlikely—whether tolerance to soluble antigens is induced by in vivo mucosal induction of class II, restricted cytotoxic (CD8+) T cells that would kill B cells in an antigen-specific fashion (134). Published evidence (31, 49, 50) that identifies reactive splenic B cells, presumably under T-cell suppression in tolerant animals, would argue against cytotoxicity representing an important mechanism for oral tolerance induction. Indeed, suppression of cytotoxic responses after oral antigen administration has been reported (40, 135).

Intraepithelial Lymphocytes in Oral Tolerance

Intraepithelial lymphocytes within the intestinal tract possess a number of unique immunological features, but their exact functional role remains unclear. Peripheral tolerance induction and thymus-independent T-cell development and selection are known to take place in the intestinal epithelium (136). IEL are of T-lymphocyte lineage (CD3+) with a majority (more than 75%) bearing the CD8 suppressor epitope. In the mouse, approximately 50% of CD8+ cells use the γ,δ T-cell receptor and are of extrathymic

origin. The number of γ,δ-positive TCR IELs is about 10% of the total found in the human epithelium. Around 60% of the CD8+ positive IEL express the homodimeric CD8$\alpha+,\beta-$ phenotype. In contrast to the common CD8$\alpha+,\beta+$ phenotypes, the CD8$\alpha+,\beta-$ phenotype is not seen in the circulation. Only scant evidence exists that they play a role in regulating oral tolerance. Their apparent ability to recognize nonpeptidic antigens is intriguing, because it could indicate a different recognition pathway from α,β T cells. Functional activities of IEL have been reported (cytotoxicity, activation) (136–146).

At a different mucosal site, Holt and colleagues, when investigating the suppression of IgE responses via an aerosol model of respiratory sensitization, identified a CD8+γ,δ-positive regulatory T cell that could suppress IgE responses on transfer (67, 147). These reports are in apparent contrast to the above-mentioned report that γ,δ cells from the gut may abrogate oral tolerance (148, 149). Clearly more work is needed to define the regulatory role of IELs in oral (mucosal) tolerance during induction, maintenance, or breakdown.

Antigen Exposure Via Breast Milk

EXPERIMENTAL MODELS

Some groups have addressed the important question of whether a qualitative difference can be discerned between antigen presented via breast milk or directly by gavage (13, 150). Direct gavage of bovine serum albumin (BSA) or ovalbumin to neonates for 1 to 3 days leads to priming of the subsequent immune response. Feeding of 20 mg/g BSA/g body weight to lactating mothers *after* birth for 1 to 3 days also

Figure 6.4

←

Effects of intestinal antigen processing and presentation on the induction of oral tolerance (hypothesis). (a) Prevention of oral tolerance induction: Antigen that bypasses "processing" by the enterocytes will be presented by conventional antigen-presenting cells (APC) to T cells (TCR/CD3) in association with class II MHC antigens in an environment conducive to activation of systemic immune responses rather than suppression. (b) Induction of oral tolerance: Foreign antigen is "processed" by enterocytes and presented directly to T cells via the TCR/CD3 complex. A second costimulatory signal via the CD28/CD8+ receptor ligand complex is not provided, and the T cell receives a tolerogenic signal. A second signal could be provided by IL-1 and antigen that may be operative in the abrogation of tolerance.

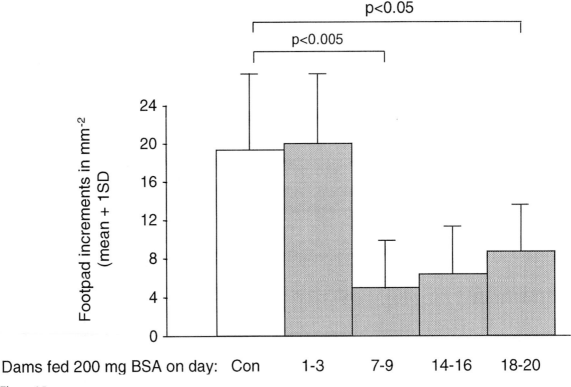

Figure 6.5

Sensitization and tolerance to bovine serum albumin (BSA) via breast milk. Suckling dams were gavaged with 200 mg BSA for 3 days while maintained on the normal (milk- and egg-free) diet at the times indicated on the graph. At the age of 4 weeks, all pups were immunized with BSA in adjuvant; their immunity was assessed 3 weeks later. Offspring of saline gavaged dams (controls, $n = 32$) demonstrated the expected cell-mediated immune response. Offspring of dams ($n = 7$) gavaged during the first 3 days of life were primed, whereas all other groups demonstrated significant specific suppression of delayed hypersensitivity. These results indicate: (1) that animals can be primed and tolerized via breast milk, and (2) that the effect on immunity is comparable to that seen with the direct feeding pattern even though the antigen was administered via breast milk. The antigen doses received differ approximately by a factor of 10^{-3} (μg versus ng). (Antibody responses were not different between experimental and control groups.)

resulted in systemic priming (Fig. 6.5) (Peng, Turner, Strobel, unpublished observation). Thus, there appears to be no quantifiable difference between the two feeding regimens. OVA administration to nursing females for 3 days before weaning (days 18, 19, and 20) resulted in 80% to 90% suppression of systemic immune responses in the offspring and was comparable to the pattern of suppression seen after antigen gavage, although specific IgG responses were not regularly suppressed.

One important difference is noted, however. The *dose* of antigen that is transmitted via suckling is several log concentrations less than that seen with gavage and in a dose range that would otherwise induce priming (32, 151). In long-term feeding experiments, one group reported priming of offspring whose mothers were maintained on a gluten-containing diet until weaning (152). Epidemiological studies in humans have clearly demonstrated that breast milk can influence subsequent host immune responses and, for example, reduce the incidence of milk allergies in childhood (153–157). Exact requirements with regard to age, dose, and nature of antigen remain to be evaluated.

STUDIES IN HUMANS

Dietary antigen excretion into breast milk seems to be a general phenomenon and has been reported for milk, egg, wheat proteins, and parasite antigens (158–160). Excreted amounts are in the range of micrograms/liter. The immunological significance of transfer of dietary antigens during breast feeding is unclear. It is generally accepted that breast feeding reduces the risk of food allergic reactions and of atopy in a population at risk (i.e., with a uni- or biparental history of atopy), but sensitizing effects in infants have also been described (161–164). Studies by Chandra (165, 166), Zeiger (157, 167), and others (168, 169) suggest that elimination of (significant) dietary antigen transfer via breast milk for six months (among other preventive measures) in a population at risk reduces the probability of a food-specific sensitization (and possibly atopic symptoms) for as long as 48 months. This effect persists even after the diet of the infant has been liberalized.

Examinations of the effects of dietary elimination in atopic mothers during pregnancy alone have failed to show a reduction of atopic symptoms in their infants. Major problems associated with such studies are the risks of sub-optimal nutrition, awkward diets, and poor compliance. Most studies combine dietary elimination during pregnancy with dietary restrictions during breast feeding. Recent research indicates a prophylactic role (delayed onset of atopic eczema) for antigen avoidance combined with delayed and staged introduction of solids in a high-risk population. Confounding factors, including smoking, pets, house dust mite, and pollutant exposure, must be taken into consideration in such investigations (169–171).

ANTIGEN HANDLING AND PROCESSING BY THE GUT

Qualitative and quantitative analysis of antigen processing and uptake by the gut is affected by method-ological and technical difficulties. This consideration is especially important in humans, where dietary antigen uptake studies must account for antigen–antibody interactions and the rapid clearance of antigen–antibody complexes by the reticulo-endothelial system at mucosal and systemic levels (Fig. 6.6) (105). To overcome these difficulties and to study mechanisms of antigen processing by the intestinal tract, we have developed an adoptive antigen transfer system in "naive" rodents that have been maintained on an OVA- and BSA-free diet. Briefly, animals are gavaged with the antigen ovalbumin (or bovine serum albumin). After one hour, serum is collected and intraperitoneally transferred into naive recipients that are systemically immunized with Freund's complete adjuvant (CFA) and antigen seven days later. Specific humoral and cell mediated immunity are assessed 21 days after immunization. CMI responses were generally suppressed by 70% to 90% compared with control responses. (Antibody suppression was variable but was often unaffected.) Appropriate controls, which included intravenous injections with native ovalbumin over a wide dose range, in vitro addition of native ovalbumin to normal serum before transfer, and filtration via other biological membranes (peritoneum) (Furrie E, Turner MW, Strobel S, 1991 unpublished observation), did not show any suppressive effects when compared with gut "processed" antigen. In vivo filtration via the liver and injection to naive recipients also failed to confer tolerance, supporting the idea that the observed effect depends on factors other than de-aggregation of the antigen by the liver (172 and our observations).

A striking time dependency of this "processing" phenomenon was identified during the studies (101). If serum was collected only five minutes after gavage, duly adjusted to comparable immunoreactive serum OVA levels, and transferred, *no* suppression of CMI (or humoral immunity) was observed (Table 6.1). This observation suggests that the antigen may have been altered (processed) in a way that would allow presentation to T lymphocytes responsible for (DTH) suppression. After affinity chromatography absorption, further immunochemical analysis of the serum containing the tolerogenic activity revealed that the suppressive activity was associated with the presence of a 21–24 kDa peptide (173) (Fig. 6.7).

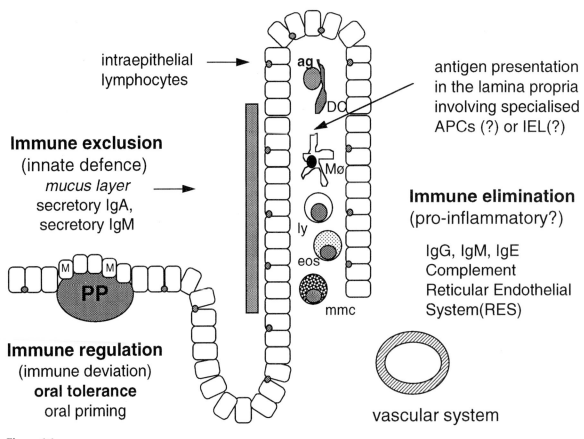

intraepithelial lymphocytes

antigen presentation in the lamina propria involving specialised APCs (?) or IEL(?)

Immune exclusion
(innate defence)
mucus layer
secretory IgA,
secretory IgM

Immune elimination
(pro-inflammatory?)

IgG, IgM, IgE
Complement
Reticular Endothelial
System(RES)

Immune regulation
(immune deviation)
oral tolerance
oral priming

vascular system

Figure 6.6

Schematic diagram of the three major functions of the intestinal epithelium and the gut-associated lymphoid tissue (GALT). **Immune exclusion** is a mostly noninflammatory process that is maintained by specific (sIgA, IgM) and non-specific innate factors (e.g., mucus, peristalsis). **Immune elimination** can be defined as a process by which potentially hazardous antigens are eliminated by specific antibody and innate defense mechanisms, such as complement, neutrophils, macrophages, mast cells, and others. **Immune regulation** or **oral tolerance** is the central process by which the major immunological organ of the body—the intestinal tract—maintains an immunological homeostasis between harmful and nonharmful processes at a local and systemic level.

APC = antigen-presenting cell
M = M cell
ag = antigen
DC = dendritic cell
Mϕ = macrophage
ly = lymphocyte
eos = eosinophil
mmc = mucosal mast cell

Table 6.1
Suppression of Delayed Hypersensitivity in Recipients of Serum Retrieved Under Different Experimental Conditions

Donor	Serum Retrieved After Feed at Antibody Responses	
	5 min	60 min
BALB/c saline	no	no
BALB/c OVA	no	yes
SCID saline	no	no
SCID OVA	no	no
BALB/c* saline	no	no
BALB/c* OVA	no	yes

are generally not suppressed and in a substantial number of experiments primed.

*Germ-free animals served to control for the possible effects of the intestinal flora. (SCID animals are kept under pathogen-free conditions.) The results indicate that the failure to generate a "tolerogen" in SCID animals was not due to colonization of the gut but more likely to the immunological abnormality of the gut-associated lymphoid tissues in those animals.
SCID = severe combined immunodeficient.

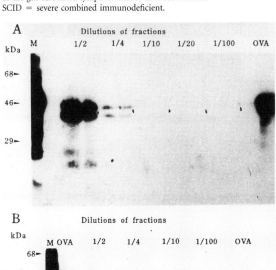

Figure 6.7

Immunoblot of affinity purified ovalbumin collected 5 and 60 minutes after an oral feed. (a) Immunoblot of fraction 2 of affinity-purified OVA derived from the serum of BALB/c mice collected 5 min after feeding OVA. (b) Immunoblot of elution fraction 2 of affinity-purified OVA derived from serum of BALB/c mice collected 60 min after feeding OVA. The OVA was detected using a polyclonal rabbit anti-OVA antibody and duplicate dilutions of the fractions were tested.

HOST IMMATURITY AND TOLERANCE INDUCTION

Experimental Studies

Soluble antigen administration intragastrically to neonatal rodents during the first 1 to 7 days of life does not lead to suppression of systemic immunity and may prime for later systemic immunity (13, 103). This observation has also been made in an experimental model of allergic encephalomyelitis in rats when myelin basic protein (MBP) was administered during the first week of life (174) (Figs. 6.8 and 6.9). "Adult type" tolerance can be achieved by feeding antigen when the animal is approximately 7 to 14 days old. Further dissection of this phenomenon indicates that this inability to induce tolerance results not only from immaturity of the digestive system or antigen handling capacity of the neonatal gut (175), but also from an as-yet-uncharacterized immunological immaturity that can partially be restored with injection of adult spleen cells immediately before intragastric gavage. Tolerance to human immunoglobulin G in rodents can be achieved in the neonatal period, possibly as a result of facilitated Fc receptor-mediated uptake (103). Studies have not determined in which way, or whether, an intestinal human (neonatal) Fc receptor contributes to tolerance induction.

A transient defect of tolerance induction occurs during weaning. The effect is related to the process of weaning and possibly related to a change in the

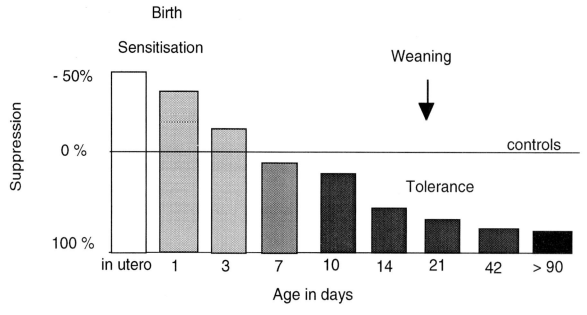

Figure 6.8

Ontogeny of oral tolerance induction after a protein feed. This graph summarizes experiments in mice investigating the effects of early antigen administration in mice. Antigen (ovalbumin at a dose of 1 mg/g body weight) administered at the days of age indicated leads to sensitization instead of tolerance if given during the first 7 to 10 days of life. Note that intrauterine injection 1 to 2 days before delivery also primes for later immune responses. All animals were immunized 4 weeks after the feed of ovalbumin and suckled by their dams as appropriate. (Weaning took place at day 20–21.)

diet and intestinal flora; it is not necessarily related to the age of the animal at weaning (176–179).

Oral Sensitization in Infants

In rare circumstances, infants experience acute anaphylactic reactions on first exposure to cow's milk after a period of presumed exclusive breast feeding (161, 180). These dramatic reports do not *prove* that the sensitization also occurred via breast milk. Other possible routes of sensitization include intrauterine exposure to antigen (13, 181), exposure to anti-idiotypic antibodies (also presented via breast milk) (24), and exposure to antigens in the neonatal nursery (11, 153, 154). In a carefully designed ongoing prospective study of 1749 Danish newborns, the authors could demonstrate that 2.2% developed cow's milk allergy. Clinical symptoms occurred in 50% of infants older than 3 months, and in 0.5% of exclusively

breast-fed infants. In tracing the records of those infants, the investigator found that *all* sensitized infants had received milk supplements during the first 3 days of life and 5 out of 9 infants had a parental history of atopy.

Early sensitization of IgE (and also for IgG) responses in human infants seems to indicate a susceptible period in early infancy (182), at least in a population at risk (i.e., with a parental or sibling history of atopy) where regulatory (suppressive) influences of the GALT are immature or may be more easily disturbed. In a prospective randomized study in humans, 250 breast-fed infants were assigned to receive either cow's milk formula (group A) or a partially hydrolyzed infant formula (group B) (whey hydrolysate) for 1 to 4 days before establishing breast feeding. After 3 months of exclusive breast feeding and supplementation with the whey hydrolysate if

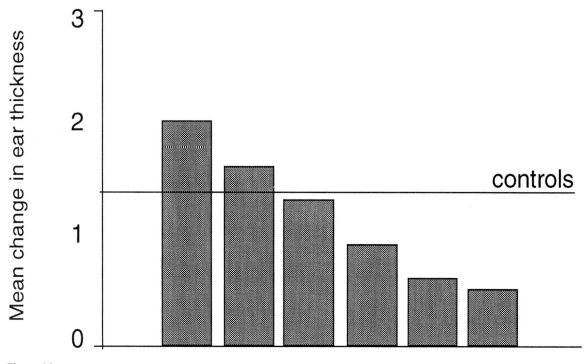

Figure 6.9

Orally induced priming and tolerance to myelin basic protein (MBP). Experimental allergic encephalomyelitis (EAE) is an acknowledged model for human multiple sclerosis (MS). In this experiment, rats were fed either MBP or saline within the first week of life and thereafter. Four to six weeks later, they were immunized with MBP in Freund's adjuvant, their skin tested, and their clinical symptoms assessed. The graph demonstrates priming for adult disease in rats that were fed in the neonatal period. Protection against EAE had been achieved in animals that were fed at around 4 weeks of age. Comparable results have been obtained with soluble proteins (see Fig. 6.8).

necessary, cow's milk formula was introduced for both groups. Infants in group A showed a significant priming effect for IgG antibody responses at 5 and 12 months, whereas their total and specific IgE responses did not differ. Nevertheless, when the amount of early post-natal milk supplementation was correlated with the IgE levels, an intake of 200 to 500 mL of cow's milk post-natally increased IgE levels at 3, 5 ($p < 0.013$), and 12 ($p < 0.06$) months (183 and unpublished observation). Although this difference in IgE levels did *not* correlate with clinical symptoms of atopy, it demonstrates the importance of giving the antigen dose at a particular time.

Basic Regulatory Mechanisms of Oral Tolerance

SUPPRESSIVE MECHANISMS

T cells with suppressive activity have been identified in the intestinal mucosa, mesenteric lymph nodes, and spleen after feeding an antigen (39, 50, 51, 57, 69, 70, 98, 184–189). Modulation of T-cell function and antigen presentation by hormones, adjuvants, immunosuppressants, and immunological immaturity can prevent tolerance induction (52, 190). Interestingly, no lymphocytes with suppressive activity can

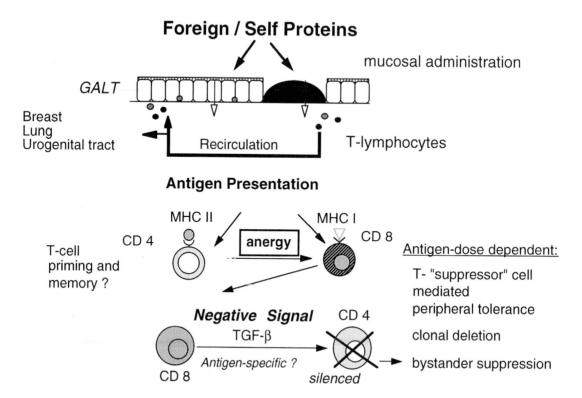

Figure 6.10

Immune deviation after administration of food and self-protein (hypothesis). Following the passage through the mucosa and processing by the GALT (including enterocytes), antigen is presented in connection with class I and/or class II molecules. Preferential presentation in association with class I antigens could lead to activation of specific CD8+ T suppressor cells. Presentation in association with class II antigens will activate CD4+ T cells and lead to memory induction. A regulatory interaction between CD4+ and CD8+ T cells in this context is conceivable. Activated CD8+ T cells can also provide a negative signal to (auto) reactive cells in affected target organs. A negative signal could be provided by TGF-β. In the absence of a costimulatory signal [e.g., via CD28-CD8+ (B7 family)], T-cell anergy (tolerance) could be induced. Other regulatory pathways are likely to exist, and the role of the CD8+ and CD4+ regulatory cell needs further clarification. These cells could play a sequential role in suppressing unwanted immune responses. The antigen dose dependency and the exact requirements remain unknown. Interestingly, neither CD4+ nor CD8+ lymphocytes are an absolute necessity for oral tolerance induction.

be identified in a tolerant host 3 to 4 weeks *after* tolerance induction, unless stimulated with IL-2, before analysis in an antigen-specific assay. Suppressive immune responses are generally thought to be antigen-specific, although this statement only partly explains the mechanisms at work (65, 191). Suppression can also be mediated by an antigen-specific trigger that leads to secretion of suppressive cytokines (e.g.,

TGF-β), which may then act on other immune cells in close proximity that are naive to the antigen (bystander suppression) (65) (Fig. 6.10).

Inhibitory serum factors (antigen–antibody complexes or antibody) have been reported for particulate antigens (192, 193). No convincing evidence exists for antibody-mediated suppression using *soluble* antigens, however.

OTHER CELLULAR MECHANISMS FOR ORAL TOLERANCE

Despite clear evidence of transferable tolerance with T cells (mostly CD8+) isolated from mesenteric lymph nodes or spleens of fed mice (possibly even isolated from the intestinal intraepithelial lymphocyte population) (194), some controversy remains about the role of clonal anergy and suppression after feeding of antigen (29, 53, 58, 64, 195, 196). Without entering into a detailed critique about the experimental details that could account for the observed differences, development of oral appears to be, at least, a two-step process in which both steps are not mutually exclusive. An early generation of T lymphocytes with suppressive activities is followed by a "tolerant" state in which other immunological mechanisms such as clonal anergy may operate.

MINIMUM HOST REQUIREMENTS

A T-dependent antigen is a prerequisite for the generation of oral tolerance. Host requirements for the induction oral tolerance are less well defined, often being dependent on the mucosal pathway selected for antigen exposure. That is, whether an antigen is administered via the conjunctival, nasal, bronchial, intestinal or any other mucosal/epithelial site determines oral tolerance (47, 97, 197, 198).

Extensive experiments have demonstrated that systemic suppression can be transferred by spleen cells (65, 68, 199) and that depletion of CD4+ cells before transfer does not interfere with the suppressive function. These findings indirectly indicate an important role for a CD8+ lymphocyte population in transfer of tolerance (40). A CD8+ TGF-β-producing cell has also been associated with phenotypic suppression in vitro. Following a similar experimental design, tolerance could be induced in CD8+ gene targeted (knock-out) mice immunized with the antigen linked to recombinant CTB subunit (Czerkinsky, Holmgren, 1996 in press) (Table 6.1).

Suppression can also be transferred when animals have been re-tolerized by antigen administration *after* prior sensitization with antigen in adjuvant (Fig. 6.11). In vivo depletion of CD4+ lymphocytes during the induction phase proved incompatible with tolerance induction, highlighting different cellular requirements at different points during the development of tolerance (40).

Specific cytokine requirements at any one point are even more difficult to determine because of their often regional activity, pleiotropy, and high interdependence. Measurement of secreted Th1 or Th2 cytokines in vitro may reveal a skewed picture. Following the Th1/Th2 paradigm (66), tolerance induction may reflect a preferential activation of Th2 cells (43, 44) with down regulation of Th1-dependent DTH responses by Th2 cytokines such as IL-4 and IL-10 (45, 200). Systemic tolerance, however, can be induced in IL-4 gene-targeted (knock-out) mice (44), and anti-IL-10 treatment does not interfere with the induction or maintenance of oral tolerance, at least in the case of tolerance to ovalbumin in rodents (45) (Table 6.2).

Summarizing from a number of reports, it seems that most, if not all, systemic immune responses are subject to "suppression" depending to a great extent on the nature of the antigen and antigen-dose chosen. Suppressed responses also include those thought to be typical Th1 responses: overall down-regulation of responses includes IgE, IgG1, IgG2a, IgG3, and cell-mediated immunity, cytotoxicity, and local mucosal immunity (secretory IgA).

Modulation of Immune Responses by Feeding the Sensitized Host

Suppression of an ongoing immune response in a sensitized host by antigen feeding has partially been achieved for humoral and cell-mediated immune responses (36, 187). Desensitization was most effective when large antigen doses were fed close to the sensitization events or on a repeated basis. The implications of these observations for human (allergic) diseases are unknown but are likely to be of great importance; as a result, research in this area is continuing. Recent reports describing the therapeutic use of orally induced suppression in the management of autoimmune diseases are encouraging (195, 201–203).

Therapeutic Applications of Oral Tolerance

In dealing with food allergies, the ultimate clinical goals are: (1) prevention of sensitization in the infant

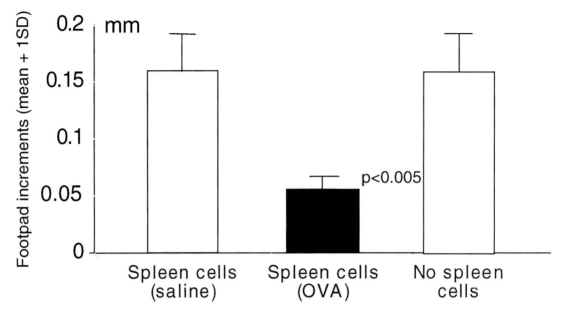

Figure 6.11

Transfer of tolerance for delayed hypersensitivity with spleen cells from animals that have been fed ovalbumin after systemic immunization. Just as in autoimmune diseases, it is also necessary to "re-tolerize food-allergic individuals after the onset of clinical symptoms." In these experiments, mice were immunized with ovalbumin in Freund's adjuvant and fed ovalbumin for 5 days at 10 mg/g body weight, with feeding taking place 7 days after systemic immunization. Spleen cells were harvested 9 days after the last feed and injected into naive recipients that were immunized with ovalbumin in adjuvant 1 week later. Only spleen cells of animals that received the antigen feeds transferred significant suppression for cell-mediated immunity. Antibody responses were not affected or primed.

Table 6.2
Oral Tolerance Requirements

Experimental Condition	Tolerance Induced	Reference
CD4, CD8 gene deletion	yes	(233)
IL-4 gene deletion	yes	(44)
depletion of CD8+ (in vivo)	yes	(40)
anti-IL-10	yes	(45)
anti-γ,δ	no	Mengel 1996, in press
graft-versus-host disease	no	(231)
depletion of CD4+ (in vivo)	no	(40)
cyclophosphamide	no (low dose)	(32, 51, 234)
estrogen + 2-deoxyguanosin	no	(190, 232)
splenectomy	no	(235)
10 Gr whole body irradiation	no	(34)
adjuvant treatment: MDP, cholera toxin/B subunit	no/yes	(52, 97, 197, 236)

(a)

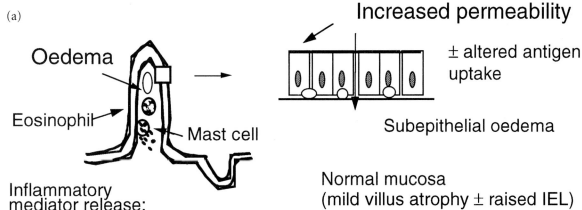

Oedema

Eosinophil

Mast cell

Increased permeability

± altered antigen uptake

Subepithelial oedema

Inflammatory
mediator release:

Prostaglandins
Leucotriens
Histamine
Eosinophilic cationic protein
etc.

Normal mucosa
(mild villus atrophy ± raised IEL)
Altered electrolyte absorption
Sucrase deficiency
Mucosal mast cell activation
Eosinophilic infiltration
Increased IgE levels in stool

(b)

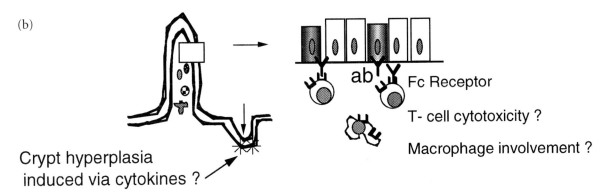

ab

Fc Receptor

T- cell cytotoxicity ?

Macrophage involvement ?

Crypt hyperplasia
induced via cytokines ?

circulating preformed IgG antibodies

Cytotoxic tissue damage in allergic gastroenteropathies remains to be
confirmed *in vivo*

Figure 6.12

(a) IgE-mediated immune responses and intestinal mucosal changes. IgE-mediated food-allergic reactions in the gut affect the mucosal physiology without changes visible at light microscopic levels. Inflammatory mediator release is able to cause immediate clinical reactions (e.g., vomiting, diarrhea) but is also able to elicit delayed reactions by recruitment of other immunocompetent cells. (b) Hypothetical effects of antibody-dependent cytotoxicity (ADCC) on intestinal morphology in food-allergic gastroenteropathies. Preformed IgG antibodies against constituents of foods may bind to epithelial cells. Cytotoxic cells via the Fc receptor may then be able to recognize and attack the enterocyte, which leads to local damage. This pathogenetic mechanism, which is also observed in vitro, has not been demonstrated in vivo.

(c)
Activation of
intestinal
pathology
through
mucosal
deposition of
Immune
complexes ?

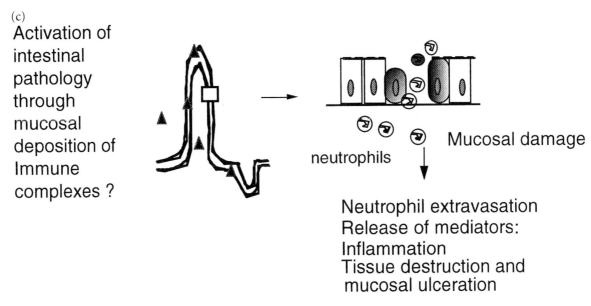

neutrophils

Mucosal damage

Neutrophil extravasation
Release of mediators:
Inflammation
Tissue destruction and
mucosal ulceration

Cell mediated delayed hypersensitivity induced mucosal pathology

(d)

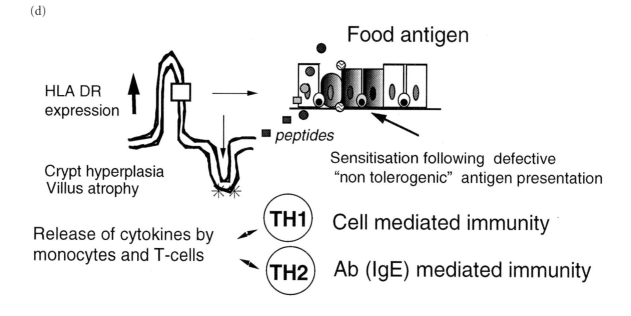

HLA DR
expression

Food antigen

peptides

Crypt hyperplasia
Villus atrophy

Sensitisation following defective
"non tolerogenic" antigen presentation

Release of cytokines by
monocytes and T-cells

TH1 Cell mediated immunity

TH2 Ab (IgE) mediated immunity

Th1 and Th2 responses are not mutually exclusive and can coexist at risk and (2) recreation of tolerance in a previously sensitized host. Figure 6.12 schematically depicts the still hypothetical effects of humoral and cell-mediated immunity on mucosal pathology. Clinical efficacy of some desensitization protocols (bee sting allergy, pollinosis, penicillin allergy) have been described (204–209). These protocols generally require injection of a more or less purified (standardized) antigen extract. Prospective well-controlled *oral* desensitization studies of *food-allergic* individuals have not yet been published (210, 211).

ORAL IMMUNOTHERAPY OF ALLERGIC DISEASES

Despite the significant regulatory effects observed in experimental models, the ultimate goal of re-tolerization via the oral route of individuals suffering from immunologically mediated adverse reactions to foods and inhalant allergens has proved elusive. The effectiveness of *subcutaneous* immunotherapy against inhalant allergies and anaphylactic reactions after bee and wasp stings is undisputed, but these therapies also carry the potential risks of serious anaphylactic reactions (204, 208, 212, 213). An advantage offered by *oral* immunotherapy might include a reduction in the risk of anaphylaxis, although the effectiveness of this approach remains controversial (210, 211, 214, 215). Several factors may explain these discrepancies. Variables like study design, route of administration and susceptibility to digestion, populations and atopic symptoms studied, preparation and administration of allergens and length of treatment may affect the outcome. In the case of gastrointestinal diseases dis-cussed in this context, it is important to consider that the affected organ will be used and then may move out of position for the induction of the "tolerizing" suppressive immune response. Nasal antigen administration (or presentation to other mucosal sites) could provide a promising alternative (198, 216). The likely therapeutic future for the mucosal route in the treatment of allergic diseases will be determined by the results of carefully controlled clinical and experimental studies. Experience gained from therapeutic studies in the management of autoimmune diseases (via mucosal autoantigen administration) may help in achieving this goal.

ORAL TOLERANCE AND AUTOIMMUNITY

The demonstration of suppression of an ongoing immune response by feeding the immunizing antigen *after* the onset of the disease is clearly an important therapeutic principle. It has been reported for both humoral and cell-mediated immune responses when ovalbumin was studied (36, 187). In those studies, immune responses were most readily suppressed when "large" antigen doses were administered close to the sensitization event, or when smaller doses were given repeatedly via drinking water.

Development of experimental autoimmune diseases (diabetes, allergic encephalomyelitis) has been linked in some rodents to the inability to induce oral tolerance to some dietary antigens; such development indicates a still poorly understood (immunoregulatory) connection between oral tolerance induction autoimmunity and age (92, 217). Treatment of human autoimmune diseases frequently involves phar-

---

6.12 (continued)

(c) Immune complex-mediated damage to the intestinal tract. Intestinal damage could theoretically be induced by immune complex deposition and activate the complement cascade. Secondary recruitment of neutrophils and other cells with subsequent release of inflammatory mediators (e.g., proteases) could then lead to mucosal ulceration and tissue destruction. Limited support for this hypothesis is provided by Ziegler 1990 #2758. (d) Cell-mediated delayed hypersensitivity reactions and IgE-mediated immunity involved in mucosal pathology. Major mucosal pathology is often caused by a cell-mediated delayed type hypersensitivity reactions. Polarization of T-cell responses toward Th1 may favor destructive responses. If the response pattern is directed versus the Th2 lymphocyte population, IgE-mediated immunity may occur. This response pattern is most often suppressed by oral antigen administration, highlighting its in vivo importance. Both responses (Th1 and Th2) are not mutually exclusive but indicate a polarization and may co-exist.

macological immune suppression. Therapeutic approaches using anti-T-cell receptor and class II MHC antibodies appear promising (reviewed 218). The development of antigen-specific (oral) therapies would appear to be far more appealing and less likely to produce systemic side effects. Because oral (mucosal) antigen administration is a powerful source of suppression, it is important and appropriate to explore this treatment avenue. A first step in delineating the treatment modalities of autoimmune diseases in animal models (7, 195, 199, 202, 219–221) and human disease (195, 201, 222–224) has been made.

Summary

The immunological outcome of antigen presented to the GALT is finely regulated by an intricate immunologic orchestra whose players, instruments, and exact order of play are only partially known. A hypothetical minimal model of GALT immunoregulation (oral tolerance) and its possible breakdown in food allergy has been outlined (Fig. 6.4). After intraluminal digestion, antigen can be processed and presented via class II-bearing enterocytes either to intraepithelial lymphocytes or lamina propria T lymphocytes (LPL) with little or no help from conventional APCs (130, 225, 226). The role of the dendritic cell in mediating tolerance in this context needs to be considered (227–230). If a loss of mucosal integrity or alteration of mucosal permeability (either primary or secondary) occurs, increased amounts of antigen bypass the tolerogenic antigen presentation of enterocytes by paracellular passage. These "unprocessed" antigens would then be "conventionally" presented by activated antigen-presenting cells to the lamina propria lymphocytes; by providing excessive help, they could prevent tolerance induction (34, 72, 231, 232).

Until the exact mechanisms underlying the mucosal-induced immunosuppression are unraveled, any hypothetical model is necessarily an oversimplification and cannot attempt to finalize the order of the key players and their instruments (cytokines). The model does, however, combine quantitative effects of altered antigen absorption and processing with its potential qualitative effects on gastrointestinal and systemic immunity, together with the lack of deliv-ering a second signal via the CD28/CD8+ pathway. The increasing scientific interest in delineating the mechanisms underlying the induction of oral tolerance and a thorough understanding of the associated powerful modulating effects are likely to yield new therapeutic, prophylactic, and vaccination strategies by using the convenient and immunologically efficient oral route.

REFERENCES

1. Dakin R. Remarks on a cutaneus affection, produced by certain poisonous vegetables. Am J Med Sci 1829;4:98–100.
2. Wells H. Studies on the chemistry of anaphylaxis. III. Experiments with isolated proteins, especially those of the hen's egg. J Infect Dis 1911;9:147–151.
3. Wells HG, Osborne T. The biological reactions of the vegetable proteins. I. Anaphylaxis. J Inf Dis 1911;8:66–124.
4. Chase M. Inhibition of experimental drug allergy by prior feeding of the sensitizing agent. Proc Soc Exp Med 1946;61:257–259.
5. Sulzberger MB. Arsphenamin hypersensitiveness in guinea pigs. II. Experiments demonstrating the role of the skin both as originator and as site of the hypersensitiveness. Arch Dermatol Syph 1930;22:839–844.
6. Nussenblatt RB, Caspi RR, Mahdi R, et al. Inhibition of S-antigen induced experimental autoimmune uveoretinitis by oral induction of tolerance with S-antigen. J Immunol 1990;144:1689–1695.
7. Weiner HL, Friedman A, Miller A, et al. Oral tolerance: immunologic mechanisms and treatment of animal and human organ-specific autoimmune diseases by oral administration of autoantigens. Ann Rev Immunol 1994;12:809–838.
8. Weiner HL, Paty DW. Diagnostic and therapeutic trials in multiple sclerosis: a new look. Summary of Jekyll Island workshop. Neurology 1989;39:972–976.
9. Whitacre CC, Gienapp IE, Orosz CG, Bitar DM. Oral tolerance in experimental autoimmune encephalomyelitis. III. Evidence for clonal anergy. J Immunol 1991;147:2155–2163.
10. Isolauri E, Suomalainen H, Kaila M, et al. Local immune response in patients with cow's milk allergy: follow up of patients retaining allergy or becoming tolerant. J Pediatr 1992;120:9–15.
11. Høst A. Importance of the first meal on the development of cow's milk allergy and intolerance. Allergy Proc 1991;12:227–232.
12. Savilahti E, Tuomikoski-Jaakkola P, Jarvenpaa AL, Virtanen M. Early feeding of preterm infants and allergic symptoms during childhood. Acta Paediatr 1993;82:340–344.
13. Strobel S, Ferguson A. Immune responses to fed protein antigens in mice. 3. Systemic tolerance or priming is related to age at which antigen is first encountered. Pediatr Res 1984;18:588–594.
14. Kajosaari M. Food allergy in Finnish children aged to 6 years. Acta Paediatr Scand 1982;71:815–819.
15. Høst A, Husby S, Osterballe O. A prospective study of cow's milk allergy in exclusively breast-fed infants. Incidence, pathogenetic role of early inadvertent exposure to cow's milk for-

mula, and characterization of bovine milk protein in human milk. Acta Paediatr Scand 1988;77:663–670.

16. Saarinen UM, Kajosaari M, Backman A, Siimes MA. Prolonged breast-feeding as prophylaxis for atopic disease. Lancet 1979;2:163–166.

17. Stintzing G, Zetterström R. Cow's milk allergy. Incidence and pathogenetic role of early exposure to cow's milk formula. Acta Paediatr Scand 1979;68:383–387.

18. Kjellman NIM, Hattevig G, Fälth-Magnusson K, Björksten B. Epidemiology of food allergy: with emphasis on the influence of maternal dietary restrictions during pregnancy and lactation on allergy in infancy. In: Hamburger RN, ed. Food intolerance in infancy: allergology, immunology and gastroenterology. New York: Raven Press, 1989, 105–114.

19. Foucard T. Development of food allergies with special reference to cow's milk allergy. Pediatrics 1985;75(suppl):S177–S181.

20. Strobel S. Food intolerance and allergy. In: Heatley RV, ed. Gastrointestinal and hepatic immunology. Cambridge: Cambridge University Press, 1994, 147–168.

21. Brandtzaeg P, Bjerke K, Kett K, et al. Production and secretion of immunoglobulins in the gastrointestinal tract. Annals of Allergy 1987;59:21–39.

22. Challacombe SJ, Tomasi TBJ. Systemic tolerance and secretory immunity after oral immunization. J Exp Med 1980;152:1459–1472.

23. Czerkinsky C, Svennerholm AM, Holmgren J. Induction and assessment of immunity at enteromucosal surfaces in humans: implications for vaccine development. Clin Infect Dis 1993;16:106–116.

24. Mellander L, Carlsson B, Hanson LA. Secretory IgA and IgM antibodies to E. coli O and poliovirus type I antigen occurs in amniotic fluid meconium and saliva from newborns. A neonatal immune response without antigenic exposure: a result of an anti-idiotypic induction? Clin Immunol 1987;63:555–561.

25. Lowney ED. Tolerance of a contact sensitiser in man. Lancet 1968;1:1377.

26. Korenblatt PE, Rothberg PM, Minden P, Farr RS. Immune responses of human adults after oral and parenteral exposure to bovine serum albumin. J Allergy 1968;41:226–235.

27. Husby S, Mestecky J, Moldoveanu Z, Holland S, Elson CO. Oral tolerance in humans. T cell but not B cell tolerance after antigen feeding. J Immunol 1994;152:4663–4670.

28. Mowat AM. The regulation of immune responses to dietary antigens. Immunol Today 1987;8:93–98.

29. Strobel S. Oral tolerance: 'Of mice and men.' Acta Paediatrica Japonica (Overseas Edition) 1995;37:133–140.

30. Thompson HS, Staines NA. Could specific oral tolerance be a therapy for autoimmune disease? Immunol Today 1990; 11:396–399.

31. Titus RG, Chiller JM. Orally induced tolerance. Definition at the cellular level. Int Arch Allergy Appl Immunol 1981;65:323–338.

32. Mowat AM, Strobel S, Drummond HE, Ferguson A. Immunological responses to fed protein antigens in mice. I. Reversal of oral tolerance to ovalbumin by cyclophosphamide. Immunology 1982;45:105–113.

33. Strobel S. Modulation of the immune response to fed antigens in mice. [Doctor of Philosophy]. Edinburgh, 1984.

34. Bruce MG, Strobel S, Hanson DG, Ferguson A. Transferable tolerance for cell mediated immunity after feeding is prevented by radiation damage and restored by immune reconstitution. Clin Exp Immunol 1987;70:611–618.

35. Kay RA, Ferguson A. The immunological consequences of feeding cholera toxin. II. Mechanisms responsible for the induction of oral tolerance for DTH. Immunology 1989;66:416–421.

36. Peng HJ, Turner MW, Strobel S. The kinetics of oral hyposensitisation to a protein antigen are determined by immune status and the timing, dose and frequency of antigen administration. Immunology 1989;67:425–431.

37. Asherson GL, Perera MA, Thomas WR, Zembala M. Contact-sensitizing agents and the intestinal tract: the production of immunity and unresponsiveness by feeding contact-sensitizing agents and the role of suppressor cells. In: Immunology of breast milk. New York: Raven Press, 1979.

38. Van Hoogstraten I, Boden D, Von Blomberg B, Kraal G, Scheper RJ. Persistent immune tolerance to nickel and chromium by oral administration prior to cutaneous sensitization. J Invest Dermatol 1992;99:608–616.

39. Van Hoogstraten I, Von Blomberg B, Boden D, Kraal G, Scheper RJ. Non-sensitizing epicutaneous skin tests prevent subsequent induction of immune tolerance. J Invest Dermatol 1994;102:80–83.

40. Garside P, Steel M, Liew FY, Mowat AM. CD4+ but not CD8+ T cells are required for the induction of oral tolerance. Int Immunol 1995;7:501–504.

41. Khoury SJ, Hancock WW, Weiner HL. Oral tolerance to myelin basic protein and natural recovery from experimental autoimmune encephalomyelitis are associated with downregulation of inflammatory cytokines and differential upregulation of transforming growth factor beta, interleukin 4, and prostaglandin E expression in the brain. J Exp Med 1992;176:1355–1364.

42. Imada M, Estelle F, Simons R, Jay FT, HayGlass KT. Allergen-stimulated interleukin-4 and interferon-gamma production in primary culture: Responses of subjects with allergic rhinitis and normal controls. Immunology 1995;85:373–380.

43. Fishman-Lobell J, Friedman A, Weiner HL. Different kinetic patterns of cytokine gene expression in vivo in orally tolerant mice. Eur J Immunol 1994;24:2720–2724.

44. Garside P, Steel M, Worthey EA, et al. T helper 2 cells are subject to high dose oral tolerance and are not essential for its induction. J Immunol 1995;154:5649–5655.

45. Aroeira LS, Cardillo F, De Albuquerque DA, Vaz NM, Mengel J. Anti-IL-10 treatment does not block either the induction or the maintenance of orally induced tolerance to OVA. Scand J Immunol 1995;41:319–323.

46. Saklayen MG, Pesce AJ, Pollak VE, Michael JG. Kinetics of oral tolerance: study of variables affecting tolerance induced by oral administration of antigen. Int Arch Allergy Appl Immunol 1984;73:5–9.

47. McMenamin C, McKersey M, Kuhnlein P, Hunig T, Holt PG. Gammadelta T cells down-regulate primary IgE responses in rats to inhaled soluble protein antigens. J Immunol 1995;154:4390–4394.

48. Holt PG. Regulation of antigen-presenting cell function(s) in lung and airway tissues. Eur Respiratory J 1993;6:120–129.

49. Richman LK, Graeff AS, Yarchoan R, Strober W. Simultaneous induction of antigen-specific IgA helper T cells and IgG suppressor T cells in the murine Peyer's patch after protein feeding. J Immunol 1981;126:2079–2083.

50. MacDonald T. Immunosuppression caused by antigen feeding. II. Suppressor T cells mask Peyer's Patch B cell priming to orally administered antigen. Eur J Immunol 1983;13:138–142.

51. Strobel S, Mowat AM, Drummond HE, Pickering MG, Fer-

guson A. Immunological responses to fed protein antigens in mice. II. Oral tolerance for CMI is due to activation of cyclophosphamide-sensitive cells by gut-processed antigen. Immunology 1983;49:451–456.

52. Strobel S, Ferguson A. Modulation of intestinal and systemic immune responses to a fed protein antigen, in mice. Gut 1986;27:829–837.

53. Mowat AM. The role of antigen recognition and suppressor cells in mice with oral tolerance to ovalbumin. Immunology 1985;56:253–260.

54. MacDonald TT. Immunosuppression caused by antigen feeding. I. Evidence for the activation of a feed-back suppressor pathway in the spleens of antigen-fed mice. Eur J Immunol 1982;12:767–769.

55. Van Hoogstraten I, Andersen KE, Von Blomberg BME, et al. Reduced frequency of nickel allergy upon oral nickel contact at an early stage. Clin Exp Immunol 1991;85:441–445.

56. Hanson DG, Miller SD. Inhibition of specific immune responses by feeding protein antigens. V. Induction of the tolerant state in the absence of specific suppressor cells. J Immunol 1982;128:2378–2381.

57. Gregerson DS, Obritsch WF, Donoso LA. Oral tolerance in experimental autoimmune uveoretinitis. Distinct mechanisms of resistance are induced by low dose vs high dose feeding protocols. J Immunol 1993;151:5751–5761.

58. Melamed D, Friedman A. Direct evidence for anergy in T lymphocytes tolerized by oral administration of ovalbumin. Eur J Immunol 1993;23:935–942.

59. Burtles SS, Hooper DC. The effect of neonatal tolerance to bovine gamma globulin (BGG) on BGG-reactive CD4+ T lymphocytes. Immunology 1992;75:311–317.

60. Teale JM, Klinman NR. Tolerance as an active process. Nature 1980;288:385–387.

61. Zacharchuk CM, Mercep M, June CH, Weissman AM, Ashwell JD. Variations in thymocyte susceptibility to clonal deletion during ontogeny. Implications for neonatal tolerance. J Immunol 1991;147:460–465.

62. Ideyama S, Hosono M, Imamura S, Tomana M, Katsura Y. Intrathymic induction of neonatal tolerance to Mls-1a determinant: clonal deletion and clonal anergy by haematolymphoid cells. Immunology 1991;74:240–245.

63. Speiser DE, Brandle R, Lees RK, Schneider R, Zinkernagel RM, MacDonald HR. Neonatal tolerance to Mls-1a determinants: deletion or anergy of V beta 6+ T lymphocytes depending upon MHC compatibility of neonatally injected cells. Int Immunol 1991;3:127–134.

64. Melamed D, Friedman A. In vivo tolerization of Th1 lymphocytes following a single feeding with ovalbumin: anergy in the absence of suppression. Eur J Immunol 1994;24:1974–1981.

65. Miller A, Lider O, Weiner HL. Antigen-driven bystander suppression after oral administration of antigens. J Exp Med 1991;174:791–798.

66. Mosman TR, Coffman RL. Th1 and Th2 cells: different patterns of cytokine excretion lead to different functional properties. Ann Rev Immunol 1989;7:145–173.

67. McMenamin C, McKersey M, Kuhnlein P, Hunig T, Holt PG. Gamma delta T cells down-regulate primary IgE responses in rats to inhaled soluble protein antigens. J Immunol 1995;154:4390–4394.

68. Lamont AG, Gordon M, Ferguson A. Oral tolerance in protein-deprived mice. II. Evidence of normal 'gut processing' of

ovalbumin, but suppressor cell deficiency, in deprived mice. Immunology 1987;61:339–343.

69. Mowat AM, Lamont AG, Parrott DM. Suppressor T cells, antigen-presenting cells and the role of I-J restriction in oral tolerance to ovalbumin. Immunology 1988;64:141–145.

70. Miller A, al Sabbagh A, Santos LM, Das MP, Weiner HL. Epitopes of myelin basic protein that trigger TGF-beta release after oral tolerization are distinct from encephalitogenic epitopes and mediate epitope-driven bystander suppression. J Immunol 1993;151:7307–7315.

71. Ding L, Shevach EM. Activation of CD4+ T cells by delivery of the B7 costimulatory signal on bystander antigen-presenting cells (trans-costimulation). Eur J Immunol 1994;24:859–866.

72. Strobel S. Food allergy role of mucosal immune regulation and oral tolerance: facts, fiction, and hypotheses. In: Walker WA, Harmatz PR, Wershil BK, eds. Immunophysiology of the gut. San Diego: Academic Press, 1993, 336–357.

73. Strobel S. Oral tolerance. In: Auricchio S, Ferguson A, Troncone R, eds. Mucosal immunity and the gut epithelium: interactions in health and disease. Basel: Karger, 1995, 65–75.

74. Strobel S, Ferguson A. Oral tolerance—induction and modulation. Klin Padiatr 1985;197:297–301.

75. David MF. Prevention of homocytotropic antibody formation and anaphylactic sensitisation by prefeeding antigens. J Allerg Clin Immunol 1977;60:180–187.

76. Riedel F, Kanter N, Schauer U, Petzoldt S, Rieger CH. Bronchial sensitization in guinea pigs following ingestion of ovalbumin. Int Arch Allergy Appl Immunol 1989;90:395–399.

77. Holt P, MacMenamin C, Nelson D. Primary sensitisation to inhalant allergens during infancy. Pediatr Allerg Immunol 1990;1:3–13.

78. Björkstén B. Risk factors in early childhood for the development of atopic diseases. Allergy 1994;49:400–407.

79. Moreau MC, Corthier G. Effect of the gastrointestinal microflora on induction and maintenance of oral tolerance to ovalbumin in C3H/HeJ mice. Infect Immun 1988;56:2766–2768.

80. Moreau MC, Coste M, Gaboriau V, Dubuquoy C. Oral tolerance to ovalbumin in mice: effect of some parameters on the induction and persistence of the suppression by systemic IgE and IgG antibody responses. Adv Exp Med Biol 1995;371:1229–1234.

81. Strobel S, Ferguson A. Persistence of oral tolerance in mice fed ovalbumin is different for humoral and cell-mediated immune responses. Immunology 1987;60:317–318.

82. Moffat M, Sharp P, Faux J, Young R, Cookson W, Hopkin J. Factors confounding genetic linkage between atopy and chromosome 1q. Clin Exp Allergy 1992;22:1046–1051.

83. Davies K. Allergy by mutation. Nature 1994;369:506.

84. Xu J, Levitt RC, Panhuysen C, et al. Evidence for two unlinked loci regulating total serum IgE levels. Am J Human Genetics 1995;57:425–430.

85. Cookson WO, Sharp PA, Faux JA, Hopkin IM. Linkage between immunoglobulin E responses underlying asthma and rhinitis and chromosome 11q. Lancet 1989;1:1292–1295.

86. Zwollo P, Ehrlich-Kautzky E, Scharf SJ, Ansaart AA, Ehrlich HA, Marsh DG. Sequencing of HLA-D in responders and nonresponders to short ragweed allergen, Amb aV. Immunogenetics 1991;33:141–151.

87. O'Hehir REO, Garman RD, Greenstein IL, Lamb JR. The specificity and regulation of T-cell responsiveness to allergens. Ann Rev Immunol 1991;9:67–95.

88. Jarrett EEE, Hall E. IgE suppression by maternal IgG. Immunology 1983;48:49–58.

89. Mowat AM, Lamont AG, Bruce MG. A genetically determined lack of oral tolerance to ovalbumin is due to failure of the immune system to respond to intestinally derived tolerogen. Eur J Immunol 1987;17:1673–1676.

90. Vaz NM, Rios MJ, Lopes LM, *et al.* Genetics of susceptibility to oral tolerance to ovalbumin. Braz J Med Biol Res 1987;20:785–790.

91. Lamont AG, Mowat AM, Browning MJ, Parrott DM. Genetic control of oral tolerance to ovalbumin in mice. Immunology 1988;63:737–739.

92. Miller ML, Cowdery JS, Laskin CA, Curtin MFJ, Steinberg AD. Heterogeneity of oral tolerance defects in autoimmune mice. Clin Immunol Immunopathol 1984;31:231–240.

93. Stokes CR, Swarbrick ET, Soothill JF. Genetic differences in immune exclusion and partial tolerance to ingested antigens. Clin Exp Immunol 1983;52:678–684.

94. Stokes CR, Newby TJ, Bourne FJ. The influence of oral immunization on local and systemic immune responses to heterologous antigens. Clin Exp Immunol 1983;52:399–406.

95. Sun JB, Holmgren J, Czerkinsky C. Cholera toxin B subunit: an efficient transmucosal carrier-delivery system for induction of peripheral immunological tolerance (see comments). Proc Natl Acad Sci USA 1994;91:10795–10799.

96. Holmgren J, Lycke N, Czerkinsky C. Cholera toxin and cholera B subunit as oral–mucosal adjuvant and antigen vector systems. Vaccine 1993;11:1179–1184.

97. Holmgren J, Czerkinsky C, Lycke N, Svennerholm AM. Strategies for the induction of immune responses at mucosal surfaces making use of cholera toxin B subunit as immunogen, carrier, and adjuvant. Am J Trop Med Hyg 1994;50.

98. Elson CO, Holland SP, Dertzbaugh MT, Cuff CF, Anderson AO. Morphologic and functional alterations of mucosal T cells by cholera toxin and its B subunit. J Immunol 1995;154:1032–1040.

99. Stokes CR, Newby TJ, Huntley JH, Patel D, Bourne FJ. The immune response of mice to bacterial antigens given by mouth. Immunology 1979;38:497–502.

100. Ermak TH, Bhagat HR, Pappo J. Lymphocyte compartments in antigen-sampling regions of rabbit mucosal lymphoid organs. Am J Tropical Med Hygiene 1994;50:14–28.

101. Peng HJ, Turner MW, Strobel S. The generation of a 'tolerogen' after the ingestion of ovalbumin is time-dependent and unrelated to serum levels of immunoreactive antigen. Clin Exp Immunol 1990;81:510–515.

102. Peng H-J, Chang Z-N, Han S-H, Won S-H, Huang H-T. Chemical denaturation of ovalbumin abrogates the induction of oral tolerance of specific IgG antibody and DTH responses in mice. Scand J Immunol 1995;42:297–304.

103. Hanson DG. Ontogeny of orally induced tolerance to soluble proteins in mice. I. Priming and tolerance in newborns. J Immunol 1981;127:1518–1524.

104. Husby S, Jensenius JC, Svehag SE. Passage of undegraded dietary antigen into the blood of healthy adults. Quantification, estimation of size distribution and relation of uptake levels of specific antibodies. Scand J Immunol 1985;22:83–92.

105. Husby S. Dietary antigens: uptake and humoral immunity in man. Acta Pathol Microbiol et Immunologica Scand 1988;96(suppl 1):1–40.

106. Husby S, Høst A, Teisner B, Svehag SE. Infants and children with cow milk allergy/intolerance. Investigation of the uptake of cow milk protein and activation of the complement system. Allergy 1990;45:547–551.

107. Kabelitz D. A large fraction of human peripheral blood g/d + T cells is activated by mycobacterium tuberculosis but not by 65-kD heat shock protein. J Exp Med 1990;171:667–679.

108. Kraft SC, Rothberg RM, M KC, Svoboda ACJM, LS, Farr RS. Gastric acid output and circulating anti-bovine serum albumin in adults. Clin Exp Immunol 1967;2:321–330.

109. Bloch KJ, Bloch DB, Stearns M, Walker WA. Intestinal uptake of macromolecules. VI. Uptake of protein antigen in vivo in normal rats and rats infected with *Nippostrongylus brasiliensis* or subjected to mild systemic anaphylaxis. Gastroenterology 1979;77:1039–1044.

110. Bloch KJ, Walker WA. Effect of locally induced intestinal anaphylaxis on the uptake of a bystander antigen. J Allergy Clin Immunol 1981;67:312–316.

111. Hanson DG, Roy MJ, Green GM, Miller SD. Inhibition of orally-induced immune tolerance in mice by prefeeding an endopeptidase inhibitor. Reg Immunol 1993;5:76–84.

112. Roberton DM, Paganelli R, Dinwiddie R, Levinsky RJ. Milk antigen absorption in the preterm and term neonate. Arch Dis Child 1982;57:369–372.

113. Axelsson I, Jakobsson I, Lindberg T, Polberger S, Benediktsson B, Räihä N. Macromolecular absorption in preterm and term infants. Acta Paed Scand 1989;78:532–537.

114. Walker WA, Sanderson IR. The enterocyte and antigen transport. In: Auricchio S, Ferguson A, Troncone R, eds. Mucosal immunity and the gut epithelium: interactions in health and disease. Basel: Karger, 1995, 18–31.

115. Walker WA. Role of mucosal barrier in antigen handling by the gut. In: Brostoff J, Challacombe SE, eds. Food allergy and intolerance, 1st ed. London: Bailliere Tindall, 1987, 209–222.

116. Stern M, Pang KY, Walker WA. Food proteins and gut mucosal barrier. II. Differential interaction of cows milk proteins with the mucous coat and the surface membrane of adult and immature rat jejunum. Pediat Res 1984;18:1252–1257.

117. Pike MG, Heddle RJ, Boulton P, Turner MW, Atherton DJ. Increased intestinal permeability in atopic eczema. J Invest Dermatol 1986;86:101–104.

118. Holm K, Savilahti E, Koskimies S, Lipsanen V, Maki M. Immunohistochemical changes in the jejunum in first degree relatives of patients with coeliac disease and the coeliac disease marker DQ genes. HLA class II antigen expression, interleukin-2 receptor positive cells and dividing crypt cells. Gut 1994;35:55–60.

119. Maki M. The humoral immune system in coeliac disease. Bailliere's Clinical Gastroenterology 1995;9:231–249.

120. Stenhammar L, K. F-M, Jansson G, Magnusson KE, Sundqvist T. Intestinal permeability to inert sugars and different-sized polyethyleneglycols in children with celiac disease. J Pediatr Gastroenterol Nutr 1989;9:281–289.

121. Collins FM, Carter PB. Development of delayed hypersensitivity in gnotobiotic mice. Int Arch Allergy Appl Immunol 1980;61:165–170.

122. Wannemuehler MJ, Kiyono H, Babb JL, Michalek SM, McGhee JR. Lipopolysaccharide (LPS) regulation of the immune response: LPS converts germfree mice to sensitivity to oral tolerance induction. J Immunol 1982;129:959–965.

123. Mayrhofer G, Spargo LDJ. Distribution of class II major histocompatibility antigens in enterocytes of the rat jejunum

and their association with organelles of the endocytic path-way. Immunology 1990;70:11–19.

124. Allison JP. CD28-B7 interactions in T-cell activation. Curr Opin Immunol 1994;6:414–419.

125. June CH, Ledbetter JA, Linsley PS, Thompson CB. The role of the CD28 receptor in T-cell activation. Immunol Today 1990;2:211–216.

126. Gelfanov V, Lai YG, Gelfanova V, Dong JY, Su JP, Liao NS. Differential requirement of CD28 costimulation for activation of murine CD8+ intestinal intraepithelial lymphocyte subsets and lymph node cells. J Immunol 1995;155:76–82.

127. Brodsky FM, Guagliardi LE. The cell biology of antigen processing and presentation. Ann Rev Immunol 1991;9:707–744.

128. Bland PW, Warren LG. Antigen presentation by epithelial cells of the rat small intestine. I. Kinetics, antigen specificity and blocking by anti-Ia antisera. Immunology 1986;58:1–7.

129. Bland PW, Warren LG. Antigen presentation by epithelial cells of the rat small intestine. II. Selective induction of suppressor T cells. Immunology 1986;58:9–14.

130. Mayer L, Panja A, Li Y, et al. Unique features of antigen presentation in the intestine. Ann NY Acad Sci 1992;664:39–46.

131. Mayer L, Shlien R. Evidence for function of Ia molecules on gut epithelial cells in man. J Exp Med 1987;166:1472–1483.

132. Trejdosiewicz LK. What is the role of human intestinal lymphocytes? Clin Exp Immunol 1993;94:395–397.

133. Trejdosiewicz LK, BadrelDin S, Smart CJ, et al. Colonic mucosal T lymphocytes in ulcerative colitis: expression of CD7 antigen in relation to MHC class II (HLA-D) antigens. Digestive Diseases and Sciences 1989;34:1449–1456.

134. Shinohara N, Watanabe M, Sachs DH, Hozumi N. Killing of antigen-reactive B cells by class II-restricted, soluble antigen-specific CD8+ cytolytic T lymphocytes. Nature 1988; 336:481–484.

135. Gautam SC, Battisto JR. Feeding trinitrochlorobenzene inhibits development of hapten-specific cytotoxic T lymphocytes by interfering with helper T-cell function. Reg Immunol 1989;2:33–41.

136. Poussier P, Julius M. Thymus independent T cell development and selection in the intestinal epithelium. Ann Rev Immunol 1994;12:521–555.

137. Cerf-Bensussan N, Guy-Grand D, Griscelli C. Intraepithelial lymphocyte of human gut: isolation, characterisation and study of natural killer activity. Gut 1985;26:81–88.

138. De Gens B, van den Enden A, Coolen C, Nagelkerken L, van der Heijden P, Rozing J. Phenotype of intraepithelial lymphocytes in euthymic and athymic mice: implications for differentiation of cells bearing a CD3 associated gamma, delta T cell receptor. Eur J Immunol 1990;20:291–298.

139. Halstensen TS, Scott H, Brandtzaeg P. Human intraepithelial T lymphocytes are mainly CD45Ra-RB+ and show increased co-expression of CD45RO in coeliac disease. Eur J Immunol 1990;20:1825–1830.

140. Guy-Grand D, Cerf-Bensussan N, Malissen B, Malassis-Seris M, Briottet C, Vassalli P. Two gut intraepithelial CD8+ lymphocyte populations with different T cell receptors: a role for the gut epithelium in T cell differentiation. J Exp Med 1991;173:471–481.

141. Sydora BC, Habu S, Taniguchi M. Intestinal intraepithelial lymphocytes preferentially repopulate the intestinal epithelium. Int Immunol 1993;5:743–751.

142. Sydora BC, Mixter PF, Holcombe HR, et al. Intestinal intra-epithelial lymphocytes are activated and cytolytic but do not proliferate as well as other T cells in response to mitogenic signals. J Immunol 1993;150:2179–2191.

143. Mowat A. Human intraepithelial lymphocytes. Springer Semi-nars in Immunopathology 1990;12:165–190.

144. Ebert EC, Roberts AI. Pitfalls in the characterization of small intestinal lymphocytes. J Immunol Methods 1995;178:219–227.

145. Blumberg RS, Yockey CE, Gross GG, Ebert EC, Balk SP. Human intestinal intraepithelial lymphocytes are derived from a limited number of T cell clones that utilize multiple V beta T cell receptor genes. J Immunol 1993;150:5144–5153.

146. Cuff CF, Cebra CK, Rubin DH, Cebra JJ. Developmental relationship between cytotoxic alpha/beta T cell receptor-positive intraepithelial lymphocytes and Peyer's patch lymphocytes. Eur J Immunol 1993;23:1333–1339.

147. McMenamin C, Schon HM, Oliver J, Girn B, Holt PG. Regulation of IgE responses to inhaled antigens: cellular mechanisms underlying allergic sensitization versus tolerance induction. Int Arch Allergy Appl Immunol 1991;94:78–82.

148. Fujihashi K, Taguchi T, McGhee JR, et al. Regulatory function for murine intraepithelial lymphocytes. Two subsets of CD3+, T cell receptor-1+ intraepithelial lymphocyte T cells abrogate oral tolerance. J Immunol 1990;145:2010–2019.

149. Fujihashi K, Kiyono H, Aicher WK, et al. Immunoregulatory function of CD3+, CD4−, and CD8− T cells. Gamma delta T cell receptor-positive T cells from nude mice abrogate oral tolerance. J Immunol 1989;143:3415–3422.

150. Troncone R, Ferguson A. Gliadin presented via the gut induces oral tolerance in mice. Clin Exp Immunol 1988;72:284–287.

151. Lamont AG, Mowat AM, Parrott DM. Priming of systemic and local delayed-type hypersensitivity responses by feeding low doses of ovalbumin to mice. Immunology 1989;66:595–599.

152. Troncone R, Ferguson A. In mice, gluten in maternal diet primes systemic immune responses to gliadin in offspring. Immunology 1988;64:533–537.

153. Halken S, Jacobsen HP, Host A, Holmenlund D. The effect of hypo-allergenic formulas in infants at risk of allergic disease. Eur J Clin Nutr 1995;49:S77–S83.

154. Høst A, Halken S. A prospective study of cow milk allergy in Danish infants during the first 3 years of life. Clinical course in relation to clinical and immunological type of hypersensitivity reaction. Allergy 1990;45:587–596.

155. Björksten B, Kjellman NI. Does breast-feeding prevent food allergy? Allergy Proc 1991;12:233–237.

156. Grulee CG, Sanford HN. The influence of breast feeding on infantile eczema. J Pediatr 1936;9:223–228.

157. Zeiger RS, Heller S, Mellon MH, Halsey JF, Hamburger RN, Sampson HA. Genetic and environmental factors affecting the development of atopy through age 4 in children of atopic parents: a prospective, randomized study of food allergen avoidance. Ped Allergy Immunol 1992;3:110–127.

158. Troncone R, Scarcella A, Danatiello A, et al. Passage of gliadin into human breast milk. 1987;76:453–456.

159. Kilshaw PJ, Cant AJ. The passage of maternal dietary proteins into human breast milk. Int Arch Allergy Appl Immunol 1984;75:8–15.

160. Petralanda I, Yarzabal L, Piessens WF. Parasite antigens are present in breast milk of women infected with *Onchocerca volvulus*. Am J Trop Med Hyg 1988;38:372–379.

161. Gerrard JW, Shenassa M. Sensitization to substances in breast milk: recognition, management and significance. Ann Allergy 1983;4738.

162. Warner JO. Food allergy in fully breast fed infants. Clin Allergy 1980;10:133–136.

163. Lindfors A, Enocksson E. Development of atopic disease after early administration of cow milk formula. Allergy 1988;43:11–16.

164. Savilahti E, Tainio VM, Salmenperä L, Siimes MA, Perheentupa J. Prolonged exclusive breast feeding and heredity as determinants in infantile atopy. Arch Dis Child 1987;62:269–273.

165. Chandra RK, Puri S, Suraiya C, Cheema PS. Influence of maternal food antigen avoidance during pregnancy and lactation on incidence of atopic eczema in infants. Clin Allergy 1986;16:563–569.

166. Chandra RK, Puri S, Hamed A. Influence of maternal diet during lactation and use of formula feeds on development of atopic eczema in high risk infants. BMJ 1989;299:228–230. (Published erratum appears in BMJ 1989;299(6704):896.)

167. Zeiger RS, Heller S, Mellon MH, et al. Effect of prenatal and postnatal dietary prophylaxis on development of atopy in early infancy: a randomised study. J Allergy Clin Immunol 1989;84:72–89.

168. Vandenplas Y, Hauser B, Van Den Borre C, et al. The long-term effect of a partial whey hydrolysate formula on the prophylaxis of atopic disease. Eur J Pediatr 1995;154:488–494.

169. Halken S, Høst A, Hansen LG, Østerballe O. Preventive effect of feeding high risk infants a casein hydrolysate formula or an ultrafiltrated whey hydrolysate formula. A prospective, randomized, comparative clinical study. Pediatr Allerg Immunol 1993;4:173–181.

170. ESPGAN committee on nutrition, Aggett PG, Haschke F, et al. Comment on antigen-reduced infant formulae. Acta Paediatr 1993;82:314–320.

171. Businco L, Dreborg S, Einarsson R, et al. Hydrolysed cow's milk formulae: allergenicity and use for treatment and prevention. An ESPACI position paper. Pediatr Allerg Immunol 1993;3:101–111.

172. Bruce MG, Ferguson A. Oral tolerance to ovalbumin in mice: studies of chemically modified and 'biologically filtered' antigen. Immunology 1986;57:627–630.

173. Furrie E, Turner MW, Strobel S. Partial characterisation of a circulating tolerogenic moiety which, after a feed of ovalbumin, suppresses delayed hypersensitivity in recipient mice. Immunology 1995;86:480–486.

174. Miller A, Lider O, Abramsky O, Weiner HL. Orally administered myelin basic protein in neonates primes for immune responses and enhances experimental autoimmune encephalomyelitis in adult animals. Eur J Immunol 1994;24:1026–1032.

175. Peng HJ, Turner MW, Strobel S. Failure to induce oral tolerance to protein antigens in neonatal mice can be corrected by transfer of adult spleen cells. Pediatr Res 1989;26:486–490.

176. Strobel S. Dietary manipulation and induction of tolerance. J Pediatr 1992;121:S74–S79.

177. Sanderson IR, Ouellette AJ, Carter EA, Harmatz PR. Ontogeny of Ia messenger RNA in the mouse small intestinal epithelium is modulated by age of weaning and diet. Gastroenterology 1993;105:974–980.

178. Miller BG, Whittemore CT, Stokes CR, Telemo E. The effect of delayed weaning on the development of oral tolerance to soya-bean protein in pigs. Br J Nutr 1994;71:615–625.

179. Heppell LM, Sissons JW, Banks SM. Sensitisation of preruminant calves and piglets to antigenic protein in early weaning diets: control of the systemic antibody responses. Res Vet Sci 1989;47:257–262.

180. Shacks SJ, Heiner DC. Allergy to breast milk. Clin Immunol Allergy 1982;2:121–136.

181. Björksten B, Kjellman NIM. Perinatal factors influencing the development of allergy. Clin Rev Allergy 1987;5:339–347.

182. Firer MA, Hosking CS, Hill DJ. Effect of antigen load on development of milk antibodies in infants allergic to milk. Br Med J 1981;283:693–696.

183. Schmitz J, Digeon B, Chastang C, et al. Effects of brief early exposure to partially hydrolyzed and whole cow milk proteins. J Pediatr 1992;121:S85–S90.

184. Sobel RA, Hafler DA, Castro EE, Morimoto C, Weiner HL. Immunohistochemical analysis of suppressor-inducer and helper-inducer T cells in multiple sclerosis brain tissue. Ann NY Acad Sci 1988;540.

185. Elson CO. Do organ-specific suppressor T cells prevent autoimmune gastritis? Gastroenterology 1990;98:226–229.

186. Miller A, Hafler DA, Weiner HL. Tolerance and suppressor mechanisms in experimental autoimmune encephalomyelitis: implications for immunotherapy of human autoimmune diseases. Faseb J 1991;5:2560–2566.

187. Lamont AG, Bruce MG, Watret KC, Ferguson A. Suppression of an established DTH response to ovalbumin in mice by feeding antigen after immunization. Immunology 1988;64:135–139.

188. Mattingly JA, Kaplan JM, Janeway CW. Two distinct antigen-specific suppressor factors induced by the oral administration of antigen. J Exp Med 1980;152:545–554.

189. Hoyne GF, Callow MG, Kuhlman J, Thomas WR. T-cell lymphokine response to orally administered proteins during priming and unresponsiveness. Immunology 1993;78:534–540.

190. Mowat AM. Depletion of suppressor T cells by 2'-deoxyguanosine abrogates tolerance in mice fed ovalbumin and permits the induction of intestinal delayed-type hypersensitivity. Immunology 1986;58:179–184.

191. Furrie E. Intestinal modification of a protein antigen and its effect on oral tolerance induction [Doctor of Philosophy]. London, 1993.

192. Kagnoff MF. Effects of antigen feeding on intestinal and systemic immune responses IV. Similarity between the suppressor factor in mice after erythrocyte-lysate injection and erythrocyte feeding. Gastroenterology 1980;79:54–61.

193. André C, Heremans JF, Vaerman J, Cambiaso CL. A mechanism for the induction of immunological tolerance by antigen feeding: antigen-antibody complexes. J Exp Med 1975;142:1509.

194. Fujihashi K, Taguchi T, Aicher WK, et al. Immunoregulatory functions for murine intraepithelial lymphocytes: gamma/delta T cell receptor-positive (TCR+) T cells abrogate oral tolerance, while alpha/beta TCR+ T cells provide B cell help. J Exp Med 1992;175:695–707.

195. Staines NA, Harper N. Oral tolerance in the control of

experimental models of autoimmune disease. Z Rheumatol 1995;54:145–154.

196. Van Hoogstraten I, Boos C, Boden D, Von Blomberg ME, Scheper RJ, Kraal G. Oral induction of tolerance to nickel sensitization in mice. J Investigative Dermatol 1993;101:26–31.

197. Czerkinsky C, Holmgren J. Exploration of mucosal immunity in humans: relevance to vaccine development. Cell Mol Biol (Noisy le grand) 1994;40.

198. Metzler B, Wraith DC. Inhibition of experimental autoimmune encephalomyelitis by inhalation but not oral administration of the encephalitogenic peptide: influence of MHC binding affinity. Int Immunol 1993;5:1159–1165.

199. Miller A, Zhang ZJ, Sobel RA, al Sabbagh A, Weiner HL. Suppression of experimental autoimmune encephalomyelitis by oral administration of myelin basic protein. VI. Suppression of adoptively transferred disease and differential effects of oral vs. intravenous tolerization. J Neuroimmunol 1993;46:73–82.

200. Friedman A, Weiner HL. Induction of anergy or active suppression following oral tolerance is determined by antigen dosage. Proc Natl Acad Sci USA 1994;91:6688–6692.

201. Trentham DE, Dynesius-Trentham RA, Orav EJ, et al. Effects of oral administration of type II collagen on rheumatoid arthritis. Science 1993;261:1727–1730.

202. Miller A, Lider O, Roberts AB, Sporn MB, Weiner HL. Suppressor T cells generated by oral tolerization to myelin basic protein suppress both in vitro and in vivo immune responses by the release of transforming growth factor beta after antigen-specific triggering. Proc Natl Acad Sci USA 1992;89:421–425.

203. Weiner HL, Mackin GA, Matsui M, et al. Double blind pilot trial of oral tolerisation with myelin antigens in multiple sclerosis. Science 1993;259:1321–1324.

204. Czarny D. Immunotherapy for allergic disorders. Modern Medicine of Australia 1994;37:80–85.

205. Berchtold E, Maibach R, Muller U. Reduction of side effects from rush-immunotherapy with honey bee venom by pretreatment with terfenadine. Clin Exp Allergy 1992;22:59–65.

206. Bauer CP. Hyposensitization treatment of inhalation-allergies in childhood. Zeitschrift fur Hautkrankheiten 1991;66:52–54.

207. Calvo M, Marin F, Grob K, et al. Ten-year follow-up in pediatric patients with allergic bronchial asthma: evaluation of specific immunotherapy. J Investigational Allerg Clin Immunol 1994;4:126–131.

208. McCormack DR, Salata KF, Hershey JN, Carpenter GB, Engler RJ. Mosquito bite anaphylaxis: immunotherapy with whole body extracts. Ann Allerg 1995;74:39–44.

209. Reisman RE. Stinging insect allergy. Medical Clinics of North America 1992;76:883–894.

210. Kay AB, Lessof MH. Allergy: conventional and alternative concepts. A report of the Royal College of Physicians Committee on Clinical Immunology and Allergy. Clinical and Experimental Allergy 1992;22(suppl):i–44.

211. Beljan JR, Bohigian GM, Estes EH J, et al. In vivo diagnostic testing and immunotherapy for allergy. Report I, Part I, of the Allergy Panel of the Council on Scientific Affairs. JAMA 1987;258:1363–1367.

212. Douglas DM, Sukenick E, Andrade WP, Brown JS. Biphasic systemic anaphylaxis: an inpatient and outpatient study. J Allergy Clin Immunol 1994;93:977–985.

213. Yunginger JW. Anaphylaxis. Ann Allergy 1992;69:87–99.

214. Björkstén B. Local immunotherapy is not documented for clinical use. Eur J Allergy Clin Immunol 1994;49:299–301.

215. Bousquet J, Michel FB, Creticos PS, et al. Sublingual immunotherapy for cat allergy [1]. J Allergy Clin Immunol 1995;95:920–921.

216. Rios MJ, Pereira MA, Lopes LM, et al. Tolerance induction and immunological priming initiated by mucosal contacts with protein antigens in inbred strains of mice. Braz J Med Biol Res 1988;21:825–836.

217. Carr RI, Tilley D, Forsyth S, Etheridge P, Sadi D. Failure of oral tolerance in (NZB × NZW) F1 mice is antigen specific and appears to parallel antibody patterns in human systemic lupus erythematosus (SLE). Clin Immunol Immunopathol 1987;42:298–310.

218. Acha-Orbea H, Steinman L, McDevitt HO. T cell receptors in autoimmune disease as targets for immune intervention. Genome 1989;31:656–661.

219. Higgins PJ, Weiner HL. Suppression of experimental autoimmune encephalomyelitis by oral administration of myelin basic protein and its fragments. J Immunol 1988;140:440–445.

220. Lider O, Santos LM, Lee CS, Higgins PJ, Weiner HL. Suppression of experimental autoimmune encephalomyelitis by oral administration of myelin basic protein. II. Suppression of disease and in vitro immune responses is mediated by antigen-specific CD8+ T lymphocytes. J Immunol 1989;142:748–752.

221. Bitar DM, Whitacre CC. Suppression of experimental autoimmune encephalomyelitis by the oral administration of myelin basic protein. Cellular Immunol 1988;112:364–370.

222. Miller A, Hafler DA, Weiner HL. Immunotherapy in autoimmune diseases. Curr Opin Immunol 1991;3:936–940.

223. Vischer TL. Oral desensitization in the treatment of human immune diseases. Z Rheumatol 1995;54:155–157.

224. Steinman L. Development of antigen-specific therapies for autoimmune disease. Mol Biol Med 1990;7:333–339.

225. Bland P. MHC class II expression by the gut epithelium. Immunol Today 1988;9:174–178.

226. Bland PW, Whiting CW. Antigen processing by isolated rat intestinal villus enterocytes. Immunology 1989;68:497–502.

227. Keren DF. Antigen processing in the mucosal immune system. Semin Immunol 1992;4:217–226.

228. Liu LM, MacPherson GG. Antigen acquisition by dendritic cells: intestinal dendritic cells acquire antigen administered orally and can prime naive T cells in vivo. J Exp Med 1993;177:1299–1307.

229. Sansom DM, Hall ND. B7/BB1, the ligand for CD28 is expressed on repeatedly activated human T cells in vitro. Eur J Immunol 1993;23:295–298.

230. Van Wilsem E, Van Hoogstraten I, Breve J, Scheper RJ, Kraal G. Dendritic cells of the oral mucosa and the induction of oral tolerance. A local affair. Immunology 1994;83:128–132.

231. Strobel S, Mowat AM, Ferguson A. Prevention of oral tolerance induction to ovalbumin and enhanced antigen presentation during a graft-versus-host reaction in mice. Immunology 1985;56:57–64.

232. Mowat AM, Lamont AG, Strobel S, Mackenzie S. The role of antigen processing and suppressor T cells in immune responses to dietary proteins in mice. Adv Exp Med Biol 1987;216A:709–720.

233. Thomas WR, Cooper D, Holt PG. Immunity at body surfaces. Immunologist 1995;5–6:201–203.

234. Hoyne GF, Callow MG, Kuo MC, Thomas WR. Differences in epitopes recognized by T cells during oral tolerance and priming. Immunol Cell Biol 1994;72:29–33.

235. Suh ED, Vistica BP, Chan CC, Raber JM, Gery I, Nussenblatt RB. Splenectomy abrogates the induction of oral tolerance in experimental autoimmune uveoretinitis. Curr Eye Res 1993;12:833–839.

236. Van der Heijden PJ, Stok W, Bianchi ATJ. Mucosal suppression by oral pre-treatment with ovalbumin and its conversion into stimulation when ovalbumin was conjugated to cholera toxin or its B subunit. Adv Exp Med Biol 1995;371:1251–1255.

237. Ziegler EE, Fomon SJ, Nelson SE, *et al.* Cow milk feeding in infancy: further observations on blood loss from the gastrointestinal tract. J Pediatr 1990;116:11–18.

7

IN VITRO DIAGNOSTIC METHODS IN THE EVALUATION OF FOOD HYPERSENSITIVITY

Carsten Bindslev-Jensen
Lars K. Poulsen

*T*he aim of this chapter is to define which laboratory tests have been demonstrated to be relevant for food hypersensitivity, and to provide a framework for evaluating new results in this area.

Introduction

The only accepted methods for establishing a firm diagnosis of food hypersensitivity are the double-blind, placebo-controlled food challenge (DBPCFC) and open the controlled challenges in young infants (2, 56). As DBPCFC constitutes the ultimate diagnostic tool, and a restricted diet represents the ultimate therapy for food hypersensitivity, it might be argued that all in vitro diagnostic methods should be considered optional rather than essential for the clinician. A diagnosis based on challenges does not, however, elucidate underlying pathogenic mechanisms or guide the clinician toward an understanding of the natural history of the reaction. On the other hand, in vitro diagnostic tests may shed light on two aspects of the disease:

1. The causative agent (i.e., the offending food item).
2. The pathophysiology of the hypersensitivity reaction.

Moreover, the two aspects may be combined when pathophysiological parameters are determined in conjunction with a placebo-controlled challenge situation.

Much effort is being directed at identifying the various cells and molecules in the immune system and discerning their possible relationships to the clinical symptoms generated when a food is ingested by a hypersensitive patient (Table 7.1). It should be emphasized, however, that the existence of an immune response to food antigens does not per se imply a symptomatic food hypersensitivity (39). Coexistence of other hypersensitivity disorders, such as asthma or dermatitis of nonfood origin (e.g., sensitization to house dust mite), may also prevent the correct interpretation of inflammatory markers.

Most of our present knowledge relates to the immediate reactions leading to clinical disease within minutes to hours after ingestion. Late reactions—perhaps immunological Type IV reactions—appear to play a role in some patients in whom a classical Type 1 reaction cannot be established. Type 1 reactions—reactions involving immunoglobulin E [IgE]—are, however, the only mechanism that has been conclusively proven to have etiological significance in food hypersensitivity.

Validation of In Vitro Diagnostic Tests

Prior to introducing diagnostic assays for new biochemical mediators into clinical practice, the following three conditions should be addressed (8):

1. Can the test measure the new mediator with sufficient specificity and precision (i.e., has the assay been technically validated)?

2. Are abnormal values of the new substance associated with clinical disease (i.e., has the assay been clinically validated) and are age- and sex-matched normal values (reference intervals) available?

3. Can other physiological or pathological conditions produce responses outside the reference interval?

When sufficient data exist to respond to the three questions, answers will often be expressed in both qualitative and quantitative terms. For example, the technical validation may demonstrate a certain interference from other substances, and the accuracy and reproducibility parameters of a biochemical test may indicate a result within ±20% of the correct value in 95% of all analyses.

In addition, the answers to questions 2 and 3 may be given qualitatively (e.g., almost all grass-allergic patients have specific IgE to cereals but no food hypersensitivity) (78) or in statistical terms, (e.g., by the concepts of sensitivity, specificity, and predictive values).

TECHNICAL VALIDATION

Despite widely varying designs for in vitro tests, some important general parameters can be applied in the technical validation (Table 7.2). Although the examples given in the table relate to tests for specific IgE, the general principle should apply to all tests. In evaluating an in vitro test, several concepts such as sensitivity and specificity can be applied. The definitions of these parameters are briefly discussed below.

Analytical Sensitivity

The analytical sensitivity (detection limit) is the smallest amount of a substance that can be determined (i.e., differentiated from zero) using the method. Depending on assay conditions, the detection limit may be defined as low as possible (e.g., as three times the standard deviation from the zero value), or it may be arbitrarily set to a higher level. Because specific IgE has been closely connected to disease, analytical sensitivity has sometimes been confused with clinical sensitivity (see below). With improved analytical sensitivities of immunological assays, it becomes increasingly important to understand that detection of any level of specific IgE does not imply pathology per se.

Related to analytical sensitivity is the *measurement range*, which defines the span between the detection limit and the largest amount that can be measured in an assay. In most cases, the measurement range can be expanded upward by dilution of the sample.

Analytical Specificity

Many in vitro tests are of immunological origin, and thus deal with the immunologically based concept of specificity; in other words, they rely on the ability of an antibody or T cell to differentiate one antigen from another. Once again, it is important to realize the difference between analytical specificity and clinical specificity. An assay for specific IgE to soybean or pea may, for example, detect IgE to peanut, whereas

Table 7.1
In Vitro Diagnostic Methods Applicable for Studies of Food Hypersensitivity

Identification of the Offending Food Items
Antibodies to food antigens:
IgE
Other isotypes: IgA, IgG, IgM
Circulating immune complexes containing food antigens

Specific cellular immune response to food antigens:
Specific T cells (determined as proliferation, cytotoxicity, etc.)
Food-induced mast cell or basophil histamine release
Food-induced leukocyte activation

The Pathophysiology of the Food Hypersensitivity
Markers of the four "classic" hypersensitivity reactions:
I. Raised IgE levels
II. ?
III. Raised complement split products
IV. ?

Markers (mediators) of inflammatory cell activation:
Lipid mediators (derived from a number of cell types) (prosta-
   glandins, leukotrienes, thromboxanes, PAF, etc.)
Mast cell (or basophil) mediators: tryptase, histamine
Eosinophil mediators: ECP, EPX/EDN, EPO
Neutrophil mediators: MPO, HNL
Cytokines, chemokines
Adhesion molecules
Complement products

Markers of decreased immunological barrier function:
Increased gastrointestinal permeability

Table 7.2
Parameters Influencing the Outcome of a Diagnostic Test

Parameter	Example: Tests for Specific IgE
Design	Choice of solid phase
	Choice of detection principle
	Time and temperature conditions of incubations (often a compromise between speed and analytical sensitivity)
	Manual–semiautomatic–automated
Reagent quality	Quality of allergen extract
	Quality of detection antibody: anti-human IgE
Apparatus	Washing of solid phase between incubations
	Raw data measurement (depending on detection principle: gamma counter, fluorometer, ELISA-reader, etc.)

The combinations of the parameters mentioned above produce the *inherent* analytical sensitivity, accuracy, and reproducibility of a diagnostic test as supplied by the manufacturer, whereas the parameters listed below add further uncertainties that will be experienced by the clinician demanding the test from the laboratory.

Human factors in laboratory	Educational background
	Experience
Quality level of laboratory	Monoplicate/duplicate determinations
	Existence of internal and external quality assurance programs
Biological factors in sample	High levels of total IgE
	High levels of specific IgG
	Cross-reactivity between different allergens

a peanut-allergic patient does not necessarily react clinically to soybean or pea (6).

Accuracy and Precision

Accuracy (correctness) describes the ability of a test to reach the target value, which is the value considered true from other assays or from consensus among a large number of assays. In contrast, precision (reproducibility) describes the ability to reach the same result in a series of multiple measurements in one assay or in a day-to-day design. An accurate test is not necessarily precise, and vice versa.

Quality Control

Tests that are analytically sensitive and specific, accurate, and precise are said to be *reliable*. The reliability of a test may be documented by the producer/supplier, but to ensure effectiveness, the standards of the

laboratory employing the tests should also be validated regularly. Suppliers of test kits and independent organizations are introducing an increasing number of quality control programs for this purpose, and major improvements are expected in the coming years (26).

CLINICAL VALIDATION

A large body of theoretical literature focuses on the clinical evaluation of diagnostic tests (reviewed in 29), so we will only briefly allude to a few concepts here (Table 7.3).

Clinical Sensitivity and Specificity

Clinical sensitivity/specificity (meaning diagnostic sensitivity/specificity, but sometimes just referred to as sensitivity/specificity) measures the fractions of

Table 7.3
Concepts in Clinical Validation of a Test

		Test Result		
		Positive	Negative	
Disease	Diseased	a	b	a+b
	Not Diseased	c	d	c+d
		a+c	b+d	a+b+c+d

True positive: a   False positive: c
True negative: d   False negative: b
Prevalence of disease in study population: $(a+b)/(a+b+c+d)$
Clinical sensitivity (SE): $a/(a+b)$
Clinical specificity: (SP): $d/(c+d)$
Positive predictive value (PPV): $a/(a+c)$
Negative predictive value (NPV): $d/(b+d)$
Concordance: $(a+d)/(a+b+c+d)$

Example 1	Example 2
Prevalence: 50%	Prevalence: 0.1%
SE = SP = 90%	SE = SP = 90%

	Pos	Neg		Pos	Neg
Disease	90	10	Disease	9	1
No disease	10	90	No disease	1000	9000

PPV = 90%	PPV = 0.9%
NPV = 90%	NPV = 99.99%

positive tests among the diseased in a study population and the fraction of negative tests among the reference population (not diseased).

Positive and Negative Predictive Values

From the clinical sensitivity and specificity, the positive and negative predictive values can be calculated according to the method in Table 7.3. From the examples given, it can be clearly seen that the prevalence of diseased persons included in a study will affect the predictive values of the test.

The True Diagnosis

Before calculating SE, SP, and predictive values for a new test, it is critical to determine "the true diagnosis." In food hypersensitivity, the "gold standard" is DBPCFC, and any new test must be validated in patients meeting this criteria (2, 8, 56). Although the procedures available for performing DBPCFC have drawbacks and limitations (9, 18) it remains the diagnostic tool to which every new test should be

compared. Knowledge of these parameters is, therefore, of utmost importance when evaluating any test used in the diagnosis of food hypersensitivity.

LEVELS OF VALIDATION

With the increasing focus on allergy and on the nature and quality of foods ingested by humans, new groups of patients have emerged—patients presenting with symptoms such as hyperactivity, muscle or joint diseases, or syndromes such as multiple chemical sensitivity, which are not classified as of atopic origin (12, 83). In these patients, our traditional diagnostic tools, such as measurement of specific IgE antibodies or prick skin tests, have little value. As a result, a number of new tests have arisen that often are used outside university settings, but that remain poorly documented and, when investigated, rarely (if ever) prove clinically valuable (8). Based on the considerations mentioned above and the information available, in vitro diagnostic tests for food hypersensitivity may be divided into three groups: (1) tests of proven value, (2) tests that must currently be classified as "not thoroughly validated," and (3) tests without value (Table 7.4). Several different methods for measurement of specific IgE (sIgE) are now available (Table 7.5). It is important to emphasize that most of these tests have been compared with another sIgE test (usually the market leader) and are therefore classified as part of the second group. Even the tests classified in the first group have been thoroughly evaluated only for the most common allergens. If such a test is used with more exotic allergens, it should be classified as "not thoroughly validated."

Strategy for the In Vitro Diagnosis of Food Hypersensitivity

The mere presence of specific IgE against a food (or the presence of any other cell or mediator) does not indicate clinical disease. Because most clinical reactions occur as immediate reactions after food ingestion, and as reactions involving IgE are the only mechanism that has been conclusively proved to be of etiological significance in food hypersensitivity, the

Table 7.4
Classification of Diagnostic Tests for In Vitro Use (Depends upon allergen measured. Examples are given. List is not all-inclusive.)

Tests that have been validated and found to be useful in the diagnosis of food hypersensitivity (Category 1)	Specific IgE: (RAST), CAP, Magic Lite, Basophil histamine release
Tests that have not been thoroughly validated (Category 2)	(RAST), CAP, Magic Lite, Basophil histamine release, Gut permeability tests, Intragastric provocation (IPEC), Patch tests, Histamine release from gut mast cells, T cells and subsets, New tests for specific IgE in serum, Specific IgE in other body fluids, IgE-complexes, IgG-complexes, Complement (or split products) Other mediators: Tryptase, Histamine in body fluids, ECP, IgG subsets, Cytokines "Probes": PEG, Lactulose/mannitol, Blood-xylose All kinds of "alternative methods" (e.g., ALCAT-test and many others)
Tests that have been validated and found *not* to be useful in the diagnosis of food hypersensitivity (Category 3)	Serum IgG

primary factor to investigate is specific IgE. When it is found, the next step is to ascertain the relevance of this finding, concluding with a DBPCFC. A negative result will necessitate reevaluation of the outcome; it may be due to insufficient sensitivity of the test with the allergen in question, or to a non-IgE-mediated reaction, either immediate or delayed (9).

Tests for Identification of the Causative Food Item

In tests attempting to identify an offending food, an extract of the food allergen in question must be utilized. If important components present in the

Table 7.5
Classification of Assays for Specific IgE with Examples of Research Procedures and Commercially Available Assays

			Detection Principle			
			Radioactivity	Enzyme Reaction	Enzyme/ Fluorescence	Chemiluminescensce
Immunochemi-cal reaction	Fluid phase			AlaStat (21)		
	Microparticles		Micro-cellulose RAST (81)			Magic Lite (46)
	Solid phase	Polystyrene	Maxisorp RAST* (71)			
		Paper	Phadebas RAST (15)	Phadezym RAST (15)		
		Cellulose "sponge"	CAP RIA (23)		CAP FEIA (23)	
		Nitrocellulose		Abbott Matrix (63)		MAST CLA (65)
		Electrophoretically separated allergen extract	CRIE* (80) Western blot* (44) 2-D blot*			

*Research analyses; not suitable for routine use.

native allergen material are missing in the extracts used for the in vitro assay, false negatives will result, lowering sensitivity of the test when compared with DBPCFC (9, 64). Use of allergenic material of optimal quality in the assay is, therefore, of primary importance.

Much attention has been drawn to the possible development of new antigens in food when processed or when ingested, but so far no convincing reports on the clinical significance of such neo-allergens have been made. It is, therefore, still advisable to use an allergenic material as close as possible to the native food, if only because the immune responses in many cases are directed toward epitopes on different proteins in the food.

Only in a limited number of foods have the allergens been sufficiently characterized and standardized to enable investigations on a single protein. The presence of labile allergens, which are destroyed during preparation of a food, is unlikely to be recognized. This lack of knowledge further hampers the use of the assays when investigating food whose quality is less well documented (Table 7.6). Because the documentation for most foods is limited or lacking, every allergen system should be evaluated as an independent entity. Thus, results from one allergen test system should never be transferred to other systems.

MEASUREMENT OF SPECIFIC IgE

Most immunochemical assays for specific IgE are based on: (1) the binding of specific IgE molecules to the allergen and (2) the binding of a detection antibody to human IgE. By combining these principles, allergen-specific IgE is selected from the total amount of IgE, as well as from other allergen-binding antibodies or proteins in the sample.

Immunochemical assays for IgE can be characterized according to the way the allergen is introduced in the assay, and according to the principle used for detection of IgE (Table 7.5). Moreover, the assay can be characterized in terms of specificity, ranging from the ability to identify panels of allergens from different foods down to single recombinant allergens (Table 7.7). Even though "screeners" and "panels" may be used initially to decide whether further testing is

Table 7.6
Allergens and Cross-Reacting Foods

Food	Cross-reactions	Reference
Allergens Well Documented and Clinically Well Established		
Cow's milk	Goat's milk, mare's milk, sheep's milk	38
Hen's egg	Goose's egg, turkey's egg, duck's egg,	53
	etc.; chicken meat, bird's feathers	49
Codfish	Plaice, mackerel, herring, other fishes	69
		5
		32
		33
Peanut*	Soy, green bean, lima bean	6
Shrimp	Crab, crayfish, lobster	16
		17
Allergens Less Well Documented		
Hazelnut	Other nuts	
	Birch (and birch cross-reacting: hazel-	30
	nut, apple, almond, tomato, po-	37
	tato, avocado, cherry)	22
Wheat*	Grasspollen, rye, sesame, maize, buck-	78
	wheat, oats	
Kiwi	Birch cross-reacting foods	79
		28
Apple	Birch and birch cross-reacting foods	66
		22
Banana	Latex, avocado, pear	51
		48
Allergens Not Documented		
Other fruits		
Other vegetables		
All kinds of meat		

* Rarely of clinical significance.

necessary, the final diagnosis should still rely on the outcome of a test for reactivity to a single food allergen. A large fraction of all patients will react to the major allergens in an extract. It seems premature to substitute "whole" allergen extracts with one to four major allergens in recombinant forms, however, even though major allergens have been cloned in a number of inhalation allergen systems, the same trend could conceivably be valid for food allergens.

The two major determinants for the quality of any assay for specific IgE must always be kept in mind (Table 7.2): (1) the assay design and performance, and (2) the quality of the allergens used in the assay.

Assay Design

As Table 7.5 shows, a large number of solid matrices exist, and theoretically based hypotheses of the opti-

Table 7.7
Types of Allergen Extracts Employed
in Assays for Specific IgE

Type	Description	Example
Screeners	Widely different allergen systems	Extracts of five different food allergens
Panels	Related allergen systems	Extracts of food allergens cross-reacting with birch pollen
Allergens	Single allergen systems	Cow's milk extract
Individual allergens	Subsystems of single allergens	rBet v1, a recombinant protein cloned from the major allergen of birch pollen

mal solid phase and ideal coupling chemistry are probably as numerous as the commercial variants. Basically, the extract included in the test should have as many of the allergenic components as possible. Each of these components should be in a sufficient surplus to bind all antibody (not only IgE antibodies) in the serum sample. Because standards for specific IgE are lacking, it is difficult to provide documentation that these demands are met. On a practical level, this lack of standards dictates that clinical trials must be performed on large and varied patient materials.

Allergen Extracts

No in vitro test for specific IgE will ever be better than the extracts it employs. Extract quality has been a driving force behind clinical and experimental advances in allergology, and revised guidelines on this issue have recently been published (20). Such major advances have been made for the important inhalation allergens and insect venoms. New allergenic materials, including foods, are constantly being reported, however, creating a gap between the desire for new tests and the available knowledge about the biochemistry and immunochemistry of these newly reported allergenic materials. Given the many new and rare allergenic materials, the lack of sera from a sufficient number of clinically well-characterized patients will limit the development of a properly validated in vitro test for specific IgE. It seems justi-

fied for a commercial supplier to categorize its IgE-based products depending on the scientific documentation of the validity of the allergen extract used in the tests. Based on the relative levels of specific IgE toward constituents in a food, it is not possible to deduce anything regarding which IgE specificity bears the most clinical relevance, another argument for the use of "native" extracts.

In most cases of foods where little or no documentation on the allergens are available, the dearth of information relates to the lack of study in a sufficient number of well-documented patients, verified by DBPCFC. Thus, a test of proven value (Table 7.4) will at best achieve this classification for a small number of allergens, where they have been investigated in a sufficient number of patients. For other allergens, the same test should be classified as "not thoroughly validated."

Quantitation

The specific IgE immune response is characterized by heterogeneity. Comparison of different sera from allergic patients has demonstrated both qualitative and quantitative differences in the reaction to individual components in an extract, as different patients react to different epitopes. Moreover, the IgE immune response is likely subject to affinity maturation, leading to changing affinity profiles over time. Accordingly, it is not surprising that defining international standards for specific IgE has not proved possible, even though international standards for allergens are emerging. In practice, two different forms of quantitation are used. The first method uses an IgE response to a model allergen for comparison to all allergen systems, assuming parallel binding curves between serum dilution curves of different allergens. In this system, quantitation is expressed in arbitrary units. A second approach is to use an assay curve from a total IgE assay, and then express specific IgE in units comparable to specific IgE units (kIU/L or ng/mL). Both methods are theoretically prone to errors (71), but given heterogeneity in the IgE immune response, a better form of quantitation is probably not possible. Comparisons between different commercial assays suggest that a reasonable correlation between different tests can be achieved in this manner (46, 63).

The Value of Specific IgE in the Diagnosis of Food Hypersensitivity

As previously noted, every allergen is unique; therefore, it is never possible to recommend a test for use with every available allergen based on data from a few foods (9, 70). Two widely investigated test systems, CAP-RAST from Pharmacia Diagnostics and Magic Lite from ALK Abello/Ciba Corning, have delivered varying results in different food allergen systems. In the diagnosis of codfish allergy, both tests demonstrate sensitivity and specificity greater than 99% (32, 33), whereas in the diagnosis of kiwi allergy, neither of the tests demonstrates a high sensitivity (58) (Table 7.8).

Several authors have tried to ascertain a "level of discrimination" between allergic patients and controls. Although it has been possible to improve the

Table 7.8
Estimation of Clinical Sensitivities and Specificities of Commercially Available IgE Tests in Adult Patient Populations Recruited to One Center [1]

Test	Allergen	SE (%)	SP (%)	Reference
RAST	Cod	100	90	31–34
CAP	Cod	100	87	31–34
Magic Lite	Cod	100	100	35
CAP	Cod	93	87	31
CAP	Mackerel	86	90	31
CAP	Herring	93	87	31
CAP	Plaice	86	94	31
RAST	Milk	100	90	61
CAP	Milk	100	87	61
Abbott	Milk	75	70	61
Magic Lite	Milk	75	90	61
RAST	Egg white	100	79	61
CAP	Egg white	100	79	61
Abbott	Egg white	89	79	61
Magic Lite	Egg white	100	72	61
RAST	Egg yolk	67	86	61
CAP	Egg yolk	89	83	61
Magic Lite	Egg yolk	89	76	61
CAP	Wheat	N.D.	68	77 [2]
CAP	Rye	N.D.	16	78 [2]
CAP	Maize	N.D.	19	78 [2]
CAP	Oats	N.D.	17	78 [2]
CAP	Buckwheat	N.D.	20	78 [2]
CAP	Sesame	N.D.	23	78 [2]
RAST	Hazelnut	43	N.D.	10 [3]
CAP	Hazelnut	67	N.D.	59 [3]
Magic Lite	Hazelnut	43	N.D.	59 [3]
CAP	Kiwi	43	N.D.	59 [3]
Magic Lite	Kiwi	0	N.D.	59 [3]
RAST	Apple	68	100	11 [4]
CAP	Apple	84	86	11 [4]
Magic Lite	Apple	6	100	11 [4]

Test:
RAST: Phadebas RAST (Pharmacia Diagnostics, Uppsala, Sweden)
CAP: Pharmacia CAP system (Pharmacia Diagnostics, Uppsala, Sweden)
Magic Lite: Magic Lite (ALK-Abello/Ciba Corning, Horsholm, Denmark)
Abbott: Abbott Matrix (Abbott Laboratories, Chicago, Illinois, United States)
[1] Food hypersensitivity was confirmed by DBPCFC if not stated otherwise.
[2] Patients with concomitant grass pollen allergy. Tolerance to cereal as reported by the patients.
[3] Patients with concomitant birch pollen allergy. Food hypersensitivity confirmed by open oral challenge.
[4] Patients with concomitant birch pollen allergy. Food hypersensitivity or tolerance as reported by the patients.

clinical sensitivity and specificity, an upper normal limit of specific IgE above which the patient is food allergic and below which he or she is not does not appear to exist (33). Consequently, most investigators have chosen high sensitivity at the expense of low specificity in the tests.

The Specificity of IgE Antibodies to Foods

Many foods share allergenic determinants—and, therefore, specific IgE molecules—against an epitope on one food that will also recognize similar epitopes on other related foods (Table 7.6). Whether such a *serological* cross-reaction will be reflected *clinically* (i.e., whether the patient will also be clinically reactive to the cross-reacting food), depends both on the nature of the food, especially the heat and acid stability, and on the way the particular food is prepared before eaten.

In codfish, the major protein, Gad c1, is extremely heat- and acid-stable; thus, the normal cooking procedure will not destroy the allergenic protein (1). A patient allergic to codfish will, therefore, also be clinically allergic to the cross-reacting fish species and should be advised to avoid all fish (5, 34). On the other hand, the frequently seen serological cross-reaction between grass pollen and wheat flour rarely has clinical importance (78).

As in the evaluation of the various test systems for specific IgE, every allergen must be evaluated separately for cross-reactions. The serological response (specific IgE) to the clinical response (DBPCFC with the food in question) must be compared for every serologically cross-reacting food (6, 13, 34, 38).

Measurement of Total IgE in Serum

Only in the case of prediction for atopy in high-risk neonates has measurement of total IgE proved to be of value (38). In other cases, even with extremely elevated serum values of IgE, no specific implications can be drawn (36).

BASOPHIL HISTAMINE RELEASE (BHR)

Theoretically, measurement of histamine released from antigen-challenged leukocyte suspensions con-

Table 7.9

Estimation of Clinical Sensitivities and Specificities of a Commercially Available Histamine Release Test in Adult Patient Populations Recruited to One Center

Method	Food	Sensitivity	Specificity	Reference
DBPCFC	Cod	0.84	0.97	32
DBPCFC	Milk[a]	0.50	1.00	62
DBPCFC	Milk[b]	1.00	0.87	64
DBPCFC	Egg[a]	0.50	0.67	62
DBPCFC	Egg[b]	0.83	0.67	64
OFC	Hazelnut	0.82	N.D.	10

[a] Commercial extracts used—no correlation to DBPCFC.
[b] Fresh extracts used—significant correlation to DBPCFC.

taining basophils would offer an advantage over measurement of specific IgE intended to quantify cell-bound IgE. On the other hand, mechanisms other than IgE measurement (such as complement activation or bypassing the IgE-molecules by lectins) may cause a basophil to degranulate and liberate histamine in vitro. Previously, the elaborate and time-consuming technique of BHR restricted its use to research settings. This limitation has been overcome by the development of the glass microfiber technique (75), which is based on whole blood and has been shown to be comparable to the standard method developed by Siraganian (45).

In studies comparing BHR to DBPCFC (Table 7.9) BHR measurement has been shown to be comparable regarding sensitivity and specificity to prick skin tests or RAST, provided that the optimal freshly prepared allergens were used. A major advantage of BHR is that freshly prepared extracts of labile foods can be used, which is impossible in IgE tests and potentially hazardous in prick skin tests. A major drawback of the BHR test is that 5% to 10% of the population have circulating basophils unresponsive to in vitro challenge with allergens and even nonspecifically to cross-linking surface IgE with anti-IgE. Therefore, the test cannot be used in these patients. Another problem is that the test requires living cells, necessitating analysis of a blood sample within 24 hours. The exact role for BHR in the diagnostic armamentarium has not been established, but it remains a suitable alternative, especially in cases of suspected food allergy to rare allergens, where a documented test for specific IgE is not available.

OTHER ANTIBODIES

Concentrations of antibodies of other isotypes, including IgG, IgM, and IgA, have been demonstrated to develop in the fetus, irrespective of the amount of food eaten by the pregnant mother (24). Conversely, the mother's intake of milk and egg during lactation affects the immunological response of the baby (24). In the search for suitable markers of clinical food hypersensitivity, much attention has been paid to changes in immunoglobulins (and their subclasses) other than IgE. Although some papers suggest a possible pathogenic role for IgA-secreting cells, which have been demonstrated to increase after challenge (42), or IgG4, which has been postulated to correlate with clinical hypersensitivity (72), no study has conclusively demonstrated a pathogenic role for these antibodies (38, 41, 52, 57, 76). In the study by Daul et al. (57), no correlation between the outcome of DBPCFC and the levels of total IgG or IgG4 was seen, and no difference between patients and controls was found. The levels of other food-specific immunoglobulins of non-IgE isotypes most likely reflect the intake of food in the individual (39) and may represent a normal phenomenon.

SPECIFIC T CELLS: LYMPHOCYTE STIMULATION TESTS

Kondo (27) has investigated two groups of patients with atopic dermatitis: a group with immediate reactions and a group with late reactions to DBPCFC. In the latter group, which reacted more than two hours after challenge, an increase in the proliferative response of peripheral blood mononuclear cells was found in vitro. Recently, increased "cutaneous lymphocyte antigen" (CLA) expression was demonstrated in children with milk-dependent eczema (3). The clinical significance of these findings remains unknown at present, and neither test should be considered a reliable diagnostic of food allergy.

Tests Related to Active Disease or Applied in a Challenge Situation

In the case of in vitro measurements of histamine release from basophils, specific IgE or other mediators from the basophil, or other leukocytes, no need exists to provoke a systemic reaction in the patient. Such an in vitro test is, therefore, useful in having the potential of rendering a challenge unnecessary. Tests where changes in the quantity of specific mediators must be elicited by a challenge may prove useful in elucidating underlying pathogenic mechanisms in food hypersensitivity or in monitoring a challenge. Some of these tests are briefly mentioned below.

PLASMA HISTAMINE

Basophils from food-allergic patients have been demonstrated to show a higher degree of spontaneous release of histamine in vitro (55). This condition probably derives from an increased secretion of a histamine-releasing factor in these patients (73). Like tryptase, plasma histamine rises following a positive food challenge (74) and can be measured in vitro. An increase in plasma histamine has been demonstrated in patients with a positive response in DBPCFC (74). The test is difficult to perform, however, in part because of histamine's short half-life in the circulation. Furthermore, at least 10% false-positive responses are generated. The major problem with the test is that it requires a clinical reaction, preferentially by DBPCFC, and will, therefore, serve as only an addendum to the clinical evaluation.

PLASMA TRYPTASE

Mast cell tryptase is, in contrast to histamine, confined to the mast cell. Simultaneous measurement of tryptase and plasma histamine might add to the knowledge of the pathogenic mechanisms underlying the clinical reaction. Unfortunately, the only clinical situation where measurement of serum tryptase has sometimes proved valuable is in the retrospective analyses of cases of anaphylaxis elicited by food allergy, where a marked rise has been demonstrated (7,

84). No significant increase has been seen in many fatal and near-fatal cases of food-induced anaphylaxis nor in DBPCFC, however. Again, the test requires a substantial clinical reaction in the patient to be positive, and therefore has little diagnostic value in the routine setting.

COMPLEMENT ACTIVATION

In the search for involvement of non-IgE mechanisms, several investigators have measured various components of the complement system in an attempt to link a clinical reaction to changes in any of the components or split products. In the time course following challenge, either no changes in the complement cascade have been found (40, 76) or the changes were so markedly heterogeneous that the authors concluded that measurement of complement levels was not useful for the clinical evaluation of a patient with suspected food hypersensitivity (54).

EOSINOPHILS AND EOSINOPHIL DEGRANULATION PRODUCTS

In a double-blind study, circulating eosinophils and an eosinophil activation product, eosinophil cationic protein (ECP), have been reported to be involved in food hypersensitivity in children (60). The authors demonstrated a decrease in circulating eosinophils immediately after challenge, followed by an increase in serum ECP eight hours after challenge. Other authors have also found a decrease in circulating eosinophils after challenge (14, 82). Thus, monitoring of eosinophils and their products may prove helpful in monitoring oral food challenge.

PERMEABILITY TESTS

In controlled studies, different groups have demonstrated increased permeability of the gastrointestinal tract to probes such as polyethylene glycol (PEG) of various sizes or to ratios of sugars such as mannitol, lactulose, or rhamnose in patients with food hypersensitivity (4, 25, 50). Intestinal permeability varies widely among healthy individuals as well as among food-sensitive patients, resulting in an almost total

overlap between the groups (25). Nevertheless, changes in intestinal permeability after challenge have repeatedly been demonstrated to correlate to positive challenge, and to be nonspecific in their inability to discriminate between patients with predominantly gastrointestinal symptoms and patients with other symptoms (25, 43).

In the future, measurement of permeability changes may prove useful in the evaluation of drugs suitable for therapy of food hypersensitivity. A decrease in the increased uptake of probes by DSCG has been demonstrated in some studies (25).

CYTOKINES

Kondo (47) has reported increased levels of IL-2 and γ-interferon following challenge. IL-4 has been demonstrated in vitro to be involved in the events leading to clinical disease (19). At the present time, more information is needed to evaluate the clinical significance of this new approach toward diagnosis.

IMMUNE COMPLEX ASSAYS

The presence of immune complexes containing IgE or IgG in serum after challenge was suggested to be a suitable tool for large-scale screening of food hypersensitivity (67, 68). Further studies, however, have not supported this contention.

Conclusions

A variety of preformed or newly generated mediators are available for in vitro measurement, as are methods for evaluation of activation of various cells involved in the immune response in food hypersensitivity. Most of these tests are allergen-nonspecific—that is, they do not give information about the possible offending food eliciting the response in the patient. The same is true for plasma histamine, tryptase, and ECP, whereas measurement of specific IgE (directly or by histamine release from basophils) demonstrates the involvement of the immune system and may help identify the offending food involved. In the future, new and more specific and sensitive assays may be developed. At present, however, no in vitro test can replace the DBPCFC in the evaluation of food allergy.

REFERENCES

1. Aas K. Antigens in food. Nutr Rev 1994;42:85–91.
2. Aas K, Bindslev-Jensen C, Bjorksten B, Bruinjzel-Koomen CAFM, Moneret Vautrin DA, Ortolani C, Wütrich B. Adverse reactions to foods. Position paper. Allergy 1995, 50: 623–635.
3. Abernathy Carver KJ, Sampson HA, Picker LJ, Leung DY. Milk-induced eczema is associated with the expansion of T cells expressing cutaneous lymphocyte antigen. J Clin Invest 1995;95:913–918.
4. Andre C, Andre F, Colin L, Cavagna S. Measurement of intestinal permeability to mannitol and lactulose as a means of diagnosing food allergy and evaluating therapeutic effectiveness of disodium cromoglycate. Ann Allergy 1987;59:127–130.
5. Bernhisel Broadbent J, Scanlon SM, Sampson HA. Fish hypersensitivity. I. In vitro and oral challenge results in fish-allergic patients. J Allergy Clin Immunol 1992;89:730–737.
6. Bernhisel Broadbent J, Taylor S, Sampson HA. Cross-allergenicity in the legume botanical family in children with food hypersensitivity. II. Laboratory correlates. J Allergy Clin Immunol 1989;84:701–709.
7. Beyer K, Niggemann B, Schulze S, Wahn U. Serum tryptase and urinary 1-methylhistamine as parameters for monitoring oral food challenges in children. Int Arch Allergy Immunol 1994;104:348–351.
8. Bindslev-Jensen C, Hansen TK, Norgaard A, Vestergaard H, Poulsen LK. In: Johansson S, ed. Progress in Allergy and Clinical Immunology, vol. III. Stockholm: Hofrege & Huber, 1995, 268–275.
9. Bindslev-Jensen C, Skov PS, Madsen F, Poulsen LK. Food allergy and food intolerance—what is the difference? Ann Allergy 1994;72:317–320.
10. Bindslev-Jensen C, Vibits A, Skov P, Weeke B. Oral allergy syndrome: the effect of astemizole. Allergy 1991;46:610–613.
11. Borici R, Poulsen LK, Nielsen L, Bindslev-Jensen C. ACI News 1994;2(suppl):445 (abstract).
12. Buchwald D, Garrity D. Comparison of patients with chronic fatigue syndrome, fibromyalgia, and multiple chemical sensitivities. Arch Intern Med 1995;154:2049–2053.
13. Businco L, Dreborg S, Einarsson R, Giampietro PG, Host A, et al. Hydrolysed cow's milk formulae. Allergenicity and use in treatment and prevention. An ESPACI position paper. European Society of Pediatric Allergy and Clinical Immunology. Pediatr Allergy Immunol 1993;4:101–111.
14. Businco L, Meglio P, Ferrara M. The role of food allergy and eosinophils in atopic dermatitis. Pediatr Allergy Immunol 1993;4:33–37.
15. Ceska M, Eriksson R, Arga JM. Radio-immunosorbent assay of allergens. J Allergy 1972;49:1–9.
16. Daul CB, Morgan JE, Lehrer SB. The natural history of shrimp hypersensitivity. J Allergy Clin Immunol 1990;86:88–93.
17. Daul CB, Morgan JE, Waring NP, McCants ML, Hughes J, et al. Immunologic evaluation of shrimp-allergic individuals. J Allergy Clin Immunol 1987;80:716–722.
18. David TJ. Hazards of challenge tests in atopic dermatitis. Allergy 1989;44(suppl 9):101–107.
19. Dorion BJ, Burks AW, Harbeck R, Williams LW, Trumble A,
20. et al. The production of interferon-gamma in response to a major peanut allergy, *Ara h* II correlates with serum levels of IgE anti-*Ara h* II. J Allergy Clin Immunol 1994;93:93–99.
20. EAACI Subcommittee on Allergen Standardization and Skin Tests. Position paper: Allergen standardization and skin test. Allergy 1993;48(suppl. 14):48–82.
21. El Sham AS, Alaba O. Liquid-phase in vitro allergen-specific IgE assay with in situ immobilization. Advances in the Biosciences 1989;74:191–201.
22. Eriksson NE. Clustering of foodstuffs in food hypersensitivity. An inquiry study in pollen allergic patients. Allergol Immunopathol Madr 1984;12:28–32.
23. Ewan PW, Coote D. Evaluation of a capsulated hydrophilic carrier polymer (the ImmunoCAP) for measurement of specific IgE antibodies. Allergy 1990;45:22–29.
24. Falth Magnusson K, Kjellman NI, Magnusson KE. Antibodies IgG, IgA, and IgM to food antigens during the first 18 months of life in relation to feeding and development of atopic disease. J Allergy Clin Immunol 1988;81:743–749.
25. Falth Magnusson K, Kjellman NI, Odelram H, Sundqvist T, Magnusson KE. Gastrointestinal permeability in children with cow's milk allergy: effect of milk challenge and sodium cromoglycate as assessed with polyethyleneglycols (PEG 400 and PEG 1000). Clin Allergy 1986;16:543–551.
26. Fifield R, Libeer J-C, Schellekens APM. Inter-laboratory external quality assessment schemes for specific IgE antibodies. The results of a European scheme for 1992. Eur J Clin Chem Biochem 1994;32:465–472.
27. Fukutomi O, Kondo N, Agata H, Shinoda S, Kuwabara N, et al. Timing of onset of allergic symptoms as a response to a double-blind, placebo-controlled food challenge in patients with food allergy combined with a radioallergosorbent test and the evaluation of proliferative lymphocyte responses. Int Arch Allergy Immunol 1994;104:352–357.
28. Gall H, Kalveram KJ, Forck G, Sterry W. Kiwi fruit allergy: a new birch pollen-associated food allergy. J Allergy Clin Immunol 1994;94:70–76.
29. Gerhardt W, Keller H. Evaluation of test data from clinical studies. Scand J Clin Lab Invest 1986;46(suppl. 181):1–74.
30. Gorchein A. Difficult asthma. BMJ 1989;299:1031–1032.
31. Hansen TK, Abrahamsen L, Bindslev-Jensen C, Poulsen LK. Results of the CAP system and immunoblotting in clinically fish allergic adults. 6th Int. symposium on immunological and clinical problems of food allergy, Lugano, Sept 24–26, 1995 (abstract).
32. Hansen TK, Bindslev-Jensen C. Codfish allergy in adults. Identification and diagnosis. Allergy 1992;47:610–617.
33. Hansen TK, Bindslev-Jensen C, Skov PS, Poulsen LK. Codfish allergy in adults. Specific tests for IgE and histamine release versus double-blind, placebo controlled challenges. Clin Exp Allergy 1995, (in press).
34. Hansen TK, Bindslev-Jensen C, Skov PS, Poulsen LK. Ann Allergy 1995, Codfish allergy in adults. IgE cross reactivity among fish species. Ann Allergy 1996 (in press).
35. Hansen TK, Poulsen LK, Bindslev-Jensen C. Assays for specific IgE in the diagnosis of codfish allergy in adults. Allergy 1993;48(suppl 16):118 (abstract).
36. Hide DW, Arshad SH, Twiselton R, Stevens M. Cord serum IgE: an insensitive method for prediction of atopy. Clin Exp Allergy 1991;21:739–743.
37. Hill SM, Milla PJ. Colitis caused by food allergy in infants. Arch Dis Child 1990;65:132–133.

38. Host A. Cow's milk protein allergy and intolerance in infancy. Pediatr Allergy Immunol 1994;5(suppl 5):5–36.
39. Husby S. Dietary antigens: uptake and humoral immunity in man. APMIS (suppl) 1998;1:1–40.
40. Husby S, Host A, Teisner B, Svehag SE. Infants and children with cow milk allergy/intolerance. Investigation of the uptake of cow milk protein and activation of the complement system. Allergy 1990;45:547–551.
41. Husby S, Schultz Larsen F, Svehag SE. IgG subclass antibodies to dietary antigens in atopic dermatitis. Acta Derm Venereol Suppl Stockh 1989;144:88–92.
42. Isolauri E, Suomalainen H, Kaila M, Jalonen T, Soppi E, et al. Local immune response in patients with cow milk allergy: follow-up of patients retaining allergy or becoming tolerant. J Pediatr 1992;120:9–15.
43. Jakobsson I. Intestinal permeability in children of different ages and with different gastrointestinal diseases. Pediatr Allergy Immunol 1993;4:33–39.
44. Jensen-Jarolim E, Poulsen LK, With H, Kieffer M, Ottevanger V, et al. Atopic dermatitis of the face, scalp, and neck: Type I reaction to the yeast Pityrosporon ovale. J Allergy Clin Immunol 1992;89:44–51.
45. Kleine Tebbe J, Werfel S, Roedsgaard D, Nolte H, Skov PS, et al. Comparison of fiberglass-based histamine assay with a conventional automated fluorometric histamine assay, case history, skin prick test, and specific serum IgE in patients with milk and egg allergic reactions. Allergy 1993;48:49–53.
46. Kleine-Tebbe J, Eickholt M, Gätjen M, Brunnée T, O'Connor A, et al. Comparison between Magic Lite- and CAP-system: two automated specific antibody assays. Clin Exp Allergy 1992;22:475–484.
47. Kondo N, Fukutomi O, Agata H, Motoyoshi F, Shinoda S, et al. The role of T lymphocytes in patients with food-sensitive atopic dermatitis. J Allergy Clin Immunol 1993;91:658–668.
48. Kurup VP, Kelly T, Elms N, Kelly K, Fink J. Cross-reactivity of food allergens in latex allergy. Allergy Proc 1994;15:211–216.
49. Langeland T. A clinical and immunological study of allergy to hen's egg white. VI. Occurrence of proteins cross-reacting with allergens in hen's egg white as studied in egg white from turkey, duck, goose, seagull, and in hen egg yolk, and hen and chicken sera and flesh. Allergy 1993;38:399–412.
50. Laudat A, Arnaud P, Napoly A, Brion F. The intestinal permeability test applied to the diagnosis of food allergy in paediatrics. West Indian Med J 1994;43:87–88.
51. Lavaud F, Prevost A, Cossart C, Guerin L, Bernard J, et al. Allergy to latex, avocado pear, and banana: evidence for a 30 kD antigen in immunoblotting. J Allergy Clin Immunol 1995;95:557–564.
52. Lilja G, Magnusson CG, Oman H, Johansson SG. Serum levels of IgG subclasses in relation to IgE and atopic disease in early infancy. Clin Exp Allergy 1990;20:407–413.
53. Mandallaz MM, de Weck AL, Dahinden CA. Bird-egg syndrome. Cross-reactivity between bird antigens and egg-yolk livetins in IgE-mediated hypersensitivity. Int Arch Allergy Appl Immunol 1988;87:143–150.
54. Martin ME, Guthrie LA, Bock SA. Serum complement changes during double-blind food challenges in children with a history of food sensitivity. Pediatrics 1984;73:532–537.
55. May CD, Remigio L. Observations on high spontaneous release of histamine from leucocytes in vitro. Clin Allergy 1982;12:229–241.
56. Metcalfe DD, Sampson HA. Workshop on experimental methodology for clinical studies of adverse reactions to foods and food additives. J Allergy Clin Immunol 1990;86:421–442.
57. Morgan JE, Daul CB, Lehrer SB. The relationships among shrimp-specific IgG subclass antibodies and immediate adverse reactions to shrimp challenge. J Allergy Clin Immunol 1990;86:387–392.
58. Nielsen L, Nolte H, Norgaard A, Voitenko V, Skov PS, et al. Allergy, Eur J Allergy Clin Immunol 1995;50(26):224 (abstract).
59. Nielsen L, Norgaard A, Skov PS, Bindslev-Jensen C. Oral allergy syndrome in pollinosis: hazelnut and kiwi. Allergy 1993;48(suppl 15):93 (abstract).
60. Niggemann B, Beyer K, Wahn U. The role of eosinophils and eosinophil cationic protein in monitoring oral challenge tests in children with food-sensitive atopic dermatitis. J Allergy Clin Immunol 1994;94:963–971.
61. Norgaard A. Type I allergy to egg and milk in adults (Ph.D. thesis). National University Hospital, University of Copenhagen, Copenhagen, 1995.
62. Norgaard A, Bindslev-Jensen C. Egg and milk allergy in adults. Diagnosis and characterization. Allergy 1992;47:503–509.
63. Norgaard A, Bindslev-Jensen C, Poulsen LK. Specific IgE in the diagnosis of egg and milk allergy in adults. Allergy 1995, 50:636–647.
64. Norgaard A, Skov PS, Bindslev-Jensen C. Egg and milk allergy in adults: comparison between fresh foods and commercial allergen extracts in skin prick test and histamine release from basophils. Clin Exp Allergy 1992;22:940–947.
65. Olsen OT, Bindslev-Jensen C, Svendsen UG. Diagnostisk sikkerhed af CLA-allergitest og RAST ved IgE-medieret allergi sammenlignet med anamnese og priktest. Ugeskrift for Læger 1989;151:3241–3245.
66. Ortolani C, Ispano M, Pastorello EA, Ansaloni R, Magri GC. Comparison of results of skin prick tests (with fresh foods and commercial food extracts) and RAST in 100 patients with oral allergy syndrome. J Allergy Clin Immunol 1989;83:683–690.
67. Paganelli R, Levinsky RJ, Atherton DJ. Detection of specific antigen within circulating immune complexes: validation of the assay and its application to food antigen–antibody complexes formed in healthy and food-allergic subjects. Clin Exp Immunol 1981;46:44–53.
68. Paganelli R, Levinsky RJ, Brostoff J, Wraith DG. Immune complexes containing food proteins in normal and atopic subjects after oral challenge and effect of sodium cromoglycate on antigen absorption. Lancet 1979;1:1270–1272.
69. Perdue MH. Food allergy: the nature of the local gastrointestinal response. J Pediatr Gastroenterol Nutr 1993;17:341–342.
70. Poulsen LK. In vitro testing for allergy. In: Basomba A, Sastre J, eds. XVI European Congress of Allergology and Clinical Immunology ECACI 1995. Postgraduate Course Syllabus. Madrid: European Academy of Allergy and Clinical Immunology, 1995, 203–210.
71. Poulsen LK, Pedersen MF, Malling H-J, Søndergaard I, Weeke B, Maxisorp RAST. A sensitive method for detection of absolute quantities of antigen-specific IgE. Allergy 1989;44:178–189.
72. Quinti I, Papetti C, D'Offizi G, Cavagni G, Panchor ML, et al. IgG subclasses to food antigens. Allerg Immunol Paris 1988;20:41–44.

73. Sampson HA, Broadbent KR, Bernhisel Broadbent J. Spontaneous release of histamine from basophils and histamine-releasing factor in patients with atopic dermatitis and food hypersensitivity. N Engl J Med 1989;321:228–232.

74. Sampson HA, Jolie PL. Increased plasma histamine concentrations after food challenges in children with atopic dermatitis. N Engl J Med 1984;311:372–376.

75. Skov PS, Norn S, Week B. A new method for detecting histamine release. Agents Actions 1984;14:414–416.

76. Tainio VM, Savilahti E. Value of immunologic tests in cow milk allergy. Allergy 1990;45:189–196.

77. Vestergaard H, Bindslev-Jensen C, Poulsen LK. Specific IgE to wheat in patients with grass pollen allergy. ACI News 1994;(suppl 2):445 (abstract).

78. Vestergaard HS, Bindslev-Jensen C, Poulsen LK. Specific IgE to cereals in patients with grass pollen allergy. Allergy, Eur J Allergy Clin Immunol 1994;(suppl. II):445 (abstract).

79. Vocks E, Borga A, Szliska C, Seifert HU, Seifert B, et al. Common allergenic structures in hazelnut, rye grain, sesame seeds, kiwi, and poppy seeds. Allergy 1993;48:168–172.

80. Weeke B, Søndergaard I, Lind P, Aukrust L, Løwenstein H. Crossed radioimmunoelectrophoresis (CRIE) for identification of allergens and determination of the antigenic specificities of patients' IgE. Scand J Immunol 1983;17:265–272.

81. Wide L, Bennich H, Johansson SGO. Diagnosis of allergy by an in vitro test for allergen antibodies. Lancet 1967; ii:1105–1107.

82. Winqvist I, Olsson I, Werner S, Stenstam M. Variations of cationic proteins from eosinophil leukocytes in food intolerance and allergic rhinitis. Allergy 1981;36:419–423.

83. Young E, Stoneham MD, Petruckevitch A, Barton J, Rona R. A population study of food intolerance (comments). Lancet 1994;343:1127–1130.

84. Yunginger JW, Nelson DR, Squillace DL, Jones RT, Holley KE, et al. Laboratory investigation of deaths due to anaphylaxis. J Forensic Sci 1991;36:857–865.

8

IN VIVO DIAGNOSIS: SKIN TESTING AND ORAL CHALLENGE PROCEDURES

S. Allan Bock

Introduction

Consideration of skin testing and oral challenge procedures may begin with two questions. The first question was posed by Charles D. May in an editorial entitled, "Are confusion and controversy about food allergy really necessary?" (1). The second question is, "By what technique can histories of adverse reactions to food be objectively and unequivocally investigated?" Most allergists are aware of the answers to both of these questions. As May explained in his editorial, this subject remains confusing only to individuals who refuse to subject their observations and claims to rigorous, unbiased examination. Such examination is properly carried out by the use of the double-blind placebo-controlled food challenge (DBPCFC).

This chapter reviews many of the studies that have been undertaken using DBPCFC. It will become clear why this procedure has become, and currently remains, the "gold standard" for the diagnosis of adverse reactions to foods. The procedure detailed in this chapter is the only technique that should be considered acceptable for scientific research conducted with patients who are being investigated for adverse reactions to food (2). Furthermore, DBPCFC is quite practical and adaptable for use by allergists in their offices or clinics (3). At the present time, all allergists should strive to confirm or refute their patients' histories of adverse reactions to food by use of this technique. In addition to describing the use of DBPCFC, this chapter discusses the role of skin testing in the evaluation of subjects with histories of adverse reactions to food.

Background

In 1986, studies of adverse reactions to foods were critically reviewed (4, 5). This section concentrates on those studies using blinded challenges.

We will begin by giving credit to the earliest pioneers of blinded challenges. May deserves credit for bringing this technique into regular and practical use both in research and clinical practice. Prior to his seminal study (6), however, blinded challenges in capsules or masked in other foods had been undertaken. At a food symposium during the sixth annual meeting of the American Academy of Allergy in 1950, F. C. Lowell began an editorial with a statement that remains true today: "There is perhaps no field of medicine in which more divergent views are held than in that of allergy to food." Lowell went on to say that to demonstrate a cause-and-effect relationship between food ingestion and symptoms, foods administered should be completely disguised, a feat perhaps best accomplished "in capsules or by stomach tube" (7).

At the same symposium, papers were presented by Loveless and by Graham and associates using blinded food challenges. Loveless used "food masking" by placing the suspected food, (milk or corn) in another food, making detection by the patient very unlikely (8, 9). Graham *et al.* presented a paper that actually represented an examination of the placebo effect as well as a study of adverse reactions to foods (10). In one of his studies, four physicians who believed that chocolate produced their own migraine headaches were challenged with chocolate or lactose in black capsules. The study did not show any relationship between chocolate and the occurrence of headaches. Other patients described in this paper underwent "reverse placebo challenges," a technique that probably could not be repeated today. Patients with definite opinions about the effect of food were challenged through a nasogastric tube. While being told that the active food was being instilled, the subject received water, in contrast, while being told that the water was being administered, challenge food was instilled. The patients in this portion of the study appeared to react more to the suggestion associated with the substance that they thought was being administered than to the true food itself. This paper is fascinating both for the physiological and placebo observations and should be reviewed by all physicians interested in this subject. Perhaps no other study better illustrates the maxim that "we should never underestimate the power of the human mind to aggravate or alleviate symptoms."

In 1971, Maslansky and Wein published a study in which eight subjects underwent DBPCFC with chocolate and an unspecified placebo in capsules (11). Three of their patients reacted to the cocoa capsules, with one patient showing symptoms of urticaria, a second experiencing fatigue and gastric bloating, and a third reporting nausea and cramps. Only one of these three patients was sensitized to cocoa as detected by allergy skin testing. None of the patients in the study reacted to placebo challenge. This study represents one of the few documented DBPCFC-confirmed reactions to chocolate in the English literature.

The most useful information to be gleaned from the literature comes from studies in the last 20 years using DBPCFC. Information based on findings from open challenge studies has been reviewed elsewhere (4, 5).

Perusal of the recent literature in which blinded food challenges have been used illustrates several interesting aspects of our current knowledge (Table 8.1). First most histories are inaccurate. Unlike other areas of medicine, the history of adverse reactions to food is more often incorrect than it is accurate. Second, when a patient does have an adverse reaction to food confirmed, typically fewer foods than were suspected can be shown to cause symptoms in any individual. Rarely do more than two or three foods cause symptoms. Third, the number of different foods

Table 8.1
General Principles Derived from Published DBPCFC Studies

1. Inaccuracy of history
2. Few foods cause most of the reactions
3. Individuals rarely react to more than three foods
4. Symptoms usually occur in the gastrointestinal, integumentary, and respiratory systems
5. Behavioral symptoms as sole symptoms are *very* unusual
6. Delayed-onset reactions outside the gastrointestinal tract are rare and difficult to reproduce

causing food reactions is largely restricted to a relatively short list. Fourth, reproducible symptoms include gastrointestinal reactions, cutaneous symptoms, and respiratory symptoms. Behavioral manifestations as the sole manifestation of an adverse reaction to food are exceedingly rare and difficult to reproduce. Fifth, despite many claims and much literature to the contrary, delayed- or late-onset reactions have proved very difficult to document, creating some doubt about the current validity of many of these claims. The exceptions to this observation include young children, in whom late- or delayed-onset reactions in the intestine have been well documented, and older subjects having gluten-sensitive enteropathy or coeliac disease (12–23). Some aspects of cutaneous reactions may truly represent late-phase reactions, and have inspired exciting and fertile research in which well-controlled observations will be correlated with laboratory measurements during future studies.

INACCURACY OF CLINICAL HISTORIES

Studies of food-allergic patients support the observation of the frequent inaccuracy of the clinical history. Of 688 patients undergoing double-blind food challenges at National Jewish, only about 40% have had a reproducible history (Table 8.2) (24, and unpublished observations). Patients counted as having an adequate clinical history included those with any symptom, any timing, and any food. A similar percentage of confirmed histories (40% to 60%) has been found by investigators at other centers studying highly selected populations (3, 25–34). If only one-half of histories can be reproduced in DBPCFC with highly selected patients, how often are they reproduced in the general

Table 8.2
Results of DBPCFC in 688 Children up to Age 19 Years

Number of children challenged	688
Number of children with positive DBPCFC	249 (36%)
Number of food challenges	1538
Number of positive food challenges	329 (21%)

population or in the population evaluated by physicians in practice? Surely the percentage must be much smaller.

REPRODUCIBILITY OF SYMPTOMS

DBPCFC studies have confirmed the reproducibility of several groups of symptoms (Table 8.3). Gastrointestinal symptoms have included nausea, vomiting, diarrhea, abdominal cramps, bloating, and gas. Documented cutaneous symptoms and signs include pruritus, atopic dermatitis, urticaria, angioedema, and nonspecific erythema that has not been characterized. Respiratory symptoms and signs include sneezing, ocular injection, serous rhinorrhea, laryngeal edema, cough, bronchorrhea, and wheezing. Interestingly, respiratory symptoms rarely appear as the sole manifestation of adverse reactions to food.

Food hypersensitivity does trigger asthma but the incidence is low enough to require rigorous confirmation before placing patients on diets that eliminate numerous foods (6, 24, 28, 30, 31, 35, 36). Sampson and James have shown increased airway reactivity in patients following food challenges (36). Their study was the first to identify this effect in a convincing number of subjects, and further research in this area is needed. Respiratory symptoms and signs occur coincident with cutaneous or gastrointestinal manifestations, or as part of an anaphylactic reaction. Similarly, cardiovascular symptoms of tachy-

Table 8.3
Symptoms Confirmed During Studies Using DBPCFC

Cutaneous: urticaria, angioedema, atopic dermatitis, erythema

Gastrointestinal: abdominal pain, nausea, vomiting, diarrhea

Respiratory: sneezing, rhinorrhea, cough, wheezing, laryngospasm, oral pruritus

Ocular: pruritus, chemosis, edema

Behavioral: headache, altered behavior (controversial)

cardia, arrhythmias, and hypotension rarely occur without symptoms and signs in another system and usually appear concurrently with severe adverse food reactions. It should be stressed that cardiovascular collapse during food ingestion can occur without other symptoms. The absence of skin manifestations does *not* eliminate the possibility of food-induced anaphylaxis; rather, the presence of skin manifestations helps to incriminate putative food offenders, and the history of urticaria and angioedema should always be sought in such cases.

The gastrointestinal symptom of "colic" was not mentioned above, as its confirmation has proved controversial due to its subjective nature and the vague definition of the condition. The studies of Jakobsson *et al.* and a few patients studied at National Jewish show unequivocally that a small percentage of children with the symptom complex termed "colic" do have an adverse reaction to foods (usually cow's milk) that is reproducible in DBPCFC (37–40). Sampson's editorial on this subject points to the likelihood of some children with colic having food allergy as well as the need for further controlled studies (41).

Patients with histories of adverse reactions to foods have incriminated almost every edible substance known to mankind. A few foods are incriminated frequently, but even fewer are confirmed. Perusing all of the well-controlled studies using DBPCFC, one finds that about 80% of all food reactions involve egg, peanut, milk, soy, and wheat. Tree nuts (nonlegume), fish, and shellfish (42, 43) account for a considerable portion of the remaining 20%. Another group of foods is reportedly associated with marked anaphylactic reactions in a few subjects. Due to the severity of these patients' histories, challenges have only occasionally been undertaken, but it seems likely that the incriminated food has been correctly identified. The most intriguing foods on this list include potato (44), banana (45), rice (46), and celery (47). Occasionally marked allergic reactions are blamed on a food, but detailed investigations usually identify the culprit as something in the food (48). Recent studies illustrate that spices (49) and food additives (50) may occasionally create significant food-induced reactions.

Two of the most common "food villains," corn and chocolate, have rarely been found to produce reactions in DBPCFC. In addition, the number of confirmed wheat reactions seems small compared with the frequency with which wheat is incriminated (excluding gluten-sensitivity enteropathy). Although strawberry, other berries, tomato, and citrus fruits have often been incriminated as the cause of urticaria and other rashes, these histories are rarely confirmed in the literature on DBPCFC. The flush occurring on the face of young children after contact with tomato is particularly easy to reproduce, but no data exist to identify the mechanism except that these children lack detectable antibody to tomato. In the absence of any data, it may be speculated that these reactions occur by some pharmacological/biochemical mechanism not related to antigen–antibody interactions and therefore arise only sporadically. It also seems plausible that this problem is most common in young children and thus its evanescence makes it difficult to study (39, 51).

CROSS-REACTIVITY BETWEEN FOODS

A number of papers have raised concerns about cross-reactivity between foods, and based on laboratory data their authors recommend that related foods be excluded from the diet of anyone reacting to one member of the family—particularly in the case of the legume family (52). These studies have not documented the clinical significance of the laboratory findings, however. Studies that have focused on this problem have rarely found clinically relevant cross-reactivity between legumes in DBPCFC (53–55). Recently, Sampson and his colleagues examined cross-reactivity among fish (56, 57) and among grains (58). The laboratory studies and the food challenge results strongly supported the conclusion that laboratory data either in vivo or in vitro cannot reliably determine the clinical relevance of cross-reactivity between foods. Thus, these general recommendations made in the absence of rigorous proof represent a serious disservice to patients who must follow these diets for themselves (or to their families, which may also exclude foods unnecessarily).

A similar problem occurs in children with milk hypersensitivity who are often assumed to be soy-sensitive. Although soy can be a sensitizing antigen, perusal of the literature does not reveal any good study using DBPCFC that proves the frequency of soy hypersensitivity in milk-hypersensitive youngsters.

Several Scandinavian groups have published studies of cross-reactivity between antigens in birch pollen and various fruits and nuts (59–64). In their studies of the relationship between watermelon and ragweed antigens, Enberg, Owenby, and their colleagues have not found immunological cross-reactions that do not seem to be necessarily related to clinical symptoms (65, 66). The clinical relevance of these reports would be greatly enhanced by DBPCFC in the subjects under investigation. These data are quite interesting because of the lack of an obvious botanical relationship between these allergens. Until more clinical research is conducted in subjects with these problems, however, prohibitions based on in vitro data may cause persons to avoid food unnecessarily.

TIMING OF ADVERSE REACTIONS

As noted earlier, documentation of the timing of reactions after administering the challenge is an area fraught with controversy. If we limit review of the literature to DBPCFC, it is rare to find reactions occurring more than a few hours after the challenge is administered except in children with protein enteropathies. Different authors define timing differently. Should the time that symptoms occur be measured from the first challenge or from the challenge nearest to the beginning of symptoms? If the initial administration of food initiates biochemical or immunologic process in the intestine but several doses over an hour (or even a few days) are required to elicit symptoms, is the reaction considered immediate or delayed? These questions have been particularly raised in studies by Hill and his colleagues with children experiencing adverse reactions to milk (67). Until we have a better understanding of the immunological/biochemical sequence of events in the intestine and elsewhere in the body, complete answers to these and other questions will remain elusive. Thus, today's authors should be required to present in detail how challenges are administered and how observations are made, especially if they report delayed-in-time reactions to foods.

History and Physical Examination

Once it is agreed that a blinded food challenge is the only reliable means by which to objectively confirm the history, the challenge must be designed. Unlike most areas of medicine where the history comprises the central component in making the diagnosis, in food hypersensitivity a thorough history is used to design the challenge that will confirm or refute the reported symptoms. The following components are essential (Table 8.4): (1) a description of the symptoms following food ingestion; (2) the time between ingestion of the food and the beginning of symptoms; (3) the approximate quantity of food required to produce the symptoms; (4) the frequency and reproducibility of the reaction; (5) the most recent occurrence of the reaction; and (6) whether exercise or some other accompanying factor is required to elicit the reaction. With this information, the physician will know the quantity with which to begin the challenge and at what intervals the challenge should be administered.

The physical examination should be directed toward the gastrointestinal, cutaneous, and respiratory systems and any particular area mentioned by the patient. The physician should look for stigmata often associated with adverse reactions to foods, including skin rashes, abnormalities of the nose, unusual chest findings, and abdominal discomfort. At the same time, the physician should closely observe the patient's behavior, and should consider other diagnostic possibilities that would move the diagnosis toward considerations other than adverse reactions to foods.

Table 8.4
History to Be Obtained

1. Description of symptoms
2. Timing of onset of symptoms
3. Quantity of food to produce symptoms
4. Frequency of reaction and reproducibility
5. Most recent occurrence
6. Accompanying factors (e.g., exercise)

Skin Testing

Many pages have been written about the utility of skin testing for foods—many of them negative. Skin testing for foods has been questioned because of problems in interpretation, and because of a questioned correlation of positive skin tests with clinical observations and with DBPCFC. Remember, however, that each food skin test extract can easily be associated with a specific food, and ingestion of that food is easily witnessed. By contrast, inhalant allergen exposure is much less clearly associated with inhalation of any specific pollen, mold, or household allergen. For example, when a patient complains of respiratory allergy symptoms in August, numerous allergens are possible depending upon the locale, including a large selection of weed pollens, mold spores, and confounding exposures to animal dander and insects. While daily allergy practice assumes that all of these allergens contribute to the symptoms, and treatment is frequently prescribed based upon this concept, practicing allergists do not have to prove which allergens are the real culprits. If challenge tests were required for each allergen to be treated, allergy therapy would become impossibly cumbersome (but more precise). This approach is required for food allergen extracts and food observations, however. It is also true that food skin tests (as well as other extracts) can have a low positive predictive accuracy. The following discussion reviews the studies that have examined the relationships between blinded food challenges and skin testing.

To approach this subject, we must ask the question: What is the correlation between positive skin tests and positive food challenges, and between negative skin tests and negative food challenges? Expressed another way: What are the positive and negative predictive accuracies of skin tests for foods? Although the information is far from complete, several studies have generated helpful data for several allergens, including egg, peanut, wheat, milk, fish, tree nuts, and soy (24, 68–73). These studies have shown that the negative predictive accuracy for these foods, except soy, approaches 100%. (It is not clear why soy represents an exception.) The positive predictive accuracies are much lower for these foods, rarely exceeding 60%. This difference arises because many subjects are sensitized (possess IgE-specific antibodies) to foods to which they do not react when the foods are ingested, perhaps because the presence of IgE is necessary but not sufficient to produce an immediate hypersensitivity reaction to food.

In addition, the predictive accuracies of skin tests are not identical in older children and in children younger than two or three years of age. Younger children are more likely to have a negative skin test and a positive challenge than are older children. In addition, it is uncommon to find a positive skin test and a negative challenge in children less than two years of age and particularly less than one year of age. Of course, in this age group skin tests are more carefully chosen, and the list of possible foods is more limited, so that a positive skin test with a good history of an immediate reaction probably has a higher positive predictive accuracy than in any other age group. Not enough data have been published to prove or disprove the veracity of this statement, but such a study could potentially appear in the future.

The size of the skin test has not been shown to correlate well with the probability of a positive food challenge. If a method could be identified that would allow correction or adjustment of the skin test response to enhance the positive predictive accuracy, thus decreasing the number of food challenges necessary, skin testing would assume far greater importance in the evaluation of food hypersensitivity.

Another issue in the consideration of food skin testing is the appropriate extract to be used. Although commercially available extracts have been used for many studies, they do have limitations. First, commercially available (in the United States) food skin test extracts have not been standardized. Thus, each bottle of extract must be viewed with caution until it has elicited a positive response in a patient known to have a symptomatic reaction to that food. Occasionally extracts may contain no material that the immune system recognizes as corresponding to the protein specified on the label. Use of such extracts could result in false-negative reactions (negative skin test, positive challenge) in subsequent skin tests.

Fruits and vegetables present another problem for extract manufacturers and allergists. Consistently potent extracts of fruits and vegetables are difficult to prepare. In recent years, clinicians have begun using fresh fruit and vegetable material to undertake food skin testing for these materials when they are suspected of causing food-induced symptoms. While this idea is gaining in popularity, it was first mentioned in the literature about 50 years ago (74, 75).

How, then, should skin testing be used in the evaluation of patients with food hypersensitivity? Skin tests for foods are most useful when a properly performed test is found to be negative. Skin tests should be applied by the prick or puncture technique using a 1 : 10 or 1 : 20 weight : volume concentration of extract. After 15 to 20 minutes, measurements are taken to determine the mean diameter of the wheal (and, in some cases, the erythema). A wheal at least 3 mm larger than the negative control is considered positive. (Appropriate positive and negative control solutions must be used.) A negative skin test almost eliminates the possibility that the food will elicit an immediate hypersensitivity reaction when ingested, as long as the reliability of the extract is certain and the history does not overwhelmingly contradict the result. If these conditions are met, then the food may usually be reintroduced openly into the diet with minimal chance that it will elicit symptoms.

A positive skin test, if properly performed, identifies the incriminated food as one that should be fed to the subject using blinded food challenge techniques. If the reported reaction was severe or involved true anaphylaxis, the skin test may be used to confirm the high probability that the correct food has been identified; under the circumstances, the need for a challenge is obviated.

To date, intradermal skin testing for food has not been shown to be useful. Until additional studies are undertaken showing their utility, it appears that intradermal skin tests carry too high a risk of producing systemic reactions without enhancing the predictive accuracy of the test. They might prove most useful in young children in whom smaller amounts of specific IgE are present in the skin. This age group tolerates the tests more poorly than any other group, however, and this speculation needs to be subjected to scientific scrutiny.

Food Challenge Administration

FOOD TO BE USED

A number of sources of foods are available to the physician wishing to undertake blinded food challenges. Dried foods are available for many incriminated allergens, with the value of these foods being related to their ability to be hidden in other foods or to be encapsulated. Grains (wheat, corn, soy, rye, rice, barley, oat, buckwheat) are readily available from grocery stores as flour or meal, making them easy to encapsulate or hide in another food. Nonfat powdered dry milk and dried egg or egg white are also readily found in grocery stores. Peanuts, beans, and tree nuts (cashew, almond, pecan, walnut) may be powdered using a mortar and pestle, a blender, a food processor, or a coffee grinder (an excellent device for creating nut flour). Preparation of fruits, some vegetables, and meats has at times proved problematic. The popularity of camping has, however, increased the availability of a wide array of freeze-dried foods, including meats, vegetable and fruits. These foods can be found in camping stores, usually in foil-wrapped packages, and contain remarkably few additives and preservatives. They can be ground to a powder and encapsulated or hidden in another food or vehicle. Baby food beef and chicken are also excellent choices for use in challenges. Fish and shellfish may be dried in a conventional or microwave oven, chopped or ground, and then hidden in a vehicle that masks their presence. Rarely will it become necessary for the allergist to employ a lyophylizer to freeze-dry some food for which no other source is available. In that unlikely event, a sufficient quantity of the food should be prepared so that it can be stored for future use.

VEHICLES

Many vehicles have been used for blinded food challenges, and the ability to disguise challenge foods is limited only by the allergist's imagination. For several investigators, capsules have offered a number of advantages. For purposes of blinding, capsules are unsurpassed because they employ a physical barrier between the challenge substance and the oral tissues, thus avoiding contact with oral taste structures. This strategy also avoids oral symptoms that may be entirely local but that may preclude accurate assessment of the systemic effect of food on the patient.

Capsules have been criticized for two major faults. First, they avoid contact of the food with the mouth, thus eliminating one common source of complaint of patients who report adverse reactions to foods. As mentioned, this approach may be desirable to assess the more important question of whether a food causes systemic symptoms. It is important for an allergist to identify foods that may cause systemic symptoms in a patient. Such reactions may have serious implications following intentional or accidental ingestion, whereas local reactions may preclude ingestion of a food because of discomfort but accidental exposure will not lead to serious consequences.

The second criticism has been that capsules limit the quantity of food that can be used in challenges as a patient can swallow only a limited number of capsules. For many foods that are available in dehydrated form, this restriction actually provides an advantage because a large amount of the offending protein can be placed in relatively few capsules. The major problem arises with grains that are available in dry form, but that may require large amounts to be ingested to test the quantity incriminated by the history. While these problems may force some compromises for practicing allergists administering food challenges, investigators choosing alternative vehicles must be certain that the challenge is truly blind.

Another vehicle with good masking properties is Tolerex that has been iced and flavored with one of the several flavors available. Several strong and distinctive food substances (e.g., vinegar, wine, and peanut oil) have been hidden in this preparation and have proved undetectable to investigator and patient alike. In addition to being distinctive gustatory substances, these foods can be difficult to encapsulate. Peanut oil has been administered in capsules in at least one study (76).

Other useful vehicles include milkshakes, a tapioca fruit mixture, infant formulas, and other foods.

Hamburger seems to be a particularly good hiding place for foods such as cereal grains. Canned tuna, which for most patients is essentially nonallergenic because the canning process denatures the allergenic proteins, has been used to hide a number of foods, including other fish. Ice cream flavored with a strong syrup (grape, for example) has been used effectively to hide strong food tastes such as shrimp (42). For young children, applesauce is a particularly good vehicle. Grains that are difficult to place in infant formulas but that are often incriminated in producing symptoms in young children can be mixed in applesauce, for example. Most liquids or soluble allergens can be mixed into infant formula in varying amounts with the assistance of a blender. Another useful vehicle that has recently been marketed in the United States is Neocate One Plus, an elemental formula designed for children. It may have a taste superior to that of many elemental infant formulas. As approximately 80% of DBPCFC documented food reactions are due to egg, peanut, milk, soy and wheat, concentrating on these substances may enable the investigator to find one or more acceptable vehicles for challenging patients of varying age and disposition.

There are two circumstances in which capsules may not be the preferred vehicle. The first occurs when the patient complains of oral symptoms following food ingestion. Such patients may actually need both capsule and non-capsule challenges to determine if their symptoms are strictly due to local contact in the mouth or if oral symptoms can also occur upon systemic absorption. This determination may be particularly crucial if the patient's symptoms include significant swelling of the oro-pharyngeal structures.

The other situation in which capsules may be contraindicated is the investigation of a patient who may experience anaphylaxis during a food challenge. Using a liquid preparation may make it easier to control the quantity ingested and avoid potential problems with slow dissolution of the capsules. Challenges in anaphylactically sensitive patients employed with extreme caution may be necessary to determine the food offender accurately and to determine, in young children, whether the problem has resolved (77).

PLACEBOS

The placebo portion of the DBPCFC is indispensable for research and extremely important in many clinical food challenges to eliminate bias on the part of the subject and the observers. When capsules are used, dextrose represents a good placebo because of its ready availability and ease of encapsulation. Another food—one that is not under suspicion—may also constitute a good placebo. The vehicle itself can be used as a placebo by giving a volume that is about the same as that containing the challenge. Some foods present a more difficult problem because they cause a distinct change in appearance of the capsules. Although chocolate has caused the greatest problem, carob has proved to be a very acceptable placebo.

PRECAUTIONS AND TREATMENT OF REACTIONS

For the practicing allergist, blinded food challenges should be considered to be a standard procedure that can be safely carried out in the office. Prior to administration of challenges, the procedure and possible outcomes should be discussed with the patient, just as any other medical procedure would be. Possible adverse outcomes should be discussed, including the chance of inducing anaphylaxis. The patient should be informed that prompt treatment is available and that, because the challenge is administered in a graded fashion, no severe symptoms are expected to occur. A physician must remain present at all times during the challenge, and the patient should be observable at all times by nursing personnel.

Any physician who administers allergy injection treatment and whose office is equipped to treat serious adverse consequences of an injection reaction, should be suitably equipped to treat a severe food reaction. Personnel should be appropriately trained and equipped in accord with the Position Statement on "Personnel and equipment to treat systemic reactions caused by immunotherapy with allergic extracts" formulated by the Executive Committee of the American Academy of Allergy and Immunology (78). For a systemic reaction that becomes severe, epinephrine (administered subcutaneously) is the initial drug of choice. Antihistamines may also be given, but their expected onset of action is too slow to be relied on for an immediate response. If shock is developing, intravenous fluids should be started and consideration should be given to transferring the patient to a hospital.* Obviously, some situations require a great deal more caution than others, and most of the challenges performed by practicing allergists are exceedingly unlikely to lead to catastrophic symptoms. Patients who have a history of anaphylaxis and who are being investigated with a food likely to cause severe reactions should probably be studied only in the hospital and with very small incremental increases in quantity of the food administered.

MEDICATION PRIOR TO CHALLENGE

Certain medications should be avoided prior to food challenge, including antihistamines (for 72–96 hours before the challenge, but longer for hydroxyzine and some newer preparations), beta agonists (12 hours), theophylline (12 hours), cromolyn (12 hours), and probably tricyclic antidepressants (96 hours or longer). Few of these medications have been studied as possible inhibitors of food reactions, and most of these recommendations represent extrapolations from skin test studies with these drugs. In any situation, it may be useful to determine that the subject reacts to a histamine skin test control.

CONDUCT OF FOOD CHALLENGES

The major purpose of a food challenge is to determine whether the food under study is responsible for the reported symptoms. To make this determination, it is optimal for the subject to be symptom-free during an elimination diet. In practice this situation often does not occur. Thus, the investigator must attempt to identify a stable baseline so that symptoms superimposed upon this baseline during food challenges will be as unequivocal as possible.

Establishment of a baseline is best accomplished by beginning with an elimination diet to observe whether the reported symptoms will resolve by removal of one or more foods from the diet. When the history specifically incriminates one or more foods, the elimination diet should concentrate on these substances. If milk is the only food identified as causing symptoms, for example, it is eliminated from the diet with the expectation that the symptoms will resolve. The resolution of symptoms with the elimination of a particular food accompanied by a positive prick or puncture skin test provides strong presumptive evidence that food hypersensitivity is present, and should be confirmed by DBPCFC in most cases (except where anaphylaxis is a concern). Many physicians have argued that remission of symptoms and a positive skin test should be sufficient to make the diagnosis and eliminate the food. Studies at different institutions have repeatedly shown, however, that even when the evidence is this strong, less than 50% of histories will be confirmed by DBPCFC. Thus, the results of diet and skin tests should still be confirmed by DBPCFC when possible.

Many patients complain that foods cause their symptoms but have no specific suspicions or report multiple suspicions. In these situations, careful questioning in an attempt to narrow the list and to determine appropriate starting doses is important. The elimination diet may be chosen from many available; a sample is found in Table 8.5. Usually, seven days on the diet is sufficient to demonstrate either remission or significant improvement of the symptoms. If the symptoms do not change, then the physician is left with three possibilities: food in

Table 8.5
Elimination Diet

Rice in any form	Asparagus
(rice cakes a helpful snack)	Beets
Pineapple	Carrots
Cranberries	Lettuce
Apricots	Sweet potato
Peaches	White vinegar
Pears	Olive oil
Apples	Honey
Chicken	Sugar (cane or beet)
Lamb	Salt

Fruits mentioned may be fresh or canned, or taken in juice form. Avoid additives, colors, or preservatives in the evaluation of subjective symptoms. Avoid any food not on this list including coffee, tea, colored beverages, and chewing gum. Take only prescribed medications.

* In the author's and H. A. Sampson's experience, both of whom have conducted more than 1500 food challenges (primarily in children) in various settings, even with patients who are anaphylactically sensitive, careful challenge has never resulted in shock that required intravenous resuscitation or in cardiopulmonary arrest.

the diet is not responsible for symptoms, some food or food in the elimination diet is triggering the symptoms, or some other factor besides an eliminated food is the cause of the problem. If the resolution of the symptoms seems equivocal to the patient, it is often advisable to return immediately to a regular diet to show a significant difference between the two diets. If the patient reports an impressive improvement in symptoms or if a baseline is easily found, oral challenges may begin. Particularly for subjective symptoms, use of the elimination diet followed by a regular diet may make the difference as clear as possible to both patient and physician.

Establishment of a stable baseline is particularly important when investigating conditions that usually have multiple precipitating factors such as atopic dermatitis or asthma. Unfortunately, few patients with these conditions will remit completely on an elimination diet. When such patients improve significantly, the stable baseline can usually be identified. The author has rarely found food diaries to be helpful in these cases, as they are cumbersome for both patient and physician. A very strict elimination diet with all infractions being recorded and an accompanying symptom diary is much more manageable and useful.

OPEN FOOD CHALLENGES

Open food challenges occasionally prove useful in the practice setting but should never be performed for investigational purposes. As noted, open challenges are actually part of the reinstitution of a regular diet following the failure of an elimination diet to produce an unequivocal result. Open challenges may also have some utility when the skin test is negative, the history doubtful, and the patient has been avoiding the food. In this situation, the food may be reintroduced into the diet with the high expectation that no reaction will occur. Ideally this reintroduction should be undertaken under observation. If no possibility of a serious reaction exists, however, then the challenge may take place at the patient's home.

In addition, open food challenges may be employed in selected situations where challenges do not reproduce the symptoms, thus refuting the history.

As the majority of challenges in clinical practice do refute the history, oral challenges may be used by the practitioner to good advantage. Whenever a positive result is obtained, the physician should perform a DBPCFC. Even the most obviously objective symptoms may not be confirmed during blind challenge. In this field, where strongly held beliefs are common, we must never underestimate the power of the central nervous system to interfere with our observations.

SINGLE-BLIND FOOD CHALLENGES

Single-blind food challenges are somewhat more useful than open food challenges because they potentially eliminate at least the bias of the subject. Therefore, they can be used to document the absence of symptoms, particularly in situations where it may be desirable to refute a history of vague or subjective symptoms without using multiple substances in the challenge. Single-blind challenges may also prove useful in certain research situations for selection of patients who will then progress to the double-blind phase of a study. Single-blind studies in patients undergoing food additive challenges have documented the observation that positive single-blind challenges cannot always be reproduced when double-blind challenges are subsequently administered.

DOUBLE-BLIND PLACEBO-CONTROLLED FOOD CHALLENGES

As indicated, the DBPCFC is the "gold standard" for the confirmation or refutation of any history of an adverse reaction to a food. At this time no good substitute exists for the DBPCFC. The primary objections to this procedure have been raised by people who have not taken the time to master the procedure; once it is mastered, DBPCFC is no more complicated to administer than any other allergy procedure or technique. It provides an immeasurable service to patients who have labored under the burden of elimination diets and faulty information. It may also help to determine the threshold of reactivity to some foods that may be tolerated in small amounts or in children who are "outgrowing" their food hypersensitivity. The physician should have available a quantity of frequently incriminated foods so that he or she does not have to begin food acquisition and preparation anew for each patient who requires challenges.

Administration of the food challenge is designed so that it will reproduce the conditions reported by the patient in the history (Table 8.6). Challenges should typically begin early in the day after an overnight fast. The starting dose should be about one-half of the minimum quantity estimated by the patient to have produced symptoms during the most recent or most severe reaction. This dose may then be doubled at time intervals slightly longer than that reported to be required for the onset of symptoms. For example, if the reaction is said to begin in about 30 minutes, then the subsequent doses may be ingested about 40 minutes following each negative challenge. If the history does not specify an interval but the reaction reportedly had a prompt onset, then an interval of 15 to 60 minutes may be used. Doubling of the dose should continue until symptoms have been elicited or until 8 to 10 g of dried food or 60 to 100 g of wet food have been administered in a single dose. By the time 8 to 10 g of dried food have been ingested by incremental challenge, the total dose may range between 15 and 20 g, a substantial amount for a dehydrated food.

Several methods are available for administering the placebo portion of the challenge. One technique is to have a separate placebo day, during which increasing numbers of placebo capsules are administered, up to the number that approximately equals the number of capsules containing 8 g of the challenge food. Another method is to intermingle the placebo

challenges with the food challenges in a random fashion, but on the same day. The patient may ingest different numbers of capsules at different times in a seemingly random manner, thereby adding to the blinding of the procedure. Some investigators suggest that all challenges should contain the same number of capsules, and thus may start with the placebo and then gradually replace some placebo capsules with food capsules. In some instances, the challenge must be altered following each dose depending on the reaction. In this situation, the investigator sends the challenge substance to the study unit to be administered by a nurse, and receives a written report prior to the next challenge so that the appropriate change can be made. By using an intermediary to transport the challenge capsules and the progress report, the investigator becomes aware of the results of each challenge without prejudicing the outcome of subsequent challenges. This procedure has proved most useful when symptoms are subjective or vague and involve the prompt onset of complaint following ingestion. For example, when studying children with headache, abdominal pain, or behavior changes, the ability to change the challenge from food to placebo, and back again, during a challenge day has clear benefits.

Challenges conducted to investigate immediate-onset symptoms may proceed with one series of challenges (active or placebo) over a 1 to 2 hour period in the morning. A second series of challenges (active or placebo not given in the morning) follows over a 1 to 2 hour period in the afternoon. For the evaluation of many symptoms and in some research protocols, this approach provides a very effective use of time and resources. Observations made by this method could be compromised by delayed or late-onset reactions.

Another approach may save time when patients are being challenged to obtain diagnostic information that is not part of a research protocol. If the challenges are arranged so that the nurses administering them never know the contents or the final interpretation, the physician may begin with the food and then omit the placebo if the challenge is unequivocally positive or negative. The physician must not have contact with the patient or the nurse during the procedure to avoid biasing the outcome.

Table 8.6
Administration of DBPCFC

Goal: To Confirm or Refute the History
1. Start with an amount about one-half the minimum expected to produce symptoms.
2. Give incremental amounts (double) at intervals slightly longer than expected to produce symptoms.
3. If multiple doses over several days are required, give the amount necessary as described by the patient two or three times per day.
4. A double-blind placebo-controlled multiple crossover may be necessary.
5. Have the patient or observer maintain a symptom score.

When the blind challenge is negative using up to about 8 g of food, then the food *must* be introduced openly into the diet in usual and customary portions prepared in a usual customary fashion, and preferably under observation. Prior to open administration of the food, the patient should be informed of the results of the blind challenge, including the type of food and the approximate quantity that was ingested. Until the food is consumed openly, the challenge procedure is considered incomplete. The ability of the patient to tolerate ingestion of the food openly will eliminate many questions about preparation, digestion, and other variables that may potentially alter the food. Although these factors have frequently been suggested as influencing food hypersensitivity, their roles have rarely been confirmed. In fact, children with food hypersensitivity to milk tend to react to any dairy preparation as long as a sufficient quantity is consumed (79). Nevertheless, the provision of an open challenge should eliminate any concerns on this front.

Rarely (in our experience) will the open challenge be positive following a negative DBPCFC. During 1014 negative DBPCFC, the subsequent open challenge has been positive in 12 cases (24). Several circumstances appear to explain this observation. First, the reaction may be due to psychological factors (that is, the patient's strongly held belief that the food under investigation will cause symptoms), and this opinion is not assuaged by the lack of symptoms during the blind portion of the challenge. Second, the blind challenge may not have achieved a sufficient dose to elicit symptoms. For example, 7 of our 12 subjects had positive open challenges following a negative blind challenge due to dose–response considerations. The blind challenge did not achieve a sufficient quantity to exceed the patient's threshold to react. This result can be achieved by repeating the blind challenge and giving a larger dose—large enough to exceed the threshold to react. Third, the challenge did not allow the food to contact the skin or mouth, which may be required to reproduce the symptoms. Five of our 12 subjects reacted only when contact with the food occurred, which did not happen during the blind portion of the challenge. As skin reactions occurred only during contact and not with systemic absorption, this observation influences the

interpretation of the challenge explained to the patient. Finally, the allergenicity of the food may be altered by challenge conditions, although this often raised concern has not been adequately documented in the literature. Some reports, using double-blind challenges, describe youngsters with hypersensitivity to milk who had severe reactions to a casein-hydrolysate formula (80, 81), and dehydration of some fish species led to negative DBPCFC that were found to elicit symptoms on open feeding (57).

The procedures described above have been directed toward evaluation of patients who report a prompt onset of symptoms. The vast majority of patients in the literature with food hypersensitivity documented by DBPCFC have experienced onset of their symptoms in minutes to hours following ingestion of the challenge. DBPCFC can also be used to evaluate subjects whose reported onset of symptoms occurs hours to days following ingestion of the suspected food.

Patients with histories of late-onset reactions report two patterns: (1) a single dose of the food causes symptoms hours to days following the challenge, or (2) multiple doses of the food over a period of hours or days are required to elicit the symptoms. The first circumstance is easier to evaluate because the challenge may be administered under observation in the office, clinic, or study unit, and the patient asked to return when symptoms begin. In this situation, use of the placebo is crucial and the challenge should be "crossed-over" two or three times to ensure that the observation is reproducible.

When the food must be given multiple times to produce the delayed symptoms, the challenge is optimally performed in the hospital under observation. Unfortunately, this approach generally requires a clinical research unit and considerable resources. Challenges for this type of problem can be performed in an outpatient setting with cooperative patients who receive capsules and will not open the capsules in order to discern their contents. This approach will be quite helpful when the history is refuted. The author has been able to help a number of adult patients determine that several foods did not cause their delayed symptoms. Because it is impractical for the patient to report to the clinic or office for each challenge, several sets of capsules are sent home with the patient. Instructions for consumption of the capsules are based upon the history. For example, if the patient indicates that ingestion of a food on three consecutive days produces symptoms on the third day, then capsules are provided in labeled containers to be taken three times per day for three days. (If once-daily administration is required, the patient might report to the clinic or office at a convenient time to take the capsules under observation, decreasing the probability of unblinding the procedure.) Thus, the food can be given one week and the placebo the next. Crossover of this technique on three occasions (six weeks), although cumbersome, is probably necessary if the challenges appear to reproduce symptoms. This procedure will not be successful with a patient who is not ready to be relieved of the problem if the challenge yields a negative finding.

As documentation of "delayed reactions" by DBPCFC remains an uncharted frontier in the study of adverse reactions to foods, a few considerations are essential. If subjective or behavioral symptoms are reproduced as "delayed reactions," the challenge should be repeated in 1 to 3 months to ensure that the observation is reproducible over time and that the problem is persistent. Identification of a homogeneous group of subjects with delayed reactions allows these patients to be studied in a controlled setting to determine the scope of the problem and the mechanisms producing these reactions.

A symptom record must be maintained during all challenges (3). If asthma is suspected, the challenges should be monitored with spirometry to detect airway obstruction at an early stage. When patients consume challenge capsules at home, they should be asked to maintain a symptom diary, and they should use a peak-flow meter if indicated.

Patients with even a remote chance of developing serious symptoms should never be challenged away from the observation of a physician and the presence of emergency equipment.

PITFALLS TO BE AVOIDED DURING FOOD CHALLENGES

Several of the problems encountered during food challenges have been covered earlier in this chapter, but a few should be emphasized. First and foremost is the failure to eliminate the bias of patient and observer by thorough blinding. This problem often arises when the patient comes to the physician to have his or her opinion confirmed. The attempt to obtain an objective result in this circumstance is doomed to failure in the vast majority of cases, and the physician is well advised to avoid challenging these patients. Some subjects are unsuitable for the procedures outlined above, and we must realize that they take little interest in the techniques and attendant information of scientific medicine.

Another problem relates to the apparent confirmation of subjective symptoms that have rarely been supported by the literature. As growing numbers of studies confirm similar symptoms attributed to a short list of foods, we must remain skeptical about extravagant claims of other kinds of responses confirmed by blinded challenges. Although the literature of allergy increasingly contains studies reporting results confirmed by DBPCFC, many of these papers contain inadequate information to analyze whether the described challenges were adequately performed. Readers of these manuscripts should retain a healthy skepticism until further confirmation is obtained. Editors and reviewers of these articles must insist that material and methods sections adequately describe the procedures used, until the body of published literature allows readers to be confident that acceptable methods have been employed.

A third common problem is the assumption that a food causing a severe food reaction is easily confirmed by the presence of a positive skin test. It is usually assumed that foods causing anaphylaxis will be associated with a positive immediate skin test, and that such a result automatically identifies the incriminated food. Too often the patient subsequently has a further episode of anaphylaxis when ingesting a different food. Conversely, patients who have apparently identified a food causing anaphylaxis may accidentally ingest the food without reaction. Thus, although regular challenge of patients with food anaphylaxis is not to be encouraged, it is important in two circumstances: (1) to be certain that the proper food has been identified (82), and (2) in young children who appear to "outgrow" their life-threatening reactions to food (77).

INTERVAL CHALLENGES

At present, no effective medical treatment exists that will enable patients with true food hypersensitivity to ingest the foods that cause symptoms without risk of manifestations. Nevertheless, allergists can be of assistance in two areas beyond diagnosis. First, they can provide emergency epinephrine to those patients with documented or potential anaphylaxis due to food ingestion. These patients should be thoroughly instructed in the appropriate use of epinephrine and impressed with the fact that if they have a reaction requiring its use, they must seek medical attention immediately to prevent a potentially fatal reaction.

Second, allergists can undertake longitudinal challenges to see if the problem is resolving. This step is especially important in children, in whom the natural history for some adverse reactions to foods involves resolution of the problem. Work with the natural history of food hypersensitivity in adults is sorely needed.

When interval challenges are planned, the interval may be determined by the severity of the initial (or most recent) reaction during DBPCFC. For some foods the interval may be as small as every one to three months, while for others an appropriate interval may be every one to two years. The initial starting dose may safely be chosen by reviewing the dose that produced the reaction at the time of the last challenge. One-half of this amount should constitute a safe starting dose. As more is learned about the natural history of different foods producing various symptoms, food-specific recommendations should gradually become possible (53, 83–85).

REFERENCES

1. May CD. Are confusion and controversy about food hypersensitivity really necessary? (editorial) J Allergy Clin Immunol 1985;75:329–333.
2. Metcalfe DD, Sampson HA. Workshop on experimental methodology for clinical studies of adverse reactions to foods and food additives. J Allergy Clin Immunol 1990;3(part 2 suppl):421–442.
3. Bock SA, Sampson HA, Atkins FM, Zeiger RS, Lehrer S, Sachs M, Bush RK, Metcalfe DD. Double-blind, placebo-controlled food challenge (DBPCFC) as an office procedure: a manual. J Allergy Clin Immunol 1988;82:986–997.
4. Bock SA. A critical evaluation of clinical trials in adverse reactions to foods in children. J Allergy Clin Immunol 1986;78:165–174.
5. Atkins FM. A critical evaluation of clinical trials in adverse reactions to foods in adults. J Allergy Clin Immunol 1986;78:174–182.
6. May CD. Objective clinical and laboratory studies of immediate hypersensitivity reactions to foods in asthmatic children. J Allergy Clin Immunol 1976;58:500–515.
7. Lowell FC. Food allergy. (editorial) J Allergy 1950;21:563–564.
8. Loveless MH. Milk allergy: a survey of its incidence; experiments with a masked ingestion test. J Allergy 1950;21:489–500.
9. Loveless MH. Allergy for corn and its derivatives; experiments with a masked ingestion test for its diagnosis. J Allergy 1950;21:500–509.
10. Graham DT, Wolf S, Wolff HG. Changes in tissue sensitivity associated with varying life situations and emotions; their relevance to allergy. J Allergy 1950;21:478–486.
11. Maslansky L, Wein G. Chocolate allergy: a double-blind study. Conn Med J 1971;35:5–9.
12. Kuitunen P, Visakorpi JK, Savilahti E, Pelkonen P. Malabsorption syndrome with cow's milk intolerance; clinical findings and course in fifty-four cases. Arch Dis Child 1975;50:351–356.
13. Savilahti E. Immunochemical study of the malabsorption syndrome with cow's milk intolerance. Gut 1973;14:491–501.
14. Lake AM, Whitington PF, Hamilton SR. Dietary protein-induced colitis in breast-fed infants. J Pediatr 1982;101:906–910.
15. Vitoria JC, Camarero C, Sojo A, Ruiz A, Rodriguez-Soriano J. Enteropathy related to fish, rice, and chicken. Arch Dis Child 1982;57:44–48.
16. Baker AL, Rosenberg IH. Refractory spruce recovery after removal of nongluten dietary proteins. Ann Int Med 1978;89:505–508.
17. Strober W, Falchuck ZM, Rogentine GN, et al. The pathogenesis of gluten-sensitive enteropathy. Ann Intern Med 1975;83:242–256.
18. Falchuck ZM, Katz AJ, Shwachman H, et al. Gluten-sensitive enteropathy: genetic analysis and organ culture study in 35 families. Scand J Gastroenterol 1978;13:839–843.
19. Falchuck ZM, Strober W. Gluten-sensitive enteropathy: synthesis of antigliadin antibody in vitro. Gut 1974;15:947–952.
20. Jos J, Labbe F, Geny B, Griscelli C. Immunoelectron microscopic localization of immunoglobulin A and secretory component in jejunal mucosa from children with coeliac disease. Scand J Immunol 1979;9:441–450.
21. Ament ME, Rubin CE. Soy protein—another cause of the flat intestinal lesion. Gastroenterology 1972;62:227–234.
22. Perkkio M, Savilahti E, Kuitunen P. Morphometric and immunohistochemical study of jejunal biopsies from children with intestinal soy allergy. Eur J Pediatr 1981;137:63–69.
23. Bock SA, Remigio LK, Gordon B. Immunochemical localization of proteins in the intestinal mucosa of children with diarrhea. J Allergy Clin Immunol 1983;72:262–268.
24. Bock SA, Atkins FM. Patterns of food hypersensitivity during 16 years of double-blind placebo-controlled food challenges. J Pediatr 1990;117:561–567.
25. Bernstein M, Day JH, Welsh A. Double-blind food challenge in the diagnosis of food sensitivity in the adult. J Allergy Clin Immunol 1982;70:205–210.
26. Atkins FM, Steinberg SS, Metcalfe DD. Evaluation of immedi-

ate adverse reactions to foods in adult patients. I. Correlation of demographic, laboratory, and prick skin test data with response to controlled oral food challenge. J Allergy Clin Immunol 1985;75:348–355.

27. Atkins FM, Steinberg SS, Metcalfe DD. Evaluation of immediate adverse reactions to foods in adult patients. II. A detailed analysis of reaction patterns during oral food challenge. J Allergy Clin Immunol 1985;75:356–363.

28. Onorato J, Merland N, Terral C, Michel FB, Bousquet J. Placebo-controlled double-blind food challenge in asthma. J Allergy Clin Immunol 1986;78:1139–1146.

29. Farah DA, Calder I, Benson L, MacKenzie JF. Specific food intolerance: its place as a cause of gastrointestinal symptoms. Gut 1985;26:164–168.

30. Bock SA, Lee W, Remigio LK, May CD. Studies of hypersensitivity reactions to foods in infants and children. J Allergy Clin Immunol 1978;62:327–334.

31. Novembre E, de Martino J, Vierucci A. Foods and respiratory allergy. J Allergy Clin Immunol 1988;81:1059–1065.

32. Pastorello EA, Stocchi L, Pravettoni V, Bigi A, Schilke ML, Incorvaia C, Zanussi C. Role of the elimination diet in adults with food allergy. J Allergy Clin Immunol 1989;84:475–483.

33. Norgaard A, Bindslev-Jensen C. Egg and milk allergy in adults. Allergy 1992;47:503–509.

34. Kivity S, Dunner K, Marian Y. The pattern of food hypersensitivity in patients with onset after 10 years of age. Clin Exp Allergy 1994;24:19–22.

35. Bock, SA. Respiratory reactions induced by food challenges in children with pulmonary disease. Pediatr Allergy Immunol 1992;3:188–194.

36. James JM, Bernhisel-Broadbent J, Sampson HA. Respiratory reactions provoked by double-blind food challenges in children. Am J Respir Crit Care Med 1994;149:59–64.

37. Jakobsson I, Lindberg T. Cow's milk proteins cause infantile colic in breast-fed infants: a double-blind crossover study. Pediatrics 1983;71:268–271.

38. Lothe L, Lindberg T. Cow's milk whey protein elicits symptoms of infantile colic in colicky formula-fed infants: a double-blind crossover study. Pediatrics 1989;83:262–266.

39. Bock SA. Prospective appraisal of complaints of adverse reactions to foods in children during the first 3 years of life. Pediatrics 1987;79:683–688.

40. Forsythe BWC. Colic and the effect of changing formulas: a double-blind multiple crossover study. J Pediatr 1989;115:521–526.

41. Sampson HA. Infantile colic and food allergy: fact or fiction. J Pediatr 1989;115:583–584.

42. Daul CB, Morgan JE, McCants ML, Hughes J, Lehrer SB. Provocation challenge studies in shrimp sensitive individuals. J Allergy Clin Immunol 1988;81:1180–1186.

43. Musmand JJ, Daul CB, Lehrer SB. Crustacea allergy. Clin Exp Allergy 1993;23:722–732.

44. Castells MC, Pascual C, Esteban MM, Ojeda JA. Allergy to white potato. J Allergy Clin Immunol 1986;78:1110–1114.

45. Linaweaver WE, Saks GL, Heiner DC. Anaphylactic shock following banana ingestion. Am J Dis Child 1976;130:207–209.

46. Strunk RC, Pinnus JL, John TJ. Rice hypersensitivity associated with serum complement depression. Clin Allergy 1978;8:51–58.

47. Stricker WE, Anohue-Lopez E, Reed CE. Food skin testing in patients with idiopathic anaphylaxis. J Allergy Clin Immunol 1986;77:526–529.

48. Tinkelman DG, Bock SA. Anaphylaxis presumed to be caused by beef containing streptomycin. Ann Allergy 1984;53:243–244.

49. Bock SA. Anaphylaxis to coriander: a sleuthing story. J Allergy Clin Immunol 1993;92:1232–1233.

50. Goodman DL, McDonnell JT, Nelson HS, Vaughan TR, Weber RW. Chronic urticaria exacerbated by the antioxidant food preservatives, butylated hydroxyanisole (BHA) and butylated hydroxytoluene (BHT). J Allergy Clin Immunol 1990;86:570–575.

51. Ratner B, Untracht S, Malone J, et al. Allergenicity of modified and processed food stuffs in orange: allergenicity of orange studied in man. J Pediatr 1953;43:421–428.

52. Barnett D, Bonham B, Howden EH. Allergenic cross-reactions among legume foods—an in vitro study. J Allergy Clin Immunol 1987;79:433–438.

53. Bock SA, Atkins FM. The natural history of peanut allergy. J Allergy Clin Immunol 1989;83:900–904.

54. Bernhisel-Broadbent J, Sampson HA. Cross-allergenicity in the legume botanical family in children with food hypersensitivity. J Allergy Clin Immunol 1989;83:435–440.

55. Bernhisel-Broadbent J, Taylor SL, Sampson HA. Cross allergenicity in the legume botanical family in children with food hypersensitivity II. Laboratory correlates. J Allergy Clin Immunol 1989;84:701–709.

56. Bernhisel-Broadbent J, Scanlon SM, Sampson HA. Fish hypersensitivity. I. In vitro and oral challenge results in fish-allergic patients. J Allergy Clin Immunol 1992;89:730–737.

57. Bernhisel-Broadbent J, Strause D, Sampson HA. Fish hypersensitivity. II. Clinical relevance of altered fish allergenicity caused by various preparation methods. J Allergy Clin Immunol 1992;90:622–629.

58. Jones SM, Magnolfi CF, Cooke SK, Sampson HA. Immunologic cross-reactivity among cereal grains and grasses in children with food hypersensitivity. J Allergy Clin Immunol 1995; 96:341–351.

59. Lahti A, Hannuksela M. Hypersensitivity to apple and carrot can be reliably detected with fresh material. Allergy 1978;33:143–146.

60. Pastorella EA, Ortolani C, Farioli L, Pravettoni V, Ispano M, Borga A, Bengtsson A, Incorvaia C, Berti C, Zanussi C. Allergenic cross-reactivity among peach, apricot, plum, and cherry in patients with oral allergy syndrome: an in vivo and in vitro study. J Allergy Clin Immunol 1994;94:669–707.

61. Dreborg S, Foucard T. Allergy to apple, carrot and potato in children with birch pollen allergy. Allergy 1983;38:167–172.

62. Hirschwehr R, Valenta R, Ebner C, Ferreira F, Sperr WR, Valent P, Rohac M, Rumpold H, Scheiner O, Kraft D. Identification of common allergenic structures in hazel pollen and hazelnuts: a possible explanation for the sensitivity to hazelnuts in patients allergic to tree pollen. J Allergy Clin Immunol 1992;90:927–936.

63. Calkhoven PG, Aalberse M, Koshite VL, Pos O, Oei HD, Aalberse RC. Cross-reactivity among birch pollen, vegetables and fruits as detected by IgE antibodies is due to at least three distinct cross-reactive structures. Allergy 1987;42:382–390.

64. Lowenstein H, Eriksson NE. Hypersensitivity to foods among birch pollen-allergic patients. Allergy 1983;38:577–587.

65. Enberg RN, Leickly FE, McCullough J, Bailey J, Ownby DR. Watermelon and ragweed share allergens. J Allergy Clin Immunol 1987;79:867–875.

66. Enberg RN, McCullough J, Ownby DR. Antibody responses in

watermelon sensitivity. J Allergy Clin Immunol 1988;82:795–800.

67. Hill DJ, Firer MA, Ball G, Hosking CS. Natural history of cow's milk allergy in children: immunological outcome over 2 years. Clin Exp Allergy 1993;23:124–131.

68. Bock SA, Buckley J, Holst A, May CD. Proper use of skin tests with food extracts in diagnosis of hypersensitivity to food in children. Clin Allergy 1977;7:375–383.

69. Bock SA, Lee W-Y, Remigio LK, Holst A, May CD. Appraisal of skin tests with food extracts for diagnosis of food hypersensitivity. Clin Allergy 1978;8:559–564.

70. Sampson HA, Albergo R. Comparison of results of prick skin tests, RAST, and double-blind placebo-controlled food challenges in children with atopic dermatitis. J Allergy Clin Immunol 1984;74:26–33.

71. Sampson HA. Comparative study of commercial food antigen extracts for the diagnosis of food hypersensitivity. J Allergy Clin Immunol 1988;82:718–726.

72. Burks AW, Mallory SB, Williams LW, Shirrell MA. Atopic dermatitis: clinical relevance of food hypersensitivity reactions. J Pediatr 1988;113:447–451.

73. Norgaard A, Skov PS, Bindslev-Jensen C. Egg and milk allergy in adults: comparison between fresh and commercial allergen extracts in skin prick test and histamine release from basophils. Clin Exp Allergy 1992;22:940–947.

74. Ancona GR, Schumacher IC. The use of raw foods as skin testing material in allergic disorders. Calif Med 1950;73:473–475.

75. Ortoloni C, Ispano M, Pastorello EA, Ansaloni R, Magri GC. Comparison of results of skin prick tests (with fresh food and commercial food extracts) and RAST in 100 patients with oral allergy syndrome. J Allergy Clin Immunol 1989;83:683–690.

76. Taylor SL, Busse WW, Sachs MI, Parker JL, Yunginger JW. Peanut oil is not allergenic to peanut sensitive individuals. J Allergy Clin Immunol 1981;68:372–375.

77. Bock SA. The natural history of severe reactions to foods in young children. J Pediatr 1985;107:676–680.

78. Executive Committee of the Academy of Allergy and reactions caused by immunotherapy with allergic extracts (position statement). J Allergy Clin Immunol 1986;77:271–273.

79. Høst A, Samuelsson EG. Allergic reactions to raw, pasteurized, and homogenized/pasteurized cow milk: a comparison. Allergy 1988;43:113–118.

80. Bock SA. Probable allergic reaction to casein hydrolysate formula. (letter) J Allergy Clin Immunol 1989;84:272.

81. Sampson HA, Bernhisel-Broadbent J, Yang E, Scanlon S. Safety of casein hydrolysate formula in children with cow milk allergy. J Pediatr 1991;118:520–525.

82. Sampson HA, Mendelson LM, Rosen JP. Fatal and near fatal anaphylactic reactions to food in children and adolescents. N Engl J Med 1992;327:380–384.

83. Bock SA. The natural history of food sensitivity. J Allergy Clin Immunol 1982;69:173–177.

84. Sampson HA, Scanlon S. Natural history of food hypersensitivity in children with atopic dermatitis. J Pediatr 1989;115:23–27.

85. Daul CB, Morgan JE, Lehrer SB. The natural history or shrimp hypersensitivity. J Allergy Clin Immunol 1990;86:88–93.

Part Two

ADVERSE REACTIONS TO FOOD ANTIGENS:
CLINICAL SCIENCE

9

IMMEDIATE REACTIONS TO FOODS IN INFANTS AND CHILDREN

Hugh A. Sampson

Introduction

Food allergic disorders comprise a group of distinct clinicopathologic entities that share abnormal or exaggerated immunologic responses to specific food proteins leading to disease. A typical classification scheme (Table 9.1) divides food hypersensitivity disorders into two categories: IgE-mediated disease, and "other," possibly immune-complex or cell-mediated, hypersensitivity-induced diseases. The IgE-mediated food hypersensitivity reactions that constitute the primary subject of this chapter generally exhibit a rapid onset, although "other" mechanisms may lead to very rapid reactions (e.g., cow's milk or soy protein-induced enterocolitis syndromes and some forms of allergic eosinophilic gastroenteritis).

The pathologic basis for IgE-mediated reactions lies in the cross-linking of antigen-specific IgE molecules on the surface of mast cells and basophils following ingestion of a specific allergen in an individual sensitive to that allergen. The resulting clinical picture may involve the gastrointestinal, cutaneous, respiratory, and/or cardiovascular systems. Symptoms provoked during gastrointestinal reactions may include itching or tingling of the mouth and throat, tightness in the throat, nausea, colicky abdominal cramps, vomiting, and diarrhea. Cutaneous signs and symptoms may include generalized erythema and pruritus, a pruritic morbilliform rash, urticaria, and angioedema. Respiratory symptoms may consist of nasal pruritus and congestion, rhinorrhea, hoarseness, dry staccato cough, dyspnea, and/or wheezing. In severe cases, cardiovascular signs include hypotension and cardiac arrhythmias (1). Some cases of food-induced anaphylaxis or urticaria are dependent upon a co-factor for exacerbation of clinical symptoms, although the only co-factor clearly demonstrated to provoke symptoms is exercise.

Two specific clinical situations—that of food-induced eczema and food-induced eosinophilic gastroenteritis—appear to involve a cellular infiltrate reminiscent of late phase IgE-mediated reactions. In individuals susceptible to these diseases, an intrinsic abnormality in the skin or gastrointestinal tract and/or selective activation of lmphocytes that "home" to these respective target organs (2) may contribute to the pathologic process. A second possibility is that these individuals suffer from frequent and recurrent mast cell degranulation, repetitive or continuous late-phase reactions, and the subsequent chronic inflammation seen in the skin of patients with atopic dermatitis and the gastrointestinal tract of patients with eosinophilic gastroenteritis.

In the second pattern of food hypersensitivity reactions, other immunopathologic mechanisms may be responsible for disease states. Gluten-sensitive enteropathy is technically a food hypersensitivity in which an abnormal immunologic response to gluten occurs. Some studies suggest that abnormal metabolism of gluten in susceptible individuals leads to an abnormal immunologic response (3). Food protein-induced enterocolitis syndromes are seen primarily in infants and young children. Although generally regarded as non-IgE mediated, the immunopathogenic mechanisms involved in these disorders remain unknown. Some children with food protein-induced enterocolitis syndromes do provide evidence for IgE-mediated phenomena, although the involvement of

Table 9.1
Food Hypersensitivity Classification

I. IgE-Mediated
   A. Immediate
      —Gastrointestinal
      —Hives, angioedema
      —Rhinitis, asthma
      —Anaphylaxis
   B. Immediate and late phase
      —Eczema
      —Allergic eosinophilic gastroenteritis
II. Immune Complex/Cell-Mediated Hypersensitivity (?)
   —Gluten-sensitive enteropathy (coeliac disease)
   —Food protein-induced enterocolitis syndromes

one immunologic mechanism does not necessarily exclude the involvement of other effector mechanisms.

Prevalence

Many members of the public perceive "food allergy" as a major health concern (4). Two prospective surveys (5, 6) found that parents reported that 23% to 28% of their children experienced at least one adverse reaction to food. When the investigators evaluated these children with suspected adverse food reactions, only about one-third of the claims could be confirmed by controlled challenge. In both studies, the prevalence of adverse food reactions was 8%; 2% to 4% of children less than 6 years of age appeared to experience food allergic reactions. In the study by Bock (6), parents reported reactions to fruits and fruit juices in 75 of 480 infants (16%), and complaints were confirmed in 56 children (12% overall) by open challenges. Symptoms developing during 60 positive challenges included skin rashes or diarrhea, and were attributed to oranges in 14 children (23%), tomatoes in 14 (23%), apples in 7 (12%), grapes in 4 (7%), and other fruits in the remaining 21 reactions (35%). Several prospective studies have evaluated the prevalence of cow's milk allergy in young infants. A study of 1759 Danish infants indicated that the prevalence of cow's milk allergy was greatest in the first year and affected 2.2% of infants (7). Similarly, a study of 1386 infants found that 2.8% of Dutch infants were affected by cow's milk allergy (8). Overall, approximately 2.5% of infants experience cow's milk allergy in the first years of life and nearly 85% of sensitive infants lose their reactivity by their third birthday (9). Parents often suspect adverse reactions to food additives in children. In a study of 4274 Dutch school children, adverse reactions to additives were suspected in 6.6% of children, but results of double-blind, placebo-controlled food challenges (DBPCFC) in a cohort of subjects suggested an overall prevalence of 1% to 2% (10). Such studies indicate that more than 500,000 children 3 years of age or younger in the United States are food allergic and that more than 1 million children between 3 years and 18 years of age experience food allergic reactions.

Pathogenesis

The vast majority of immediate allergic reactions to foods are due to IgE-mediated hypersensitivity. The primary effector cells in these reactions are mast cells and basophils, although other IgE-bearing cells (e.g., macrophages, monocytes, dendritic cells) are likely to be activated as well. When considering IgE-mediated responses, three critical elements should be considered: the allergen, the gastrointestinal tract barrier, and the patient's predisposition to develop an IgE response.

In general, studies in children implicate a limited number of foods in the pathogenesis of allergic reactions (6, 11–16); these foods include egg, milk, peanut, soy, wheat, nuts, and fish. The eating patterns of a society influence the prevalence of a specific food hypersensitivity. For example, peanut hypersensitivity is relatively common in children in the United States but virtually nonexistent in Sweden, where peanut butter is rarely consumed. On the other hand, rice hypersensitivity is extremely rare in the United States but not uncommon in Japan.

In general, food allergens appear to have some unique properties that make them allergenic. The allergenic fractions of these substances share several characteristics: they are predominantly water-soluble, heat- and acid-stable glycoproteins with molecular weights in the range of 15,000 to 60,000 daltons.

The average individual's gastrointestinal tract will process an estimated 100 tons or more of food during a lifetime. Consequently, food represents the largest antigenic load confronting the human immune system. Infants ingest proteins from fewer sources than adults; their food sources consist of mother's milk or commercial formulas based on bovine milk and soybean protein. Dietary proteins ingested by older children are derived from meat, poultry, and fish (42.3%); dairy products (21.2%); flour and cereal products (18.6%); dry beans, peanut, and soya products (5.4%); vegetables (6.7%); eggs (4.9%); and fruits and miscellaneous sources (1.4%) (17). Commercially processed proteins used as food ingredients include casein and whey from bovine milk, gelatin and collagen from animal tendons and hides, soy protein isolates from soybean, and gluten from the flour of wheat, corn, and oats.

The human organism incorporates both nonspecific and specific barrier systems that limit the ingress of intact proteins and that indirectly or directly decrease the immune responsiveness to food proteins. Ingested food is initially acted on by stomach acid and pepsins, pancreatic enzymes, and intestinal peptidases. Many large proteins are broken down into small peptides and amino acids, which are then absorbed by the mucosal endothelial cells. Mucosal endothelial cell lysosomes further degrade these absorbed peptides into smaller peptides and amino acids.

Antigenic proteins and peptides that traverse the mucosal endothelial barrier elicit an immune response that leads to active secretion of antigen-specific antibodies into the gut. Secretory IgA is the predominant immunoglobulin that forms complexes with respective antigens and prevents their absorption. Circulating IgA probably plays some role in clearing antigenic components that penetrate the gastrointestinal barrier. Abnormalities in any of these systems (e.g., achlorhydria, cystic fibrosis, selective IgA deficiency, or immaturity) can increase antigenic penetration of the gastrointestinal barrier. In addition, exogenous substances such as alcohol may reduce gastric mucus and contribute to the disruption of the epithelial barrier.

Despite these physiologic and immunologic barriers to antigen absorption, clear documentation exists that food antigens penetrate the normal gastrointestinal tract. Seventy-four percent of children sensitized with serum from an egg-allergic subject (Prausnitz–Küstner test) developed a positive wheal-and-flare response within 15 to 60 minutes of ingesting egg (18). Similarly, 65 adults sensitized with serum from a fish-allergic individual were fed raw fish and 94% of these subjects developed a wheal-and-flare response at the sensitized site, but not at a control site (19). Furthermore, Walzer (20) demonstrated that only minute quantities of allergen are necessary to elicit an IgE-mediated response. The protein nitrogen equivalent of 1/44,000 of a peanut kernel injected intravenously was sufficient to elicit a wheal-and-flare response at a passively sensitized skin site. In addition, food allergens have been shown to be readily absorbed from all sections of the gastrointestinal tract and the nasal airway. In these and other studies, it was demonstrated that specific factors could affect the amount of antigen absorbed and alter the timing of symptom onset; these factors include the amount of antigen ingested, whether the antigen is consumed alone or with other foods, the degree of cooking necessary to render proteins less soluble, and the presence of gastrointestinal disturbances (e.g., inflammation) which may render the mucosal wall more permeable. Consequently, such factors must be taken into account when evaluating the history of a patient with a possible food hypersensitivity.

The third factor that contributes to the development of food allergic reactions is an individual's genetic predisposition to develop an IgE-mediated response. Research suggests that some individuals may inherit an imbalance between Th2 and Th1 leading to increased levels of IgE, increased FcE receptors on many cell types, and production of cytokines favoring the attraction of allergic inflammatory cells (21). In addition, various factors such as viral infection and other allergen exposures, may influence an individual's ability to promote or inhibit an IgE-antibody response.

Clinical Manifestations

The clinical signs and symptoms linked to immediate food hypersensitivity and reported in clinical trials are listed in Table 9.2. Systemic anaphylaxis is an acute, potentially fatal reaction involving multiple

Table 9.2
Presumed IgE-Mediated Food-Hypersensitivity
Reactions Reported in Blinded Challenges

Generalized reactions
Anaphylaxis
Food-dependent, exercise-induced anaphylaxis

Cutaneous reactions
Urticaria/angioedema
Food-dependent, exercise-induced urticaria/angioedema
Atopic dermatitis

Respiratory reactions
Rhinoconjunctivitis
Laryngeal edema
Asthma

Gastrointestinal reactions
Gastrointestinal anaphylaxis (abdominal pain, nausea, vomiting,
    and diarrhea)
Colic
Allergic eosinophilic gastroenteritis (with gastroesophageal reflux)

organ systems. Its symptoms may include tongue swelling and itching, palatal itching or tingling, throat itching and tightness, nausea, colicky abdominal pain, vomiting, diarrhea, dyspnea, wheezing, cyanosis, chest pain, urticaria, angioedema, hypotension, and shock. Anaphylactic reactions secondary to food proteins are well recognized and have been confirmed in several studies. The number of fatal food allergic reactions that occur in the United States each year is unknown, but is estimated to exceed 100 deaths per year. In fact, a recent survey suggested that food allergy is the most common cause of severe anaphylaxis treated in U.S. emergency departments, occurring more than twice as frequently as insect sting-induced anaphylaxis (22).

Although fatal food-induced anaphylaxis appears to occur more often in adults, fatal and near-fatal cases occur in children as well, especially among teenagers. In reviewing six fatal and seven near-fatal food-induced anaphylactic reactions that occurred in children (aged 2 to 17 years) from three metropolitan areas over a 14-month period (23), several common risk factors were noted. In particular, all patients had asthma (although it was generally well controlled); all patients were unaware that they were ingesting the food allergen; all patients had experienced previous allergic reactions to the incriminated food; and all patients had immediate symptoms, with about half

experiencing a quiescent period prior to a major respiratory collapse. No patient who died received adrenalin immediately, although three patients with near-fatal reactions received adrenalin within 15 minutes of developing their first symptoms and still developed respiratory collapse and hypotension requiring mechanical ventilation and vasopressor support for 12 hours to 3 weeks. Unlike children with other forms of anaphylaxis (e.g., bee sting, drug allergy), children investigated with life-threatening food-induced anaphylaxis had no significant increase in serum tryptase, raising some questions about the exact mechanism of food-induced anaphylaxis. Severe life-threatening reactions in children and adolescents are most often associated with the ingestion of peanuts, nuts, and seafood, while milk, egg, soy, and wheat appear less likely to provoke fatal reactions. Patients sensitive to these foods should be warned that mild symptoms may, in fact, represent a harbinger of more serious symptoms. Health care professionals must realize that fatal reactions do not necessarily happen immediately but may progress over 1–2 hours depending upon the amount of allergen ingested.

The prevalence of the diagnosis of food-dependent exercise-induced anaphylaxis or urticaria appears to be increasing in teenagers and young adults, possibly due to the growing popularity of exercising in the past decade. Two forms of food-dependent exercise-induced anaphylaxis have been described: reactions following the ingestion of specific foods and (rarely) reactions following the ingestion of any food (24–26). Anaphylaxis typically occurs when a patient exercises within 2–4 hours of ingesting the food, but otherwise he or she can ingest the food without any apparent reaction and can exercise without any apparent reaction as long as the specific food (or any food in the case of nonspecific reactors) has not been ingested within the past several hours. Patients with specific food-dependent exercise-induced anaphylaxis usually have positive prick skin tests to the food that provokes symptoms and occasionally have a history of reacting to the food when they were younger. Specific management of this disorder involves identifying the food that causes the reaction (i.e., DBPCFC with exercise) and completely avoiding the food prior to any anticipated exercise.

Food-induced anaphylaxis occasionally may be

misdiagnosed as idiopathic anaphylaxis (27, 28). In an evaluation of 102 patients with presumed idiopathic anaphylaxis, prick skin tests to a battery of food antigens were used to identify seven patients with food-induced anaphylaxis.

IgE-mediated hypersensitivity has been demonstrated to be a pathogenic factor in some patients with atopic dermatitis (13, 14, 29). In this series of patients referred for evaluation of severe atopic dermatitis, approximately 60% of the children were found to have IgE-mediated food-hypersensitivity reactions. Many foods that exacerbate skin symptoms in patients who have significant eczematous lesions do not provoke obvious immediate symptoms when the patient consumes the food on a regular basis. In the initial controlled oral food challenge following 10–14 days of allergen elimination from the diet, however, the vast majority of patients will develop a pruritic, morbilliform rash within 60–90 minutes of ingesting the test allergen. Typical urticaria is uncommon. Interestingly, once a child has avoided a food allergen for 6–12 months and skin symptoms have largely resolved, blinded challenges will often produce an urticarial skin response instead of the morbilliform rash.

Respiratory reactions may occur secondary to

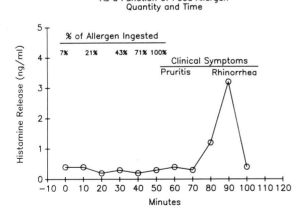

Figure 9.1

Histamine concentration in nasal lavage fluids obtained every 10 minutes in an adolescent experiencing a positive blinded food challenge. The subject ingested 8 g of the test food prior to the onset of nasal symptoms.

food hypersensitivity. Figure 9.1 depicts nasal lavage histamine concentrations from a 15-year-old patient experiencing a positive food challenge. Within minutes to 2 hours of ingestion, food allergens may induce typical signs and symptoms of rhinoconjunctivitis, although upper airway symptoms rarely appear alone (30). Signs and symptoms demonstrated in blinded food challenges include periocular erythema, pruritus and edema, and tearing, as well as nasal pruritus, congestion, rhinorrhea, and sneezing. Nasal lavage fluid histamine was found to increase up to 10-fold (31) and ECP rose significantly (unpublished) during positive DBPCFCs with the onset of nasal symptoms in some children. These studies confirmed reports that ingested allergens circulate rapidly to the nasal mucosa and activate mast cells, thereby provoking typical allergic rhinitis symptoms.

Some degree of laryngeal edema occurs in the majority of food allergic reactions, but fortunately it is generally mild. Symptoms may consist of a sensation of tightness or a "lump" in the throat, itchiness in the throat, a dry "staccato" cough, dysphonia, or a sensation of pruritus in the ear canals (presumably referred pruritus). In a review of 323 children and adolescents with atopic dermatitis undergoing DBPCFC for the evaluation of food allergy, significant changes in pulmonary function studies were documented in a subgroup of patients (32). Fifty-five percent of the patients had a history of asthma, and 45% presented with both asthma and allergic rhinitis. Food hypersensitivity was confirmed by DBPCFC in 205 (64%) patients, and 121 (59%) of these experienced immediate respiratory symptoms ranging from nasal and laryngeal symptoms to wheezing in 34 (17%). In addition, 88 patients were monitored with spirometry during DBPCFCs; 13 (15%) of these patients developed pulmonary symptoms including wheezing during DBPCFC, although only 6 patients (7.5%) had a decrease of more than 20% in their FEV_1. Figure 9.2 depicts the spirometric values of a 9-year-old male experiencing a positive blinded challenge to both egg and barley; only the latter leads to significant bronchospasm in this subject.

More recently, the pathogenic role of food allergy in provocation of airway hyperresponsiveness was demonstrated (33). Spirometry and standardized methacholine inhalation challenges (MICs) were per-

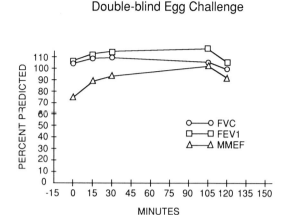

PULMONARY FUNCTION STUDIES
Double-blind Egg Challenge

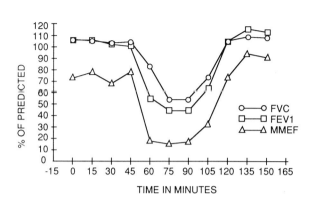

Pulmonary Function Tests During A
Positive DBPCFC To Barley

Figure 9.2

(a) Spirometric values from a 9-year-old male experiencing a positive blinded food challenge to egg, with no evidence of pulmonary involvement. (b) Spirometric values from the same child experiencing a positive reaction to barley with marked bronchospasm. After the patient was treated with nebulized metaproterenol, pulmonary functions returned to baseline.

FVC = forced vital capacity
FEV_1 = forced expiratory flow at 1 second
MMEF = maximal mid-expiratory flow

formed before and after DBPCFCs in 26 asthmatic children and adolescents with documented food hypersensitivity. Twelve patients experienced chest symptoms (nine had coughing, two had wheezing, and one experienced both cough and wheezing). Significant increases in airway reactivity, defined as a twofold or greater decrease in the $PD_{20}FEV_1$, were documented in seven patients who experienced chest symptoms during positive DBPCFC. Overall, the study demonstrated that food-induced allergic reactions could induce both immediate brochospasm and an increase in airway reactivity.

Oehling (34) reported that 8.5% of 284 asthmatic children followed in a pulmonary clinic had food-induced bronchospasm. In a similar study, Novembre *et al.* (35) screened 140 children followed in a pediatric asthma clinic by history, prick skin tests, RASTs, and blinded food challenges. Overall, 5.7% of the patients demonstrated wheezing secondary to a food challenge. Interestingly, most children with food-induced wheezing had atopic dermatitis or a history of atopic dermatitis. More recently, Bock reported

that 67 (24%) of 279 children referred to an asthma center with histories of food-induced wheezing had positive DBPCFCs with wheezing as one of their symptoms (36). No late-phase reactions were documented and isolated wheezing (i.e., pulmonary symptoms only) was present in only five patients. Evaluation of food-induced respiratory disease may need to be undertaken in the absence of a suggestive history in patients with chronic asthma and includes appropriate skin testing or RAST analyses to food antigens, and DBPCFCs following strict elimination of suspected food allergens. Because many factors can exacerbate wheezing, elimination diets alone generally have little use.

The oral allergy syndrome (OAS) is a form of IgE-mediated contact urticaria confined to the lips and oropharynx, and by definition does not involve other target organs. OAS is most often seen in patients with allergic pollenosis (37) and must be distinguished from oral symptoms that represent the harbinger of a more generalized anaphylactic reaction. Symptoms may include the rapid onset of pruritus and mild angioedema of the lips, tongue, palate, and throat, generally followed by a rapid resolution of symptoms. OAS may also result from cross-reactivity between specific epitopes in pollens and various fresh fruits and vegetables. Clinical cross-reactivity has been described among fruits in the *Prunoideae* subfamily (peach, cherry, apricot, and plum) (38).

DBPCFCs have frequently produced immediate hypersensitivity reactions of the gastrointestinal tract (gastrointestinal anaphylaxis) in sensitized individuals leading to nausea, vomiting, abdominal pain, and diarrhea (39). In addition, 10% to 15% of cases of infantile colic have been attributed to an IgE-mediated hypersensitivity (40–43). Infants with cow's milk or soy protein-induced enterocolitis syndrome often present in the first 3 months of life with severe vomiting and diarrhea, followed by hypotension and shock in approximately 15% of infants (44, 45). The immunologic mechanism of this disorder is unknown, but recent research suggests that antigen-induced secretion of tumor necrosis factor-α (TNF-α) from local mononuclear cells (i.e., lymphocytes and monocytes) may account for the secretory diarrhea and hypotension (46). Allergic eosinophilic gastroenteritis is characterized by pronounced infiltration of the stomach and/or small intestinal mucosa, muscular layer, and/or serosa with eosinophils; clinical symptoms are generally correlated with the degree of eosinophil infiltration of the bowel wall. In children—especially those experiencing gastroesophageal reflux—food hypersensitivity may be a more common cause of allergic eosinophilic gastroenteritis than previously appreciated. Recently, a group of 10 children with post-prandial abdominal pain (colic), early satiety (or food refusal), vomiting (frequently with thick, "stringy" mucus), occasionally diarrhea, and failure to thrive were reported (47). These children proved refractory to all standard medical therapy, and 6 of the 10 children had undergone Nissen fundoplication but continued to have symptoms (retching instead of vomiting) and failure to thrive. Following 6–8 weeks of an amino acid-based elemental diet (Neocate plus rice), symptoms completely resolved in 8 of 10 children; subsequent biopsies revealed marked reduction or clearing of the eosinophilic infiltrate in the esophagus. Symptoms promptly recurred (often within minutes to hours) following

challenges with specific foods. Both IgE-mediated and non-IgE-mediated hypersensitivity reactions appeared to be responsible for the reactions.

Exacerbation of migraine headaches has been reported in a small number of highly selected children undergoing a double-blind crossover trial (48), although this finding has not been confirmed by other investigators (49). A large variety of other symptoms have been attributed to food allergy, but controlled studies have not supported a role for IgE-mediated allergies in these disorders (50). Two recent studies have rekindled interest in allergy as one potential mechanism for the sudden infant death syndrome (SIDS). In one study, 20 out of 50 (40%) infants dying of SIDS had an elevated serum tryptase level (51). β-lactoglobulin-specific IgE antibodies were present in 15 of 38 infants with SIDS compared with only 1 of 9 normal controls, suggesting that infants with detectable β-lactoglobulin IgE were at higher risk for SIDS. In a second study, SIDS was also associated with higher serum concentrations of tryptase compared with control cases (52), again suggesting the possibility of anaphylaxis occurring around the time of death in some cases of SIDS.

Diagnosis

As in most diagnostic exercises, history, physical examination, and laboratory studies provide the basic tools for evaluating IgE-mediated food hypersensitivity disorders. A medical history and a detailed account of the suspected reactions should be obtained from each patient. The severity of the reaction may be gauged by the duration of symptoms and the treatment required for control. All reactions must be carefully evaluated both to identify suspect foods and to eliminate other causes of reactions resembling those of true food allergy. This investigation includes the consideration of a number of conditions including: enzyme deficiencies; various gastrointestinal diseases; anatomical defects; reactions to additives, toxins, and contaminants; collagen vascular diseases; endocrine disorders; and psychological factors (Table 9.3).

In infants and young children, a variety of gastrointestinal disorders may have symptoms suggestive

Table 9.3
Differential Diagnosis of Food Hypersensitivity

Enzyme deficiencies
Transient fructose/sorbital malabsorption
Lactase deficiency
Sucrase deficiency
Phenylketonuria

Gastrointestinal disease
Post-infectious malabsorption
  Viral, bacterial, parasitic
Hiatal hernia
Peptic ulcer
Gall bladder disease
Post-surgical dumping syndrome
Neoplasia
Inflammatory bowel disease
Pancreatic insufficiency

Additives and contaminants
Dyes
  Tartrazine
Exogenous chemicals
  Nitrates and nitrites
  Monosodium glutamate
  Sulfiting agents
  Antibiotics

Endogenous chemicals
Caffeine
Histamine
Tyramine
Phenylethylamine
Alcohol
Theobromine
Tryptamine

Toxins
Bacterial toxins
  Aflatoxin
  Botulism
  Ergot
  Fungi
  Staphylococcal toxin
  Toxigenic *E. coli*
  Vibrio cholerae
Endogenous toxins
  Certain mushrooms-α-amanitine
  "Shellfish"—saxitoxin

Psychological reactions
Bulimia
Anorexia nervosa

of food hypersensitivity reactions: abdominal pain, vomiting, diarrhea, and occasionally cough, wheezing, and pulmonary infiltrates. As many structural abnormalities and enzymatic deficiencies present in

this age group and an infant has 6 to 8 feedings per day, it is not difficult to understand how "milk allergy" may be misdiagnosed. Overfeeding and chalazia, which occur in as many as 50% of newborns, may result in vomiting after feeding. Chronic cough and wheezing may occur secondary to recurrent aspiration or structural abnormalities such as hiatal hernia with gastroesophageal reflux, pyloric stenosis, and (rarely) an H-type tracheoesophageal fistula. Hirschsprung's disease, or congenital aganglionic megacolon with partial intestinal obstruction, often presents with diarrhea, vomiting, tachypnea secondary to abdominal distention, and irritability.

Various enzyme deficiencies may mimic or complicate coeliac disease or other food-induced enteropathies. For example, disaccharidase deficiencies are frequently associated with bloating, abdominal cramps, and diarrhea secondary to foods containing specific sugars. Although congenital lactase, sucrase, and isomaltase deficiencies are rare, secondary disaccharidase deficiencies are frequently seen following bacterial or viral gastroenteritis. Other enzyme deficiencies such as galactose-4-epimerase (galactosemia) may present in infancy with vomiting and diarrhea after milk ingestion. In addition, pancreatic enzyme deficiency (e.g., cystic fibrosis) may initially be confused with one of the food-induced malabsorption syndromes.

A variety of toxins may produce symptoms that appear indistinguishable from immediate hypersensitivity reactions. In scombroid poisoning, ingestion of unusually high levels of histamine lead within minutes to a variety of symptoms that usually last for a few hours, but that may occasionally last for several days (53). Scombroid fish most commonly implicated in histamine poisoning include tuna, skipjack, and mackerel; non-scombroid fish most frequently involved include mahi-mahi, sardines, anchovies, and herring. Swiss cheese has also been involved in histamine poisoning (54). Ciguatera poisoning represents a substantial problem in the Caribbean and Pacific areas; it may lead to tingling of the lips, tongue, and throat, followed by nausea, vomiting, dryness of the mouth, abdominal cramps, diarrhea, headache, and sometime chills, fever, and myalgia (55). The toxin involved is a lipid-soluble, heat-stable chemical produced by algae that is, in turn, consumed by reef fish (grouper, snapper, sea bass, and more than 300 other species).

Suspected food allergens are identified primarily by their ingestion in some proximity to the time of a reaction. Such foods are more likely to be identified if they are consumed infrequently. Factors such as whether the food was raw, cooked, or otherwise processed influence the reaction, especially in the case of some fruits and vegetables.

Occasionally a suspected food allergen may fail to provoke an allergic reaction consistently. Reasons for this inconsistency are unclear but may include the consumption of a quantity below the threshold amount likely to induce a reaction, the need to associate exercise with specific food ingestion, the presence of other simultaneously ingested foods that interfere with absorption (e.g., fats), the physical state of the food (e.g., raw fruits), and the ability of concomitant medications such as antihistamines to mask mild reactions.

Foods may also be contaminated by other foods. Cross-contamination of one food by another may take place prior to processing, during processing, and during food preparation. The last problem is often seen in restaurants where different foods may be prepared using the same utensils. In several cases, non-dairy desserts (tofu ice cream and rice ice cream) have been found to be contaminated with cow's milk protein secondary to processing in dairy plants where machinery was inadequately cleaned (56).

Certain foods themselves may cause problems resembling adverse food reactions. Prunes, soybeans, and onions can produce gastroenteric symptoms via irritation or pharmacologic activity. Amines such as tyramine and phenylethylamine, nitrates and nitrites, and alcohol may cause headaches in susceptible individuals. Methylxanthines (caffeine, theobromine, and theophylline) are variably found in coffee, tea, cola, and chocolate. In large amounts, these substances cause nervousness, tremor, and tachycardia. Vasoactive amines (epinephrine, norepinephrine, tyramine, dopamine, histamine, and 5-hydroxy tryptamine) are found in bananas, tomatoes, avocados, cheeses, pineapples, and wines. Chocolate also contains phenylethylamine. Symptoms from these foods, however, are rarely confused with "classical" allergic reactions.

Following the history, physical examination, and laboratory tests used to eliminate other diseases in the differential diagnosis, the evaluation may continue with the use of diet diaries and elimination diets, if the clinical history remains uncertain. A 10- to 14-day diet diary may clarify the relationship between symptoms and specific food ingestion. During this time, the patient records the type and amount of foods ingested and the occurrence and character of adverse reactions. This record may prove useful in searching for suspect foods and in establishing baseline symptoms against which to measure the success or failure of elimination diets. If symptoms fail to occur within this period, the elicitation of symptoms may be too infrequent to appreciate a change in their occurrence during the period of an elimination diet. Although they are sometimes helpful, more often diet diaries match the initial history in confusion by failing to establish a recognizable relationship between certain foods and symptoms. On the other hand, they may help confirm the suspicion that no relationship exists between a clinical condition such as hives and foods.

If only one or several foods emerge as prime suspects, the initial elimination diet can consist simply of removing these foods. Care must be taken that suspected foods are not inadvertently consumed while hidden in other foods. For example, a common food such as milk is found in a large variety of processed foods such as baked goods, processed meats, non-dairy creamers, and canned tuna fish.

The success of an elimination diet depends upon the identification of the correct allergen(s), the implementation of a comprehensive allergen-exclusion diet, the ability of the patient to maintain a diet completely free of all forms of the offending allergen, and the assumption that other factors do not provoke similar symptoms during the period of study. If the offending food is removed from the diet of the affected individual, the food-induced illness should resolve. In practice, the likelihood of establishing a diagnosis using elimination diets is greater when only one or two foods are responsible for the symptoms. Elimination diets alone should not be considered diagnostic of food allergy, especially in chronic disorders (e.g., asthma, atopic dermatitis). Consequently, without a highly knowledgeable physician (and usually a dietitian), the elimination diet can be highly misleading, resulting in both false-positive and false-negative diagnoses. Throughout the diet testing procedure, it should be remembered that changing the type and amount of foods may also alter symptoms of such diseases as disaccharidase deficiency, gluten-sensitive enteropathy, and cystic fibrosis.

Elimination diets are not usually necessary in the diagnosis of food-induced anaphylaxis where the identity of the offending food is often obvious. In cases of anaphylaxis where the offending food is not well delineated, however, the patients should be advised not to eat foods suspected of causing the anaphylactic reaction. In addition, elimination diets should be followed by reintroduction of suspect foods to the diet only in situations where symptoms are not life-threatening, such as in chronic hives or rhinitis.

If removal of one or several foods from the diet does not successfully eliminate symptoms, if multiple food sensitivities are suspected, or if symptoms are unlikely to be due to foods (e.g., as in chronic urticaria), initiation of a severely limited diet may be warranted. Severe elimination diets, especially in children, should be used for only short periods of time—i.e., no longer than 1 to 2 weeks. Extensive elimination diets include the following: infants under 3 months of age—milk substitute alone (casein hydrolysates such as Alimentum or Nutramigen, or amino acid-derived formulas such as Neocate or Vivonex); 3 to 6 months—milk substitute and rice cereal, applesauce, pears, carrots, squash, and lamb (57); older children and adolescents—Neocate 1 Plus, rice or corn, and applesauce. Casein hydrolysate formulas or commercial elemental diets such as Neocate 1 Plus or Vivonex should be used under a physician's guidance to replace defined foods. Caution must be taken to instruct the patient to take nothing by mouth but the foods on the diet and water. Both oral and topical medications, including aspirin, vitamins, laxatives, and creams, must be avoided when possible.

Continuation of symptoms while on restricted diets indicates that symptoms are not due to foods or other substances. The unlikely possibility that individual foods on the restricted diets themselves cause symptoms may be ruled out by substituting other foods known not to correlate with symptoms. If symptoms resolve on the restricted diet, resumption of a normal diet should be accompanied by a return of symptoms, and subsequent resumption of the restricted diet should once again alleviate these symptoms. Such cycling should reproducibly eliminate or provoke symptoms to allow the conclusion that symptoms are secondary to foods. In most cases, some form of blinded challenge should be conducted to confirm the causative role of the suspect food.

Once a relationship to diet has been established, foods representing "safe" food groups eaten by the patient during the control period should be individually returned to the diet in normal amounts at intervals of 3 to 4 days. Foods reinstituted into the diet without the induction of symptoms may remain in the diet. Foods provoking symptoms should be removed until the procedure is completed and an oral food challenge can be conducted. Although this procedure is lengthy, it is direct and applicable to either inpatient or outpatient evaluations with a minimum of confusion.

Although skin tests and RASTs are often dismissed as unhelpful, they can rule out other causes of adverse food reactions and may provide clues as to specific foods leading to IgE-mediated reactions. Prick skin testing with food extracts, and in some cases fresh foods (e.g., fruits, vegetables), has been shown to be valuable in excluding IgE-mediated food hypersensitivity, but only suggestive in predicting the presence of symptomatic food allergy (58–61). Positive skin tests emerge in the absence of symptomatic food allergy about 60% to 65% of the time (false positives). Allergic reactions to foods appear in less than 5% of cases with negative skin tests (false negatives) if such tests are properly performed. Consequently, skin testing is best utilized to support a clinical impression that one or more foods in a given individual are capable of causing Type I hypersensitivity. Pediatric studies (58, 60) have shown that food extracts in a concentration of 1 : 20 weight to volume (w/v) applied by the puncture technique give wheals that are 3 mm or greater than the negative control wheals within 10 to 30 minutes in virtually all subjects having allergic reactions to foods verified by oral food challenge. It may be advisable to examine the reaction sites 12 to 24 hours later because of the possibility of a late-phase component of Type I hypersensitivity reaction, although this condition has rarely been observed in controlled studies.

RAST is slightly less sensitive than the skin test (60) but may aid in the evaluation of certain cases of eczema or dermatographism where the skin condition would interfere with skin testing or support a diagnosis of food anaphylaxis where the risk of skin testing is considered too great. Peripheral blood basophils from individuals with suspected food allergies can be examined in vitro to determine if they degranulate in the presence of dilute suspensions of food antigens; such degranulation requires the presence of IgE on the basophil specific to the suspected food. Basophil histamine release assays do not establish a diagnosis of food allergy, and appear to offer no advantage over skin testing (62, 63). They may, however, prove useful in evaluating patients with extensive eczema or dermatographism, or in instances where skin testing may represent a risk to the patient. A high, spontaneous in vitro release of histamine from basophils taken from subjects allergic to foods has been reported (58, 64).

Double-blind placebo-controlled food challenges remain the "gold standard" for diagnosing adverse reactions to foods. DBPCFC is unnecessary if the medical history indicates a potentially life-threatening reaction following the isolated ingestion of a food, which is supported by the presence of tests for food-specific IgE. The use of oral challenge to reproduce symptoms should especially be avoided in cases involving a recent history of life-threatening anaphylaxis to a definite food allergen. No food challenge is entirely without risk of side effects, and the patient must be apprised of these dangers. Such procedures should be performed only under the supervision of a physician.

A single unequivocal positive reaction such as hives or asthma to a food tested in a DBPCFC may be taken as reasonable evidence of an adverse reaction to food. In cases of subjective complaints, a number of positive tests to a suspect food and a comparable number of negative placebo tests are necessary to substantiate the diagnosis. Acceptance of a positive test does not prove that an immunological mechanism is responsible, as adverse reactions may also be due to diseases such as disaccharidase deficiency.

In spite of every precaution taken, potentially severe adverse reactions may occur following challenge. Personnel and equipment must be available to treat anaphylactic reactions (see the American Academy of Allergy and Immunology Position Statement, J Allergy Clin Immunol 1986;77:271).

Therapy

Once food hypersensitivity is diagnosed, the only proven therapy is avoidance of the specific food allergen. No scientific evidence supports the use of rotational diets or immunotherapy with food antigens in the treatment of food hypersensitivity. A number of studies have been published on the use of cromolyn sodium taken orally to treat adverse food reactions (65). These studies often involved patients without documented food hypersensitivity or used inadequate study designs to evaluate the target drug. Not surprisingly, these studies have generated contradictory results. In one double-blind crossover trial of patients with food hypersensitivity documented by DBPCFCs, for example, cromolyn sodium was found to be no more beneficial than the placebo control in blocking hypersensitivity reactions (66).

Fortunately, food hypersensitivity is not always a life-long affliction, especially in young patients (67–69). In follow-up studies of children with primarily atopic respiratory disease (67), 44% of patients followed for 1 to 7 years lost their food hypersensitivity by historical report. Similarly, 37 patients with gastrointestinal symptoms secondary to milk hypersensitivity were studied by repeat challenges 1 and 4 years after the initial diagnosis (68), and a loss of mild hypersensitivity was reported in 12 of the 37 (32%) children. In a study of children with atopic dermatitis and food hypersensitivity (69), 19 of 75 children (25%) lost all evidence of clinical reactivity when rechallenged after 1 year on an appropriate elimination diet. After 2 years on elimination diets, 23 of the children (31%) had lost their symptomatic reactivity to all antigens previously eliciting positive clinical responses. Loss of clinical hypersensitivity was observed more frequently with soy and foods other than peanut, wheat, egg, and milk. Prick skin test and RAST results remained positive and virtually unchanged in children who became clinically tolerant.

Even the most careful patient may inadvertently ingest clinically significant amounts of the food to which he or she is sensitive. In a follow-up study of children with severe peanut allergy (70), one-half (16 of 32 subjects) had accidentally ingested peanut within the year prior to follow-up and only one-fourth of patients had been able to completely avoid peanuts for several years, despite their best efforts.

When the symptoms of this exposure involve sites distant from the gastrointestinal tract, the treatment for each specific symptom does not differ from that employed when other causative factors are involved. For example, the treatment for food-induced urticaria is the same as the treatment for idiopathic urticaria. Patients experiencing laryngeal or pulmonary symptoms should receive immediate epinephrine and/or bronchodilator therapy. Laryngeal symptoms are often relieved by spraying epinephrine (Primatene Mist®) or injecting epinephrine subcutaneously. Pulmonary symptoms are often relieved by administering nebulized beta-adrenergic agents, although injection of epinephrine is the treatment of choice in anaphylaxis. If any question of hypotension arises, subcutaneous epinephrine must be administered and intravenous fluids provided if necessary. Gastrointestinal symptoms after inadvertent food ingestion are frequently treated with antihistamines. Both protein-induced enterocolitis and IgE-mediated food hypersensitivity may result in protracted vomiting, dehydration, and hypotension in children, however, and a need for intravenous fluids must be anticipated.

The treatment for food-induced anaphylaxis differs only slightly from the treatment for idiopathic anaphylaxis. If the patient does not respond to epinephrine administration and other initial resuscitative measures, gastric lavage may be indicated to decrease further antigen absorption. The patient with potential anaphylactic reactivity (i.e., patients with a history of a previous anaphylactic reaction or patients with asthma and food allergy) should be taught how to self-administer epinephrine and should have an epinephrine-containing syringe and antihistamine available at all times. An identification Medi-Alert bracelet stating the patient's sensitivity is also advised. In addition, daycare centers, schools, and other caretakers should have a list of emergency numbers (with back-ups) to be called if a food-allergic child should accidentally receive a food allergen.

It must be appreciated that a patient may experience some mild symptoms in the first few minutes (e.g., tongue or throat tingling, mild abdominal discomfort) followed by a 10- to 60-minute period with no significant change before experiencing further symptoms, particularly in the case of peanut and nut hypersensitivities. If a patient realizes that an allergen has been ingested, he or she should immediately take a loading dose of liquid diphenhydramine. Asthmatic patients may also be advised to administer an aerosolized beta-agonist by medi-dose inhaler or nebulizer. Children with food allergy do not generally develop more severe reactions with each subsequent ingestion, although peanut and nut hypersensitivity may prove an exception to this rule. Patients with a history of life-threatening anaphylaxis or hypersensitivity to peanuts, nuts, fish, or shellfish who do not have injectable epinephrine (e.g., Epi-Pen or ANA Kit) should seek medical attention immediately. If patients have epinephrine (two doses), do not have a history of previous life-threatening anaphylaxis, and are within 15 to 20 minutes of medical help, they may wait to see if further symptoms develop. If any laryngeal or pulmonary symptoms occur, the patient should administer one dose of subcutaneous epinephrine and seek medical attention immediately. As in bee sting hypersensitivity, the early administration of epinephrine appears to greatly reduce the likelihood of a fatal outcome.

All patients with IgE-mediated food allergy should be warned about the possibility of developing a severe anaphylactic reaction and should be educated in the appropriate treatment measures to be taken in case of an accidental ingestion.

Conclusion

The true prevalence of immediate food hypersensitivity reactions in the pediatric population is approximately 5% in children less than 4 years of age and 1% to 2% in older children. Food allergy is clearly a leading cause of life-threatening anaphylaxis outside the hospital, and many people die each year from food-allergic reactions, although the actual morbidity and mortality rates are unknown. Complacency on the part of the medical community, largely inspired by the plethora of inaccurate information on the subject, has contributed to this dearth of data. In the United States, societal eating patterns have changed in the last 10 to 20 years, with highly allergenic foods (e.g., peanuts, nuts, fish) being readily available and introduced to children at a young age. No good means of treating (i.e., curing) food hypersensitivity is available. Research in the area of food allergic reactions has been intensified, but the number of unanswered questions remains formidable.

REFERENCES

1. Sampson HA, Mendelson L, Rosen JP. Fatal and near-fatal food-induced anaphylaxis in children. N Engl J Med 1992; 327:380–384.
2. Abernathy-Carver KJ, Sampson HA, Picker LJ, Leung DYM. Milk-induced eczema is associated with the expansion of T cells expressing cutaneous lymphocyte antigen. J Clin Invest 1995;95:913–918.
3. Cornell HJ. Amino acid composition of peptides remaining after in vitro digestion of a gliadin sub-fraction with duodenal mucosa from patients with coeliac disease. Clin Chimica Acta 1988;176:279–290.
4. Sloan AE. A perspective on popular perceptions of adverse reactions to foods. J Allergy Clin Immunol 1986;78:127–132.
5. Kayosaari M. Food allergy in Finnish children aged 1 to 6 years. Acta Paediatric Scand 1982;71:815–819.
6. Bock SA. Prospective appraisal of complaints of adverse reactions to foods in children during the first 3 years of life. Pediatr 1987;79:683–688.
7. Host A, Halken S. A prospective study of cow milk allergy in Danish infants during the first 3 years of life. Allergy 1990;45:587–596.
8. Schrander JJP, van den Bogart JPH, Forget PP, Schrander-Stumpel CTRM, Kuijten RH, Kester ADM. Cow's milk protein intolerance in infants under 1 year of age: a prospective epidemiological study. Eur J Pediatr 1993;152:640–644.
9. Host A. Cow's milk protein allergy and intolerance in infancy. Pediatr Allergy Immunol 1994;5:5–36.
10. Fuglsang G, Madsen C, Saval P, Osterballe O. Prevalence of intolerance to food additives among Danish school children. Pediatr Allergy Immunol 1993;4:123–129.
11. May CD. Objective clinical and laboratory studies of immediate hypersensitivity reactions to foods in asthmatic children. J Allergy Clin Immunol 1976;58:500–515.
12. Bock SA, Lee Y, Remigio LK, May CD. Studies of hypersensitivity reactions to foods in infants and children. J Allergy Clin Immunol 1978;62:327–334.
13. Sampson HA. Role of immediate hypersensitivity in the pathogenesis of atopic dermatitis. J Allergy Clin Immunol 1983;71:473–480.
14. Sampson HA, McCaskill CM. Food hypersensitivity and atopic dermatitis: evaluation of 113 patients. J Pediatr 1985;107:669–675.
15. Sampson HA. Food allergy. J Allergy Clin Immunol 1989;84:1061–1067.
16. Burks AW, Mallory SB, Williams LW, Shirrell MA. Atopic dermatitis: clinical relevance of food hypersensitivity reactions. J Pediatr 1988;113:447–451.
17. Alison RG, ed. An evaluation of the potential for dietary proteins to contribute to systemic diseases. Bethesda, MD: Life Sciences Research Office, Federation of American Societies for Experimental Biology, 1982, 2.
18. Wilson SJ, Walzer M. Absorption of undigested proteins in human beings. IV. Absorption of unaltered egg protein in infants. Am J Dis Child 1935;50:49–54.
19. Brunner M, Walzer M. Absorption of undigested proteins in human beings: the absorption of unaltered fish protein in adults. Arch Intern Med 1928;42:173–179.
20. Walzer M. Absorption of allergens. J Allergy 1942;13:554–562.
21. Vercelli D, Geha R. Regulation of IgE synthesis in humans: a tale of two signals. J Allergy Clin Immunol 1991;88:285–295.
22. Yocum MW, Khan DA. Assessment of patients who have experienced anaphylaxis: a 3-year survey. Mayo Clin Proc 1994;69:16–23.
23. Sampson HA, Mendelson LM, Rosen JP. Fatal and near-fatal anaphylactic reactions to food in children and adolescents. N Engl J Med 1992;327:380–384.
24. Romano A, Di Fonso M, Giuffreda F, Quaratino D, Papa G, Palmieri V, Venuti A. Diagnostic work-up for food-dependent, exercise-induced anaphylaxis. Allergy 1995;50:817–824.
25. Dohi M, Suko M, Sugiyama H, Yamashita N, Tadokoro K, Juji F, Okudaira H, Sano Y, Ito K, Miyamoto T. Food-dependent exercise-induced anaphylaxis: a study on 11 Japanese cases. J Allergy Clin Immunol 1991;87:34–40.
26. Kushimoto K, Toshiyuki A. Masked type I wheat allergy. Relation to exercise-induced anaphylaxis. Arch Dermatol 1985;121:355–360.
27. Stricker WE, Anorve-Lopez E, Reed CE. Food skin testing in patients with idiopathic anaphylaxis. J Allergy Clin Immunol 1986;77:516–519.
28. Bock SA. Anaphylaxis to coriander: a sleuthing story. J Allergy Clin Immunol 1993;91:1232–1233.
29. Jones SM, Sampson HA. The role of allergens in atopic dermatitis. Clinical Reviews in Allergy 1993;11:471–490.
30. Bock SA, Atkins FM. The natural history of peanut allergy. J Allergy Clin Immunol 1989;83:900–904.
31. Silber G, Sampson H. Nasal mediator release following double-blind placebo-controlled oral food challenges. J Allergy Clin Immunol 1988;81:241 (abstr).
32. James JM, Bernhisel-Broadbent J, Sampson HA. Respiratory reactions provoked by double-blind food challenges in children. Am J Respir Crit Care Med 1994;149:59–64.
33. James JM, Eigenmann PA, Eggleston PA, Sampson HA. Airway reactivity changes in food-allergic, asthmatic children undergoing double-blind placebo-controlled food challenges. Am J Respir Crit Care Med 1996 (in press).
34. Oehling A, Cagnani CEB. Food allergy and child asthma. Allergol Immunopathol 1980;8:7–14.
35. Novembre E, de Martino M, Vierucci A. Foods and respiratory allergy. J Allergy Clin Immunol 1988;81:1059–1065.
36. Bock SA. Respiratory reactions induced by food challenges in children with pulmonary disease. Pediatr Allergy Immunol 1992;3:188–194.
37. Ortolani C, Ispano M, Pastorello EA, Ansaloni R, Magri GC. Comparison of results of skin prick tests (with fresh foods

and commercial food extracts) and RAST in 100 patients with oral allergy syndrome. J Allergy Clin Immunol 1989;83:683–690.

38. Pastorello E, Ortolani C, Farioli L, Pravettoni V, Ispano M, Borga A, Bengtsson A, Incorvaia C, Berti C, Zanussi C. Allergenic cross-reactivity among peach, apricot, plum, and cherry in patients with oral allergy syndrome: an in vivo and in vitro study. J Allergy Clin Immunol 1994;94:699–707.

39. Sampson HA. Clinical manifestations of adverse food reactions. Pediatr Allerg Immunol 1995;6:29–37.

40. Sampson HA. Infantile colic and food allergy; fact or fiction? J Pediatr 1989;115:583–584.

41. Jakobsson I, Lindberg T. Cow's milk proteins cause infantile colic in breast-fed infants: a double-blind crossover study. Pediatr 1983;71:268–271.

42. Lothe L, Lindberg T. Cow's milk whey protein elicits symptoms of infantile colic in colicky formula-fed infants: a double-blind crossover study. Pediatr 1989;83:262–266.

43. Forsyth BWC. Colic and the effect of changing formulas: a double-blind, multiple-crossover study. J Pediatr 1989;115:521–526.

44. Goldman AS, Anderson DW, Sellars WA, *et al.* Milk allergy. I. Oral challenge with milk and isolated milk proteins in allergic children. Clin Allergy 1963;32:425–443.

45. Powell GK. Milk- and soy-induced enterocolitis of infancy. J Pediatr 1978;93:550–560.

46. Heyman M, Darmon N, Dupont C, Dugas B, Hirribaren A, Blaton M, Desjeux J. Mononuclear cells from infants allergic to cow's milk secrete tumor necrosis factor alpha, altering intestinal function. Gastroenterol 1994;106:1514–1523.

47. Kelly KJ, Lazenby AJ, Rowe PC, Yardley JH, Perman JA, Sampson HA. Eosinophilic esophagitis attributed to gastroesophageal reflux: improvement with an amino-acid based formula. Gastroenterology 1995;109:1503–1512.

48. Egger J, Wilson J, Carter CM, Turner MW, Soothill JF. Is migraine food allergy? a double-blind controlled trial of oligoantigenic diet treatment. Lancet 1983;2:865–869.

49. Salfield SAW, Wardley BL, Houlsby WT, Turner SL, Spalton AP, Beckles-Wilson NR, Herber SM. Controlled study of exclusion of dietary vasoactive amines in migraine. Arch Dis Child 1987;62:458–460.

50. Sampson HA. Differential diagnosis in adverse reactions to foods. J Allergy Clin Immunol 1986;78:212–219.

51. Platt M, Yunginger J, Sekula-Perlman A, Irani A, Smialek J, Mirchandani H, Schwartz L. Involvement of mast cells in sudden infant death. J Allergy Clin Immunol 1994;94:250–256.

52. Holgate ST, Walters C, Walls A, Lawrence S, Shell D, Variend S, Fleming P, Berry P, Gilbers R, Robinson C. The anaphylaxis hypothesis of sudden infant death syndrome (SIDS): mast cell degranulation in cot death revealed by elevated concentrations of tryptase in serum. Clin Exper Allergy 1994;24:1115–1122.

53. Taylor SL, Hui JV, Lyons DE. Toxicology of scombroid poisoning. In: Ragelis EP, ed. Seafood toxins. Washington, DC: American Chemical Society, 1984, 417–430.

54. Taylor SL, Keefe TJ, Windham ES, Howell JF. Outbreak of histamine poisoning associated with consumption of Swiss cheese. J Food Protect 1982;45:455–457.

55. National Research Council Committee on Food Protection. Toxicants occurring naturally in foods. Washington, DC: National Academy of Sciences, 1973.

56. Gern JE, Yang EY, Evrard HM, Sampson HA. Allergic reactions to milk-containing "dairy-free" products. J Allergy Clin Immunol 1990;85:273.

57. Crawford LV. Allergy diets. In: Bierman CW, Pearlman DS, eds. Allergic diseases of infants, childhood, and adolescence. Philadelphia: W.B. Saunders, 1980, 394–406.

58. Bock SA, Buckley J, Holst A, *et al.* Proper use of skin tests with food extracts in diagnosis of hypersensitivity to food in children. Clin Allergy 1977;7:375–383.

59. Aas K. The diagnosis of hypersensitivity to ingested foods. Clin Allergy 1978;8:39–50.

60. Sampson HA, Albergo R. Comparison of results of skin tests, RAST, and double-blind placebo-controlled food challenges in children with atopic dermatitis. J Allergy Clin Immunol 1984;74:26–33.

61. Sampson HA. Comparative study of commercial food antigen extracts for the diagnosis of food hypersensitivity. J Allergy Clin Immunol 1988;718–726.

62. Hirsch SR, Zastrow JE. Basophil degranulation: a new method of observation and its correlation with skin testing. J Allergy Clin Immunol 1972;50:338–347.

63. May CD, Alberto R. In vitro responses of leukocytes to food proteins in allergic and normal children: lymphocyte stimulation and histamine release. Clin Allergy 1972;2:335–344.

64. Sampson HA, Broadbent KR, Bernhisel-Broadbent J. "Spontaneous" basophil histamine release and histamine releasing factor in patients with atopic dermatitis and food hypersensitivity. N Engl J Med 1989;321:228–232.

65. Sogn DD. Medications and their use in treatment of adverse reaction to foods. J Allergy Clin Immunol 1986;78:238–242.

66. Burks AW, Sampson HA. Double-blind placebo-controlled trial of oral cromolyn sodium in children with documented food hypersensitivity. J Allergy Clin Immunol 1988;81:417–423.

67. Bock SA. The natural history of food sensitivity. J Allergy Clin Immunol 1982;69:173–177.

68. Businco L, Benincori N, Cantani A, *et al.* Chronic diarrhea due to cow's milk allergy. A 4- to 10-year follow-up. Ann Allergy 1985;55:844–847.

69. Sampson HA, Scanlon S. Natural history of food hypersensitivity in children with atopic dermatitis. J Pediatr 1989;115:23–27.

70. Bock SA, Atkins FM. The natural history of peanut allergy. J Allergy Clin Immunol 1989;83:900–904.

10

FOOD ALLERGY IN ADULTS

Dean D. Metcalfe

Introduction

Adverse reactions to food and drink have appeared in writings for centuries. Not until 1921, however, did Prausnitz and Kustner demonstrate that the factor responsible for an "allergic" reaction to a food was present in serum and could be transferred to a non-sensitive individual (1). This observation serves as the basis of the P-K test, which is now understood to involve the passive transfer of IgE. In 1950, blinded and placebo-controlled food challenges on individuals suspected of having mild food allergy were reported (2). The physicians conducting these tests were among the first to correlate clinical reactions to foods to abnormal in vivo responses, which are now accepted to have an immunologic basis.

Food allergy (hypersensitivity) is an abnormal reaction resulting from heightened immunologic responses to glycoprotein components within foods (1). The term *food intolerance* is often applied to any abnormal response to an ingested food. Food intolerance may also result from a toxic or pharmacologic property of a food; alternatively, it may represent an abnormal metabolic response of the host to a food component. Hypersensitivity to food in adults may be divided into two general subgroups based on the presumptive immunologic mechanisms involved: food allergen-specific IgE responses, and non-IgE-dependent immunologic responses corresponding respectively to immediate and delayed-in-time reactions (Table 10.1). IgE-dependent reactions are further classified as to symptom complexes developed in the primary target organs. Delayed reactions do not include food protein-induced colitis and enterocolitis, as such diseases have been described in infants and children but are not generally recognized in adults.

Whether such pathologic entities exist in adults but are hidden within the spectrum of inflammatory bowel diseases remains to be demonstrated.

Prevalence

Data on the prevalence of food hypersensitivity reactions in specific adult populations are limited. The public's perception of the number of food-allergic individuals is clearly far greater than carefully controlled studies have demonstrated. As an example, a Dutch study examining the prevalence of food allergy and food intolerance in adults using questionnaires, clinical follow-ups, and double-blind, placebo-controlled food challenges (DBPCFC) estimated the prevalence of food allergy and intolerance together to be 2.4% (3). As adults suffer from food allergies less than children, a consensus has developed that less than 1% to 2% of adults have food allergies (4). The prevalence of food additive intolerance appears to be even lower, an estimated 0.01% to 0.23% (5).

IGE-Mediated Immediate Reactions

IgE-mediated immediate hypersensitivity reactions to food occur rapidly following ingestion or inhalation of a food antigen to which an individual is sensitive. A number of target organs may be affected. Reactions include urticaria, angioedema, rhinoconjunctivitis, laryngeal edema, asthma, oral allergy syndrome (6), vomiting, diarrhea, and systemic anaphylaxis (Table 10.1). In some instances, urticaria or anaphylaxis is dependent on a costimulus to exacerbate symptoms such as in food-dependent exercise-induced anaphylaxis (7–10). The presumption is that the threshold

Table 10.1
Categorization of Immunologically Mediated Reactions to Foods in Adults

Disease	Primary Target Organs	Effector Systems
Immediate Reactions		
Rhinoconjunctivitis	Eyes, upper respiratory tract	IgE: Basophils/mast cells
Oral allergy syndrome	Mouth	IgE: Mast cells
Urticaria/angioedema	Skin	IgE: Basophils/mast cells
Atopic dermatitis	Skin	IgE: Mast cells, eosinophils
Asthma	Lower respiratory tract	IgE: Mast cells, eosinophils, lymphocytes
Gastrointestinal reactions	Gastrointestinal mucosa	IgE: Mast cells
Systemic anaphylaxis	Skin, respiratory tract, gastrointestinal tract, cardiovascular system	IgE: Basophils/mast cells
Delayed Reactions		
Allergic eosinophilic gastroenteritis	Gastrointestinal mucosa, submucosa	IgE: Mast cells, eosinophils, lymphocytes
Gluten-sensitive enteropathy	Gastrointestinal mucosa	IgA, IgG: Lymphocytes
Dermatitis herpetiformis	Skin	IgA: Lymphocytes, neutrophils

for mast cell activation is lowered by the accessory stimulus, although no data have been gathered as yet to support this hypothesis.

PATHOGENESIS

Mast cells, basophils, and IgE all play major roles in immediate hypersensitivity reactions to food. A rise in plasma histamine has been associated with the development of urticaria, laryngeal edema, wheezing, vomiting, diarrhea, and hypotension after blinded food challenges (11). Interaction between IgE on mast cell surfaces with food extracts has been demonstrated by immediate wheal and erythema reactions in the dermis after local injection of these extracts (11, 12). Gastrointestinal mucosal reactions similar to those that follow mast cell degranulation in human skin have been reported in both in vivo and in vitro studies (13, 14). Food antigen-specific IgE has been demonstrated to lead to the degranulation of gastrointestinal mast cells after passive sensitization (16).

Upon high-affinity IgE receptor (FcεRI) aggregation, mast cells exert their effects on tissues by releasing preformed mediators such as histamine, tryptase, and tumor necrosis factor, as well as newly synthesized arrays of mediators such as prostaglandins, leukotrienes, and cytokines that may contribute to the IgE-mediated late-phase response (15, 16). Basophils release histamine and other mediators in response to FcεRI cross-linking; they also respond to histamine-releasing factors that increase their releasability or even induce degranulation (17, 18). The amino acid and cDNA sequences of one such molecule have recently been identified at the molecular level (17). This molecule may possibly react with unique IgEs produced by atopic individuals.

Increased intestinal mucosal permeability following mast cell activation facilitates the entry and distribution of a food antigen to other target organs, initiating degranulation of mast cells at those sites. Nevertheless, an alteration in mucosal permeability is not necessary and does not serve as the underlying defect in food allergy. This observation is consistent with clinical data that have failed to demonstrate defects in IgA synthesis, find associated gastrointestinal diseases including achlorhydria, or generate evidence of immune complex diseases in patients with immediate reactions to foods.

The most reliable clinical correlates of immediate reactions to foods are a family and personal history of atopy and the presence of positive skin tests to foods and inhalants. This evidence indicates that the basis of the production of IgE in response to foods relates to inherited patterns of IgE synthesis and regulation (19). Patients with IgE-mediated food allergy, however, do not consistently give a family history of hypersensitivity to specific foods, suggesting that the development of IgE directed to food antigens is multifactorial. It has been suggested that some individuals inherit an isotype-specific defect, which leads to an inability to down-regulate an IgE-mediated response (19). Other factors, including viral infections and environment, may also influence the regulation of an IgE-antibody response.

Allergens in Foods

Almost every major food antigen identified is a protein or glycoprotein with a molecular weight between 10,000 and 40,000 daltons. These allergens tend to resist denaturation by heat or acid and degradation by proteases. In adults, the most common food allergens causing systemic reactions are peanuts, tree nuts, crustaceae, fish, and egg (4, 20).

Peanuts are one of the most allergenic foods. They are responsible in many reports of fatal and near-fatal anaphylaxis (21, 22). Using crossed-radio-immunoelectrophoresis, 16 allergenic fractions have been identified in raw peanuts (23). Peanut I is a major peanut allergen that is isolated from raw, defatted, peanut meal. It consists of two major bands of 20,000 and 30,000 daltons identified by SDS-PAGE (24). Soybeans are also a major crop of the legume family. In one instance, an allergic reaction to soybeans was traced to a reaction to Kunitz soybean trypsin inhibitor (25). Other members of the legume family include a variety of green beans, kidney beans, garbanzo beans, garden peas, black-eyed peas, and lentils. Significant cross-reactivity among members of this family has been demonstrated in vitro and by skin test reactivity. Results of DBPCFC, however, demonstrate that clinically important cross-reactivity to legumes is rare (28). Clinical hypersensitivity to one legume does not warrant dietary elimination of all legumes (26).

Shrimp antigens have also been isolated (27–30). The major allergen designated previously as antigen II (28) or Sa II (29), now referred to as *Pen i* I, is a heat-stable protein with a molecular weight of approximately 34,000 daltons. Amino acid sequence analysis of *Pen i* I indicates it has significant homology with the muscle protein tropomyosin from *Drosophila melanogaster* (32, 33). Isolated shrimp tropomyosin also binds Sa II-specific IgE. T-cell epitopes have been described. Tropomyosin is thought to be the allergen responsible for cross-reactivity between members of the crustacea (shrimp, lobster, crab, and crawfish) (30, 31).

Fish are among the most common causes of food-allergic reactions in adults (20). Allergen M (*Gad c* I) from codfish, the first extensively studied allergen, is a parvalbumin found in the muscle of fish and amphibians. *Gad c* I is a heat-stable, partially protease-resistant, single-polypeptide-chain protein with a molecular weight of approximately 12,000 daltons (32–34). Synthetic peptides corresponding to regions 13–32, 49–64, and 88–103 have been shown to bind IgE from cod-allergic subjects (35). One study utilizing SDS-PAGE and immunoblot analyses showed immunologic cross-reactivity between *Gad c* I and other 10 common fish species (36). In this study, two of 11 patients who had multiple positive skin tests to various fish reacted to three fish upon DBPCFC, and one patient reacted to two fish. Unlike many other food allergens, fish allergens appear to be relatively susceptible to degradation during food processing (37). Canned tuna and canned salmon are sometimes tolerated by patients who are allergic to fresh-cooked tuna and salmon (12).

Chicken egg may also cause food allergic reactions in adults. The egg white is more allergenic than egg yolk. The major egg allergens appear to be ovalbumin, ovomucoid, and conalbumin (38–42). Ovomucoid is heat-stable. In some individuals, IgE can be found directed to egg yolk proteins (43). Cross-allergenicity has been demonstrated among eggs from different birds (43).

Clinical Patterns of Target Organ Responses

IgE-mediated immediate reactions to ingested food may involve one or more target organs, including the skin, respiratory tract, gastrointestinal tract, and cardiovascular system. Oropharyngeal reactions, which are often observed first, are typically characterized by pruritus and urticaria in and around the mouth. Uvular edema may also be present. Only rarely does the initial exposure to antigen result in obstructed airflow. This development of oropharyngeal symptoms with food ingestion, termed the *oral allergy syndrome,* is most commonly the result of ingestion of fresh fruits and vegetables (6, 20). Patients sensitive to birch pollen have been reported to develop the syndrome after the ingestion of raw potatoes, celery, carrots, apples, hazelnuts, and kiwi fruit (6, 12, 44), while ragweed-sensitive patients may develop symptoms after contact with melons and bananas (6, 12).

Gastrointestinal manifestations of immediate food reactions are commonly seen and may sometimes be the only problem noted. Entry of the food allergen into the stomach and the intestine may result in nausea, vomiting, cramping pain, abdominal distention, flatulence, and diarrhea.

Systemic anaphylaxis is the constellation of signs and symptoms that result from systemic IgE-mediated mast cell and basophil activation. It occurs within minutes, but occasionally has been reported to occur hours after ingestion of an offending food (45). Patients develop pruritus, urticaria, angioedema, laryngeal edema, bronchospasm, cramping abdominal pain, diarrhea, hypotension, vascular collapse, and cardiac dysrhythmias. Early recognition of the problem and a prompt intervention are the keys to treatment. In one study, a common occurrence was a failure to administer epinephrine immediately (23). Systemic anaphylactic reactions in adults are most often associated with the ingestion of peanuts, treenuts, fish, and crustacea.

In addition to foods, other factors such as exercise may be necessary to uncover a reaction. Anaphylaxis has been reported following ingestion of certain foods such as shrimp, wheat, and celery when exercising (46–49). In some patients, attacks are associated with meals, but no specific foods are implicated.

Cutaneous manifestations of IgE-mediated food allergy, which include acute urticaria and angioedema, are common. Chronic urticaria is much less frequent. In one report of 554 adults with urticaria, food allergy was demonstrated in only 1.4% (50).

Respiratory symptoms including asthma have been observed during oral challenge with suspected foods. Although rhinitis and asthma are frequently suspected to have a food-related origin, the frequency of such reactions appears to be low (51) and rarely occurs without other organ involvement (52, 53).

Relatively few studies have analyzed immediate reactions to foods in adults and/or employed protocols that examine the entire clinical picture. In one comprehensive study, however, 45 patients with a history of immediate reactions to foods were evaluated by history, physical examination, laboratory studies, skin testing, and DBPCFC (52, 53). Of the patients studied, 56% reported an allergic reaction to one food, while 84% reported that as many as three foods could elicit a reaction. Allergic reactions to foods had an average age of onset of 19.8 years. All occurred in patients with an allergic history, although few had histories of reactions in childhood. Most reactions had persisted over an average of 14.8 years. Reactions generally involved the gastrointestinal tract alone or in combination with the skin or respiratory tract. Twenty-five patients participated in DBPCFC. All challenges with placebo were negative; positive challenges were observed most frequently to crustacea and peanuts. Doses of challenge foods provoking symptoms ranged from 5 to 100 g. The clinical signs and symptoms noted on food challenge reproduced those reported by history. Reactions were usually mild and self-limited.

ATOPIC DERMATITIS

Atopic dermatitis is an inflammatory condition of the skin that is characterized by a chronic relapsing course, extreme pruritus, age-related dermal distribution patterns, and association with allergic rhinitis and asthma (54, 55). The role of food hypersensitivity in atopic dermatitis has been investigated primarily in children. Approximately one-third of children with atopic dermatitis seen in university dermatology and allergy clinics have been observed to have food hypersensitivity contributing to their skin symptoms (54). Far fewer adults with atopic dermatitis appear to benefit from food elimination diets, although comparable studies to those done in children need to be performed in adults.

Diagnostic Tests

The diagnosis of an immediate IgE-mediated reaction to a food is dependent on the history, an appropriate exclusion diet, skin testing or antigen-specific IgE in vitro tests, and blinded provocation. Food-specific IgG or IgG4 antibody levels, food antigen–antibody complexes, or lymphocyte responses to food antigen have no convincing diagnostic value in predicting or verifying immediate food hypersensitivity.

IN VITRO TESTS

Examples of in vitro tests to measure antigen-specific IgE include the radioallergosorbent test (RAST), the enzyme-linked immunosorbent assay (ELISA), and the basophil histamine release assay. In vitro tests are considered somewhat less sensitive than skin testing (56). Although modifications of the RAST have been developed, all involve antigens coupled to a solid phase such as a paper disk. Patient sera are allowed to react with this solid phase. Following washing, the amount of bound antigen-specific IgE antibodies is calculated by adding labeled anti-human IgE antibodies. The ELISA represents a variation of this methodology. Antigen may be quantified using these assays by measuring the ability of an extract to inhibit binding of specific antibody to the solid phase.

IN VIVO TESTS

Skin testing with food extracts provides a simple and reliable method of demonstrating food allergen-specific IgE antibodies. The negative predictive value of food allergen skin testing is greater than 95%, whereas the positive predictive value is low (56). Skin testing to food antigen is usually performed by the prick skin test, in which a drop of 1 : 10 or 1 : 20 glycerinated food extract, a positive histamine control, and a negative saline control are placed on the skin. The skin is then punctured through the drop with a sterile needle. Skin testing using appropriately diluted extracts may be performed by the intradermal technique. Such testing is more likely to produce clinically irrelevant positive tests (57), however, and is associated with a higher frequency of systemic

reactions. IgE-mediated food allergy is unusual when skin tests prove negative. The use of extracts of fresh fruits and vegetables is often necessary to exclude the oral allergy syndrome in cases where the allergen is extremely labile. In patients with extensive skin disease, patients with significant dermatographism, or patients in whom exposure to minute quantities of a specific food resulted in a life-threatening reaction, in vitro diagnostics are used to demonstrate food allergen-specific IgE.

ORAL CHALLENGE

DBPCFC is another diagnostic procedure commonly used to evaluate a variety of food-related complaints and clinical correlations of food allergy (58). Suspect foods should be eliminated for 10 to 14 days prior to DBPCFCs, and antihistamines should be discontinued and other medications minimized. The food challenge is administered in a fasting state, starting with a dose unlikely to provoke symptoms. The dose is then doubled every 30 to 60 minutes (or more), depending upon the type of reaction suspected and the length of time required to produce symptoms. After the patient has tolerated 10 g of lyophilized food blinded in capsules or liquid, the food should be given openly in usual quantities under observation to verify lack of sensitivity (12). A randomized challenge with an equal number of placebo and food antigens is necessary to control for a variety of confounding factors. DBPCFCs should be conducted in a clinic or hospital setting only if trained personnel and equipment for treating systemic anaphylaxis are present, and only with the patient's informed consent. Patients with a convincing history of systemic anaphylaxis to a specific food should not be challenged with that food. In adults, blinded challenge is often used to convince a patient that the food of concern to them is not associated with symptoms.

Management

Strict elimination of offending foods is the mainstay of therapy, as it prevents immediate food hypersensitivity reactions. Severe elimination diets may lead to malnutrition and should be instituted with nutritional guidance. Patients must be instructed on how to read food labels to detect hidden food allergens. In addition, patients with specific food allergies must exercise extreme caution when eating in restaurants. Even after a patient asks restaurant employees about the presence of a specific food, experience demonstrates that a reaction can still occur because the ingredients are not known or recognized by the chef. No appropriately designed trial has demonstrated clear efficacy and indications for the use of prophylactic medications, oral desensitization, and injection immunotherapy in the management of allergic reactions to foods.

The treatment of food-induced anaphylaxis is essentially the same as that for anaphylaxis due to a medication or insect sting (4). A patient with potential anaphylactic reactivity must be taught to self-administer epinephrine, and must keep an epinephrine-containing syringe and an antihistamine available at all times. A patient may sometimes inadvertently ingest a food to which he or she is sensitive. Laryngeal or pulmonary symptoms appearing after such an inadvertent food exposure should be treated immediately with epinephrine or bronchodilator therapy, or both. Patients may exhibit only mild symptoms in the first few minutes after ingestion, followed 10 to 60 minutes later by hypotension and other severe problems. Following self-medication for systemic reactions, the patient should immediately seek medical attention. Besides eliminating food allergens that provoke symptoms in atopic dermatitis, control of pruritus may be attempted with antihistamines and/or a brief application of a topical steroid in severe cases. Maintenance of skin hydration is an important component of therapy. When an infection is suspected, an anti-staphylococcal antibiotic may be prescribed.

Delayed Reactions to Foods

ALLERGIC EOSINOPHILIC GASTROENTERITIS

Eosinophilic gastroenteritis is a relatively rare chronic digestive disease that is characterized by peripheral eosinophilia and eosinophilic infiltration of the stomach or the small intestine. It is seen more frequently during the third decade of life. Clinical symptoms reflect the extent of eosinophilic infiltration in the bowel wall. When a significant eosinophilic infiltration is present in the mucosa, symptoms correspond to those of malabsorption. The clinical picture resembles that seen with obstruction if the infiltration predominantly occurs in the muscular layer. Serosal involvement produces ascites containing eosinophils.

The immunopathogenic mechanisms involved in allergic eosinophilic gastroenteritis are unclear. The disease may be due to severe food allergies that lead to repeated immediate hypersensitivity reactions in the gastrointestinal mucosa. Patients often are atopic, have an elevated serum IgE level, and have specific IgE antibodies for 15 to 40 food antigens (59, 60). T cells from patients with this disease produce high amounts of IL-4 and IL-5, which are Th2-type cytokines (61). Gamma-interferon mRNA could not be detected by RT-PCR in biopsies from patients with allergic eosinophilic gastroenteritis, but was present in normal biopsies (61).

Current treatments for eosinophilic gastroenteritis remain unsatisfactory. Dietary avoidance of incriminated foods may be tried, but the number of foods involved may preclude the long-term use of such a diet. Patients who respond poorly to dietary restrictions and those without evidence of food hypersensitivity may require oral corticosteroid therapy. While this course of action usually results in clinical improvement, long-term treatment with corticosteroids is frequently required (6).

GLUTEN-SENSITIVE ENTEROPATHY (COELIAC DISEASE)

Gluten-sensitive enteropathy is a mucosal disease of the small intestine precipitated by the alcohol-soluble portion of gluten, gliadin, in susceptible individuals. The HLA-DR3DQ2 haplotype has the strongest disease associations (62). The onset of symptoms, which may consist of intermittent diarrhea, abdominal pain, and irritability, typically occurs 6 to 12 months after introduction of gluten into the diet. Extensive mucosal injury may lead to malabsorption with a clinical picture including steatorrhea, peripheral edema from protein loss, anemia, bleeding diathesis, tetany, and growth failure. A subsequent increase in the incidence of gastrointestinal lymphoma has been reported (63). The acute reaction of the intestinal mucosa consists of edema, an increase in vascular permeability, and an eosinophil and neutrophil infiltration. Gliadin has been separated by gel electrophoresis into four proline- and glutamine-rich fractions, each of which precipitates small bowel injury in vitro (64). Blunting of the mucosal surface, villous atrophy, and a dense infiltration of the lamina propria with plasma cells, B cells, and T cells is observed in chronic disease.

Diagnosis depends on biopsy evidence of small intestinal mucosa injury upon gluten challenge. Treatment is directed at elimination of gluten from the diet (e.g., elimination of gluten-containing wheat, barley, rye, and oats). Improvement in symptoms is seen as soon as 2 weeks after the institution of a gluten-free diet, although histologic improvement may take 2 to 3 months. Growth usually returns to normal once the small intestinal mucosa has healed. Strict gastrointestinal rest, and in some instances the use of steroids, is necessary to suppress diarrhea in cases of severe inflammation.

Dermatitis Herpetiformis

Dermatitis herpetiformis is a chronic papulovesicular skin disorder frequently associated with asymptomatic gluten-sensitive enteropathy. The histologic appearance of skin lesions resembles a granulocytic infiltration at the dermoepidermal junction associated with edema and blister formation. Granular IgA deposits with associated J-chains are found in the papillary dermis. Complement-mediated injury is implicated. The histology of intestinal lesions is similar to coeliac disease, although it is generally less severe.

Skin lesions are symmetrically distributed on extensor surfaces of elbows, knees, and buttocks. Most patients have little or no gastrointestinal complaints. The diagnosis rests on the typical appearance of these skin lesions and histologic findings of IgA deposits in the perilesional or uninvolved skin. Fifteen percent of patients will have a normal small intestinal mucosa on histologic evaluation. Treatment consists of the removal of gluten from the diet and the use of dapsone or sulfapyridine.

Natural History of Food Allergies

Some adults (65) may lose their sensitivity if the responsible food allergen is completely eliminated from the diet. Thus, after 1 to 2 years of allergen avoidance, as many as one-third of children and adults lose their clinical sensitivity (65, 66). Patients with an allergy to peanut, tree nut, fish, or shellfish rarely lose their clinical reactivity, however (65–67). Loss of sensitivity correlates with allergen avoidance, but whether reintroduction and repeated exposure to the same allergen will cause the sensitivity to reappear is unknown.

REFERENCES

1. Prausnitz C, Kustner H. Studien uber die Ueberempfindliehkeit. Zentralbl Bakteriol Parasitenlzd Infektionskr Hyg 1921;86:160.
2. Loveless MH. Milk allergy: a survey of its incidence; experiments with a masked ingestion test. J Allergy 1950;21:489.
3. Jansen JJN, Kardiaal AFM, Huijbers G, *et al.* Prevalence of food allergy and intolerance in the adult Dutch population. J Allergy Clin Immunol 1994;93:446.
4. Sampson HA, Metcalfe DD. Food allergies. JAMA 1992;268:2840.
5. Young E, Patel S, Stoneham M, Rona R, Wilkinson JD. The prevalence of reaction to food additives in a survey population. J Royal College of Physicians of London 1987;21:241.
6. Enberg RN. Food-induced oropharyngeal symptoms: the oral allergy syndrome. In: Anderson JA, ed. Food allergy: immunology and allergy clinics of North America. Philadelphia: WB Saunders, 1991, 767–772.
7. Kidd JM 3d, Cohen SH, Sosman AJ, *et al.* Food-dependent exercise-induced anaphylaxis. J Allergy Clin Immunol 1983;71:407–411.
8. Maulitz R, Pratt DS, Schocket AL. Exercise-induced anaphylactic reaction to shellfish. J Allergy Clin Immunol 1979;63:433–434.
9. Kushimoto H, Aoki T. Masked type I wheat allergy. Arch Dermatol 1985;121:355.
10. Schocket AL. Exercise- and pressure-induced syndromes. In: Metcalfe DD, Sampson HA, Simon RA, eds. Food allergy: adverse reactions to foods and food additives. Oxford: Blackwell Scientific Publications, 1991, 199–206.
11. Sampson HA, Jolie PL. Increased plasma histamine concentrations after food challenges in children with atopic dermatitis. N Engl J Med 1984;311:372–376.
12. Sampson HA. Adverse reactions to foods. In: Middleton E Jr, Reed CE, Ellis EF, Adkinson NF Jr, Yunginger JW, Busse WW, eds. Allergy: principles and practice. St. Louis: Mosby-Year Book, 1993, 1661–1686.

13. Gray I, Harten M, Walzer M. Studies in mucous membrane hypersensitiveness. IV. The allergic reaction in the passively sensitized mucous membranes of the ileum and colon in humans. Am J Intern Med 1940;13:2050.

14. Selbekk BH, Aas K, Myren J. In vitro sensitization and mast cell degranulation in human jejunal mucosa. Scand J Gastroenterol 1978;13:87.

15. Barrett KE. Mast cells, basophils, and immunoglobulin E. In: Metcalfe DD, Sampson HA, Simon RA, eds. Food allergy: adverse reactions to foods and food additives. Oxford: Blackwell Scientific Publications, 1991, 13–35.

16. Sampson SA. Mast cell involvement in food allergy. In: Kaliner MA, Metcalfe DD, eds. The mast cell in health and disease. New York: Marcel Dekker, 1993, 609–626.

17. MacDonald SM, Rafnar T, Langdon J, et al. Molecular identification of an IgE-dependent histamine-releasing factor. Science 1995;269:688–690.

18. Sampson HA, Broadbent KR, Bernhisel-Broadbent J. "Spontaneous" basophil histamine release and histamine releasing factor in patients with atopic dermatitis and food hypersensitivity. N Engl J Med 1989;321:228–232.

19. Geha R. Human IgE. J Allergy Clin Immunol 1985;74:109.

20. Metcalfe DD. Allergic gastrointestinal diseases. In: Rich RR, Fleisher TA, Schwartz BD, Shearer WT, Strober W, eds. Clinical immunology: principles and practice. St. Louis: Mosby-Year Book, 1995, 966–975.

21. Sampson HA, Mendelson L, Rosen JP. Fatal and near-fatal food anaphylactic reactions to food in children and adolescents. N Engl J Med 1992;327:380–384.

22. Yunginger JW, Sweeney KG, Sturner WQ, et al. Fatal food-induced anaphylaxis. JAMA 1988;260:1450–1452.

23. Barnett D, Baldo BA, Howden MEH. Multiplicity of allergens in peanuts. J Allergy Clin Immunol 1983;72:61–68.

24. Sachs MI, Jones RT, Yunginger JW. Isolation and partial purification of a major peanut allergen. J Allergy Clin Immunol 1981;67:27.

25. Moroz LA, Yung WH. Kunitz soybean trypsin inhibitor. N Engl J Med 1980;302:1126.

26. Bernhisel-Broadbent J, Sampson HA. Cross-allergenicity in the legume botanical family in children with food hypersensitivity. J Allergy Clin Immunol 1989;83:435–440.

27. Nagpal S, Metcalfe DD, Subba Rao PV. Identification of a shrimp-derived allergen as tRNA. J Immunol 1987;138:4169.

28. Hoffman DR, Day ED Jr, Miller JS. The major heat stable allergen of shrimp. Ann Allergy 1981;47:17.

29. Nagpal S, Rajappa L, Metcalfe DD, Subba Rao PV. Isolation and characterization of heat stable allergens from shrimp (Penaeus indicus). J Allergy Clin Immunol 1989;83:26.

30. Shanti KN, Martin MB, Nagpal S, Metcalfe DD, Subba Rao PV. Tropomyosin as the major shrimp allergen and characterization of its IgE binding epitopes. J Immunol 1993;151:5354.

31. Daul CB, Slattery M, Reese G, Lehrer SB. Identification of the major brown shrimp (Penaeus aztecus) allergen (Pen a I) as the muscle protein tropomyosin. Int Arch Allergy Appl Immunol 1994;105:49.

32. Aas K, Jebsen JW. Studies of hypersensitivity to fish. Partial purification and crystallization of a major allergenic component of cod. Int Arch Allergy Appl Immunol 1967;32:1.

33. Elsayed S, Aas K. Isolation of purified allergens (cod) by isoelectric focusing. Int Arch Allergy Appl Immunol 1971;40:428.

34. Elsayed S, Bennich H. The primary structure of allergen M from cod. Scand J Immunol 1975;4:203.

35. Elsayed S, Apold J. Immunochemical analysis of cod fish allergen M: locations of the immunoglobulin binding sites as demonstrated by the native and synthetic peptides. Allergy 1983;38:449.

36. Bernhisel-Broadbent J, Scanlon SM, Sampson HA. Fish hypersensitivity. I. In vitro results and oral challenge in fish allergic patients. J Allergy Clin Immunol 1992;89:730.

37. Bernhisel-Broadbent J, Sampson HA. Fish hypersensitivity. II. Clinical relevance of altered fish allergenicity secondary to various preparation methods. J Allergy Clin Immunol 1992;90:622–629.

38. Bleumink E, Young E. Studies on the atopic allergen in hen's egg. I. Identification of the skin-reactive fraction in egg white. Int Arch Allergy Appl Immunol 1969;35:1.

39. Bleumink E, Young E. Studies on the atopic allergen in hen's eggs. II. Further characterization of the skin-reactive fraction in egg-white; immuno-electrophoretic studies. Int Arch Allergy Appl Immunol 1971;40:72.

40. Hoffman DR. Immunochemical identification of the allergens in egg white. J Allergy Clin Immunol 1983;71:481.

41. Anet J, Back JF, Baker RS, Barnett D, Burley RW, Howden MEH. Allergens in the white and yolk of hen's egg. A study of IgE binding by egg proteins. Int Arch Allergy Appl Immunol 1985;77:364.

42. Langeland T. A clinical and immunological study of allergy to hen's egg white. III. Allergens in hen's egg white studied by crossed radioimmunoelectrophoresis (CRIE). Allergy 1982;37:521.

43. Langeland T. A clinical and immunological study of allergy to hen's egg white. VI. Occurrence of proteins cross-reacting with allergens in hen's egg white as studied in egg white from turkey, duck, goose, seagull, and in hen egg yolk, and hen and chicken sera and flesh. Allergy 1983;38:399.

44. Gall H, Kalveram KJ, Forck G, Sterry W. Kiwi fruit allergy: a new birch pollen-associated food allergy. J Allergy Clin Immunol 1994;94:70–76.

45. Golbert TM, Patterson R, Pruzansky JJ. Systemic allergic reactions to ingested antigens. J Allergy 1969;44:96.

46. Kidd J, Cohen SH, Sosman AJ, Fink JN. Food dependent exercise induced anaphylaxis. J Allergy Clin Immunol 1982;69:103–111.

47. Maulitz RM, Pratt DS, Schocket AL. Exercise induced anaphylactic reaction to shellfish. J Allergy Clin Immunol 1979;63:433–434.

48. Kushimoto H, Aoki T. Masked type I wheat allergy. Arch Dermatol 1985;121:355.

49. Schocket AL. Exercise and pressure-induced syndromes. In: Metcalfe DD, Sampson HA, Simon RA, eds. Food allergy: adverse reactions to foods and food additives. Oxford: Blackwell Scientific Publications, 1991, 199–206.

50. Champion RH, Roberts SO, Carpenter RG, Roger JH. Urticaria and angioedema: a review of 554 patients. Br J Dermatol 1969;81:588–597.

51. Bousquet J, Chanez P, Michel F-B. The respiratory tract and food hypersensitivity. In: Metcalfe DD, Sampson HA, Simon RA, eds. Food allergy: adverse reactions to foods and food additives. Oxford: Blackwell Scientific Publications, 1991, 139–149.

52. Atkins FM, Steinberg SS, Metcalfe DD. Evaluation of immedi-

ate adverse reactions to foods in adults. I. Correlation of demographic, laboratory, and prick skin test data with response to controlled oral food challenge. J Allergy Clin Immunol 1985;75:348.

53. Atkins FM, Steinberg SS, Metcalfe DD. Evaluation of immediate adverse reactions to foods in adults. II. A detailed analysis of reaction patterns during oral food challenge. J Allergy Clin Immunol 1985;75:356.

54. Burks AW, Mallory SB, Williams LW, Shirrell MA. Atopic dermatitis: clinical relevance of food hypersensitivity reactions. J Pediatr 1988;113:447.

55. Blaylock WK. Atopic dermatitis: diagnosis and pathobiology. J Allergy Clin Immunol 1976;57:62–79.

56. Sampson HA. In vitro diagnosis and mediator assays for food allergies. Allergy Proc 1993;14:259–261.

57. Bock SA, Buckley J, Holst A, May CD. Proper use of skin tests with food extracts in diagnosis of hypersensitivity to food in children. Clin Allergy 1977;7:375.

58. Bock SA, Sampson HA, Atkins FM, Zeiger RS, Lehrer S, Sacks M, Bush RK, Metcalfe DD. Double-blind placebo-controlled food challenge as an office procedure: a manual. J Allergy Clin Immunol 1988;82:986.

59. Thounce JQ, Tanner MS. Eosinophilic gastroenteritis. Arch Dis Child 1985;60:1186.

60. Min K-U, Metcalfe DD. Eosinophilic gastroenteritis. In: Ander-son JA, ed. Food allergy. Immunology and allergy clinics of North America (vol II). Philadelphia: WB Saunders, 1991, 799–813.

61. Jaffe JS, James SP, Mullins GE, et al. Evidence for an abnormal profile of IL-4, IL-5, and γ-IFN in peripheral blood T cells from patients with allergic eosinophilic gastroenteritis. J Clin Immunol 1994;14:299–309.

62. Sollid LM, Markussen G, Ek J, et al. Evidence for a primary association of celiac disease to a particular HLA-DQ α/β heterodimer. J Exp Med 1989;169:345–349.

63. Harris OD, Cooke WT, Thompson H, Waterhouse JAN. Malignancy in adult celiac disease and idiopathic steatorrhea. Am J Med 1967;42:899.

64. Howdle PD, Ciclitire PJ, Simpson FJ, et al. Are all gliadins toxic to coeliac disease? An in vitro study of alpha, beta, gamma and omega gliadins. Scand J Gastroenterol 1984;19:41.

65. Pastorello EA, Stocchi L, Pravettoni V, et al. Role of the elimination diet in adults with food allergy. J Allergy Clin Immunol 1989;84:475.

66. Businco L, Benincori N, Cantani A, et al. Chronic diarrhea due to cow's milk allergy: a 4- to 10-year follow-up study. Ann Allergy 1985;55:844.

67. Bock SA, Atkins FM. The natural history of peanut sensitivity. J Allergy Clin Immunol 1989;83:900.

11

ECZEMA AND FOOD HYPERSENSITIVITY

Hugh A. Sampson

Atopic dermatitis is a form of eczema that generally begins in early infancy and is characterized by extreme pruritus, chronically relapsing course, and distinctive distribution. The rash is generally an erythematous, papulovesicular eruption, frequently with weeping and crusting in early life, that eventually progresses to a scaly, lichenified rash (1). The distribution of the rash typically varies with age (2); it involves the cheeks and extensor surfaces of the arms and legs in infants, the flexor surfaces in the young child, and flexor surfaces, hands, and feet in the teenage patient and young adult. Unlike most dermatoses, atopic dermatitis does not include a primary skin lesion, but rather is identified by a constellation of symptoms. The diagnostic criteria of Hanifin and Rajka (3) provide an internationally accepted standard for diagnosing atopic dermatitis, and the SCORAD Index (4) adapted by the European Task Force on Atopic Dermatitis provides a standardized method for gauging severity.

Libellus de Aegretudinibus Infantium (Handbook of Diseases of Children), a pediatric textbook written in 1472 by an Italian physician, Paolo Bagellardo, contains the first known scientific discussion of eczema. The chapter on skin provides advice on lubrication of skin and prevention of scratching in children having this skin disorder. In the early 1600s, Helmont discussed the association between a pruritic skin rash and asthma, and von Hebra described the flexural distribution of a chronic itchy skin disease in 1884 (5). Besnier, a French physician, is credited with the first comprehensive description of atopic dermatitis nearly a century ago (6). He emphasized the hereditary nature of this disorder, its chronically recurring course, and its association with hayfever and asthma. Initially the disorder was called "prurigo diathesique," but later became known as "prurigo Besnier." Wise

and Sulzberger (7) further emphasized the relationship between atopic eczema, asthma, and hayfever by coining the term "atopic dermatitis," the term generally used today. The incidence of atopic dermatitis has been increasing over the past 40 years, and the condition is now estimated to affect between 10% and 12% of the pediatric population (8).

The pathogenic role of allergy in atopic dermatitis has been debated since Besnier's original description. A number of observations have suggested a significant role for IgE-mediated mechanisms in atopic dermatitis:

1. Approximately 80% of children have positive immediate skin tests and RASTs to various dietary and environmental allergens (9, 10).
2. 80% to 90% of children have elevated serum IgE concentrations (11).
3. 65% to 85% of patients have a positive family history of atopy (12).
4. 50% to 80% of children develop other atopic disorders such as allergic rhinitis and asthma (13, 14).
5. Eczema can develop in recipients of bone marrow transplants from atopic donors (15, 16) and may resolve in patients with Wiskott-Aldrich syndrome following successful bone marrow transplantation and engraftment (17).

The pathogenic role of IgE in atopic dermatitis is further supported by studies delineating the immunopathogenic role of the IgE-mediated cutaneous late-phase response and of IgE-bearing antigen-presenting cells (APCs), especially Langerhans' cells, in establishing the Th2 lymphocytic response. Previously, skin biopsies from patients with atopic dermatitis were considered inconsistent with an IgE-mediated mechanism because they revealed a nonspecific dermatitis characterized by a lymphocytic infiltrate that appeared indicative of a classical Type IV, cell-mediated response. Acute skin lesions of atopic dermatitis are described histologically as having spongiosis, epidermal hyperplasia, and ballooning of the keratinocytes secondary to intracellular edema. Mast cell and basophil numbers are normal, while eosinophils are sparse (18). Chronic skin lesions exhibit moderate to marked hyperplasia of the epidermis, elongation of the rete ridges, and prominent hyperkeratosis. Spongiosis is variable, and the numbers of mast cells and Langerhans' cells are significantly increased. Demyelination and fibrosis of cutaneous nerves are observed at all levels of the dermis. Capillary numbers are often increased, and capillary walls may be thickened. Although this pattern is not considered typical of the Type I, IgE-mediated response, it is consistent with an end-stage cutaneous IgE-dependent "late-phase" reaction and the preferential activation of Th2 cells by IgE-bearing Langerhans' cells (19, 20).

IgE-Mediated Cutaneous Late-Phase Reaction

Dolovich and coworkers (21) were first to describe the cutaneous late-phase reaction of IgE-mediated hypersensitivity. These investigators and others (22–24) have demonstrated that within minutes of encountering an allergen, mast cells and basophils become activated by antigen-induced bridging of IgE molecules, which are bound to the cell membrane by high-affinity FcE receptors. An initial flare (vasodilation) and wheal (capillary leakiness) appear when mast cell mediators are released. This response peaks within 15 to 30 minutes, and then fades over time. Approximately 90 minutes after contact with allergen, the lesion is diffuse, and only slightly erythematous and edematous, but largely asymptomatic. Clinically, mild pruritus may begin by 4 hours, but distinctive erythema, tenderness, and warmth of the involved skin develops by 6 to 12 hours. The symptoms then slowly resolve over 24 to 48 hours.

Histologically, the late-phase lesion begins with an influx of neutrophils and eosinophils that takes place 2 to 4 hours after the immediate reaction. This influx is promoted by cytokines released from mast cells, endothelial cells, and possibly other cell sources. Once present, the neutrophils and eosinophils release other mediators of inflammation (e.g., platelet activating factor, prostaglandins, leukotrienes, major basic protein, O_2^-) that perpetuate the response. After 6 to 8 hours, primarily mononuclear cells and eosinophils are observed, and lesser numbers of neutrophils, basophils, and mast cells are seen. During the ensuing 24 to 48 hours, the infiltrating cell population again changes, and later biopsies show primarily a mononuclear cell infiltrate, which appears virtually indistinguishable from the classic Type IV, cell-mediated response.

In the last several years, research has shown that the IgE-mediated response is far more complex than that suggested by the classification of hypersensitivity by Gell and Coombs (25), and that the role played by IgE antibodies in the pathogenesis of atopic dermatitis involves a number of cell types. Receptors for IgE antibodies have been identified on B cells, T cells, monocytes, macrophages, eosinophils, and platelets (26–28). Langerhans' cells, the "professional" APCs in the skin, are increased in atopic dermatitis lesions, possess allergen-specific IgE antibodies on their surface (29), and promote Th2 responses to allergens (19, 20). Utilizing in situ hybridization, it has been shown that lymphocytes infiltrating the skin of early and late eczematous skin lesions are primarily Th2-type cells, expressing mRNA for IL-4 and IL-5 but not IFN-γ (30). This situation is in distinct contrast to lymphocytes found in classic delayed-type hypersensitivity reactions, such as PPD, where infiltrating lymphocytes are of the Th1-type, expressing mRNA for IFN-γ and IL-2 but not IL-4 and IL-5 (31). In addition, cutaneous vascular endothelial cells in patients with atopic dermatitis express abnormally high levels of VCAM-1, E-selectin, and ICAM-1 (32)—a sign of IL-4 and TNF-α stimulation—whereas no class II MHC antigens are expressed on kerotinocytes—a sign of IFN-γ stimulation that is typically seen in delayed-type cell mediated reactions (33).

Previously, eosinophils were not considered to play a pathogenic role in the skin lesions of atopic dermatitis because they are not abundant in routine hematoxylin-eosin stained histologic sections of eczematous lesions. A more major role is suggested by the presence of eosinophil major basic protein (MBP), the major protein of eosinophilic granules, in active eczematous lesions, however. MBP is a cytolytic protein secreted almost exclusively by eosinophils; it is known to damage skin epithelial cells (34) and promote further mast cell degranulation (35). Utilizing an antibody specific for MBP and an indirect fluorescein-staining technique, biopsies of eczematous skin lesions from patients with atopic dermatitis have been shown to demonstrate extensive extracellular MBP deposition in a fibrillar pattern in the superficial dermis (36). MBP was not found in biopsy specimens from uninvolved skin sites in these same patients, indicating that this eosinophil product resulted from specific deposition—not nonspecific sequestration. Control studies on patients with contact dermatitis revealed no dermal deposition of MBP. This study provided further evidence that the typical mononuclear cell infiltrate in lesions of atopic dermatitis may result from IgE-induced cutaneous late-phase reactions, with subsequent eosinophil degranulation and dermal deposition of MBP. Infiltrating lymphocytes are capable of releasing a variety of interleukins that may promote mast cell proliferation (IL-3), cell surface expression of FcE receptors, IgE synthesis (IL-4), and eosinophil proliferation (IL-5).

Food Hypersensitivity and Atopic Dermatitis

By the turn of the twentieth century, physicians were suggesting that reactions to food proteins could cause eczematous skin rashes. Schloss was among the first to present evidence that food allergy could play a pathogenic role in atopic dermatitis (37). He provided several case reports of patients who experienced improvement in their eczema after avoiding specific foods. Shortly thereafter, Talbot (38) and Blackfan (39) each described a series of patients who had positive skin tests to certain foods and who later experienced clearing of their skin when the foods were removed from their diets. Since then, other

reports have appeared in the literature implicating food allergy in the pathogenesis of atopic dermatitis (40, 41). After openly challenging eczema patients with foods, however, other investigators discounted these findings (42–44). At a Symposium on Atopic Dermatitis in 1965, it was concluded that food allergy led to urticarial lesions in some patients with atopic dermatitis, but not eczema (45).

In a series of experiments, Walzer and his colleagues (46, 47) unequivocally demonstrated that ingested food antigens readily penetrate the gastrointestinal barrier and are transported in the circulation to mast cells in the skin. To demonstrate this process, 65 normal adults were passively sensitized by intracutaneous injection of serum (i.e., P-K test) from a patient with severe fish allergy and a normal control (46). The following day the volunteers were fed fish; 61 of the 65 subjects developed a wheal and flare reaction within 90 minutes at the sensitized site but not the control site. A series of experiments conducted in 66 normal children with serum from an egg-allergic subject found similar results (47). Walzer and his colleagues studied the absorption of food antigens from various locations in the gastrointestinal tract and other sites, such as the nose, eye, and urinary bladder, and concluded that "the absorption of unaltered protein into the circulation is a normal, physiologic phenomenon occurring in nonatopic as well as atopic individuals, at all ages, and with many allergens" (48). In addition, Walzer's group was able to show that the intravenous injection of the protein nitrogen equivalent of 1/44,000 of one peanut kernel was sufficient to induce wheal and flare at a passively sensitized skin site. In 1936, Engman et al. (49) reported a child with atopic dermatitis and allergy to wheat such that ingestion of a wheat cracker would produce intense itching. To demonstrate the role of scratching and rubbing in the development of eczema, they admitted the patient to the hospital when his skin was clear and bandaged his left arm and leg in a thick, stiff crinoline bandage. Within 2 hours after the child was given two wheat crackers, he was itching and scratching. The following morning the boy had typical eczematous lesions, except under the bandages, where the skin remained clear. Engman reportedly repeated this experiment in several other cases. Taken together, these studies conducted more than

50 years ago clearly showed that ingested food allergens were readily accessible to cutaneous mast cells and the "skin-associated lymphoid tissue," and that they could produce intense pruritus, scratching, and rubbing that led to typical eczematous lesions in the sensitized host.

In the late 1970s, Hammar reported the induction of eczematous skin lesions in 15 of 81 hospitalized children less than 5 years of age after 2 to 3 days of ingesting 100 mL of milk daily (50). The significance of these findings was questioned, however, because the challenges were done openly and a repeat challenge 18 months later produced similar symptoms in only 4 of 15 patients (51). Atherton et al. (52) reported that two-thirds of children with atopic dermatitis between the ages of 2 and 8 years showed marked improvement during a double-blind crossover trial of egg and milk exclusion that was conducted over a 12-week period in the patients' homes. In this study, 45% of the patients enrolled dropped out or were excluded from analysis, controls were not instituted for environmental and other triggers of atopic dermatitis, and a significant order effect was found, all of which raised questions about the authors' conclusions. Utilizing a similar trial design, Nield et al. (53) demonstrated improvement in some patients during the milk and egg exclusion phase, but overall no significant difference was seen in 40 patients completing the crossover trial. Juto et al. (54) reported that 7 of 20 infants with eczema healed and 12 of 20 improved on a highly restricted elimination diet. Nonblinded challenges to cow's milk reportedly resulted in increased itching and rash in 12 of 20 infants. Hill et al. (55) treated 8 children with severe atopic dermatitis with Vivonex for 2 weeks followed by the addition of two vegetables and two fruits for 3 months. All patients experienced improvement in their eczema while maintaining the diet but relapsed within weeks of discontinuing it. While supporting a role for food intolerance in the exacerbation of atopic dermatitis, most of these studies failed to control for other trigger factors, placebo effect, or observer bias. A double-blind study in 23 hospitalized adults on an antigen-free diet (Vivasorb) failed to show any significant difference between the antigen-free and placebo groups (56). The study groups were too small to conclude "no significant difference (type II statistical error), however, and some adults with markedly elevated serum IgE concentrations appeared to respond to the antigen-free diet.

In their studies of children who were suspected of having food hypersensitivity and respiratory allergy, May and Bock (57) reported that 4 of 7 children with a history of eczematous reactions to foods developed skin rashes within 2 hours of administration of a double-blind, placebo-controlled oral food challenge (DBPCFC). Using a similar challenge protocol, the author has systematically studied 470 patients referred for evaluation of severe atopic dermatitis, as reviewed below. Burks et al. (58) has also employed an oral DBPCFC to study 46 children with mild to severe atopic dermatitis presenting to a university dermatology and allergy clinic. As seen in other controlled oral challenge studies, children experienced cutaneous, respiratory, and gastrointestinal symptoms. One-third of the children developed symptoms during the blinded food challenges. No correlation was seen between the likelihood of a positive food challenge and the severity of the skin symptoms.

In the past 15 years, the author's studies have addressed the etiologic role of IgE-mediated food hypersensitivity in atopic dermatitis (56–62). Using oral DBPCFC, 470 patients with atopic dermatitis have been evaluated for food hypersensitivity. Subjects ranged in age from 3 months to 24 years, with a median age of 4.1 years. The median clinical score for the group was 15 (range 0 to 30) at the time of the first Clinical Research Unit admission, based upon the clinical scoring system depicted in Table 11.1. Family history was positive for atopic disease in 91% of subjects. One hundred fifty-seven patients (39%) had allergic rhinitis and asthma at the time of initial evaluation, and only 94 (20%) had neither allergic rhinitis nor asthma. In 376 (80%) patients, serum total IgE concentration was elevated, with a median of 3410 IU/mL and a range of 1.5–45,000 IU/mL.

Any patient with chronic severe eczema fulfilling the criteria of Hanifin and Rajka (3) for the diagnosis of atopic dermatitis was eligible for the study, regardless of whether clinical history or previous allergy tests suggested a diagnosis of food hypersensitivity. All patients were admitted to the Clinical Research Unit to provide a stable, low-allergen environment. Foods administered during DBPCFCs were selected

Table 11.1
Clinical Scoring System

Characteristics	Score	Characteristics	Score
Extension		*Intensity—Night Pattern*	
Infantile Stage (less than 2 yrs of age)		Absent, sleeps through night without attention	0
Absent	0	Occasionally awakens scratching, but back to sleep with minimal attention	2
Less than 20% involvement	2		
20%–50% of skin involved	4	Awakens scratching 1–2 times each night	4
More than 50% of skin involved	6		
Childhood and Adult Stages		Requires frequent rubbing during the night to retard scratching, sleeps very little	6
Absent	0		
Not more than 2 predilection sites involved	2	**Antihistamine Use**	
		None or occasional prednisone use	0
Involvement more than 2 but less than 6	4	Daily bedtime use	1
Dermatitis including and extending beyond predilection areas, >25% involvement	6	Daily bedtime use plus 1–2 daytime doses on most days	2
		Daily bedtime use plus daytime usage to limit allowed	3
Course (remission = eczema not completely absent, but confined to typical areas)		**Antibiotic/Prednisone Use (for Skin in Past 3 Months)**	
Absent	0	None	0
More than 2 months' remission during quarter	1	1 course with noninflamed periods	1
Remissions less than 2 months	2	2 courses with noninflamed periods	2
Continuous course	3	3 or more courses, or no clearing	3
Scratching		**School Missed or Parents Missing Work due to Skin Symptoms**	
Intensity–Day Pattern		None	0
Absent	0	Average 1 day missed per quarter	1
Scratches when tired/anxious, easily distracted	2	Average 2 days missed per quarter	2
Evaluated as greater than 2 but less than 6	4	Average 3 or more days missed per quarter	3
Almost constant, scratching to point of excoriation: school and play concentration impossible	6	**Total** [Possible total = 30]	

on the basis of skin test (and RAST) results or a strongly suggestive history of food hypersensitivity. Foods selected for the challenge protocol were excluded from the patient's diet for 7 to 10 days prior to admission. In addition, the following medications were withheld: oral corticosteroids for at least 1 month prior to admission, antihistamines for at least 7 to 10 days, and inhaled and oral beta-adrenergic drugs for 8 hours prior to the challenge. Subjects were allowed to continue on inhaled cromolyn sodium and oral theophylline.

The initial 220 patients were skin-tested to a battery of 20 food extracts (Greer Laboratories, Lenoir, N.C.) on the day of admission to confirm previous results, standardize skin test data, and determine

which foods would be used in the DBPCFC (Table 11.2). Treatment consisted of an aggressive topical regimen consisting of two to three soaking baths (or wet wraps) per day, followed by the application of a lubricating cream to the entire body and topical corticosteroid (1% hydrocortisone cream for the face and 0.025% to 0.1% triamcinolone ointment for the trunk and extremities) to active eczematous areas. Anti-staphylococcal antibiotics were generally administered and chloral hydrate was used for sedation. Utilizing this regimen, control of erythema and pruritus could generally be achieved in 3 to 4 days. Once a stable baseline was established, a venous line was placed prior to initiating challenges to provide an "open line" in case of a major anaphylactic reaction

Table 11.2
Foods Eliciting Positive Prick Skin Tests in 220 Children with Atopic Dermatitis

Food	Number of Patients	% of Tests	Food	Number of Patients	% of Tests
egg	124	20%	beef	42	7%
milk	54	9%	chicken	33	5%
peanut	98	16%	pork	40	6%
soy	58	9%	potato	16	3%
wheat	34	5%	rye	20	3%
green pea	34	5%	others	66	11%

and to provide access for atraumatic serial blood sampling.

During a 1-week admission, three to four DBPCFCs would be conducted (63). The Clinical Research Unit Dietician determined the order of all challenges using a randomization scheme on the Unit's computer (CLINFO). Only the dietitian was aware of the contents of the challenge until the code was broken at the end of the study week. Two challenges were performed each day—one containing the test food antigen and one containing placebo. Over a 60- to 90-minute period, as much as 10 g of dehydrated powdered food was administered in opaque capsules (14 to 18 "00" capsules, depending upon the food antigen) or in 100 mL of juice. Challenges in the past several years all have been camouflaged in juices or blenderized food. The initial challenge dose of 100 mg to 500 mg was increased in a stepwise fashion at 15-minute intervals until the entire 10 g was consumed or a reaction occurred. Each challenge was evaluated and scored using a previously published symptom sheet (59).

All negative DBPCFCs were confirmed by feeding the food openly to the patient prior to discharge to ensure the accuracy of the blinded challenge and to reassure the patient (and parent) that the food could be ingested safely. In the initial 1000 food challenges performed, five reactions occurred during the open feeding following negative DBPCFCs (<1% false-negative results). Three children—two aged 4 years and one aged 2 years—developed symptoms after drinking milk. One of these patients developed cutaneous, nasal, and respiratory symptoms after consuming approximately 100 mL of milk, one child developed cutaneous symptoms and periocular

edema after ingesting about 80 mL, and the third child developed cutaneous, upper respiratory, and gastrointestinal symptoms after ingesting about 10 mL of milk. The fourth child, aged 5 years, developed cutaneous, gastrointestinal, nasal, and respiratory symptoms after eating a standard portion of peas. A fifth child, aged 3 years, developed scattered urticaria following the ingestion of one teaspoon of peanut butter.

In the initial evaluation of 470 children with atopic dermatitis, a total of 1776 DBPCFCs were conducted (Table 11.3). DBPCFCs were not conducted in 193 instances because clinical history indicated a convincing account of a major anaphylactic reaction (mostly to peanuts and nuts). History was considered "convincing" when a patient experienced severe respiratory symptoms (laryngeal edema or wheezing) or hypotension within minutes of ingesting an isolated food and required emergency care by a physician. In each case where the challenge was not performed, the patients had a markedly positive prick skin test to the food in question. No patient experienced a severe anaphylactic reaction during DBPCFC,

Table 11.3
Food Challenges in 470 Patients with Atopic Dermatitis

Total number of food challenges	1776
Negative challenges	1062
Positive by history	193
(majority peanut and nut)	
Positive challenges	714
• Cutaneous symptoms	529 (74%)
Skin only	195 (27%)
• Gastrointestinal symptoms	358 (50%)
• Respiratory symptoms	322 (45%)

although roughly half of the patients required oral diphenhydramine for severe pruritus, and several patients required subcutaneous epinephrine for respiratory symptoms. Of the 1776 DBPCFCs performed to date, 714 had positive results and 1062 were interpreted as negative. Cutaneous reactions developed in 529 cases (74%), with the responses consisting of a pruritic, erythematous, macular, or morbilliform rash primarily in previous predilection sites. Symptoms confined exclusively to the skin occurred in only 30% of the reactions. Typical urticarial lesions were rarely seen and generally consisted of only a few lesions. Intense pruritus and scratching frequently resulted in superficial excoriations and occasionally bleeding. Gastrointestinal symptoms were seen in 358 of the reactions (50%), even though such a history was rarely elicited from the patients. These symptoms consisted of nausea or abdominal pain (or both), plus vomiting or diarrhea (or both). Respiratory symptoms, which most frequently involved the upper respiratory tract, were seen in 322 of the positive DBPCFC (45%). Respiratory symptoms included nasal congestion, rhinorrhea, sneezing, tightness of the throat, hoarseness, or wheezing.

Virtually all symptoms secondary to the blinded food challenges developed between 5 minutes and 2 hours after initiating the challenge. Symptoms associated with the immediate response were generally abrupt in onset, marked, and lasted 1 to 2 hours. Several patients experienced a second episode of increased cutaneous pruritus and transient morbilliform rash 6 to 10 hours after the initial positive challenge. Symptoms associated with the late response were less prominent than the immediate symptoms and tended to last for several hours. Only one child (3 years of age) developed an isolated "delayed" reaction; a pruritic, erythematous rash developed approximately 4 hours after the child ingested egg.

Although many reports have suggested that children with atopic dermatitis are sensitive to a large number of foods, most patients (80%) developed symptoms to only one to three foods by DBPCFC. Most children in this study had positive prick skin tests to several foods (mean: 3.5; range: 0–10), although only about one-third of positive skin tests correlated with positive food challenges. One hundred sixty-nine children (36%) reacted to only one food,

122 (26%) reacted to two foods, 85 (18%) reacted to three foods, 47 (10%) reacted to four foods, and another 47 (10%) reacted to five or more different foods. Five foods (egg, peanut, milk, wheat, and soy) accounted for approximately 80% of the positive clinical responses (Table 11.4).

Allergic reactions to foods appear to be very specific. Although patients frequently have positive skin tests (and RASTs) to several members of a botanical family or animal species, indicating immunologic cross-reactivity, only two patients in one study had symptomatic intra-botanical cross-reactivity and only two subjects exhibited symptomatic intra-species cross-reactivity as determined by DBPCFC. Legume cross-reactivity was evaluated in 69 children with atopic dermatitis utilizing prick skin tests, in vitro measurements of specific IgE antibodies (immunodot blot), and Western blot analyses (64, 65). Although extensive immunologic cross-reactivity was demonstrated in many patients via these tests, only 2 patients proved symptomatic to more than one legume when challenged orally. Both of these patients had a history of severe allergic reactions to peanut and mild reactions to a soy challenge. In addition, both "outgrew" their reactivity to soy in 1 to 2 years. Similar studies with cereal grains showed significant IgE antibody cross-reactivity between grains and grass pollens but little clinical cross-reactivity (66). Consequently, the practice of avoiding all foods within a botanical family when one member is suspected of provoking allergic symptoms appears to be unwarranted.

As noted earlier, patients experiencing positive DBPCFCs develop a pruritic, morbilliform rash instead of the classical urticarial lesion. To demonstrate that the ingestion of food antigens led to IgE-medi-

Table 11.4

Five Major Food Allergens in 470 Patients with Atopic Dermatitis

Food	Challenge +	Hx +	Total	%
Egg	178	35	213	57
Milk	96	47	143	38
Peanut	28	82	110	29
Soy	55	4	59	16
Wheat	43	0	43	11

ated reactions, researchers sought markers of mast cell activation. Thirty-three patients undergoing DBPCFCs were monitored for changes in circulating plasma histamine (67). Histamine concentration was measured prior to initiating the challenge and following the ingestion of the test antigen. Following the blinded challenge, patients experiencing clinical symptoms developed a rise in their plasma histamine (mean: 296 ± 80 pg/mL to 1055 ± 356 pg/mL; $p <$ 0.001). As shown in Figure 11.1, subjects ingesting placebo or a food, which did not provoke clinical symptoms, had no demonstrable rise in their plasma histamine concentration.

Blood samples were also obtained to determine whether basophils had been activated during the challenge and were, therefore, contributing to the rise in plasma histamine. Samples were obtained prior to the challenge, both immediately following and 30 minutes after the development of the first objective symptoms (68). Each sample was evaluated for basophil number and total histamine content of the leukocyte preparation. No difference was observed in basophil number or total histamine content of the basophils at any time point. This finding suggests that circulating basophils do not account for the rise in plasma histamine observed.

Circulating food antigen–antibody complexes have been reported by several investigators (69–71). To rule out the possibility that mast cells were being activated by complement, a sensitive radioimmunoas-

say was used to quantitate C3a des-arg and C5a des-arg prior to DBPCFC and immediately, 15 minutes, and 30 minutes following the development of objective symptoms. Measurement of the anaphylatoxins, C3a and C5a, provides a sensitive indicator of complement activation (72). No significant change was observed in plasma C3a des-arg concentrations following positive DBPCFCs in 18 patients. C5a des-arg was undetectable in all samples examined (73). Thus, no evidence exists that the complement cascade is activated (or in turn activates mast cells) during allergic reactions to food in children experiencing positive challenges.

Studies utilizing the DBPCFC clearly demonstrate an immediate, IgE-mediated food hypersensitivity reaction in some children with atopic dermatitis. Under normal circumstances, such distinct reactions are rarely seen because foods are generally not ingested following prolonged avoidance of the food antigen and then taken in isolation on an empty stomach. The second onset of pruritus and rash in some children following DBPCFC suggests a "late-phase" component of an IgE-mediated response. Two food allergic patients who had experienced clearing of their eczema after maintaining an appropriate food allergen avoidance diet were rechallenged to establish that ingestion of an allergen during a DBPCFC could induce a late-phase response (73). Both patients developed a pruritic morbilliform skin rash within 30 to 60 minutes that cleared in 45 to 60 minutes. Skin biopsies obtained from the involved sites 4 and 14 hours later revealed an infiltration of eosinophils and deposition of major basic protein (MBP). The dermal infiltrate contained more eosinophils and less prominent MBP deposition than were seen with the chronic lesions. In three other food-allergic patients who had experienced clearing of their eczema after maintaining an appropriate food allergen avoidance diet, the author found a change in the "density profiles" of circulating eosinophils from normodense (nonactivated) to hypodense (activated) following a positive food challenge (74). Suomalainen *et al.* (75) found a rise in plasma ECP levels in milk-allergic children experiencing skin symptoms following a milk challenge, but not in children experiencing only gastrointestinal symptoms. These studies indicate that ingestion of a food allergen by an allergic patient leads

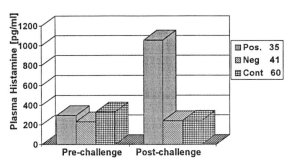

Figure 11.1

Mean plasma histamine levels in patients prior to and following DBPCFCs. Overall, 35 challenges were considered clinically positive and 101 negative. Of the negative DBPCFCs, 41 were negative to food allergens and 60 were negative to placebo.

to activation of circulating eosinophils, which may infiltrate the skin of patients with atopic dermatitis.

The exact pathogenic role of eosinophils in eczematous skin lesions remains to be established. Leiferman *et al.* evaluated skin biopsies from active AD lesions (36) and found MBP in the dermis of active skin lesions but not in skin with a normal appearance. Once recruited, eosinophils may release mediators (e.g., LTC_4), several cationic proteins (e.g., MBP, ECP, EDN) that contribute to the pathogenesis of the allergic reaction, and cytokines that may contribute to the inflammatory response (e.g., IL-1β, IL-6, TNF-α, MIP-1) or perpetuate chronic inflammation (e.g., IL-3, IL-5, GM-CSF) (76). MBP is toxic to many cell types and can cause histamine release from mast cells (77, 78). EDN, a powerful neurotoxin, may account for the demyelination of nerves in the dermal layer seen in eczematous skin. These and other mediators (e.g., leukotrienes, prostaglandins, and platelet-activating factor) have been reported as prominent in AD and support a pathogenic role for IgE-mediated late-phase reaction (73).

Children with atopic dermatitis and newly diagnosed food hypersensitivity have been found to have high "spontaneous" basophil histamine release (SBHR) from peripheral blood basophils in vitro compared with patients with atopic dermatitis and no food allergy, and normal controls (mean: 35.1% + 3.9% versus 1.8% + 0.2% versus 2.3% + 0.2%, $p < 0.001$) (68). When these food-allergic patients followed an appropriate elimination diet for at least 1 year, they experienced good clearing of their eczema and experienced a significant fall in SBHR (Fig. 11.2). Unstimulated peripheral blood mononuclear cells from food-allergic subjects with high SBHR produced a histamine-releasing factor in vitro that could activate basophils from other food-sensitive individuals, but not non-food-sensitive subjects. When food-allergic patients were maintained on an appropriate food allergen-free diet for 9 to 12 months, mononuclear cells no longer "spontaneously" generated HRF (Fig. 11.2). It was postulated that ingestion of food allergens leads to histamine-releasing factor production in vivo, which can then activate, or lower the "threshold" of activation, of mast cells. It could also account for the increased basophil "releasability" reported in some patients with atopic dermatitis (79, 80) and the

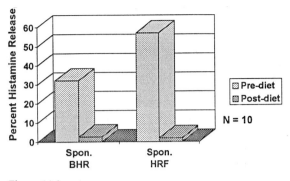

Figure 11.2

The mean percentage of "spontaneous" basophil histamine release (Spon. BHR) and "spontaneously" generated "histamine-releasing factor" (Spon. HRF) in 10 atopic dermatitis patients with food allergy prior to and approximately 1 year after the initiation of an appropriate allergen exclusion diet.

high SBHR seen in food-sensitive subjects in vitro. The loss of "spontaneously" generated histamine-releasing factor appeared to correlate with the loss of "cutaneous hyperreactivity" (increased pruritus due to a variety of minor stimuli such as heat, stress, or irritants) and inversely with the improvement in the patients' skin.

Several investigators have demonstrated an influx of mononuclear cells in tissue biopsies from eczematous lesions—primarily CD4+ Th2-type lymphocytes (81). It has also been shown that T cells migrating into skin blisters overlying cutaneous delayed-type hypersensitivity reactions are highly enriched for the homing receptor, "cutaneous lymphocyte antigen" (CLA), whereas lymphocytes isolated from the lungs of asthmatics are predominantly CLA-negative (82). Thus, the propensity to develop AD may depend on the skin- or lung-seeking characteristics of memory T cells. Peripheral blood mononuclear cells (PBMCs) from 7 AD patients with milk allergy, 10 with milk-induced gastroenteropathies, and 8 normal controls were stimulated in vitro with casein and then evaluated for expression of homing receptors (83). As seen in Figure 11.3, only patients with atopic dermatitis and milk allergy demonstrated a significant increase in CLA+ T cells, suggesting that the homing receptor expression on antigen-specific T cells plays a role in

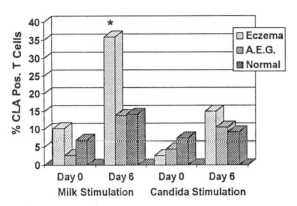

Figure 11.3

Milk-allergic patients with atopic dermatitis have significantly increased numbers of lymphocytes bearing the "cutaneous lymphocyte antigen" (CLA) in vitro compared with patients having gastrointestinal milk allergy and normal controls. No similar increase is observed in CLA+ cells to an irrelevant antigen, *Candida albicans*.

determining which tissues are involved in allergic responses.

Diagnosing Food Hypersensitivity in Patients with Atopic Dermatitis

As discussed elsewhere, the oral DBPCFC is the "gold standard" for diagnosing food hypersensitivity and is essential for clinical research. In an office practice, a 2- to 3-week trial elimination diet may be implemented if a few foods are suspected after obtaining a careful history and evidence of food antigen-specific IgE antibodies (e.g., through prick skin tests or RASTs). Symptoms are recorded in a diary during the trial period. If unequivocal improvement is documented, foods believed least likely to be responsible (e.g., foods other than egg, peanut, milk, soy, and wheat) are added back to the diet. Any food suspected of causing a severe anaphylactic reaction should never be administered at home, however, because of its potential for inducing anaphylactic shock (84). If a clear deterioration in the patient's atopic dermatitis should occur, the food should be removed from the diet. If cause and effect can be established in this manner, the patient should remain on the avoidance diet unless it requires elimination of more than one "major" food (egg, milk, soy, wheat) or two or more "minor" foods (all others). If severe symptoms persist on the elimination diet and food allergy remains in question, a brief trial (1 to 2 weeks) of a severely restricted diet may be undertaken. If elimination diet results are equivocal or several foods are implicated, blinded oral food challenges should be performed once the patient's symptoms have been sufficiently cleared (this process may require hospitalization) to establish the diagnosis. Multiple dietary restrictions are rarely necessary. Other modalities for diagnosis of food hypersensitivity, such as sublingual provocation with drops of antigen extracts, subcutaneous provocation with varying concentrations of food extracts, and measurements of IgG or IgG4 specific antibody, have never been shown to be useful or effective in controlled studies (85).

In a recent study (submitted), the author compared the outcome of DBPCFCs in 196 patients with atopic dermatitis and food allergy to specific levels of food antigen-specific IgE as determined by the Pharmacia CAP System RAST FEIA. As shown in Table 11.5, concentrations of food antigen-specific IgE antibody were found above when patients had a likelihood greater than 95% of experiencing a positive food challenge—that is, positive predictive value (PPV). Patients with egg, milk, peanut, or fish-specific IgE concentrations exceeding the 95% PPV may not need to be challenged to diagnose food allergy. Patients with specific IgE values less than the 95% PPV may still react to the food in question, as indicated by the low sensitivity of the test at this value. A food challenge would, therefore, be necessary to establish the diagnosis. As shown in Table 11.5, even at IgE

Table 11.5
Pharmacia CAP-RAST 95% Positive
Predictive Accuracy Values

Food	Cut-off	Sensitivity	Specificity
Egg	5.5 U/mL	61%	92%
Milk	31.5 U/mL	51%	98%
Peanut	15.0 U/mL	73%	92%
Fish	19.5 U/mL	40%	99%

Wheat > 100 IU/mL = 60% PPV
Soy > 100 IU/mL < 50% PPV

levels greater than 100 IU/mL, the 95% PPVs for wheat and soy are never attained.

Once food hypersensitivity is diagnosed, therapy is straightforward. The patient is placed on a diet meticulously eliminating all forms of the offending food allergen. Instructing the patient and family to read food labels to avoid "hidden" sources of the suspect food is critical. While antihistamines and epinephrine may modify the symptoms of an immediate food hypersensitivity reaction after an accidental ingestion, they have no prophylactic role in the treatment of food allergy. Although some investigators advocate prevention of food allergen-induced symptoms with oral cromolyn, a controlled, blinded trial of oral cromolyn in patients with "challenge-proven" food hypersensitivity demonstrated no benefit (86). Treatment of food hypersensitivity with oral desensitization, immunotherapy, and rotational diets also has not been proven effective in controlled trials.

With the initiation of an appropriate food allergen elimination diet, food-allergic patients generally experience significant improvement in their eczematous symptoms. In follow-up over 3 to 4 years, such patients typically have significant improvement in their clinical symptoms compared with patients without food allergy or who fail to comply with the allergen elimination diet (87) (Fig. 11.4). In addition, several immunologic parameters normalize—that is, there is loss of "spontaneous" basophil histamine release, loss of "spontaneous" generation of histamine-releasing factor, normalization of circulating eosinophil (74) and basophil (88) activation, decrease in total serum IgE levels (87), and, in many cases, loss of clinical food reactivity.

Natural History of Food Hypersensitivity in Atopic Dermatitis

Approximately one-third of children with atopic dermatitis and food allergy "lost" (or "outgrew") their clinical reactivity over a period of 1 to 3 years (87). Three factors appeared to have the greatest importance in determining the probability of patients losing their clinical reactivity: the food to which the patient was allergic (i.e., patients allergic to peanuts, nuts,

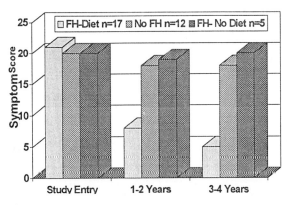

Figure 11.4

Food-allergic, atopic dermatitis patients placed on an appropriate food allergen elimination diet (FH-Diet) experienced significant improvement in their eczema over 3 to 4 years follow-up compared with atopic dermatitis patients without food allergy (no FH) and food-allergic, atopic dermatitis who did not maintain their food allergen elimination diet (no Diet).

fish, and shellfish were unlikely to lose their clinical reactivity, whereas those allergic to soy, wheat, milk, and egg were much more likely to develop clinical tolerance); the level of specific IgE antibody to a particular food (i.e., the higher the level of food antigen-specific IgE, the less likely that clinical tolerance would develop in the subsequent few years [88]); and the degree to which the patient adhered to the elimination diet (i.e., patients ingesting small amounts of allergen or having frequent accidental ingestions were less likely to develop clinical tolerance). Prick skin test results did not correlate with loss of clinical reactivity and remained positive for 5 or more years after the food had been reintroduced into the diet. Therefore, it is recommended that patients be rechallenged intermittently (e.g., egg: every 2–3 years; milk, soy, wheat: every 1–2 years; foods other than peanut, nuts, fish, and shellfish: every 1–2 years) to determine whether their food allergies persist, so that restriction diets may be discontinued as soon as possible. No patient had a recurrence of allergic symptoms or worsening of eczema once food hypersensitivity was "lost." The immunologic changes associated with loss of symptomatic food hypersensitivity are under intensive study.

Prevention of Food Hypersensitivity and Atopic Dermatitis

Prevention of allergic disease by manipulation of the infant's diet and environment has generated intense interest. Since Grulee and Sanford reported a decrease in the incidence of atopic dermatitis in breast-fed infants in the 1930s (89), numerous conflicting reports have surfaced about the relative benefit of breast-feeding infants to prevent or delay the onset of atopic disease (90–92). The potential benefit of breast feeding is complicated by transmission of food antigens in maternal breast milk (93, 94). Six infants (aged 2.5 to 6 months) who developed classic infantile atopic dermatitis while being exclusively breast-fed were evaluated. All infants had positive prick skin tests to egg and showed complete clearing of their skin when their mothers' egg-containing foods were completely excluded from their diet. Four of the six infants were challenged on the research unit by first feeding eggs to their mothers and then having the mothers breast-feed their babies. Each infant developed an eczematoid rash within 4 to 36 hours after its mother ingested eggs. This evidence and findings from other studies support the recommendation of placing selected mothers on diets that avoid highly allergenic foods during the period of lactation.

Several investigators have evaluated the effect of eliminating certain foods from the maternal diet during lactation (95–97). In two series, infants from atopic families whose mothers excluded egg, milk, and fish from their diets during (prophylaxis group) lactation had significantly less atopic dermatitis and food allergy at 18 months compared with infants whose mothers' diets were unrestricted (98, 99). At 4 years, the prophylaxis group had less atopic dermatitis, but no difference was observed in food allergy or respiratory allergy (99) (Fig. 11.5). A study by Lindfors and Enocksson (100) has also suggested a possibility of developing high dose tolerance. These investigators concluded that initial and early regular feedings with a cow's milk formula, followed by a gradual replacement with prolonged breast feeding, reduced the development of allergic symptoms in 112 infants in the first 18 months of age to 18%, com-

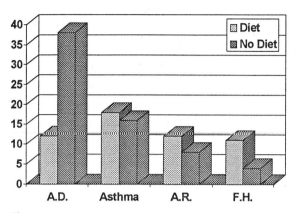

Figure 11.5

Infants from atopic families whose mothers eliminated egg, milk, and fish during lactation had less atopic dermatitis at 4 years compared with similar infants whose mothers had no dietary restrictions during lactation (99). No similar decrease was seen for asthma, allergic rhinitis, or food allergy.

pared with 33% in the 104 exclusively breast-fed infant group.

A prospective, nonrandomized study of 1265 unselected neonates evaluated the effect of solid food introduction over a 10-year period (101, 102). A significant linear relationship was found between the number of solid foods introduced into the diet by 4 months of age and subsequent atopic dermatitis, with a threefold increase in recurrent eczema noted at 10 years of age in infants receiving four or more solid foods compared with infants receiving no solid foods prior to 4 months of age. No relationship was found between asthma and the introduction of solid foods. A prospective, nonrandomized study comparing breast-fed infants who first received solid foods at 3 months or 6 months of age revealed reduced atopic dermatitis and food allergy at 1 year of age in the group avoiding solids for the 6-month period (103), but no significant difference in these parameters at 5 years (104). As neither series randomized patients, these studies must be considered suggestive until an appropriate randomized trial confirms the benefit of delaying solid food introduction.

In the most comprehensive, prospective, randomized allergy prevention trial, Zeiger *et al.* compared the benefits of maternal and infant food allergen avoidance on the prevention of allergic disease in infants at high risk for such disease (105–108). Breast feeding was encouraged in both prophylaxis and control groups. In the prophylaxis group, the diets of lactating mothers were restricted in terms of egg, cow milk, and peanut, a casein hydrolysate formula was utilized for supplementation or weaning, and solid food introduction was delayed. The control infants received a cow's milk formula for supplementation and the American Academy of Pediatrics recommendations for infant feeding were followed (peanuts, nuts, and fish are not recommended in the first 2 years). The prevalence of food allergy, cow's milk sensitization, and atopic dermatitis in the prophylaxis group were reduced significantly during the first 2 years compared with the control group, but no significant differences were observed in the period prevalence of atopic dermatitis beyond 2 years. The cumulative prevalence of food allergy remained lower in the prophylaxis group when followed up at 4 and 7 years. The investigators concluded that maternal and infant food allergen avoidance compared with standard feeding practices reduces food allergy and atopic dermatitis in the first 2 years, but failed to modify allergic disease prevalence after 2 years of age. Consequently, they suggested that the benefits of food allergy preventive measures have limited duration because of the frequent remission of food allergy in early childhood (108).

Because studies to date are inconclusive, it is difficult to make firm recommendations regarding prevention strategies for food allergy and atopic dermatitis. In families at high risk for atopic disorders, however, it would seem prudent to avoid exposing young infants to food allergens that provoke "lifelong" sensitization (e.g., peanuts, nuts, fish, shellfish) for the first 2 to 3 years of life. In highly motivated, "high-risk" families, avoidance of cow milk for the first year and egg for the first 2 years may prevent some atopic dermatitis and food allergy. It might also be wise for mothers of such "high-risk" infants to avoid peanuts, nuts, fish, and shellfish while breast feeding, and perhaps even during the third trimester of pregnancy, as these foods do not generally constitute a major part of most diets. Whether all lactating mothers in "high-risk" families should avoid milk and eggs remains an open question.

Other Nutritional Factors Implicated in the Pathogenesis of Atopic Dermatitis

More than 50 years ago, Hansen (109) reported that essential fatty acid levels were depressed in the blood of patients with atopic dermatitis and that supplementation with corn oil (high in linoleic acid) resulted in improvement of the eczema. Conflicting reports followed (110–112), but the advent of topical steroids displaced this form of therapy. Interest was renewed when two studies (113, 114) demonstrated the beneficial effect of administering evening primrose oil, which is rich in cis-linoleic acid (18:2n6) and gamma-linolenic acid (18:3n6). Human breast milk is also rich in linoleic and gamma-linolenic acids, and claims have been made that its beneficial effect on infantile eczema relates to the presence of these essential fatty acids (115, 116). The purported beneficial effect is secondary to changes in arachidonic metabolism brought about by normalization of fatty acid levels. Studies disagree on whether these levels differ in patients with atopic dermatitis compared with normal controls (117, 118). A large-scale study conducted in the United States could demonstrate no beneficial effects from evening primrose oil (119). A study with fish oil supplementation (120) claimed mild beneficial effects, but its evidence was unconvincing.

Decreased concentration of selenium in the whole blood of patients with atopic dermatitis has been reported (121) and the possibility of benefits from supplementation was suggested. A recent study could find no difference in total-body exchangeable and plasma selenium concentrations, nor did it identify a difference in selenium pharmacokinetics in atopic dermatitis patients compared with normal controls (122). In children with biotinidase deficiency, cutaneous manifestations resemble those noted with atopic dermatitis (123). A recent study reported depressed biotinidase activity in four children with atopic dermatitis (and no neurological symptoms) who responded to oral biotin treatment (124). Further studies on the role of biotinidase activity in children with atopic dermatitis are necessary before this form of therapy can be recommended.

Several investigators have reported abnormal absorption of non-metabolizable sugars in some children with atopic dermatitis, indicating abnormal gut permeability in these patients (125, 126). In children with atopic dermatitis, all subjects with food hypersensitivity confirmed by DBPCFC were found to have abnormal lactulose absorption (127) that normalized when the responsible allergen was eliminated from the diet. Similarly, Dupont and colleagues (128) demonstrated a threefold rise in the lactulose/mannitol urinary ratio in atopic dermatitis patients following a positive oral allergen provocation test. These studies indicate that gastrointestinal changes (often subclinical) are present in most children with atopic dermatitis and food hypersensitivity; they may also account for the low percentile weights seen in many children with atopic dermatitis.

Conclusion

Despite years of debate, it is now apparent that food hypersensitivity plays a significant pathogenic role in atopic dermatitis in as many as one-third (58) of children with atopic dermatitis. The significance of food allergy in adults with atopic dermatitis remains to be established, however. The study of this subset of atopic dermatitis patients with food-induced inflammation should provide an excellent human model with which to study the IgE-mediated hypersensitivity reaction.

REFERENCES

1. Blaylock WK. Atopic dermatitis: diagnosis and pathobiology. J Allergy Clin Immunol 1976;57:62–79.
2. Hill LW, Sulzberger MG. Evaluation of atopic dermatitis. Arch Dermatol Syph 1935;32:451–463.
3. Hanifin JM, Rajka G. Diagnostic features of atopic dermatitis. Acta Dermatol Venereol 1980;92(suppl):44–47.
4. European Task Force on Atopic Dermatitis. Severity scoring of atopic dermatitis: the SCORAD index. Dermatology 1993;186:23–31.
5. Hanifin JM. Atopic dermatitis. In: Middleton E, Reed CE, Ellis EF, Adkinson NF, Yunginger JW, eds. Allergy: principles and practice. St. Louis: C.V. Mosby, 1988, 1404.
6. Besnier E. Premiere note et observations preliminaries pour sevir d'introduction a l'etude des pruriqos diathesiques. Ann de Dermatol Syphil 1892;23:634–637.
7. Wise F, Sulzberger MB. Yearbook of dermatology and syphilology. Chicago: Yearbook Medical Publishers, 1933, 59.
8. Hanifin JM. Epidemiology of atopic dermatitis. Monographs in Allergy 1987;21:116–131.
9. Sampson HA. Atopic dermatitis. Ann Allergy 1992;69:469–481.
10. Hoffman DR, Yamamoto FY, Sellar B, Haddad Z. Diagnosis of IgE-mediated reactions to food antigens by radioimmunoassay. Clin Immunol 1975;55:256–267.
11. Johnson E, Irons J, Patterson R, Roberts M. Serum IgE concentration in atopic dermatitis. J Allergy Clin Immunol 1974;54:94–99.
12. NIAID Task Force Report: Dermatologic Allergy. Asthma and the Other Allergic Diseases. NIH Publication #79-387, May 1979, 375.
13. Pasternack B. The prediction of asthma in infantile eczema. J Pediatr 1965;66:164–165.
14. Stifler WC. A twenty-one year follow-up of infantile eczema. J Pediatr 1965;66:166–167.
15. Saarinin UM. Transfer of latent atopy by bone marrow transplantation? A case report. J Allergy Clin Immunol 1984;74:196–200.
16. Agosti JM, Sprenger JD, Lum LG, et al. Transfer of allergen-specific IgE-mediated hypersensitivity with allogeneic bone marrow transplantation. N Engl J Med 1988;319:1623–1627.
17. Saurat J-H. Eczema in primary immune-deficiencies. Acta Derm Venereol (Stockh) 1985;114:125–128.
18. Tong AKF, Mihm MC. The pathology of atopic dermatitis. Clin Rev Allergy 1986;4:27–42.
19. Mudde G, van Reijsen F, Boland G, de Gast G, Bruijnzeel P, Bruijnzeel-Koomen C. Allergen presentation by epidermal Langerhans cells from patients with atopic dermatitis is mediated by IgE. Immunol 1990;69:335–341.
20. Mudde G, Bheekha R, Bruijnzeel-Koomen C. Consequences of IgE/CD23-mediated antigen presentation in allergy. Immunol Today 1995;16:380–383.
21. Dolovich J, Hargreave FE, Chalmers R, et al. Late cutaneous allergic responses in isolated IgE-dependent reactions. J Allergy Clin Immunol 1973;52:38–46.
22. Solley GO, Gleich GJ, Jordan RE, Schroeter AL. Late phase of the immediate wheal and flare skin reaction: its dependence on IgE antibodies. J Clin Invest 1976;58:408–420.
23. Atkins PC, Zweiman B. The IgE-mediated late-phase skin response-unraveling the enigma. J Allergy Clin Immunol 1987;79:12–15.
24. Gleich GJ. The late phase of the immunoglobulin E-mediated reactions: a link between anaphylaxis and common allergic disease? J Allergy Clin Immunol 1982;70:160–163.
25. Gell P, Coombs R. Classification of allergic reactions responsible for hypersensitivity and disease. In: Gell P, Coombs R, Lachmann P, eds. Clinical aspects of immunology. Oxford: Blackwell, 1975, 761–781.
26. Spiegelberg HL. Structure and function of Fc receptors for IgE on lymphocytes, monocytes and macrophages. Adv Immunol 1984;35:61–88.

27. Joseph M, Capron A, Ameisen J-C, et al. The receptors for IgE on blood platelets. Eur J Immunol 1986;16:306–312.

28. Capron M, Capron A, Joseph M. IgE receptors on phagocytic cells and immune response to Schistosome infection. Monogra Allergy 1983;18:33–44.

29. Bruynzeel-Kooman C, VanWicker DF, Toonstra J, et al. The presence of IgE molecules on epidermal Langerhans cells in patients with atopic dermatitis. Arch Dermatol Res 1986;297:199–205.

30. Hamid Q, Boguniewicz M, Leung DYM. Differential in situ cytokine gene expression in acute versus chronic atopic dermatitis. J Clin Invest 1994;94:870–876.

31. Tsicopoulos A, Hamid Q, Varney V, Ying S, Moqbel R, Durham S, et al. Preferential messenger RNA expression of Th-1-type cells (IFN-gamma, IL-2) in classical delayed-type (tuberculin) hypersensitivity reactions in human skin. J Immunol 1992;148:2058–2061.

32. Wakita H, Sakamoto T, Tokura Y, Takigawa M. E-selectin and vascular cell adhesion molecule-1 as critical adhesion molecules for infiltration of T lymphocytes and eosinophils in atopic dermatitis. J Cutan Pathol 1994;21:33–39.

33. Barker J, MacDonald D. Epidermal class II human lymphocyte antigen expression in atopic dermatitis: a comparison with experimental allergic contact dermatitis. J Am Acad Dermatol 1987;16:1175–1179.

34. Gleich GJ, Frigas E, Loegering DA, et al. Cytotoxic properties of eosinophilic major basic protein. J Immunol 1979;123:2925–2927.

35. O'Donnell MC, Ackerman SJ, Gleich GJ, Thomas LL. Activation of basophil and mast cell histamine release by eosinophil granule major basic protein. J Exp Med 1983;157:1981–1991.

36. Leiferman KM, Ackerman SJ, Sampson HA, et al. Dermal deposition of eosinophil granule major basic protein in atopic dermatitis. Comparison with onchocerciasis. N Engl J Med 1985;313:282–285.

37. Schloss OM. Allergy to common foods. Trans Am Pediatr Soc 1915;27:62–68.

38. Talbot FB. Eczema in childhood. Med Clinics N Am 1918;1:985–996.

39. Blackfan KD. A consideration of certain aspects of protein hypersensitiveness in children. Am J Med Sci 1920;160:341–350.

40. Flood JM, Perry DJ. Role of food allergy in eczematoid dermatitis. Arch Dermatol Syph 1947;55:493–506.

41. Rowe A, Rowe AH. Atopic dermatitis in infants and children. J Pediatr 1951;39:80–86.

42. Cooke RA. A consideration of some allergy problems I. Allergic dermatitis (eczema). J Allergy 1944;15:203–211.

43. Freedman SS. Milk allergy in infantile atopic eczema. Am J Dis Child 1961;102:76–81.

44. Holt LE. Conference on infantile eczema. Some challenge studies with foods. J Pediatr 1965;66:235–241.

45. Meara RH. Skin reactions in atopic eczema. Br J Dermatol 1955;67:60–64.

46. Brunner M, Walzer M. Absorption of undigested proteins in human beings: the absorption of unaltered fish protein in adults. Arch Intern Med 1928;42:173–179.

47. Wilson SJ, Walzer M. Absorption of undigested proteins in human beings. IV. Absorption of unaltered egg protein in infants. Am J Dis Child 1935;50:49–54.

48. Walzer M. Absorption of allergens. J Allergy 1942;13:554–562.

49. Engman WF, Weiss RS, Engman MF. Eczema and environment. Med Clin N Am 1936;20:651–663.

50. Hammar H. Provocation with cow's milk and cereals in atopic dermatitis. Acta Dermato Vener (Stockh) 1977;57:159–163.

51. David TJ, Waddington E, Staton RHJ. Nutritional hazards of elimination diets in children with atopic eczema. Arch Dis Child 1984;59:323–325.

52. Atherton DJ, Soothill JF, Sewell M, Wells RS, Chilvers CED. A double-blind controlled crossover trial of an antigen-avoidance diet in atopic eczema. Lancet 1978;1:401–403.

53. Neild VS, Marsden RA, Bailes JA, Bland JM. Egg and milk exclusion diets in atopic eczema. Br J Dermatol 1986;114:117–123.

54. Juto P, Engberg S, Winberg J. Treatment of infantile atopic dermatitis with a strict elimination diet. Clinical Allergy 1978;8:493–500.

55. Hill DJ, Lynch BC. Elemental diet in the management of severe eczema in childhood. Clin Allergy 1982;12:313–315.

56. Munkvad M, Danielsen L, Hoj L, Povlsen CO, et al. Acta Derm Venereol (Stockh) 1984;64:524–528.

57. Bock SA, Lee WY, Remigio LK, May CD. Studies of hypersensitivity reactions to foods in infants and children. J Allergy Clin Immunol 1978;62:327–334.

58. Burks AW, Mallory SB, Williams LW, Shirrell MA. Atopic dermatitis: clinical relevance of food hypersensitivity reactions. J Pediatr 1988;113:447–451.

59. Sampson HA. Role of immediate food hypersensitivity in the pathogenesis of atopic dermatitis. J Allergy Clin Immunol 1983;71:473–480.

60. Sampson HA, McCaskill CM. Food hypersensitivity and atopic dermatitis: evaluation of 113 patients. J of Pediatr 1985;107:669–675.

61. Sampson HA. Atopic dermatitis. Ann Allergy 1992;69:469–481.

62. Jones SM, Sampson HA. The role of allergens in atopic dermatitis. Clinical Reviews in Allergy 1993;11:471–490.

63. Leinhas JL, McCaskill C, Sampson HA. Food allergy challenges: guidelines and implications. J Am Dietetic Assoc 1987;87:604–608.

64. Broadbent JB, Sampson HA. Cross-allergenicity in the legume botanical family in children with food hypersensitivity. J Allergy Clin Immunol 1989;83:435–440.

65. Bernhisel-Broadbent J, Taylor SL, Sampson HA. Cross-allergenicity in the Legume botanical family in children with food hypersensitivity. II. Laboratory correlates. J Allergy Clin Immunol 1989;84:701–709.

66. Jones SM, Magnolfi CF, Cooke SK, Sampson HA. Immunologic cross-reactivity among cereal grains and grasses in children with food hypersensitivity. J Allergy Clin Immunol 1995;96:341–351.

67. Sampson HA, Jolie PL. Increased plasma histamine concentrations after food challenges in children with atopic dermatitis. N Engl J Med 1984;311:372–376.

68. Sampson HA, Broadbent KR, Bernhisel-Broadbent J. "Spontaneous" basophil histamine release and histamine releasing factor in patients with atopic dermatitis and food hypersensitivity. N Engl J Med 1989;321:228–232.

69. Paganelli R, Levinsky RJ, Brostoff J, Wraith DG. Immune complexes containing food proteins in normal and atopic subjects after oral challenge and effect of sodium cromoglycate on antigen absorption. Lancet 1979;1:1270–1272.

70. Brostoff J, Carini C, Wraith DG, Johns P. Production of IgE complexes by allergen challenge in atopic patients and the effect of sodium cromoglycate. Lancet 1979;1:1268–1272.

71. Paganelli R, Atherton DJ, Levinsky R. Differences between normal and milk allergic subjects in their immune responses after milk ingestion. Arch Dis Child 1983;58:201–206.

72. Chenowith DE, Hugli TE. Biologically active peptides of complement: techniques and significance of C3a and C5a measurement. In: Nakamura RM, Tucker ES, eds. Immunoassays: Clinical Laboratory Techniques for the 1980's. New York: Alan R. Liss, 1981, 443–461

73. Sampson HA. The role of food allergy and mediator release in atopic dermatitis. J Allergy Clin Immunol 1988;81:635–645.

74. Jones SM, Cooke SB, Sampson HA. Alteration in eosinophil activation in food allergic children with atopic dermatitis. Pediatr Allergy Immunol (submitted).

75. Suomalainen H, Soppi E, Isolauri E. Evidence for eosinophil activation in cow's milk allergy. Pediatr Allergy Immunol 1994;5:27–31.

76. Gleich GJ, Leiferman KM. Eosinophils and hypersensitivity disease. In: Reed CE, ed. Proceedings of the XII International Congress of Allergology and Clinical Immunology. St. Louis: C.V. Mosby 1986, 124–130.

77. Leiferman KM, Peters MS, Gleich GJ. The eosinophil and cutaneous edema. J Am Acad Dermatol 1986;15:513–517.

78. Gleich GJ, Frigas E, Loegering DA, Wassom DL, Steinmuller D. Cytotoxic properties of eosinophil major basic protein. J Immunol 1979;123:2925–2927.

79. Marone G, Giugliano R, Lembo G, Ayala F. Human basophil releasability. II. Changes in basophil releasability in patients with atopic dermatitis. J Invest Dermatol 1986;87:19–23.

80. James JM, Kagey-Sobotka A, Sampson HA. Severe atopic dermatitis patients have activated circulating basophils. J Allergy Clin Immunol 1993;91:1155–1162.

81. Leung DYM. Atopic dermatitis: the skin as a window into the pathogenesis of chronic allergic diseases. J Allergy Clin Immunol 1995;96:302–318.

82. Picker LJ, Martin RJ, Trumble A, Newman LS, Collins PA, Bergstresser PR, et al. Differential expression of lymphocyte homing receptors by human memory/effector T cells in pulmonary versus cutaneous immune effector sites. Eur J Immunol 1994;24:1269–1277.

83. Abernathy-Carver K, Sampson H, Picker L, Leung D. Milk-induced eczema is associated with the expansion of T cells expressing cutaneous lymphocyte antigen. J Clin Invest 1995;95:913–918.

84. David TJ. Anaphylactic shock during elimination diets for severe atopic dermatitis. Arch Dis Child 1984;59:983–986.

85. Reisman RE. American Academy of Allergy position statement controversial techniques. J Allergy Clin Immunol 1981;67:333–338.

86. Burks AW, Sampson HA. Double-blind placebo-controlled trial of oral cromolyn sodium in children with documented food hypersensitivity. J Allergy Clin Immunol 1988;77:417–423.

87. Sampson HA, Scanlon S. Natural history of food hypersensitivity in children with atopic dermatitis. J Pediatr 1989;115:23–27.

88. James JM, Sampson HA. Immunologic changes associated with the development of tolerance in children with cow's milk allergy. J Pediatr 1992;121:371–377.

89. Grulee CG, Sanford HN. The influence of breast and artificial feeding on infantile eczema. J Pediatr 1936;9:223–225.

90. Kramer MS, Moroz B. Do breast-feeding and delayed introduction of solid food protect against subsequent atopic eczema? J Pediatr 1981;98:546–550.

91. Chandra RK, Puri S, Cheema PS. Predictive value of cord blood IgE in the development of atopic disease and role of breast-feeding in its prevention. Clin Allergy 1985;15:517–522.

92. Van Asperen PP, Kemp AS, Mellis CM. Relationship of diet in the development of atopy in infancy. Clin Allergy 1984;14:525–532.

93. Jakobsson I, Lindberg T, Benediktsson B, et al. Dietary bovine β-lactoglobulin is transferred to human milk. Acta Pediatr Scand 1985;74:342–345.

94. Husby S, Jensenius J, Svehag S. Passage of undegraded dietary antigen into the blood of healthy adults. Quantification, estimation of size distribution and relation of uptake to levels of specific antibodies. Scand J Immunol 1985;22:83–92.

95. Host A. Cow's milk protein allergy and intolerance in infancy. Pediatr Allergy Immunol 1994;5:5–36.

96. Zeiger RS. Development and prevention of allergic disease in childhood. In: Middleton E, Reed C, Ellis E, Adkinson N, Yunginger J, Busse W, eds. Allergy: principles and practice. 4th ed. St. Louis: Mosby, 1993, 1137–1171.

97. Chandra R, Shakuntla P, Hamed A. Influence of maternal diet during lactation and use of formula feeds on development of atopic eczema in high risk infants. Br Med J 1989;299:228–230.

98. Hattevig G, Kjellman B, Bjorksten B, Kjellman N. Effect of maternal avoidance of eggs, cow's milk and fish during lactation upon allergic manifestations in infants. Clin Exper Allergy 1989;19:27–32.

99. Sigurs N, Hattevig G, Kjellman B. Maternal avoidance of eggs, cow's milk, and fish during lactation: effect on allergic manifestation, skin-prick tests, and specific IgE antibodies in children at age 4 years. Pediatr 1992;89:735–739.

100. Lindfors A, Enocksson E. Development of atopic disease after early administration of cow milk formula. Allergy 1988;43:11–16.

101. Fergusson D, Horwood L, Shannon F. Asthma and infant diet. Arch Dis Child 1983;58:48–51.

102. Fergusson DM, Horwood LJ, Shannon FT. Early solid feeding and recurrent eczema: a 10-year longitudinal study. Pediatrics 1990;86:541–546.

103. Kajosaari M, Saarinen UM. Prophylaxis of atopic disease by six months; total solid food elimination. Arch Paediatr Scand 1983;72:411–414.

104. Kajosaari M. Atopy prophylaxis in high-risk infants: prospective 5-year follow-up study of children with six months exclusive breastfeeding and solid food elimination. Adv Exp Med Biol 1991;310:453–458.

105. Zeiger R, Heller S, Mellon M, Forsythe A, O'Connor R, Hamburger R. Effect of combined maternal and infant food-allergen avoidance on development of atopy in early infancy: a randomized study. J Allergy Clin Immunol 1989;84:72–89.

106. Zeiger R. Prevention of food allergy in infancy. Ann Allergy 1990;65:430–441.

107. Zeiger R, Heller S, Mellon M, Halsey J, Hamburger R, Sampson H. Genetic and environmental factors affecting the development of atopy through age 4 in children of atopic parents: a prospective randomized study of food allergen avoidance. Pediatr Allergy Immunol 1992;3:110–127.

108. Zeiger R, Heller S. The development and prediction of atopy

in high-risk children: follow-up at seven years in a prospective randomized study of combined maternal and infant food allergen avoidance. J Allergy Clin Immunol 1995;95:1179–1190.

109. Hansen AE. Serum lipid changes and therapeutic effects of various oils in infantile eczema. Proc Soc Exp Biol Med 1933;31:160–161.

110. Cornbleet T. Use of maize oil (unsaturated fatty acids) in the treatment of eczema. Arch Dermatol Syphilol 1935;31:224–226.

111. Finnerud CW, Kesler RL, Weise HF. Ingestion of lard in the treatment of eczema and allied dermatoses. Arch Dermatol Syphilol 1941;44:849–861.

112. Taub SJ, Zakon SJ. Use of unsaturated fatty acids in the treatment of eczema. JAMA 1935;105:1675.

113. Lovell CR, Burton JL, Horrobin DF. Treatment of atopic dermatitis with evening primrose oil. Lancet 1981;1:278.

114. Wright S, Burton JL. Evening primrose seed oil improves atopic eczema. Lancet 1982;2:1120–1122.

115. Matthew DJ, Taylor B, Norman AP, et al. Prevention of eczema. Lancet 1977;1:321–324.

116. Chandra RK. Prospective studies of the effect of breast feeding on the incidence of infection and allergy. Acta Paed Scand 1979;68:691–694.

117. Manku MS, Horrobin DF, Morse NL, et al. Essential fatty acids in the plasma phospholipids of patients with atopic eczema. Br J Dermatol 1984;110:643–648.

118. Schalin-Karrila M, Mattila L, Jansen CT, Uotila P. Evening primrose oil in the treatment of atopic eczema: effect on clinical status, plasma phospholipid fatty acids and circulating blood prostaglandins. Br J Dermatol 1987;117:11–19.

119. Bamford JTM, Gibson RW, Renier CM. Atopic eczema unresponsive to evening primrose oil. J Am Acad Dermatol 1985;13:959–965.

120. Bjorneboe A, Soyland E, Bjorneboe GA, et al. Effect of dietary supplementation with eicosapentaenoic acid in the treatment of atopic dermatitis. Br J Dermatol 1987;117:463–469.

121. Hinks LJ, Young S, Clayton B. Trace element status in eczema and psoriasis. Clin Exp Dermatol 1987;12:93–97.

122. Fairris GM, Perkins PJ, Lawson AD, Blake GM. The pharmacokinetics of selenium in psoriasis and atopic dermatitis. Acta Derm Venereol 1988;68:434–436.

123. Wolf B, Grier RE, Allen RJ, et al. Phenotypic variation in biotinidase deficiency. J Pediatr 1983;103:233–236.

124. Iikura Y, Odajima Y, Nagakura T, et al. Oral biotin treatment is effective for atopic dermatitis in children with low biotinidase activity. Acta Paediatr Scand 1988;77:762–763.

125. Jackson PG, Baker RWR, Lessof MH, et al. Intestinal permeability in patients with eczema and food allergy. Lancet 1981;1:1285–1286.

126. Pike MG, Heddle RJ, Boulton P, et al. Increased intestinal permeability in atopic eczema. J Invest Dermatol 1986;86:101–104.

127. Flick JA, Sampson HA, Perman JA. Intestinal permeability to carbohydrates in children with atopic dermatitis and food hypersensitivity. Pediatr Res 1988;23:303A.

128. Dupont C, Barau E, Molkhou P, et al. Food-induced alterations of intestinal permeability in children with cow's milk sensitive enteropathy and atopic dermatitis. J Pediatr Gastroenterology Nutr 1989;8:459–465.

12

FOOD-INDUCED URTICARIA

Fred M. Atkins

Urticaria, a common skin reaction pattern occurring at some time in the life of approximately 15% to 20% of the population, is characterized by transient erythematous, well-demarcated, raised skin lesions that may exhibit central clearing and that are usually intensely pruritic (1). The lesions result from inflammatory reactions that cause localized transudation of fluid from dilated small blood vessels and capillaries in the superficial dermis. Individual urticarial lesions are short-lived, rarely persisting longer than 24 hours; new lesions may continue to develop and subside over periods varying in duration from days to years. Urticaria of less than 6 weeks' duration is arbitrarily considered "acute," while urticaria recurring frequently for longer than 6 weeks is referred to as "chronic" (2). Approximately one-fourth of patients presenting with urticaria will at some time develop chronic urticaria (3). Comparisons of populations of patients with acute versus chronic urticaria reveal differences in characteristics other than just the duration of urticaria. For example, acute urticaria is more common in younger patients, while chronic urticaria occurs more frequently in middle-aged women (4). Although the occurrence of acute urticaria is increased in atopic patients, evidence in support of a higher incidence of atopic disease in patients with chronic urticaria is lacking (5, 6). In addition, the search for an underlying cause is more often successful in cases of acute urticaria than in chronic urticaria (7). The reported incidence of the identification of the agent or mechanism responsible in patients with chronic urticaria varies markedly, but in most studies is less than 20% (5).

Foods are recognized as a common etiologic agent in a number of studies evaluating patients with urticaria; however, the role of foods is considered to be more important in acute than in chronic urticaria (7–13). For example, Sehgal and Rege reported foods as an etiologic agent in approximately 20% of 158 subjects with urticaria or angioedema (7). In a study of 215 subjects with urticaria, Nizami and Baboo reported foods as the cause in 12 of 21 subjects (57%) with acute urticaria and in 25 of 194 subjects (13%) with chronic urticaria (8). In 1969 Champion and associates reported foods responsible for only 1.4% of 554 subjects with chronic urticaria (11). Twenty years and 1756 patients later, Warin reported foods as the cause of chronic urticaria in 2.2% of the patients (12). Similarly, Harris and coworkers reported that foods were implicated in approximately 2% of 94 children with chronic urticaria evaluated retrospectively (13). In another retrospective study of 226 children with chronic urticaria, the cause was attributed to foods in 4% and food additives in 2.6% (14). Although studies of different populations of patients with urticaria provide estimates, the exact prevalence of food-induced acute or chronic urticaria in the general population remains unknown. Evaluations in various centers of highly selected populations of patients with histories of adverse reactions to foods reveal that reproducible reactions to foods are noted in only approximately 60% or fewer of such patients (15). These findings suggest that estimates obtained from questionnaires or by taking histories in selected populations of patients without performing food challenges may overestimate the prevalence of such reactions. Food challenges are needed to prove the association between ingestion of the suspected food and the development of urticaria and to eliminate physician or patient bias. Relying solely on the reporting of food-related urticaria to medical personnel may underestimate the frequency of such reactions.

Many individuals, particularly those with acute urticaria, identify the association, avoid the suspected food, and do not seek further evaluation.

Mechanisms

Knowledge of the various mechanisms by which foods have been documented to produce adverse reactions is fundamental to the evaluation of the patient with a history suggestive of food-induced urticaria. One simplistic, but practical means of categorizing adverse reactions to foods by mechanism depends on the involvement of the immune system in the pathogenesis of the reaction (16). Reactions in which the immune system plays a prominent role are examples of "food allergy" or "food hypersensitivity." Of documented allergic reactions to foods resulting in urticaria, mast-cell-dependent reactions mediated by immunoglobulin E (IgE) are the most common. Urticarial reactions to foods may result from exposure by ingestion, injection, direct contact with the skin, or inhalation. Egg, peanut, milk, nuts, soy, wheat, fish, and shellfish are the foods most often implicated in allergic reactions, but apparent IgE-mediated reactions to numerous other foods, or contaminating substances in foods such as molds, antibiotics, latex, or dust mites have been reported (15, 17–21). Studies involving the characterization and isolation of food allergens suggest that the majority are glycoproteins (22). In allergic reactions to foods manifested by urticaria, the onset of the reaction is usually within minutes to hours after exposure to the offending food. Studies of the natural history of allergic reactions to foods in children suggest that some who experience urticaria following exposure to certain foods such as milk, egg, soy, or wheat early in life may later tolerate these foods without difficulty (23). Loss of sensitivity to other foods such as peanuts, nuts, or fish may occur less frequently (23–25).

Reactions resulting from idiosyncratic, metabolic, toxic, or pharmacologic responses to food substances rather than immunologic mechanisms are referred to collectively by the term food intolerance (16). Numerous food dyes, additives, and other ingredients such as tartrazine, other azo and nonazo dyes, natural salicylates, benzoic acid derivatives, and meta-

bisulfites have been reported as capable of provoking urticaria through mechanisms that are not completely understood (26–30). Certain foods such as egg white, strawberries, and shellfish have been demonstrated to contain substances that are direct liberators of histamine through a nonimmunologic mechanism (31, 32). The ingestion of foods that contain large amounts of histamine, either naturally or as a result of spoilage, has also been demonstrated to cause acute urticaria (33). Consideration of the different mechanisms by which foods are capable of producing urticaria aids the clinician in obtaining a complete history, recognizing potential provocateurs of urticaria, selecting appropriate diagnostic tests, and designing a logical, individualized approach to evaluation and treatment.

Diagnosis of Food-Induced Urticaria

Cutaneous symptoms and signs in addition to urticaria confirmed by double-blind, placebo-controlled food challenges include angioedema, generalized pruritus caused by eczema, and nonspecific macular erythematous rashes (15). Cutaneous symptoms may be the sole manifestation of an adverse reaction to a food; gastrointestinal, respiratory, and less frequently cardiovascular symptoms may also accompany or precede cutaneous reactions. The diagnostic tools available to determine whether foods play a role in the production of urticaria in a patient include the history, physical examination, skin testing or radioallergosorbent test (RAST), diet and symptom diaries, elimination diets, and food challenges. The diagnostic approach to the patient with apparent food-related urticaria parallels that used in the diagnosis of other adverse reactions to foods with emphasis on the exclusion of other potential causes of urticaria.

HISTORY AND PHYSICAL EXAMINATION

A thorough history is the obvious first step in the evaluation of the patient with apparent food-induced urticaria. Although patients may experience urticaria only as a result of a reaction to a food, a careful history searching for other potential precipitants of urticaria such as physical causes, infectious agents, drugs, inhalant allergens, insect stings, systemic diseases, and psychogenic factors is important. For each food suspected of causing urticaria, a complete description of previous reactions must be obtained. Information to be elicited includes: (1) the amount of food required to produce urticaria, (2) simultaneously ingested foods, (3) the timing of the onset of urticaria following food ingestion, (4) accompanying symptoms in other organ systems, (5) the reproducibility of the reaction, (6) the most recent suspected occurrence, and (7) the severity of the urticaria as well as the approximate duration and response to treatment. When possible it is practical to suggest that the patient record at least a portion of this information prior to the physician interview because the process of focusing on reactions in an effort to record them occasionally provides important supplemental information.

The severity of reported food-induced reactions that include urticaria ranges from mild to life-threatening (34–38). In many cases urticaria alone is noted; however, other cutaneous symptoms, such as angioedema, or symptoms in other organ systems may be observed as well. Useful information in determining the degree of sensitivity of the subject to the offending food includes the amount of food necessary to provoke urticaria, the severity of accompanying symptoms in other organs, the degree of urticaria or angioedema observed in previous reactions, and the response of the symptoms to medical intervention. In exquisitely sensitive subjects ingestion of milligram amounts of food may provoke life-threatening anaphylaxis (36).

Foods suspected of causing acute urticaria are often identified by their ingestion on several occasions in proximity to the development of urticaria. In most documented food-related episodes of acute urticaria, symptoms begin within minutes to several hours after ingestion of the suspected food. The recognition and substantiation of a direct relationship between food ingestion and the onset of urticaria becomes more difficult as the time between ingestion of the suspected food and onset of urticaria increases. Preliminary evidence suggests that foods may play a previously unrecognized role in specific urticarial syndromes. Davis and colleagues reported that five of six patients with delayed pressure urticaria, an urticarial syndrome in which patients develop symptoms at a site hours after pressure has been applied, developed delayed cutaneous reactions to skin tests to specific foods (39). Removal from the diet of foods causing a delayed cutaneous reaction on skin testing resulted in a negative pressure challenge, whereas a positive pressure challenge was observed after these patients ate foods that elicited a delayed cutaneous response on skin testing. Further clinical investigation to evaluate these findings is needed.

Exposure to foods by routes other than ingestion has been demonstrated to provoke urticaria in food-sensitive patients. Crespo and associates reported their evaluation of 21 children who experienced allergic reactions upon the accidental inhalation of fish odors or fumes (40). Urticaria and angioedema were the most common manifestation, occurring in 19 of the 21 children evaluated. The ability of foods upon contact with the skin to provoke urticaria and even anaphylaxis has also been reported (41). The food-induced contact urticaria syndrome is well documented in children with atopic dermatitis, but is also seen in individuals without this disorder (42, 43). Thus, potential exposures to foods other than by ingestion must be considered when evaluating the food-sensitive patient with acute urticaria.

Foods commonly implicated in challenges as capable of provoking urticaria in sensitive subjects include egg, peanut, milk, nuts, soy, wheat, fish, and shellfish: case histories of reactions to numerous other foods also suggest that virtually any protein-containing food may be allergenic (15). For this reason, discounting a suggestive history solely on the basis of the suspected food is not advised. When exposure to a suspected food inconsistently produces urticaria, attention should be directed to differences in either the method of preparation or the amount consumed. Denaturation of food allergens by heating, addition of unsuspected additives or spices, or cross-contamination of one food with another may account for apparent discrepancies. Reports of allergic reactions to foods that include urticaria occurring only when ingestion is followed by strenuous exercise underscore the necessity of completely reviewing the circumstances surrounding a reaction (44–47). Aspirin-induced urticarial reactions or reactions to other medications should be excluded by reviewing all medications including over-the-counter preparations taken prior to the reaction.

The physical examination of the patient with a history suggestive of food-induced urticaria should be thorough and should include a search for findings associated with systemic diseases known to cause urticaria. The appearance and distribution of any urticarial lesion should be noted. Although the physical examination of most patients with food-induced acute urticaria is unremarkable between exposures to the offending food, findings characteristic of allergic disease are often encountered.

LABORATORY TESTS

Unless information obtained by the history and physical examination leads to suspicion of causes other than foods, an extensive laboratory evaluation of patients with apparent food-induced acute urticaria is not indicated. Since attacks of food-induced acute urticaria remit soon after the offending food has been withdrawn from the diet, the clinical evaluation focuses on accurate identification of the offending food by using the techniques discussed below. An evaluation of 125 patients with chronic urticaria by Nelson and associates using 11 commonly recommended studies yielded abnormal results in only 26 (20.8%) patients, but the majority of the abnormal findings were expected based upon the history and physical examination (48). Thus, extensive testing of patients with chronic urticaria is not warranted unless indicated by the initial evaluation.

SKIN TESTING

Skin testing with extracts of foods suggested by the history is an important part of the evaluation of the patient with apparent food-induced urticaria. Epicutaneous skin testing using food extracts at weight–volume ratios of 1 : 10 or 1 : 20 have been demonstrated to detect food antigen-specific IgE antibody in sensitized subjects (49–52). Skin test sites that exhibit a wheal larger by 3 mm or more than that of the negative diluent control at 10 to 30 minutes after placement are considered positive. Rather than performing skin tests to a large standard panel of food extracts, the selection of foods for

skin testing is based on information obtained by the history. Statistical analysis of data obtained by epicutaneous skin testing with food extracts suggests that the negative predictive accuracy of properly performed tests is excellent (51). Thus, if a properly performed food skin test is negative, the likelihood of an IgE-mediated reaction occurring upon food challenge is markedly reduced. Substances that produce urticaria by nonimmunologic mechanisms are not detected by skin testing, however, and should be considered if the skin test is negative and the history suggests a strong link between ingestion of the suspected food and the onset of urticaria. The positive predictive accuracy of epicutaneous food skin tests is less reliable, as illustrated by the finding that persons with positive food skin tests can often eat foods to which they are skin test positive without experiencing an adverse reaction (15). For this reason, the permanent removal of a food from the diet on the basis of skin test results alone is not recommended. Intradermal skin testing to foods is generally avoided because of the increased likelihood of nonspecific irritant reactions, the increased potential for systemic reactions, and the absence of information suggesting a high degree of clinical correlation (49, 50).

RADIOALLERGOSORBENT TESTING

Skin testing is the preferred method for identifying antigen-specific IgE in patients with food-induced urticaria; however, RAST is an acceptable means of identifying circulating allergen-specific IgE and can be used as an adjunct to, or under certain circumstances in place of, skin testing (53). Although the major advantage of RAST is the lack of risk to the patient, the risk of properly performed skin testing is not so great as to suggest the clinical preference of the RAST over skin testing. RAST is more expensive and takes longer to give results than skin testing. It may be helpful in the patient in whom widespread urticaria, other skin disease, dermatographia, or the need for the continuous administration of medications may affect skin testing. As with skin testing, RAST does not identify substances that produce urticaria by means other than IgE-mediated mechanisms, and individual tests should be selected on the basis of the history rather than by the performance of testing to a standard panel of foods. The enzyme-linked immunosorbent assay (ELISA), a more recently developed test, can be used in similar situations as the RAST for the identification of food antigen-specific IgE (54).

DIET/SYMPTOM DIARY

The purpose of the diet/symptom diary in evaluating the patient with food-induced urticaria is to provide detailed information about the patient's regular diet and an accurate record of the frequency, timing, and duration of urticarial reactions. The information is often collected over a period of weeks and thoroughly reviewed for an apparent temporal association between the ingestion of a specific food and the onset of urticaria. Alternatively, information obtained from the diet/symptom diary may reveal that ingestion of a previously suspected food is not reproducibly associated with the onset of urticaria. For example, some patients are unaware that they frequently ingest foods that contain as an ingredient significant amounts of other foods to which they consider themselves sensitive. The advantage of the diet/symptom diary is that useful information may be obtained at little expense. In addition, the information obtained may establish a baseline of symptoms that can be used to gauge the success of attempted therapeutic maneuvers such as elimination diets.

ELIMINATION DIETS

The premise on which the elimination diet is based in the evaluation of the patient with food-induced urticaria is that elimination of the offending food will result in resolution of the urticaria and reintroduction of the food will cause a recurrence. The degree of restriction of the diet depends on the number of foods thought to provoke urticaria or the prevalence of the suspected food in the diet. Reintroduction of suspected foods into the diet is preferably performed by controlled challenge in an office setting if few foods are suspected and the history suggests a close temporal association between ingestion of the suspected food and onset of urticaria. The performance of food challenges or reintroduction of a suspected food into the diet should be reserved

for a period when the patient is free of urticaria or at least until its occurrence is infrequent.

Evaluations in various centers of highly selected populations of patients with histories of adverse reactions to foods reveal that most subjects with allergic reactions to foods are sensitive to three or fewer foods; thus, extensive elimination diets or elemental diets are rarely necessary and should be used only for limited periods (15). When multiple foods are thought to be involved, or if episodes of urticaria are considered related to food ingestion but a specific food has not been identified, one of several standard elimination diets may be introduced (15, 55, 56). The success of the elimination diet is measured by comparing the frequency of episodes of urticaria on an elimination diet to the frequency noted over an appropriate period on the patient's regular diet. Interference by other factors that may exacerbate urticaria and lack of patient compliance must be taken into consideration. If improvement of the clinical course is noted on the elimination diet, other foods are introduced individually into the diet at appropriate intervals and an association between the introduction of foods and the occurrence of urticaria is noted. Any food thought to provoke urticaria is removed from the diet, and reintroduction is attempted again at a later date either openly or by blinded food challenge.

Several studies have implicated food dyes and other additives as causes of chronic urticaria and have suggested that diets to exclude these substances may induce remission (26–30, 57, 58). Suspected additives include azo dyes, benzoates, butylated hydroxyanisole (BHA), butylated hydroxytoluene (BHT), sodium nitrite, sodium nitrate, sodium glutamate, sorbic acid, yeast, and sodium metabisulfite (31, 57, 58). The mechanisms responsible for reactions to these substances remain undetermined. Although aspirin has been demonstrated to aggravate chronic urticaria, challenges of aspirin-sensitive subjects with sodium salicylate that occurs naturally have not been shown to provoke urticaria (59). A lack of in vitro methods to identify additive sensitivity leaves improvement on a diet free of the suspected additive, followed by provocation of urticaria on blinded challenge, as the only reliable means of establishing the diagnosis. The reported success of elimination diets combined with oral challenges to diagnose food additives as a cause of chronic urticaria varies markedly. A review of selected studies examining the response to diets free of dyes and benzoates by Juhlin revealed remission rates ranging from 21% to 80% (57). Other studies suggest that the reason for the resolution of symptoms on elimination diets may not always be easily identified by oral additive challenges. For example, Kemp and Schembri reported marked remission in 7 of 18 children (40%) placed on an elimination diet; the incidence of reactions to oral challenges with tartrazine, sodium benzoate, and yeast was not significantly higher than that of reactions to placebo, however (56). Similarly, Hannuksela and Lahti challenged 44 patients with chronic urticaria with benzoic acid butylhydroxytoluene, butylhydroxanisole β-carotene, β-8-apo-carotenal, and sodium metabisulfite in a double-blind, placebo-controlled fashion and observed only one reaction to benzoic acid and one to placebo (60).

FOOD CHALLENGE

Food challenge may be performed in an open, single-blind, or double-blind, placebo-controlled manner. A thorough review of the methods and benefits of the performance of food challenges as an office procedure has been published (15). Open challenges are useful when the skin test is negative and the likelihood of a reaction to a specific food is considered doubtful. In addition, open challenges may help in the evaluation of the reliable patient with an objective symptom such as urticaria and without a fixed belief that a particular food will cause symptoms. In the single-blind challenge only the subject is unaware of the contents of the challenge, whereas in the double-blind challenge neither the observer nor the patient knows whether the challenge material to be ingested contains the suspected food or a placebo. Challenges are performed by administering dried foods in opaque capsules or masking foods within other foods. The initial dose of food administered depends on the suspected sensitivity of the patient, as judged by the severity of previous reactions, and the information obtained regarding the amount of food that must be ingested to provoke urticaria. If the initial dose does

not induce a reaction after an appropriate period of observation, gradually increasing doses of the food are administered at intervals until either urticaria develops or a normal portion of the food has been ingested. A negative blind challenge is followed by administration of a normal portion of the food in an open fashion. The absence of the development of urticaria after ingestion of a normal portion of the suspected food virtually eliminates the suspected food as cause of acute urticaria. The onset of urticaria after challenge with the suspected food to which the subject was skin test positive supports the conclusion that the acute urticaria resulted from an IgE-mediated reaction. A food challenge resulting in urticaria in the patient with a negative skin test to the challenge food suggests that a form of food intolerance was involved in the production of the reaction, or the skin test was improperly performed, or the urticaria occurred coincidentally during food challenge or due to some other unrecognized precipitant. Challenges may have to be repeated if the results are equivocal. The possibility of unexpected severe reactions must always be considered, and the challenge carefully designed to provide maximum safety to the patient.

Treatment

Because episodes of food-induced acute urticaria are limited to exposure to the offending food, an individualized diet eliminating foods or substances in foods to which the patient has been proved sensitive results in remission of the urticaria. Avoidance of the offending food is best accomplished by thoroughly instructing the patient about the elimination diet and reviewing hidden sources of suspected foods or additives. If episodes of urticaria continue on the individualized elimination diet, the patient's diet should be reviewed for unrecognized sources of exposure. If no inadvertent exposure to an offending food is identified and the patient is considered compliant, then efforts to uncover other offending foods or to identify other causes of urticaria must be considered. In patients with chronic urticaria, removal of offending foods may lead to a reduction of the frequency of urticarial episodes rather than complete remission, as factors other than foods may provoke urticaria. Lingering questions about the role of foods may be answered by using a strict elimination diet for short periods. Occasionally, patients with chronic urticaria become convinced that foods alone are the cause of their symptoms and restrict foods from their diet for which no evidence of sensitivity exists. Continued counseling and encouragement to reintroduce these foods are necessary to avoid diets with nutritional or caloric deficiencies.

A plan for pharmacologic management of unexpected exposures to offending foods is important because even the most careful patients occasionally accidentally ingest a food to which they are sensitive. H_1 antihistamines such as diphenhydramine hydrochloride or chlorpheniramine may be used for acute treatment. In patients with food-induced acute urticaria, treatment of the acute episode may suffice; occasionally patients may benefit from treatment with antihistamines for 24 to 72 hours after a reaction. Although patients with chronic urticaria are often taking antihistamines regularly, additional doses are frequently administered acutely upon exposure to an offending food. If sedation that often accompanies the use of H_1 antihistamines poses a problem, a nonsedating H_1 antihistamine such as terfenadine can be used (61). Patients who develop angioedema in addition to urticaria or experience accompanying symptoms in other organs should be taught how to self-administer epinephrine and should have antihistamines and an epinephrine-containing syringe available at all times. Identification bracelets or tags stating the patient's sensitivities are also advisable.

A proven method for the prevention of food-induced urticaria by means other than avoidance of the offending food is presently not available. Desensitization to offending foods by either the oral or parenteral administration of dilute extracts is not currently recommended due to a lack of evidence to support its efficacy (62, 63). The search continues for pharmacologic agents that can be used prophylactically to prevent food-induced urticaria. Although H_1 antihistamines may alter food-induced urticarial reactions, complete inhibition of reactions is infrequently achieved. The efficacy of cromolyn sodium in preventing reactions to foods remains to be established (63, 64). Although ketotifen, an antihistamine with mast-cell-stabilizing properties, has been claimed to have a protective effect, further carefully controlled clinical trials to determine efficacy are needed (64, 65).

REFERENCES

1. Sheldon JM, Matthews KP, Lovell RG. The vexing urticaria problem: present concepts of etiology and management. J Allergy 1954;25:525–560.
2. Guin JD. The evaluation of patients with urticaria. Dermatol Clin 1985;3:29–49.
3. Greaves MW. Chronic urticaria. N Engl J Med 1995;332:1767–1772.
4. Monroe EW, Jones HE. Urticaria: an updated review. Arch Dermatol 1977;113:80–90.
5. Kaplan AP. Urticaria and angioedema. In: Middleton E, Reed CE, Ellis EF, eds. Allergy, principles and practice. 3rd ed. St. Louis: CV Mosby, 1988, 1377–1401.
6. Matthews KP. Urticaria and angioedema. J Allergy Clin Immunol 1983;71:1.
7. Sehgal VN, Rege VL. An interrogative study of 158 urticaria patients. Ann Allergy 1973;31:279–283.
8. Nizami RM, Baboo MT. Office management of patients with urticaria: an analysis of 215 patients. Ann Allergy 1974;33:78–85.
9. Kauppinen K, Juntunen K, Lanki H. Urticaria in children: retrospective evaluation and follow-up. Allergy 1984;39:469–472.
10. Halpern SR. Chronic hives in children: an analysis of 75 cases. Ann Allergy 1965;23:589–599.
11. Champion RH, Roberts SOB, Carpenter RG, Roger JH. Urticaria and angioedema: a review of 554 patients. Br J Dermatol 1969;81:588–597.
12. Champion RH. Urticaria: then and now. Br J Dermatol 1988;119:427–436.
13. Harris A, Twarog FJ, Geha RF. Chronic urticaria in childhood: natural course and etiology. Ann Allergy 1983;51:161–165.
14. Volonakis M, Katsarou-Katsari A, Stratigos J. Etiologic factors in childhood chronic urticaria. Ann Allergy 1992;69:61–65.
15. Bock SA, Sampson HA, Atkins FM, et al. Double-blind, placebo-controlled food challenge as an office procedure: a manual. J Allergy Clin Immunol 1988;82:986–997.
16. Anderson JA. The establishment of a common language concerning adverse reactions to foods and food additives. J Allergy Clin Immunol 1986;178:140–144.
17. Rockwell WJ. Reactions to molds in foods. In: Chiaramonte LT, Schneider AT, Lifshitz F, eds. Food allergy: a practical approach to diagnosis and management. New York: Marcel Dekker, 1988, 153–170.
18. Boonk WJ, Van Ketel WG. The role of penicillin in the pathogenesis of chronic urticaria. Br J Dermatol 1982;106:183–190.
19. Wicher K, Reisman RE. Anaphylactic reaction to penicillin (or penicillin-like substance) in a soft drink. J Allergy Clin Immunol 1980;66:155–157.

20. Schwartz HJ. Latex: a potential hidden "food" allergen in fast food restaurants. J Allergy Clin Immunol 1995;95:139–140.

21. Erben AM, Rodriguez JL, McCullough J, Ownby DR. Anaphylaxis after ingestion of beignets contaminated with *Dermatophagoides farinae*. J Allergy Clin Immunol 1993;92:846–849.

22. Metcalfe DD. Food allergens. Clin Rev Allergy 1985;3:331–349.

23. Bock SA. Natural history of severe reactions to foods in young children. J Pediatr 1985;107:676–680.

24. Bock SA. The natural history of food sensitivity. J Allergy Clin Immunol 1982;69:173–177.

25. Bock SA, Atkins FM. The natural history of peanut allergy. J Allergy Clin Immunol 1989;83:900–904.

26. Lockey SD. Reactions to hidden agents in foods, beverages and drugs. Ann Allergy 1971;29:461–466.

27. Juhlin L, Michaelsson G, Zetterstrom O. Urticaria and asthma induced by food and drug additives in patients with aspirin sensitivity. J Allergy Clin Immunol 1972;50:92–98.

28. Ros AM, Juhlin L, Michaelsson G. A follow-up study of patients with recurrent urticaria and hypersensitivity to aspirin, benzoates and azo dyes. Br J Dermatol 1976;95:19–24.

29. Juhlin L. Recurrent urticaria: clinical investigation of 330 patients. Br J Dermatol 1981;104:369–381.

30. Goodman DL, McDonnell JT, Nelson HS, Vaughan TR, Weber RW. Chronic urticaria exacerbated by the antioxidant food preservatives butylated hydroxyanisole (BHA) and butylated hydroxytoluene (BHT). J Allergy Clin Immunol 1990;86:570–575.

31. Schachter M, Talesnik J. The release of histamine by egg-white in nonsensitized animals. J Physiol 1952;118:258–263.

32. Anderson JA, Sogn DD, eds. Adverse food reactions that involve or are suspected of involving immune mechanisms: an anatomical categorization. In: American Academy of Allergy and Immunology Committee on Adverse Reactions to Foods. Washington, DC: National Institute of Allergy and Infectious Diseases, 1984, 43–102.

33. Uragoda CG. Histamine poisoning in tuberculosis patients after ingestion of tuna fish. Am Rev Respir Dis 1980;121:157–159.

34. Bock SA, Lee W, Remigio LK, May CD. Studies of hypersensitivity reactions to foods in infants and children. J Allergy Clin Immunol 1978;62:327–334.

35. Sampson HA, Albergo R. Food hypersensitivity and atopic dermatitis; evaluation of 113 patients. J Pediat 1985;107:669–675.

36. Atkins FM, Wilson M, Bock SA. Cottonseed hypersensitivity: new concerns over an old problem. J Allergy Clin Immunol 1988;82:242–250.

37. Squillace BA, Sweeney KG, Jones RT, Yunginger JW, Helm RM. Fatal food-induced anaphylaxis. JAMA 1988;260:1450–1454.

38. Sampson HA, Mendelson L, Rosen JP. Fatal and near fatal food enaphylaxis reactions in children. J Allergy Clin Immunol 1991;87:176.

39. Davis KC, Mekori YA, Kohler PF, Schocket AL. Possible role of diet in delayed pressure urticaria—preliminary report. J Allergy Clin Immunol 1986;77:566–569.

40. Crespo JF, Pascual O, Dominguez O, Munoz FM, Estaban MM. Allergic reactions associated with airborne fish particles in IgE-mediated fish hypersensitive patients. Allergy 1995;50:257–261.

41. Jarmoc LM, Primack WA. Anaphylaxis to cutaneous exposure to milk protein. Clin Pediatr 1987;26:154–156.

42. Oranje AP, Van Gysel D, Mulder PGH, Dieges PH. Food-induced contact urticaria syndrome (CUS) in atopic dermatitis: reproducibility of repeated and duplicate testing with a skin provocation test, the skin application food test (SAFT). Contact Dermatitis 1994;31:314–318.

43. Fisher AA. Contact urticaria from handling meats and fowl. Cutis 1982;30:726–729.

44. Maulitz RM, Pratt DS, Schocket AL. Exercise-induced anaphylactic reaction to shellfish. J Allergy Clin Immunol 1979;63:433–434.

45. Kushimoto H, Aoki T. Masked type I wheat allergy. Arch Dermatol 1985;121:355–360.

46. Kivity S, Sneh E, Greif J, Topilsky M, Mekori YA. The effect of food and exercise on the skin response to compound 48/80 in patients with food-associated exercise-induced urticaria-angioedema. J Allergy Clin Immunol 1988;81:1155–1158.

47. Martin Munoz F, Lopez Cazana JM, Villas F, Contreras JF, Diaz JM, Ojeda JA. Exercise-induced anaphylactic reaction to hazelnut. Allergy 1994;49:314–316.

48. Jacobson KW, Branch LB, Nelson HS. Laboratory tests in chronic urticaria. JAMA 1980;243:1644–1646.

49. Bock SA, Lee Y, Remigio LK, May CD. Studies of hypersensitivity reactions to foods in infants and children. J Allergy Clin Immunol 1978;62:327–334.

50. Bock SA, Buckley J, Holst A, May CD. Proper use of skin test with food extracts in diagnosis of hypersensitivity to food in children. Clin Allergy 1977;7:375–383.

51. Sampson HA, Albergo R. Comparison of results of skin tests, RAST, and double-blind, placebo-controlled food challenges with atopic dermatitis. J Allergy Clin Immunol 1984;74:26–33.

52. Atkins FM, Steinberg SS, Metcalfe DD. Evaluation of immediate adverse reactions to foods in adult patients. I. Correlation of demographic, laboratory, and prick skin test data with response to controlled oral food challenge. J Allergy Clin Immunol 1985;75:348–355.

53. Chua YY, Bremmer K, Lakdawalla N, et al. In vivo and in vitro correlates of food allergy. J Allergy Clin Immunol 1976;58:299–307.

54. Kettelhut BV, Metcalfe DD. Adverse reactions to foods. In: Middleton E, Reed LE, Ellis EF, eds. Allergy, principles and practice, 3rd ed. St. Louis: CV Mosby, 1988, 1481–1502.

55. Atkins FM, Metcalfe DD. The diagnosis and treatment of food allergy. Ann Rev Nutr 1984;4:233–255.

56. Kemp AS, Schembri G. An elimination diet for chronic urticaria of childhood. Med J Aust 1985;143:234–235.

57. Juhlin L. Additives and chronic urticaria. Ann Allergy 1987;59:119–123.

58. Gibson A, Clancy R. Management of chronic idiopathic urticaria by the identification and exclusion of dietary factors. Clin Allergy 1980;10:699–704.

59. Samter M, Beers RF. Concerning the nature of intolerance to aspirin. J Allergy 1967;40:281–293.

60. Hannuksela M, Lahti A. Peroral challenge tests with food additives in urticaria and atopic dermatitis. Int J Dermatol 1986;25:178–180.

61. Ciprandi G, Scordamaglia A, Bagnasco M, Canonica GW. Pharmacologic treatment of adverse reactions to foods: comparison of different protocols. Ann Allergy 1987;58:341–343.

62. Sampson HA. Adverse reactions to foods. In: Middleton E, Reed CE, Ellis EF, Adkinson FN, Yunginger JW, Busse WW,

eds. Allergy: principles and practice. St. Louis: Mosby, 1993, 1661–1686.

63. Kettelhut BV, Metcalfe DD. Food allergy in adults. In: Lichtenstein LM, Fauci AS, eds. Current therapy in allergy, immunology and rheumatology–3. Toronto: BC Decker, 1988, 56–59.

64. Sogn D. Medications and their use in the treatment of adverse reactions to foods. J Allergy Clin Immunol 1986;78:238–243.

65. Neffen H, Oehling A, Subira ML. A study of the protective effect of ketotifen in food allergy. Allergol Immunopathol 1980;8:97–104.

13

ORAL ALLERGY SYNDROME

Elide Anna Pastorello
Claudio Ortolani

Definition

The term *oral allergy syndrome (OAS)* is currently used to indicate a complexity of clinical symptoms caused by an IgE-mediated reaction that arises in the oropharyngeal mucosa when it comes in direct contact with a culprit food in a sensitized subject (1). The name used to identify OAS focuses on the need for direct contact of the oral mucosa with the offending food to trigger local symptoms, usually in the form of oral itching, lip swelling, and labial angioedema, but also glottis edema or, in even rarer cases, systemic anaphylactic reactions. The syndrome is mainly caused by sensitization to fresh fruits and vegetables in subjects with hypersensitivity to pollens (2–6); it has also been described in subjects allergic to shrimps and eggs (1), where it may represent the beginning of a more severe, systemic reaction. OAS was first described in 1942 for apple and hazelnut in patients allergic to birch pollen (2). Since then, many other kinds of allergic reactions to various fruits and vegetables have been described in association with pollen allergy (3–13). The association between OAS and allergy to pollen has prompted the initiation of many studies aimed at clarifying its immunochemical cause.

The identification of allergenic components sharing common structures in various pollens and foods has given a solid scientific basis to clinical observations. As a result, OAS to fresh fruits and vegetables is one of the best-characterized models of an IgE-mediated allergic reaction to food.

Epidemiology

Only a few studies have addressed the prevalence of OAS, all of which have concentrated on OAS from fruits and vegetables. Recently, a study from Switzerland (13) reported that approximately 35% of patients allergic to pollens shared allergic symptoms and skin prick test (SPT) positivity to fresh fruits and vegetables. Pastorello *et al.* observed a similar prevalence among 300 patients allergic to pollens (14). Allergy to fruits and vegetables occurs most frequently in subjects with hayfever from birch allergen. In 1977, Hannuksela and Lahti reported positive skin tests for fresh fruits and vegetables in 35% of patients with birch allergy (4). Another Scandinavian study, based on 2626 hayfever subjects, found that 63% of birch-allergic patients presented with hypersensitivity to one or more fruits or vegetables (15). Similar findings have been reported in Austria by Ebner *et al.*, who noted that more than 75% of birch-allergic patients complained of allergic symptoms after eating apples (11).

Adults appear to develop OAS to fresh fruits and vegetables more frequently than children. A study from Israel found that fruits and vegetables were the most frequent source of food allergy for patients over the age of 10 (16).

Clinical Features

The main clinical features of OAS are the following: (1) a clinical picture characterized by erythema, pruritus, and edema at the oral mucosal sites and, less frequently, associated systemic symptoms; (2) clinical reactions to multiple allergenic sources that give rise to "clusters of hypersensitivity"; and (3) an association with rhinitis or asthma due to allergy to pollens of different kinds (17).

SYMPTOMS

Symptoms are characteristically elicited in allergic subjects while and/or shortly after eating fresh fruits and vegetables. They are immediate and arise in the lining of the lips, the oropharynx, and the gastrointestinal tract, which comes into direct contact with the offending food (Table 13.1). The symptoms consist of intra-oral and lip irritation, angioedema, papulae, and, more rarely, blisters, which appear within a few minutes after contact with the offending food. Systemic symptoms such as urticaria, rhinitis, asthma, or occasionally even anaphylactic shock may appear after contact with the culprit food, especially if the patient ingests the culprit food despite the local disturbance (Table 13.2).

Local symptoms clearly prevail, as has been well documented by various studies on patients with allergic reactions to fresh fruits and vegetables (5–7, 10, 12). In a study of 90 patients suffering from ragweed allergic rhinitis and allergy to melon and banana, Anderson et al. (7) found that all of the subjects experienced oropharyngeal symptoms. Similarly, Eriksson et al. (5) reported that 78% of 255 patients allergic to birch and related foods (e.g., apple, peach, cherry, pear, and carrot) complained of symptoms localized in the oral mucosa. Ortolani et al. reported that local symptoms occurred in 83.6% of 262 patients allergic to fresh fruits and vegetables (6). In a subsequent study on a larger population, the same authors found that 93.9% of 706 patients had local oral symptoms (12).

The most severe local symptom of OAS is glottic edema. This symptom appears particularly frequently in relation to allergy to celery, a vegetable known to induce severe allergic reactions (18). In a first study of

Table 13.1
Skin-Mucosal Contact Provoked Symptoms Observed in 706 OAS Patients (12)

Symptoms	Number of Patients	%
Only oral	596	84.4
Oral + gastrointestinal	67	9.5
Only gastrointestinal	29	4.1

Table 13.2
Systemic Symptoms Associated with Oral/Gastrointestinal Contact Symptoms Observed in 706 OAS Patients (12)

Symptoms	Number of Patients	%
Urticaria/angioedema	191	27.0
Rhinitis	63	8.9
Asthma	50	7.1
Conjunctivitis	25	3.5
Anaphylactic shock	15	2.1

262 patients with OAS from fresh fruit and vegetables, Ortolani et al. observed 62 cases (26%) of glottic edema after ingestion of several fresh foods (6). In a subsequent study, the same authors reported that 98 of 706 OAS patients (13.9%) presented at least one well-documented episode of glottic edema (12). Ortolani et al. (6) analyzed the onset of local symptoms in 43 patients, and noted that the symptoms developed within 5 minutes in the majority of cases, and within 10 to 30 minutes in all but 3 cases. In the three remaining cases symptoms developed 90 minutes after ingestion of the food (Fig. 13.1).

In the study by Eriksson et al. (17), most patients complained of both systemic and local symptoms. The authors described cases with urticaria/angioedema, eczema, asthma, conjunctivitis, and rhinitis. None of the patients experienced anaphylactic shock. In the study by Pauli et al. (18), 4 out of 20 patients (20%) who were allergic to celery presented with anaphylaxis. In the study by Ortolani et al., 1.5% of patients developed anaphylactic shock after ingestion of apricot, lentil, peach, or tomato (6). In a second study, the same authors found that 2.1% of patients had anaphylactic shock after ingestion of peach, apricot, walnut, cherry, tomato, apple, hazelnut, or pear (Table 13.3) (12).

"CLUSTERS OF HYPERSENSITIVITY"

Sensitization to certain fruits or vegetables may be significantly associated with sensitization to other foods belonging to the same botanical family and with sensitization to unrelated foods as well. Clinically this phenomenon has been defined as a "cluster

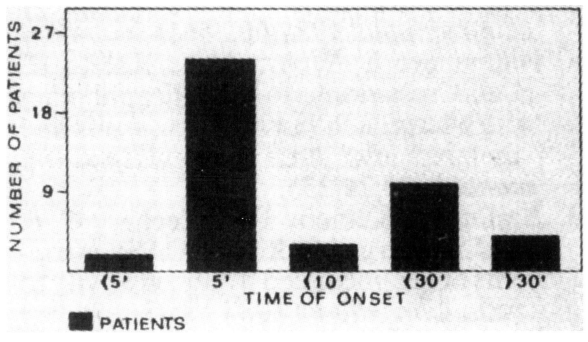

Figure 13.1

Onset of symptoms after culprit food ingestion in 43 OAS patients. (Reprinted from Ortolani C, *et al.* Ann Allergy 1988;61(part two):47–52.)

Table 13.3
Food that Provoked Anaphylactic Shock 23 Times in 15 out of 706 Investigated Patients

Food	Number with Anaphylactic Shock	Number of Patients Allergic to This Food
Peach	4	330
Apricot	3	189
Walnut	2	216
Cherry	2	188
Tomato	2	188
Apple	1	385
Hazelnut	1	237
Pear	1	171
Fennel	1	130
Plum	1	123
Pea	1	47
Chestnut	1	40
Maize	1	25
Lettuce	1	23
Lentil	1	4

From Ortolani C, Pastorello EA, Farioli L, *et al.* Ann Allergy 1993; 71:470–476. Reprinted by permission.

of hypersensitivity" (19). The following clusters have been described by Eriksson (19):

1. Hazelnut, walnut, brazil nut, almond, and dessert almond reciprocally, and even nuts combined with apple and stone fruits.
2. Stone fruits reciprocally and in combination with apple and pear.
3. Apple and pear.
4. Kiwi fruit and avocado.
5. Potato and carrot.
6. Parsley and celery.

Other "clusters" have also been described: celery, carrot, mugwort, and spices (20); apple, carrot, and potato (21); fennel and celery (6); cherry and apple (6); melon, watermelon, and tomato (6); fennel, celery, and carrot (22); lettuce and carrot (23); tomato and peanut (24); and celery, cucumber, carrot, and

Table 13.4
Oral Food Challenges Findings, History (Pollens), SPTs, and RAST Results in 21 Patients with (1–19) and without (20, 21) OAS to Prunoideae

Patient Numbers	OFC				Symptoms		SPT						RAST					
	P	C	A	PL	G	B	P	C	A	PL	G	B	P	C	A	PL	G	B
1	OP	—	—	OP	—	—	++	+++	++	++	—	—	2	1	2	2	0	0
2	OP	—	—		+		++++	++	++	++	++++	—	3	2	3	3	3	0
3	OP	—	—	—	—	—	++	++	++++	+++	—	—	3	2	3	2	0	0
4	OP	—	—	—	—	—	+++	+++	+++	++	—	—	3	2	2	2	0	0
5	OP	OP	—	—	—	—	++++	++	++	++	—	—	3	2	3	3	0	0
6	OP	OP	OP	OP	+	—	++	++	++	++	+++	—	3	1	3	3	3	0
7	OP	OP	OP	OP	—	—	++	++	++	+++	—	—	4	3	4	4	4	0
8	GI	OP	—	—	+	+	++	++	++	++	+++	++++	3	2	3	3	4	4
9	OP	OP	OP	—	+	—	+++	+++	++	+++	++	++	3	2	3	3	4	3
10	OP	—	—	—	+	—	++	++	++	++	++	+++	2	3	3	2	2	3
11	OP	OP	OP	OP	+	+	++	++	++	++	++++	++++	2	2	2	2	3	2
12	OP	OP	—	OP	+	+	++	+++	++	++	++++	++++	3	2	3	3	4	4
13	OP	GI	—	OP	—	—	++	++	++	++	++	++	2	2	2	2	3	3
14	OP	—	—	—	+	+	++	++	++	+++	++++	+++	4	3	4	4	4	2
15	GI	GI	—	—	+	—	++++	++	+++	+++	++++	++	2	1	2	2	4	2
16	OP	OP	OP	OP	+	+	++	+++	+++	+++	+++	+++	3	2	3	3	3	4
17	OP	—	—	—	+	—	+++	++	+++	++	+++	+++	3	2	3	3	4	4
18	OP	OP	OP	OP	+	+	++++	+++	+++	++	+++	+++	4	3	3	3	3	3
19	OP	—	—	—	+	+	+++	++	++	++	+++	++	3	3	3	3	4	2
20	—	—	—	—	+	+	+++	+++	++	++	+++	+++	2	3	3	3	3	4
21	—	—	—	—	—	+	+++	++	++	++	++	++	2	2	2	2	2	4

SPT results are expressed in number of pluses compared with the wheal flare elicited by histamine 10 mg (considered +++). RAST results are expressed as classes of positivity: 0, <0.35 PRU; 1, 0.35–0.7 PRU; 2, 0.7–3.5 PRU; 3, 3.5–17.5 PRU; 4, >17.5 PRU.
P, peach; C, cherry; A, apricot; PL, plum; G, grass; B, birch; OP, oropharyngeal symptoms (oral irritation, local itching and tingling, angioedema, throat tightness, lip tightness/swelling, oral mucosal papules or blisters); GI, gastrointestinal symptoms (abdominal pain, vomiting); PRU, Phadebas RAST units.
From Pastorello EA, Ortolani C, Farioli L, *et al.* J Allergy Clin Immunol 1994;94:699–707. Reprinted by permission.

watermelon (25). Many of these associations have been established by skin tests or RASTs and have not been confirmed by oral challenge. In a recent study (26), Pastorello *et al.* used the oral open food challenge test (OFC) to check for clinical cross-reactivity in members of the Prunoideae subfamily such as peach, apricot, plum, and cherry. Nineteen out of 23 patients allergic to peach presented a positive OFC for at least one other prunoid: 10 (52.6%) for cherry, 8 (42.1%) for plum, and 6 (31.5%) for apricot (Table 13.4). Sometimes these clusters of hypersensitivity include fruits and vegetables belonging to different botanical families, as in the association of tomato and peanut allergies (24). This cluster is reported only in patients allergic to pollen and is probably caused by the sensitization to common epitopes.

ASSOCIATION WITH RHINITIS OR ASTHMA DUE TO POLLEN ALLERGY

In the majority of cases, OAS to fresh fruits and vegetables is associated with allergy to different pollens. In 1942, the first report of the association allergy to birch and allergy to apple was published (2). Since that time, this kind of association has been widely confirmed, and many others have been described involving pollens such as grasses, ragweed, and mugwort (Table 13.5) (5, 12, 20). Hayfever often occurs before OAS with a significant difference in the timing of occurrence (6). The geographic prevalence of the local flora often represents the most influential environmental factor in inducing the common sensitization to fruits and vegetables. In Italy, where hayfever

Table 13.5
Associations Between Pollinosis and Allergy to Fresh Fruits and Vegetables

Author	Year	Pollen	Fruit/Vegetable
Tuft, Blumstein (2)	1942	birch	apple
Juhlin-Danfelt (3)	1948	birch	apple, hazelnut
Anderson *et al.* (7)	1970	ragweed	melon, banana
Eriksson (5)	1978	birch	apple, hazelnut, carrot, potato
Wüthrich (8)	1981	mugwort	celery
Pauli *et al.* (9)	1982	mugwort	celery
Wüthrich (20)	1985	mugwort	celery, carrot, spices
Pauli *et al.* (38)	1985	birch, mugwort	celery
Enberg *et al.* (10)	1987	ragweed	watermelon, gourd family
Ortolani *et al.* (6)	1988	grass	tomato, melon, watermelon
De Martino *et al.* (24)	1988	grass	tomato, peanut
Ebner *et al.* (11)	1991	birch	apple
Ortolani *et al.* (12)	1992	birch	celery, fennel

mainly derives from grass pollen, Ortolani *et al.* found an association between grass allergy and food allergy to tomato, melon, watermelon, and orange, all of which are widely consumed (6). More recently, the association between birch allergy and OAS to fennel was also described (22). Finally, the association between kiwi fruit allergy and grass pollen allergy was also reported in Italy (12), while kiwi fruit allergy has been described only in association with birch pollen allergy in Scandinavia and in the United States (27, 28). In the United States, an association between ragweed allergy and allergy to melon and banana has been reported (7). Ragweed allergy was also found to be associated to allergy to members of the gourd family (i.e., watermelon, cantaloupe, honeydew, zucchini, and cucumber) (10). Another known association exists between allergy to hazelnut and allergy to hazel pollen (29, 31).

A common finding in these studies is a statistically significant relationship between the presence of symptoms to fresh fruits and vegetables and high levels of specific IgE to related pollens. In the study by Enberg *et al.* (10), only those patients with the highest RAST levels to ragweed presented symptoms to fruits of the gourd family. Similarly, Eriksson *et al.* (32) found that high levels of birch specific IgE antibodies in serum were closely related to the occurrence of allergy to fruits and vegetables. Ebner *et al.* (11) confirmed a higher incidence of apple allergy

in subjects having high levels of birch specific IgE compared with subjects having lower values.

Etiopathogenesis

LOCAL ORAL SYMPTOMS

Amlot *et al.* (1) suggested that local oral symptoms are caused by a high concentration of mast cells in the oropharyngeal mucosa. This condition would lead to a stronger interaction between the allergens rapidly released from the fruit or vegetable and the specific IgE bound on the cell surface. This interaction, in turn, might explain the early onset of OAS symptoms. Local oral symptoms are also caused by a high concentration of allergens on the oral mucosa, which are rapidly released from the fruit or vegetable as they come in contact with the saliva of the allergic subject. This kind of reaction resembles that seen with pollens, which react in their intact form with the IgE antibodies bound to mast cells in the mucosa of the upper and lower airways.

IMMUNOCHEMICAL BASIS OF CLINICAL CROSS-REACTIVITY

All of the reported clinical associations are likely to be based on the presence of cross-reacting allergens in pollens and in foods; cross-reactivity between foods of the same class or family may also generate such symptoms. This cross-reactivity has been functionally demonstrated first by RAST inhibition experiments using birch and apple extracts, celery and birch extracts, ragweed, melon, and banana extracts, as well as between other pollens and fruits or vegetables (Table 13.6) (10, 24, 33–40). Other cross-reacting allergens have been identified using immunoelectrophoretic techniques and still others using immunoblotting techniques (10, 11). Ebner *et al.* first demonstrated the immunologic basis of cross-reactivity between apple and birch using Western blot experiments (11). They identified corresponding IgE binding in birch and apple extracts in the molecular weight region of 17 kD. In inhibition experiments, sera pre-incubated with minimal amounts of birch pollen extract completely lost reactivity against apple allergens with a molecular weight of 17 to 18 kD, although the reverse was not observed for apple allergens. Furthermore, immunoblotting with a Bet v 1 monoclonal specific antibody detected a 17 kD protein in apple extract. Finally, employing a Northern blotting technique with a Bet v 1 cDNA clone as a probe, the authors demonstrated cross-hybridization of birch and apple allergen-coding nucleic acids, suggesting homology at the nucleic acid level (Figs. 13.2 and 13.3). Ebner *et al.* provided the first conclusive demonstration that antigens in birch pollen and apple share allergenic epitopes. These epitopes lead to

IgE cross-reactivity that may account for the clinical symptoms induced by birch and apple.

Hirschwehr *et al.* found a 17 kD allergen similar to Bet v 1 in hazel pollen, which is known to cross-react with birch pollen and hazelnut (30). Bet v 1 appears to be an important pan-allergen, being widely distributed in nature and capable of influencing sensitization. Similar amino acid sequences were found within the major tree pollen allergen group (Bet v 1, Aln g 1, and Cor a 1) and within a certain family of pathogenesis-related proteins encoded by "disease resistance response" genes from bean, parsley, pea, and potato. In stressful environmental conditions, these allergens could be overexpressed, thereby influencing the rate of sensitization to Bet v 1 (40).

Profilin, another birch allergen defined as Bet v 2, plays a key role in sensitization to foods and is extremely widespread in the vegetable and animal kingdom (41). Profilins are proteins of approximately 14 kD molecular weight that regulate actin polymerization and participate in signal transduction as actin-sequestering proteins. Vallier *et al.* demonstrated the presence of profilin in birch and celery and identified cross-reacting IgE in sera of patients allergic to both of these allergenic sources (42). Profilins present in grasses, mugwort, and birch share amino acid sequences, thus leading to complex features of cross-reactivity between pollens and foods. These proteins probably play a role in plant fertilization, and, given their highly allergenic nature, they will presumably

Table 13.6
Allergenic Cross-Reactivity Between Fruits/Vegetables and Pollens as Assessed by in Vitro Techniques

Author	Year	Fruit/Vegetable	Pollen	Technique
Andersen *et al.* (29)	1978	hazelnut	birch	CLIE
Lahti *et al.* (33)	1980	apple	birch	RAST-inhibition
Halmepuro *et al.* (34)	1984	apple, carrot, celery	birch	RAST-inhibition
Pauli *et al.* (38)	1985	celery	birch, mugwort	RAST-inhibition
Calkhoven *et al.* (35)	1987	apple, cherry peach, potato	birch grass	RAST-inhibition SDS-Page immunoblotting
Enberg *et al.* (10)	1987	watermelon	ragweed	ELISA-inhibition, IEF
De Martino *et al.* (24)	1988	tomato, peanut	grass	RAST-inhibition
Vallier *et al.* (36)	1988	celery	mugwort, birch	Immunoblotting
Wüthrich *et al.* (50)	1990	celery	mugwort	RAST-inhibition
Ebner *et al.* (11)	1991	apple	birch	Immunoblotting
Hirschwehr *et al.* (30)	1992	hazelnut	hazel	Immunoblotting
Pastorello *et al.* (26)	1994	peach, cherry, apricot, plum	birch, grass	Immunoblotting

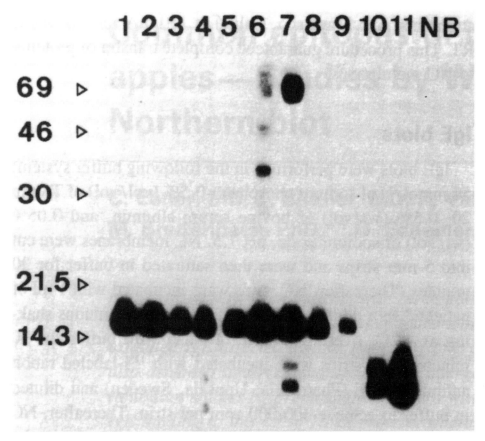

Figure 13.2

IgE immunoblots with sera from 11 selected patients on birch-pollen extract-coated nitrocellulose strips. *Patients 1–5, 8, 9:* IgE binding to the major allergen, Bet v 1; *Patients 6, 7:* IgE binding to Bet v 1 and to minor allergens; *Patients 10, 11:* reaction with a minor allergen in the molecular weight range of 13 kD, exclusively. (Reprinted from Ebner C, *et al.* J Allergy Clin Immunol 1991;88:588–594.)

be identified as one of the important pan-allergens (43).

The clinical cross-reactivity between members of the same botanical family is easy to understand, despite the fact that only a few allergens common to analogous foods have been identified. Recently, the basis of the allergic cross-reactivity between the members of the Prunoideae family (peach, apricot, plum, and cherry) has been demonstrated (26). Using SDS-Page and immunoblotting techniques on the sera of patients with a clinically evident reaction to one or more of these fruits, Pastorello *et al.* identified an IgE reactive component of about 13 kD against which 95% of sera reacted (Fig. 13.4). The authors observed 100% inhibition of peach blotting by cherry, plum, and apricot extracts. Peach blotting was not inhibited by birch and grass extracts, however (Fig. 13.5). Other allergenic components of molecular weight 14 kD, 20 kD, and higher were inhibited by both pollen extracts. Patients with positive RAST for peach but who lacked clinical symptoms did not react to the 13 kD component. Thus, this component seems to be strictly associated with clinical reactivity. In contrast, the IgE response to other allergens is not associated with

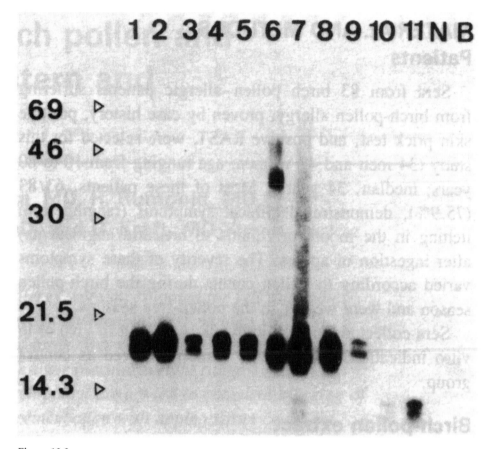

Figure 13.3

IgE immunoblots with sera from 11 selected patients on apple extract-coated nitrocellulose strips. *Patients 1–5, 8, 9:* IgE binding in the molecular weight range 17 to 18 kD; *Patients 6, 7:* IgE binding to the major allergen and to minor allergens; *Patients 10, 11:* patients reacting with a minor allergen in the region 13 kD, exclusively. (Reprinted from Ebner C, *et al.* J Allergy Clin Immunol 1991;88:588–594.)

clinical reactivity but is only a consequence of a cross-sensitization to birch or grass pollen.

Similarly, Vocks *et al.* observed that a relevant allergen of kiwi fruit is a 30 kD molecule (44). In the study conducted by Pravettoni *et al.*, all sera of 27 patients tested with a positive open challenge to kiwi fruit reacted to a 30 kD allergen (45). Immunoblotting after inhibition by grass and birch extract showed only a small decrease in the IgE binding to the 30 kD band, but a major drop in IgE binding to all of the other allergenic proteins.

An important future task will involve the identi-fication the nature of these allergens to understand their wide dispersion in the vegetable kingdom. For example, a 30 kD allergen has been found in latex, banana, and avocado (46). This allergen could be an important constituent of cellular lutoids.

Diagnosis

Diagnosis of OAS is based on the generally accepted procedures for the diagnosis of IgE-mediated food allergy (47, 48). Due to its features, however, OAS

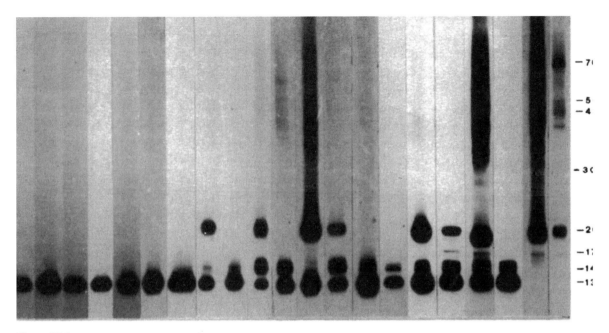

Figure 13.4

Autoradiographs of IgE-immunoblot analysis of peach extract with sera from 21 patients, presenting specific IgE to peach. The molecular weight of some of the allergens are given. Patients' numbers are reported in the lower part of the figure. Patients 1 to 19 presented OAS to peach. (Reprinted from Pastorello EA, *et al.* J Allergy Clin Immunol 1994;94:699–707.)

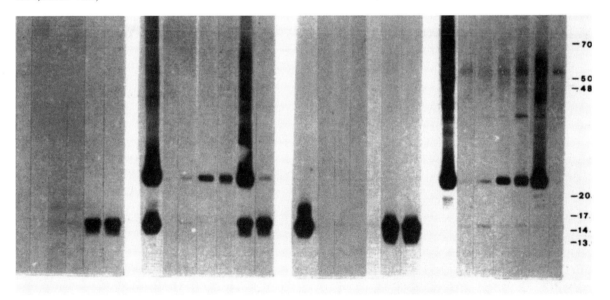

Figure 13.5

Immunoblotting inhibition in the sera of four patients. P, peach; C, cherry; A, apple; PL, plum; G, grass; B, birch. (Reprinted from Pastorello EA, *et al.* J Allergy Clin Immunol 1994;94:699–707.)

requires a slightly different diagnostic approach (49).

The clinical history plays a substantial role in diagnosis. In most cases, the relationship between the contact of a food with the oral mucosa and the occurrence of symptoms is evident. Most patients manifest symptoms within 5 minutes, and almost all patients within 30 minutes after contact with the offending food (Fig. 13.1) (6). The occurrence of symptoms immediately after oral contact pinpoints the role of the food as a causal agent. In those cases where symptoms are always manifested after any contact with a particular food, the diagnosis becomes particularly clear.

Other elements of the clinical history may support the diagnosis of OAS: the localization of the symptoms to the mouth, lips, pharynx, and glottis, and the co-presence of allergic rhinitis. The diagnosis is backed by the presence of known associations between the causal agents of hayfever and food allergy (i.e., birch and apple or mugwort and celery).

Positive skin and in vitro tests for specific IgE antibodies to food confirm a diagnostic suspicion of IgE-mediated food allergy. The reliability of these tests is questionable in OAS, however, due to the lability of some food allergens, which lose their allergenicity during the preparation of the extracts. This lability is illustrated by the fact that many patients suffering from severe OAS can eat a cooked version of the offending food without presenting any symptoms. In a study of 70 patients with positive skin tests to birch and/or mugwort pollens and celery, 94% of the patients gave a positive SPT to raw celery but only 36% to the cooked vegetable (50).

SPT with commercial extracts of fruits (e.g., apple) have poor reliability (4, 49). Some modifications of the skin test technique have been proposed, including a scratch test with fresh foods, a direct SPT based on pricking the skin with the lancet through the food, and the prick + prick technique (the lancet is inserted into the vegetable, withdrawn, and then used to prick the patient's skin) (20, 29, 51, 52). The prick + prick technique combines reliability with simplicity, increases diagnostic sensitivity, and shows good reproducibility when testing different botanical varieties of the same fruit or different parts of the fruit, such as the peel or pulp (21). In one study, SPT sensitivity using a commercial apple extract increased from 0.02 to 0.82 when prick + prick was used with fresh apple, although SPT specificity fell from 100 to 65 (49). A recent study reported that the prick + prick technique with foods such as milk, egg, nuts, and seafood was more sensitive than SPT with commercial extracts (53).

Even the reliability of specific IgE determinations is affected by the loss of allergenicity during the preparation of commercial extracts (34, 39, 54). Moreover, lectins in vegetables are theoretically able to give false-positive results in vitro because of specific bonds with the solid phase (55). Fresh foods—particularly fresh apple—have been proposed as coating material for the RAST disk (53). RAST prepared with this technique showed concordance with both clinical history and skin tests. Björkstén et al. were able to increase apple RAST diagnostic sensitivity to 90% by inhibition of reactions with phenolic compounds during apple extract preparation (54). Poor results obtained with a commercial specific IgE determination for celery significantly improved after coating the disk with fresh celery, particularly celery roots (38). Use of fresh fruits and vegetables for routine specific IgE determination is impractical, however. For these reasons it is important to establish the reliability of the current diagnostic procedures.

The diagnostic accuracy of skin tests using commercial extracts, of skin tests using fresh foods, and of specific IgE determination to foods was evaluated by Ortolani et al., who compared the results of these tests in 100 patients suffering from OAS (Table 13.7) (49). Skin tests with the prick + prick technique proved to be the most sensitive for fruits and vegetables such as carrot, celery, cherry, apple, tomato, orange, and peach, all of which contain unstable allergens; in contrast, SPT with commercial extracts were the most sensitive options for foods with stable allergens such as peanut, nut, and pea. Commercial specific IgE determinations offered good sensitivity for only apple and celery. The specificity of these three tests for different foods varied widely, ranging from 40 (pea) to 100 (apple) for commercial SPT; from 42 (carrot) to 93 (peanut) for prick + prick; and from 61 (peanut) to 87 (carrot) for RAST. The overall specificity was unsatisfactory, because most false-positive results could be related to cross-reactivity. In this study, the three tests exhibited comparable

Table 13.7
Sensitivity, Specificity, and Predictive Indices for Seven Food Antigens in 100 OAS Patients

Food	N	P		FFSPT	CSPT	RAST
Apple	73	60	SE	82	2	70
			SP	65	100	72
			PPV	78	100	79
			NPV	71	40	62
Peanut	52	46	SE	12	67	42
			SP	93	46	61
			PPV	59	51	48
			NPV	55	62	55
Orange	52	29	SE	67	27	20
			SP	73	97	81
			PPV	50	79	30
			NPV	84	76	71
Carrot	50	20	SE	100	80	50
			SP	42	65	87
			PPV	30	36	49
			NPV	100	93	87
Tomato	44	36	SE	75	25	31
			SP	61	79	86
			PPV	52	40	55
			NPV	81	65	69
Hazelnut	47	57	SE	41	22	48
			SP	80	85	75
			PPV	73	66	72
			NPV	51	45	52
Pea	18	44	SE	62	75	50
			SP	50	40	80
			PPV	49	50	66
			NPV	63	67	67

(From Ortolani C, *et al.* J Allergy Clin Immunol 1989;83:683–690. Reprinted by permission.)
N, number of patients studied; P, prevalence; FFSPT, fresh food skin prick test; CSPT, commercial skin prick test; RAST, radioallergosorbent test; SE, sensitivity; SP, specificity; PPV, predictive positive value; NPV, negative predictive value.

overall diagnostic accuracy for only peanut, hazelnut, carrot, and pea.

Another factor influencing the sensitivity of SPT with fresh fruits and vegetables is the ripeness of the fruit or vegetable used in the diagnostic procedure. Allergenic potency may increase during the material's maturation as shown for Golden Delicious apples by Vieths *et al.* (56). This increase in the allergenic properties of mature fruits is due to an 18 kD allergen. In another study, Vieths *et al.* showed that the different allergenic potencies of 16 apple strains were related to the occurrence of this 18 kD allergen (57). The role of single allergenic proteins is further stressed by Pastorello *et al.*'s study, which showed that Prunoideae include a common 13 kD allergen that appears to be related to the occurrence of symptoms (26). These results strongly suggest that improvement

in diagnosis will be obtained only when the appropriate purified allergens for skin tests and specific IgE determination are employed.

False-positive results of SPT and specific IgE determination are frequently obtained among allergic patients with OAS and/or birch hayfever. False-positive SPT do not occur in non-allergic controls when either commercial extracts or fresh foods are used, however (49). This finding suggests that the false-positive allergic tests so frequently observed in these patients may indicate asymptomatic hypersensitivity caused by cross-reactivity.

At this stage, it is evident that tests used for diagnosis of food allergy lack reliable allergens. SPT using fresh vegetables is an improvement in diagnosis, but the allergens employed are not standardized.

Oral food provocation tests are rarely required

for clinical diagnostic purposes. The patient's history and allergy tests are typically sufficient for an almost certain diagnosis (47, 49). A patient does not usually need to undergo a provocation test. In selected cases (i.e., polysensitization or associated systemic reactions), food provocation tests may be necessary. The design of double-blind, placebo-controlled food challenges must consider the lability of allergens and the difficulty of masking the taste and consistency of each food. The food must be administered to the patient in its natural form—not dried, lyophilized, or in capsules—because it needs to come in contact with the oral mucosa to induce symptoms.

Future research should be directed at identifying the major food allergens, particularly in fresh fruits and vegetables. The use of standardized food allergens will greatly improve our understanding of the OAS syndrome.

REFERENCES

1. Amlot PL, Kemeny DM, Zachary C, Parks P, Lessof MH. Oral allergy syndrome (OAS): symptoms of IgE mediated hypersensitivity to foods. Clin Allergy 1987;17:33–38.
2. Tuft L, Blumstein GI. Studies in food allergy. II. Sensitization to fresh fruits: clinical and experimental observations. J Allergy 1942;13:574–581.
3. Juhlin-Danfelt C. About the occurrence of various forms of pollen allergy in Sweden. Acta Med Scand 1948;26:563–577.
4. Hannuksela M, Lahti A. Immediate reaction to fruits and vegetables. Contact Dermat 1977;3:79–84.
5. Eriksson NE. Food sensitivity reported by patients with asthma and hay fever. Allergy 1978;33:189–196.
6. Ortolani C, Ispano M, Pastorello EA, Bigi A, Ansaloni R. The oral allergy syndrome. Ann Allergy 1988;61:47–52.
7. Anderson BL, Dreyfuss E, Logan S, Shonstane ED, Glaser S. Melon and banana sensitivity coincident with ragweed pollinosis. J Allergy 1970;45:310–319.
8. Wüthrich B. Nahrungsmittelallergie. Allergologie 1981;4:320–328.
9. Pauli G, Bessot JC, Kopferschmidtt-Kuber MC, et al. Allergie au céleri, allergie au pollen d'amoise, une nouvelle entité? Revue Fr Allerg 1982;22:36.
10. Enberg RN, Leickly FE, McCullough S, Bailey J, Ownby DR. Watermelon and ragweed share allergens. J Allergy Clin Immunol 1987;79:867–875.
11. Ebner C, Birkner T, Valenta R, et al. Common epitopes of birch pollen and apples. Studies by Western and Northern blot. J Allergy Clin Immunol 1991;88:588–595.
12. Ortolani C, Pastorello EA, Farioli L, et al. IgE mediated allergy from vegetable allergens. Ann Allergy 1993;83:683–690.
13. Bircher AJ, Van Melle G, Haller E, Curty B, Frei PC. IgE to food allergens are highly prevalent in patients allergic to pollens, with and without symptoms of food allergy. Clin Exper Allergy 1994;24:367–374.
14. Pastorello EA, Ispano M, Pravettoni V, et al. Clinical aspects

15. Eriksson NE. Birch pollen allergy associated with food hypersensitivity. An inquiry study. Nordic Aerobiology 1984;66–69.
16. Kivity S, Dunner K, Marian Y. The pattern of food hypersensitivity in patients with onset after 10 years of age. Clin Exper Allergy 1994;24:19–22.
17. Eriksson NE, Formgren H, Svenonius E. Food hypersensitivity in patients with pollen allergy. Allergy 1982;37:437–443.
18. Pauli G, Bessot JC, Braun PA, Dieterman-Molard A, Kopferschmidt-Kubler MC. Celery allergy: clinical and biological study of 20 cases. Ann Allergy 1988;60:243–246.
19. Eriksson NE. Clustering of foodstuffs in food hypersensitivity. An inquiry study in pollen allergic patients. Allergol Immunopathol 1984;12:28–32.
20. Wüthrich B, Dietschi R. Das "Selleri-Karotten-Beifuss-Gewürz-syndrom: hauttest- und Rast-ergebnisse. Schweiz Med Wschr 1985;45:310–364.
21. Dreborg S, Foucard T. Allergy to apple, carrot and potato in children with birch pollen allergy. Allergy 1983;38:167–172.
22. Farioli L, Pravettoni V, Ispano M, et al. Allergenic cross-reactivity between fennel and celery. ACI News 1994:446 (abstr).
23. Hebling A, Schwartz HJ, Lopez M, Lehrer SB. Lettuce and carrot allergy: are they related? Allergy Proc 1994;15:33–38.
24. De Martino M, Novembre E, Cozza G, et al. Sensitivity to tomato and peanut allergens in children monosensitized to grass pollen. Allergy 1988;43:206–213.
25. Jordan-Wagner DL, Whisman BA, Goetz DW. Cross-allergenicity among celery, cucumber, carrot and watermelon. Ann Allergy 1993;71:70–79.
26. Pastorello EA, Ortolani C, Farioli L, et al. Allergenic cross-reactivity among peach, apricot, plum, and cherry in patients with oral allergy syndrome: an in vivo and in vitro study. J Allergy Clin Immunol 1994;94:699–707.
27. Gall H, Kalveram KJ, Fork G, Sterry W. Kiwi fruit allergy: a new birch pollen associated food allergy. J Allergy Clin Immunol 1994;94:70–76.
28. Freye HB. Life-threatening anaphylaxis to kiwi fruit and prevalence of kiwi fruit sensitivity in the United States. Allergologie 1989;12:89–90.
29. Andersen KE, Lowenstein H. An investigation of the possible immunological relationship between allergen extracts from birch pollen, hazelnut, potato and apple. Contact Dermatitis 1978;4:73–79.
30. Hirschwehr R, Valenta R, Ebner C, et al. Identification of common allergenic structures in hazel pollen and hazelnuts: a possible explanation for sensitivity to hazelnuts in patients allergic to tree pollen. J Allergy Clin Immunol 1992;90:927–936.
31. Belin L. Immunological analysis of birch pollen antigens, with special reference to the allergenic components. Int Arch Allergy 1972;42:300–322.
32. Eriksson NE, Wihl JA, Arrendhal H. Birch pollen-related food hypersensitivity: influence of total and specific IgE levels. Allergy 1983;38:353–357.
33. Lahti A, Björkstén F, Hannuksela M. Allergy to birch pollen and apple, and cross-reactivity of the allergens studied with the RAST. Allergy 1980;35:297–300.
34. Halmepuro L, Vountela K, Kalimo KK, Björkstén F. Cross-reactivity of IgE antibodies with allergens in birch pollen, fruits and vegetables. Int Arch Allergy Appl Immunol 1984;74:235–240.

of food allergy. Proc XVI European Congress of Allergology and Clinical Immunology, 1995;883–888.

35. Calkhoven PG, Aalbers M, Koshte VL, Pos O, Oei HD, Aalbersee RC. Cross-reactivity among birch pollen, vegetables and fruits as detected by IgE antibodies is due to at least three distinct cross-reactive structures. Allergy 1987;42:382–390.

36. Vallier P, Dechamp C, Vial O, Deviller P. A study of allergens in celery with cross-reactivity to mugwort and birch pollen. Clin Allergy 1988;18:491–500.

37. De la Hoz B, Fernandez-Rivas M, Quirce S, et al. Swiss chard hypersensitivity: clinical and immunologic study. Ann Allergy 1991;67:487–492.

38. Pauli G, Bessot JC, Dieterman-Molard A, Braun PA, Thierry R. Celery sensitivity: clinical and immunological correlations with pollen allergy. Clin Allergy 1985;15:273–279.

39. Pastorello EA, Farioli L, Pravettoni V, et al. A RAST inhibition study of cross-reactivity between peach, plum, apricot, birch and timothy. Schweiz Wschr 1991;121:80.

40. Pettenburger K, Breiteneder H, Valenta R, et al. Distribution of allergens and mRNAs coding for allergens isolated from various tissues of white birch. In: Sehon A, Kraft D, Kunkel G, eds. Epitopes of atopic allergens. Brussels: The UCB Institute of Allergy, 1990, 65–69.

41. Valenta R, Duchêne M, Pettenburger K, et al. Identification of profilin as a novel pollen allergen; IgE autoreactivity in sensitized individuals. Science 1991;253:557–560.

42. Vallier P, Dechamp C, Valenta R, Vial O, Deviller P. Purification and characterization of an allergen from celery immunochemically related to an allergen present in several other plant species. Identification as a prolifin. Clin Exp Allergy 1992;22:774–782.

43. Valenta R, Duchene M, Ebner C, et al. Profilins constitute a novel family of functional plant pan-allergens. J Exp Med 1992;2:377–385.

44. Vocks E, Borga A, Saliska C, et al. Common allergenic structures in hazelnut, rye grass, sesame seeds, kiwi and poppy seeds. Allergy 1993;48:168–172.

45. Pravettoni V, Farioli L, Ispano M, et al. Allergenic patients of kiwi and cross-reactivity with grass pollen. ACI News 1994 (suppl 2):74.

46. Lavad F, Prevost A, Cossart G, et al. Allergy to latex, avocado pear and banana: evidence for a 30kd antigen in immunoblotting. J Allergy Clin Immunol 1995;95:557–564.

47. Sampson HA. Adverse reactions to food. In: Middleton E Jr, Reed CE, Ellis EF, Adkinson NF Jr, Yunginger JW, Busse WW, eds. Allergy. Principles and practice. vol 2. 4th ed. St Louis: Mosby—Year Book, 1993, 1661–1704.

48. Aas K, Bindslev-Jensen C, Björkstén, et al. Position paper of the European Academy of Allergology and Clinical Immunology on adverse reactions to food. Allergy 1995;12:357–378.

49. Ortolani C, Ispano M, Pastorello EA, Ansaloni R, Magri A. Comparison of results of skin prick tests (with fresh foods and commercial extracts) and RAST in 100 patients with oral allergy syndrome. J Allergy Clin Immunol 1989;83: 683–690.

50. Wüthrich B, Staeger J, Johansson SGO. Celery allergy associated with birch and mugwort pollinosis. Allergy 1990;45:566–571.

51. Lahti A, Hannuksela M. Hypersensitivity to apple and carrot can be reliably detected with fresh material. Allergy 1978;33:143–146.

52. Wüthrich B, Hofer T. Nahrungsmittelallergie: das "Sellerie-Beifuß-Gewürz-Syndrom." Assoziation mit einer Mangofrucht-Allergie? Dtsch Med Wschr 1984;109:981–986.

53. Rosen JP, Selcow JE, Mendelson LM, Grodovsky MP, Factor JM, Sampson HA. Skin testing with natural foods in patients suspected of having food allergies: is it a necessity? J Allergy Clin Immunol 1994;93:1068–1070.

54. Björkstén F, Halmepuro L, Hannuksela M, Lahti A. Extraction and properties of apple allergens. Allergy 1980;35:671–677.

55. Barnet D, Howden MEH. Lectins and radioallergosorbent test. J Allergy Clin Immunol 1987;80:558–561.

56. Vieths S, Schöning B, Jankiewicz A. Occurrence of IgE binding allergens during ripening of apple fruits. Food Agric Immunol 1993;5:93–105.

57. Vieths S, Jankiewicz A, Schöning B, Aulepp H. Apple allergy: the IgE binding potency of apple strains is related to the occurrence of the 18-kD allergen. Allergy 1994;49:262–271.

14

THE RESPIRATORY TRACT AND FOOD HYPERSENSITIVITY

Jean Bousquet
Pascal Chañez
François-B. Michel

Adverse reactions to foods can be classified on the basis of the mechanisms of the reaction. Allergic or food hypersensitivity reactions are those that result from an immune event (1); the best-known example of such a reaction is IgE-mediated food anaphylaxis. Other types of hypersensitivity reactions have also been associated with food allergy. Nonimmunologic adverse reactions are often classified as food intolerance, as is the case for sulfite or aspirin-induced asthma.

Food hypersensitivity reactions induce several types of pulmonary responses, although the vast majority of reactions appear to be IgE-mediated.

Asthma Induced by Food Allergy

Food allergy has always posed a difficult problem, especially in asthma, where some investigators deny its existence even as others tend to overestimate its prevalence. In IgE-mediated food asthma, the difficulties not only derive from the concept that ingested allergens may not be able to cause immune reactions or trigger mast cells present in the airways, but also relate to the diagnosis of food allergy, which often creates problems. Double-blind food challenges should thus be performed in many patients to confirm the diagnosis of food-induced asthma. Moreover, the mechanisms of a reaction should be characterized as foods trigger airway obstruction by both allergic and nonallergic mechanisms, for which the ensuing treatments may differ.

CLINICAL CASES DEMONSTRATING ASTHMA INDUCED BY FOOD ALLERGY

Several cases demonstrate that asthma may be triggered by foods (2–7) and that an appropriate diet is able to control asthma. Many of these are cases merely speculative, however. It is always extremely difficult to ascribe an asthma attack to food allergy when the delay between the ingestion and symptoms exceeds more than 24 hours owing to the great variability of the airway obstruction in chronic asthmatics. The best demonstration of this variation is observed in double-blind food challenges (Fig. 14.1). In some highly allergic individuals or in occupational allergy (bakers), inhalation challenges with foods can lead to immediate bronchial responses. Elimination diets can also produce striking results (Fig. 14.2), but their interpretation may be difficult when patients are allergic to both foods and inhalants (8).

MECHANISMS OF ASTHMA TRIGGERED BY FOOD ALLERGENS

Mechanisms underlying food-induced asthma are not always easy to characterize and may relate to immediate allergic responses (IgE-mediated and possibly IgG-mediated), immune-complex reactions, and lymphocyte activation. The best recognized reactions remain, however, the IgE-mediated immune responses (9). IgG or IgG4 might also be involved, but no definite evidence exists to prove that these immunoglobulin isotypes are important in food allergy. Some anecdotal cases have, however, been published.

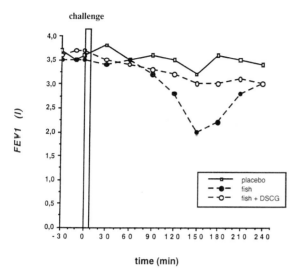

Figure 14.1

Oral provocative challenge in a patient allergic to fish. DSCG, disodium cromoglycate. From Bousquet *et al.* (8).

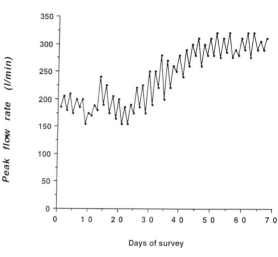

Figure 14.2

Evolution of peak flow rates in a patient allergic to eggs after an egg-free diet. From Bousquet *et al.* (8).

When foods are ingested, several hypothetical mechanisms may be envisaged. Intact foods are absorbed in the alimentary tract, and gastrointestinal absorption may be increased by enhanced permeability due to minor anaphylactic reactions that may not be clinically evident. Foods may also be handled differently by patients than by nonallergic individuals. It has been speculated that in normal subjects foods are complexed by IgA and then rapidly cleared by the reticuloendothelial system (10). In allergic patients, either foods in greater amounts may reach the lungs and stimulate airway mast cells or immune complexes made from foods and IgE may lead to some pathological changes (11) (Fig. 14.3). These complexes are not yet demonstrated, however, and their role remains putative. Early symptoms often include oral irritation and/or throat tightness (12) with wheezing. During food allergic reactions, anaphylactic mediators are released (13, 14). They may possibly reach the lungs and trigger asthma, even though they are rapidly metabolized in the bloodstream.

Food-induced asthma may also be triggered by the inhalation of volatile food antigens, directly stimulating airway mast cells, especially in highly allergic individuals or in occupational allergy.

In addition to allergen-specific mechanisms, many nonspecific mechanisms may aggravate respiratory symptoms due to food allergy, such as exercise (15, 16), cold drinks (17, 18), aspirin (19), or concomitant intake of alcohol.

CLINICAL PRESENTATION

Respiratory symptoms due to an IgE-mediated food allergic reaction can occur suddenly if the food is not routinely ingested and may be associated with other symptoms of generalized anaphylaxis. These acute attacks of asthma may be extremely severe, even leading to death (20, 21). On the other hand, if the food is ingested routinely, the patient rather may present with chronic asthma, which is often associated with atopic dermatitis. The severity of chronic asthma varies widely and may take only the form of a persistent cough (22). It has also been observed that foods may increase the nonspecific bronchial hyperreactivity without causing frank wheezing in some (18, 23) but not all patients (24).

In infants, symptoms may take the form of classical asthma, or may also present as intermittent attacks of dyspnea, tachypnea, and occasionally fever. Other symptoms of food allergy are often present concomitantly (25).

DIAGNOSIS OF FOOD ALLERGY INDUCING ASTHMA

Although most immune mechanisms may induce a food allergic reaction, besides coeliac disease, the IgE-mediated allergic reaction is more easily diagnosed than others. The diagnosis of food allergy is sometimes made more difficult because currently available allergen extracts are not standardized, and their stability is poorly determined (26, 27). For allergen extracts that are rapidly degraded (e.g., allergen extracts of fruits and vegetables) (28), skin tests may produce false-negative results in food allergic individuals. Even more so than in inhalant allergy, the presence of food-specific IgE in serum or a positive skin test to a foodstuff does not always correlate with a food allergy because many patients outgrow their allergy with age (29, 30) and not all patients with food-specific IgE demonstrate a clinical sensitivity. In many instances, the diagnosis must be confirmed by a double-blind food challenge that should be carried out under precisely specified conditions and by trained investigators.

Patients who develop acute urticaria or anaphylaxis often make the diagnosis of "food intolerance" by themselves, and the presence of positive skin tests or serum specific IgE correlating with the claims of the patient makes possible a diagnosis without performing a food challenge. Food challenge may cause severe reactions in patients with anaphylaxis and should be performed only with great care and

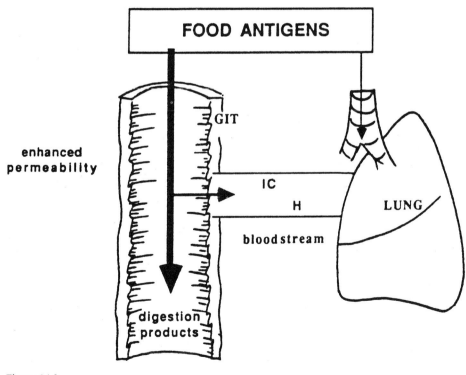

Figure 14.3

Putative mechanisms of food allergy in asthma. IC, immune complexes formed by foods and specific antibodies; H, histamine and other mediators released during the allergic reaction in the gut; GIT, gastrointestinal tract. Adapted from Atherton (98).

under close supervision. In asthma, however, patients rarely incriminate a food as a cause of wheezing, so it may fall to the investigator to suspect a food allergy. This suspicion may be confirmed by double-blind food challenges (31).

Suspicion of Food Allergy in Asthma

Food allergy should be suspected in four cases: (1) when asthma started early in life, especially if the patient has had or currently presents with atopic dermatitis (31, 32); (2) when total serum IgE exceeds 1000 IU/L by the PRIST (31); (3) in patients having presented with anaphylactic symptoms or acute urticaria due to food allergy; and (4) in any patient with poorly controlled asthma and elevated total serum IgE levels.

Skin Tests and Serum Specific Antibodies

The diagnosis of IgE-mediated food asthma should begin with a detailed clinical history and the performance of skin prick tests with food allergens. If possible, positive skin tests should be confirmed by the titration of serum specific IgE. With fruits and vegetables, the test should involve fresh food. Some investigators have proposed to use intradermal skin tests when prick tests are negative, but they cause a greater number of nonspecific positive reactions and may induce systemic reactions. The presence of a positive skin prick test or serum specific IgE does not guarantee the positivity of a food challenge, as only one-third of patients presenting with positive skin prick tests or serum specific IgE are identified as having asthma during food challenge (31). Thus, a diet should not be started before food challenges have been performed (33). The titration of serum food specific IgG or IgG4 has no proven value in the routine diagnosis of food allergy.

Food Challenge

Food challenges should be performed in a manner similar to that reported by Bock and May (34), or Sampson *et al.* (32, 35, 36). The food suspected as causing symptoms should be eliminated from the diet for a minimum of 2 weeks before testing. The selection of foods for administration is based upon positive skin tests or specific IgE, or on a strongly positive history despite negative skin prick tests or RAST.

As much as possible, patients should discontinue anti-asthma medications that might modify the performance of the test. Medication withdrawal may induce a deterioration of lung function, however, making evaluation difficult. Moreover, in patients with severe asthma, it is not possible to discontinue all medications. Occasionally the challenge must be conducted with a patient receiving β-agonists and/or theophylline. In such a case, the medications should be identical on placebo and test days.

When possible, lyophilized foods should be placed in size 0 dye-free opaque capsules. If administered as a liquid, foods should be mixed in a broth or in a juice to disguise the taste. Fresh foods can also be used (37, 38). Although patients who present with anaphylactic symptoms should not routinely be tested, it is nevertheless advised to increase the doses slowly from 100 mg to 10 g. Ideally, challenges should be done in a double-blind manner. If several foods are incriminated, however, a screening with single-blind challenges may be performed first. In the case of food-induced asthma, pulmonary function tests should be serially performed for up to 8 hours as late reactions can occur (31). During challenge, a physician should follow up with the patient, as some systemic reaction might develop. The challenge is only considered to be positive if the $PD_{20}FEV_1$ is reached on a test day, without any such drop in FEV_1 during the placebo day (Fig. 14.1), or if the patient presents a clinically demonstrable exacerbation of asthma. A minority of patients have a significant drop in FEV_1 during challenge (32). For asthma, the test with placebo is critical, given the great variability of pulmonary function that is characteristic of the disease. In young children, pulmonary function tests are not easily performed and interpreted without the use of sophisticated equipment. Thus, the diagnosis of asthma may be based on only clinical examination. Some patients develop systemic symptoms such as acute urticaria or atopic dermatitis without any airway response. Most patients developing an airway response present nonrespiratory symptoms during challenge (39). Food challenges may be improved by measuring the release of mediators in peripheral blood (13) or an increase in gut permeability (40, 41).

The measure of nonspecific bronchial responsiveness before and after an oral challenge has been proposed. Some patients develop an increase of bronchial responsiveness to histamine only after a food challenge without exhibiting any change in baseline pulmonary function (18, 23).

A positive food challenge does not necessarily imply that the patient has an IgE-mediated allergy, but that he or she is intolerant to foods. If specific IgE or prick tests to this food generate positive results, an IgE-mediated mechanism is likely involved (42). When oral cromoglycate is commercially available, a further food challenge may be performed to test the efficacy of this drug in the patient. The results of double-blind food challenge in asthma are similar to those observed with other food-induced symptoms, in that only one-third to one-half of patients with positive skin tests or specific IgE have a positive oral challenge (31, 32, 34, 43).

Elimination Diet

Elimination diets are used primarily for the diagnosis of chronic diseases such as eczema, asthma, and rhinitis. In the case of asthma, the diagnosis of food allergy by elimination diets often proves difficult for many reasons (31, 43): (1) food allergy is almost constantly associated with inhalant allergy and possibly with other triggers, and variations in airway obstruction may be due to factors unrelated to foods; (2) both food and inhalant allergens aggravate nonspecific bronchial hyperreactivity, and it may take days or even weeks to observe an improvement of asthma; and (3) the great variability of airway obstruction in chronic asthmatics may obscure the benefits of dietary manipulations. When a patient is highly allergic to a given food, however, significant improvement or even complete remission of asthma can be observed.

As for other forms of food allergy, unproven and controversial techniques should be avoided (44).

PREVALENCE OF FOOD ALLERGY IN ASTHMA

Although food allergy is better recognized today, its real prevalence has been investigated in only a few studies. Prospective, population-based studies are required to assess the true incidence of food-allergic diseases. The rate of food allergy obtained depends on the methods used. In response to a questionnaire, the number of people who think they have experienced adverse reactions to foods may be as high as 33% (45). When appropriate tests are used, this percentage decreases sharply (46–48). Double-blind food challenges indicate that the prevalence of food allergy is less than 1% in adults but is greater in children (49). This estimate may be low as food challenge may not identify the entire population of food-allergic individuals. Some genetic and environmental factors can also increase the prevalence of food allergy.

Asthma due to foods may be caused by both immunologic and non-immunologic mechanisms. IgE-mediated allergy may be a less common trigger of asthma than food intolerance. Reports of a high prevalence of food allergy in asthma did not differentiate between the mechanisms of food-induced asthma (50–52).

Most cases of food-induced asthma are observed in early infancy and are often related to cow's milk hypersensitivity. Asthma has been noted in 7% to 29% of this group (53–59) according to the definition of cow's milk allergy. In their study, Hill *et al.* (59) surveyed 100 children (mean age 16 months) presenting with manifestations of cow's milk intolerance. Among these subjects, 27 had early manifestations after cow's milk challenge, with urticaria or angioedema noted as well as cow's milk specific IgE. In this group, 48% experienced wheezing, and challenge induced cough or wheeze in 29%. In a second group of 53 patients presenting with mainly digestive symptoms, the prevalence of wheezing was low (13%) and milk challenge induced wheezing in 4%. A third group consisted of 20 infants with late-onset symptoms after milk ingestion. Members of this group with atopic dermatitis had an IgE-mediated allergic reaction to cow's milk, and asthma was frequently observed.

The prevalence of food allergy peaks in children and decreases with age (Fig. 14.4). Differences in the disappearance rate depend on the allergen involved and on individual factors (29, 30, 60–63). Most children with cow's milk allergy tolerate at least small amounts of cow's milk at 3 years of age. Egg allergy usually subsides before puberty, but tends to persist

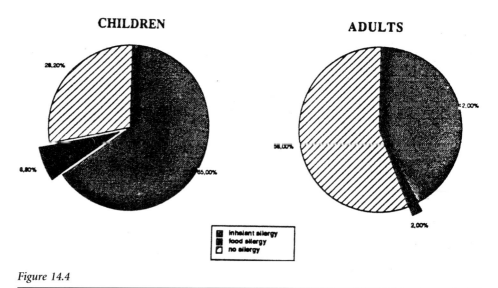

Figure 14.4

Prevalence of food allergy in asthmatic patients according to their age. From Onorato *et al.* (31).

if it started early or if atopic symptoms are severe. On the other hand, allergy to fish, shellfish, nuts, and peanut does not disappear in most patients, although it may be less severe.

Although some investigators have proposed that many intrinsic adult asthmatics may, in fact, be allergic to foods (64), controlled studies performed by food challenges (31, 65, 66) or skin tests (67) do not substantiate this assertion. In areas where mugwort and birch pollens are rare, food allergy represents only a minor cause of perennial asthma, being present in 4% to 9% of asthmatic children (68, 69) and in 1% to 4% of asthmatic adults (Fig. 14.1) (31, 70, 71).

Patients with allergic rhinitis/conjunctivitis to birch—and to a lesser extent to other Betulaceae (hazel, alder) pollen—frequently prove hypersensitive to nuts, apples, carrots, and potatoes (72). Some birch or hazel pollen allergens cross-react with allergens of apple, other fruits (73), or various nuts (74). Most patients with food hypersensitivity exhibit a severe allergy to pollens (72). Some Compositeae pollen allergens (mugwort) cross-react with foods of the Ombelliferae family (celery in particular) (75). Although IgEs to food allergens are extremely common in patients allergic to Betulaceae and Compositeae pollens, only a portion of these individuals present

with symptoms of food allergy (76). Ragweed (*Ambrosia* pollen)-sensitive individuals may develop symptoms when eating banana or melon. Most patients present mild symptoms, but anaphylaxis may occur with these cross-reacting foods. Gastrointestinal and dermatologic symptoms appear more frequently than asthma. Asthma due to food allergy, however, is two to three times more common in areas where birch and mugwort pollens are present than in comparable areas without such pollinoses (77).

In non-Caucasian populations, the prevalence of food allergy may be greater (78). According to the regular diet of a given country, differences may be observed, such as dye allergy that was reported to be more frequent in Great Britain.

TREATMENT OF ASTHMA INDUCED BY FOOD ALLERGY

The presence of a positive skin prick test or RAST to a given food should not itself lead to an elimination diet, because only 30% to 40% of patients have asthma when they are challenged orally with the offending food. A positive food challenge favors dietary avoidance (79, 80) but the nutritive value of a diet must always be maintained—especially calcium intake in a diet planned for cow's milk avoidance (81). In addition, the reintroduction of a food—whether accidental or intentional—may be associated with anaphylaxis or severe respiratory obstruction, as individual patients tend to continue to react with the same symptoms as they had before use of the elimination diet.

The efficacy of oral sodium cromoglycate is not completely established, but this drug was found in some studies to prevent asthma due to food allergy (Fig. 14.1) (31, 82, 83). Only a fraction of patients appear to benefit from this treatment but, when available and effective, it may be used to decrease the reactivity of the gastrointestinal tract to dietary allergens and to allow a less restrictive diet. Ketotifene has also been used and seemed to have value in the treatment of skin symptoms, even though it is also used in the treatment of mild asthma (84).

At present, no evidence supports specific immunotherapy for food allergens by either the oral or the parenteral route, as efficacy data are also lacking. There is also the potential severity of anaphylactic reactions with which to contend (85, 86). In any case, asthma is a disease of the airways, and patients should always be treated for bronchial inflammation and obstruction as well as for food allergy.

The prevention of food allergy may be attempted in newborns at high risk for allergy (87). There is no clear demonstration that breast feeding, even when prolonged, may prevent the onset of allergy in later life (88).

Rhinitis Induced by Food Allergy

Chronic rhinitis is another respiratory tract manifestation of food allergy, and this symptom may occur during food challenges (89, 90). It may occur alone or in association with other manifestations (91). The mechanisms of food-induced rhinitis do not differ from those of food-induced asthma. The acute onset of rhinitis (and conjunctivitis) may represent a manifestation of an IgE-mediated allergic reaction caused by any allergen, including foods (inhaled or ingested). Chronic rhinitis is more commonly manifested by chronic nasal obstruction associated with paroxysmal sneezing and rhinorrhea. Food-induced rhinitis more

typically occurs in children than in adults. Although milk allergy is often described as a cause of rhino-conjunctivitis (22, 54, 55, 92), other food allergens may produce this effect as well. The prevalence of food-induced rhino-conjunctivitis is probably overestimated, as double-blind food challenges give positive results in only one-third to one-fourth of tests. The treatment of food-induced rhino-conjunctivitis includes eye drops of disodium cromoglycate as available, as well as other therapy.

Serous Otitis Media

The involvement of food allergy in serous otitis media has been proposed (93). It does not, however, appear to be a common trigger, although double-blind food challenges have demonstrated its reality. Moreover, nasal congestion aggravates otitis, and foods may, therefore, be indirectly involved.

Alveolitis

RECURRENT PNEUMONIA

In 1958, Heiner and Sears described a syndrome induced by milk, associating chronic or recurrent pulmonary disease, allergic rhinitis and/or asthma, anorexia, gastrointestinal symptoms, eosinophilia, and serum precipitins to cow's milk constituents (94). Symptoms disappeared with a milk-free diet. This syndrome is rare, and no evidence suggests a similar disease in adults. The possible contribution of milk aspiration in this syndrome should be considered. In a group of children with asthma and recurrent pneumonia, Euler *et al.* (95) observed an increased incidence of dysfunction of the lower esophageal sphincter. The immunological mechanisms of this syndrome do not favor the role of reaginic antibodies, but rather an antigen–antibody reaction or cell-mediated immunity.

Milk-induced primary pulmonary hemosiderosis may occur in 10% of children with milk-related pulmonary infiltrates. It may be related to the deposition of immune complexes containing milk in the lung parenchyma (96). In adults with idiopathic pulmonary hemosiderosis, no direct evidence suggests an association with food hypersensitivity.

RELATIONSHIPS BETWEEN GLUTEN ENTEROPATHY AND FOOD ALLERGY

Patients with gluten enteropathy may become sensitized and develop antibodies to a component of egg yolk (97). These patients also seem to be particularly prone to develop bird fancier's lung.

REFERENCES

1. Anderson J, Sogn D. Adverse reactions to foods. In: Coartfa, ed. Bethesda, MD: NIH Publication 84-2442 (NIAID A), 1984.
2. Hoigné R, Scherrer M. An attack of bronchial asthma produced by egg-white and studied by means of lung function tests. Int Arch Allergy 1960;17:152–158.
3. Bousquet J, Dhivert H, Clauzel AM, Hewitt B, Michel FB. Occupational allergy to sunflower pollen. J Allergy Clin Immunol 1985;75:70–74.
4. Axelsson IG, Ihre E, Zetterstrom O. Anaphylactic reactions to sunflower seed. Allergy 1994;49:517–520.
5. Blanco C, Carrillo T, Castillo R, Quiralte J, Cuevas M. Avocado hypersensitivity. Allergy 1994;49:454–459.
6. Quirce S, Diez-Gomez ML, Hinojosa M, et al. Housewives with raw potato-induced bronchial asthma. Allergy 1989;44:532–536.
7. Martin JA, Compaired JA, de-la-Hoz B, et al. Bronchial asthma induced by chick pea and lentil. Allergy 1992;47:185–187.
8. Bousquet J, Chanez P, Michel F. The respiratory tract and food hypersensitivity. In: Metcalfe D, Sampson H, Simon R, eds. Food allergy, adverse reactions to foods and food additives. Boston: Blackwell Scientific Publications, 1991, 139–149.
9. Sampson H. Adverse reactions to foods. In: Middleton E Jr, Reed C, Ellis E, Adkinson N Jr, Yunginger J, Busse W, eds. Allergy: principles and practice. 4th ed. St Louis: Mosby, 1992, 1661–1705.
10. Mestecky J, McGhee JR. Immunoglobulin A (IgA): molecular and cellular interactions involved in IgA biosynthesis and immune response. Adv Immunol 1987;40:153–245.
11. Dannaeus A, Inganas M, Johansson SG, Foucard T. Intestinal uptake of ovalbumin in malabsorption and food allergy in relation to serum IgG antibody and orally administered sodium cromoglycate. Clin Allergy 1979;9:263–270.
12. Amlot PL, Kemeny DM, Zachary C, Parkes P, Lessof MH. Oral allergy syndrome (OAS): symptoms of IgE-mediated hypersensitivity to foods. Clin Allergy 1987;17:33–42.
13. Sampson HA, Jolie PL. Increased plasma histamine concentrations after food challenges in children with atopic dermatitis. N Engl J Med 1984;311:372–376.
14. Sampson HA, Broadbent KR, Bernhisel-Broadbent J. Spontaneous release of histamine from basophils and histamine-releasing factor in patients with atopic dermatitis and food hypersensitivity. N Engl J Med 1989;321:228–232.
15. Maulitz RM, Pratt DS, Schocket AL. Exercise-induced anaphylactic reaction to shellfish. J Allergy Clin Immunol 1979; 63:433–434.
16. Kidd J, Cohen SH, Sosman AJ, Fink JN. Food-dependent exercise-induced anaphylaxis. J Allergy Clin Immunol 1983; 71:407–411.
17. Wilson NM, Chudry N, Silverman M. Role of the oesophagus in asthma induced by the ingestion of ice and acid. Thorax 1987;42:506–510.
18. Wilson NM, Dixon C, Silverman M. Increased bronchial responsiveness caused by ingestion of ice. Eur J Respir Dis 1985;66:25–30.
19. Cant A, Gibson P, Dancy M. Food hypersensitivity made life-threatening by ingestion of aspirin. Br Med J 1984;288:755–756.
20. Yunginger JW, Sweeney KG, Sturner WQ, et al. Fatal food-induced anaphylaxis. Jama 1988;260:1450–1452.
21. Sampson HA, Mendelson L, Rosen JP. Fatal and near-fatal anaphylactic reactions to food in children and adolescents. N Engl J Med 1992;327:380–384.
22. Clein NW. Cow's milk allergy in infants. Pediatr Clin North Am 1954;4:949–962.
23. James J, Eigenmann P, Eggleston P, Sapson H. Airway reactivity changes in food-allergic, asthmatic children undergoing double-blind placebo-controlled food challenges. Am J Respir Crit Care Med 1995 (in press).
24. Zwetchkenbaum JF, Skufca R, Nelson HS. An examination of food hypersensitivity as a cause of increased bronchial responsiveness to inhaled methacholine. J Allergy Clin Immunol 1991;88:360–364.
25. Bock SA, Sampson HA. Food allergy in infancy. Pediatr Clin North Am 1994;41:1047–1067.
26. Metcalfe DD. Food allergens. Clin Rev Allergy 1985;3:331–349.
27. Yunginger J. Food antigens. In: Metcalfe D, Sampson H, Simon R, eds. Food allergy. Adverse reactions to foods and food additives. Boston: Blackwell Scientific Publications, 1991, 36–51.
28. Bjorksten F, Halmepuro L, Hannuksela M, Lahti A. Extraction and properties of apple allergens. Allergy 1980;35:671–677.
29. Dannaeus A, Inganas M. A follow-up study of children with food allergy. Clinical course in relation to serum IgE- and IgG-antibody levels to milk, egg and fish. Clin Allergy 1981;11:533–539.
30. Bock SA. The natural history of adverse reactions to foods. N Engl Reg Allergy Proc 1986;7:504–510.
31. Onorato J, Merland N, Terral C, Michel FB, Bousquet J. Placebo-controlled double-blind food challenge in asthma. J Allergy Clin Immunol 1986;78:1139–1146.
32. James JM, Bernhisel-Broadbent J, Sampson HA. Respiratory reactions provoked by double-blind food challenges in children. Am J Respir Crit Care Med 1994;149:59–64.
33. Yunginger JW. Proper application of available laboratory tests for adverse reactions to foods and food additives. J Allergy Clin Immunol 1986;78:220–223.
34. Bock SA. A critical evaluation of clinical trials in adverse reactions to foods in children. J Allergy Clin Immunol 1986;78:165–174.
35. Sampson HA, Albergo R. Comparison of results of skin tests, RAST, and double-blind, placebo-controlled food challenges in children with atopic dermatitis. J Allergy Clin Immunol 1984;74:26–33.
36. Bock SA, Sampson HA, Atkins FM, et al. Double-blind, placebo-controlled food challenge (DBPCFC) as an office procedure: a manual. J Allergy Clin Immunol 1988;82:986–997.

37. Norgaard A, Bindslev-Jensen C. Egg and milk allergy in adults. Diagnosis and characterization. Allergy 1992;47:503–509.

38. Hansen TK, Bindslev-Jensen C. Codfish allergy in adults. Identification and diagnosis. Allergy 1992;47:610–617.

39. Bock S. Respiratory reactions induced by food challenges in children with pulmonary disease. J Pediatr Allergy Immunol 1992;3:188–194.

40. Falth-Magnusson K, Kjellman NI, Odelram H, Sundqvist T, Magnusson KE. Gastrointestinal permeability in children with cow's milk allergy: effect of milk challenge and sodium cromoglycate as assessed with polyethyleneglycols (PEG 400 and PEG 1000). Clin Allergy 1986;16:543–551.

41. Andre F, Andre C, Feknous M, Colin L, Cavagna S. Digestive permeability to different-sized molecules and to sodium cromoglycate in food allergy. Allergy Proc 1991;12:293–298.

42. Metcalfe DD. Food hypersensitivity. J Allergy Clin Immunol 1984;73:749–762.

43. Atkins FM, Steinberg SS, Metcalfe DD. Evaluation of immediate adverse reactions to foods in adult patients. I. Correlation of demographic, laboratory, and prick skin test data with response to controlled oral food challenge. J Allergy Clin Immunol 1985;75:348–355.

44. Van-Metre T Jr. Critique of controversial and unproven procedures for diagnosis and therapy of allergic disorders. Pediatr Clin North Am 1983;30:807–813.

45. Bender AE, Matthews DR. Adverse reactions to foods. Br J Nutr 1981;46:403–407.

46. Jansen JJ, Kardinaal AF, Huijbers G, Vlieg-Boerstra BJ, Martens BP, Ockhuizen T. Prevalence of food allergy and intolerance in the adult Dutch population. J Allergy Clin Immunol 1994;93:446–456.

47. Burr ML, Merrett TG. Food intolerance: a community survey. Br J Nutr 1983;49:217–219.

48. Young E, Stoneham M, Petruckevitch A, Barton J, Rona R. A population study of food intolerance. Lancet 1994;343:1127–1130.

49. Anderson JA. The clinical spectrum of food allergy in adults. Clin Exp Allergy 1991;1:304–315.

50. Eriksson NE. Food sensitivity reported by patients with asthma and hay fever. A relationship between food sensitivity and birch pollen-allergy and between food sensitivity and acetylsalicylic acid intolerance. Allergy 1978;33:189–196.

51. Zetterstrom O. Food and asthma II. Eur J Respir Dis 1984;65(suppl 136):169–173.

52. Rowe A. Food allergy. Its manifestations and control and the elimination diets. A compendium. Springfield: CC Thomas, 1972.

53. Gerrard J. Familial recurrent rhinorrhea and bronchitis due to cow's milk. JAMA 1966;198:605–607.

54. Buisseret PD. Common manifestations of cow's milk allergy in children. Lancet 1978;1:304–305.

55. Bahna S, Heiner D. Allergies to milk. New York: Grune and Stratton, 1980.

56. Bachman K, Dees S. Milk allergy. I. Observations on incidence and symptoms in "well" babies. Pediatrics 1957;20:393–399.

57. Goldman A, Anderson D, Selles W, et al. Milk allergy. I. Oral challenge with milk and isolated milk proteins in allergic children. Pediatrics 1963;20:400–407.

58. Savilahti E. Cow's milk allergy. Allergy 1981;36:73–88.

59. Hill DJ, Firer MA, Shelton MJ, Hosking CS. Manifestations of milk allergy in infancy: clinical and immunologic findings. J Pediatr 1986;109:270–276.

60. Daul CB, Morgan JE, Lehrer SB. The natural history of shrimp hypersensitivity. J Allergy Clin Immunol 1990;86:88–93.

61. Bishop JM, Hill DJ, Hosking CS. Natural history of cow milk allergy: clinical outcome. J Pediatr 1990;116:862–867.

62. Hill DJ, Firer MA, Ball G, Hosking CS. Natural history of cow's milk allergy in children: immunological outcome over 2 years. Clin Exp Allergy 1993;23:124–131.

63. Kjellman N. Natural course of asthma and allergy in childhood. Pediatr Allergy Immunol 1994;5(suppl 1):13–18.

64. Wraith D. Asthma. Clin Immunol Allergy 1982;2:101–112.

65. Oehling A. Importance of food allergy in childhood asthma. Allergol Immunopathol Madr 1981;9:71–73.

66. Ganderton M. Diet and asthma. Br Med J 1978;i:1624.

67. Hendrick D, Davies R. An analysis of skin prick test reactions in 656 asthmatic children. Thorax 1975;30:2–8.

68. Anderson H, Palmer J, Brailey P, Cooper J, West S. A community survey of asthma and wheezing illness in 8–10 year old children. Report to SW Thames Regional Health Authority, 1981.

69. Novembre E, de-Martino M, Vierucci A. Foods and respiratory allergy. J Allergy Clin Immunol 1988;81:1059–1065.

70. Van-Metre T Jr, Anderson S, Barnard J, et al. A controlled study of the effects of manifestations of chronic asthma of a rigid elimination diet based on Rowe's cereal-free diet 1, 2, 3. J Allergy 1968;41:195–208.

71. Burr ML, Fehily AM, Stott NC, Merrett TG. Food-allergic asthma in general practice. Hum Nutr Appl Nutr 1985;39:349–355.

72. Eriksson NE, Formgren H, Svenonius E. Food hypersensitivity in patients with pollen allergy. Allergy 1982;37:437–443.

73. Ebner C, Birkner T, Valenta R, et al. Common epitopes of birch pollen and apples—studies by Western and Northern blot. J Allergy Clin Immunol 1991;88:588–594.

74. Hirschwehr R, Valenta R, Ebner C, et al. Identification of common allergenic structures in hazel pollen and hazelnuts: a possible explanation for sensitivity to hazelnuts in patients allergic to tree pollen. J Allergy Clin Immunol 1992;90:927–936.

75. Pauli G, Bessot JC, Dietemann-Molard A, Braun PA, Thierry R. Celery sensitivity: clinical and immunological correlations with pollen allergy. Clin Allergy 1985;15:273–279.

76. Bircher AJ, Van-Melle G, Haller E, Curty B, Frei PC. IgE to food allergens are highly prevalent in patients allergic to pollens, with and without symptoms of food allergy. Clin Exp Allergy 1994;24:367–374.

77. Moneret-Vautrin D, Mohr N, Gérard H, Nicolas J, Lacoste J, Grilliat J. Incidence de l'allergie alimentaire IgE-dépendante dans la maladie asthmatique. Méd & Hig 1986;44:926–933.

78. Wilson NM. Food related asthma: a difference between two ethnic groups. Arch Dis Child 1985;60:861–865.

79. Hoj L, Osterballe O, Bundgaard A, Weeke B, Weiss M. A double-blind controlled trial of elemental diet in severe, perennial asthma. Allergy 1981;36:257–262.

80. Ogle K, Bullock J. Children with allergic rhinitis and/or bronchial asthma treated with elimination diet. Ann Allergy 1977;39:8–11.

81. McGowan M, Gibney MJ. Calcium intakes in individuals on diets for the management of cow's milk allergy: a case control study. Eur J Clin Nutr 1993;47:609–616.

82. Dannaeus A, Foucard T, Johansson S. The effect of orally administered sodium cromoglycate on symptoms of allergy. Clin Allergy 1977;7:109–115.

83. Dahl R. Oral and inhaled sodium cromoglycate in challenge test with food allergens or acetylsalicylic acid. Allergy 1981;36:161–165.

84. Ellul-Micallef R. Effect of oral sodium cromoglycate and ketotifen in fish-induced bronchial asthma. Thorax 1983;38:527–530.

85. Oppenheimer JJ, Nelson HS, Bock SA, Christensen F, Leung DY. Treatment of peanut allergy with rush immunotherapy. J Allergy Clin Immunol 1992;90:256–262.

86. Sampson HA. Food allergy and the role of immunotherapy. J Allergy Clin Immunol 1992;90:151–152.

87. Michel FB, Bousquet J, Dannaeus A, *et al*. Preventive measures in early childhood allergy. J Allergy Clin Immunol 1986;78:1022–1027.

88. Arshad SH, Matthews S, Gant C, Hide DW. Effect of allergen avoidance on development of allergic disorders in infancy. Lancet 1992;339:1493–1497.

89. Atkins FM, Steinberg SS, Metcalfe DD. Evaluation of immediate adverse reactions to foods in adult patients. II. A detailed analysis of reaction patterns during oral food challenge. J Allergy Clin Immunol 1985;75:356–363.

90. Pelikan Z, Pelikan-Filipek M. Bronchial response to the food ingestion challenge. Ann Allergy 1987;58:164–172.

91. Pastorello E, Ortolani C, Luraghi MT, *et al*. Evaluation of allergic etiology in perennial rhinitis. Ann Allergy 1985;55:854–856.

92. Nichaman MZ, McPherson RS. Estimating prevalence of adverse reactions to foods: principles and constraints. J Allergy Clin Immunol 1986;78:148–154.

93. Lim D, Bluestone C, Klein J, Nelson J. Recent advances in otitis media with effusion. In: Bluestone C, Klein J, Nelson J, eds. Proceedings of an International Symposium. Philadelphia: BC Dekker, 1984.

94. Heiner D, Sears J. Chronic respiratory disease associated with multiple circulating precipitins to cow's milk. Am J Dis Child 1960;100:200–202.

95. Euler AR, Byrne WJ, Ament ME, *et al*. Recurrent pulmonary disease in children: a complication of gastroesophageal reflux. Pediatrics 1979;63:47–51.

96. Heiner D. Pulmonary siderosis. In: Gellis S, Kagan D, eds. Current pediatric therapy. vol. 5. Philadelphia: WB Saunders, 1971, 139–141.

97. Faux JA, Hendrick DJ, Anand BS. Precipitins to different avian serum antigens in bird fancier's lung and coeliac disease. Clin Allergy 1978;8:101–108.

98. Atherton D. Atopic eczema. Clin Immunol Allergy 1982;2:77–100.

15

ANAPHYLAXIS AND FOOD ALLERGY

A. Wesley Burks
Hugh A. Sampson

Introduction

Although fatal allergic reactions have been recognized for more than 4500 years (1), not until this century was the syndrome of anaphylaxis fully characterized. In their classic studies, Portier and Richet (1902) described the rapid death of several dogs that they were attempting to immunize against the toxic sting of the sea anemone (2). Because this reaction represented the opposite of their intended "prophylaxis," they coined the term "anaphylaxis," or "without or against protection." From these studies, Portier and Richet concluded that anaphylaxis required a latent period for sensitization and reexposure to the sensitizing material. Shortly thereafter, Schlossman (1905) reported a patient who developed acute shock after the ingestion of cow's milk (3). The first series of modern-day descriptions of food anaphylaxis in man was published in 1969 by Golbert and colleagues (4). They described 10 cases of anaphylaxis following the ingestion of various foods, including different legumes, fish, and milk.

Definition

Clinical anaphylaxis is a syndrome of diverse etiology and dramatic presentation of symptoms associated with the classic features of Type I, IgE-mediated hypersensitivity (5). Typically, the term *anaphylaxis* connotes an immunologically mediated event that occurs after exposure to certain foreign substances; in contrast, the term *anaphylactoid* indicates a clinically indistinguishable reaction that is not believed to be immunologically mediated but probably involves many of the same mediators (e.g., histamine). The syndrome results from the generation and release of a variety of potent biologically active mediators and their concerted effects on various target organs. Anaphylaxis is recognized by cutaneous, respiratory, cardiovascular, and gastrointestinal signs and symptoms occurring either singly or in combination. This chapter focuses on allergic reactions to foods that manifest as signs and symptoms involving multiple target organs or the cardiovascular system alone.

Prevalence

The prevalence of anaphylaxis is unknown because, unlike with many disorders, physicians are not required to report such reactions to a national register. In addition, many cases are likely misdiagnosed. Also contributing to this lack of scientific data is the fact that many patients who experience a mild anaphylactic reaction recognize the causative relationship to a specific food and simply avoid that food rather than consult a physician. Sorensen and colleagues reviewed all cases of anaphylactic shock occurring outside the hospital in the Thisted Hospital catchment area in Denmark (6). Twenty cases of anaphylaxis were identified, or 3.2 cases per 100,000 inhabitants per year, of which 5% were fatal. If similar rates occur in the United States (and anaphylaxis may be slightly more common in the United States), about 8300 cases of anaphylaxis could be anticipated each year, with about 415 deaths attributed to this cause. As suggested above, these investigators found that 8 of the 20 cases (40%) had been given an incorrect *International Classification of Diseases* code at the time of discharge. In this series, drugs, food, and insect stings accounted for virtually all of the anaphylactic reactions.

Unfortunately, no *International Classification of Diseases* code has been developed for food-induced anaphylaxis, so it is extremely difficult to obtain any reliable information regarding the prevalence, incidence, or mortality rates for these reactions. In a retrospective survey, Yocum and Khan (7) reviewed all cases of anaphylaxis treated in the Mayo Clinic Emergency Department (United States) over a 3.5-year period. Records were reviewed on all patients experiencing respiratory obstructive symptoms and/or cardiovascular symptoms plus evidence of allergic mediator release (e.g., urticaria). Overall, 179 patients were identified; 66% were female, 49% were atopic, and 37% had experienced an immediate reaction to the responsible allergen in the past. A probable cause was identified in 142 cases (Table 15.1): food—59 cases (33%); bee sting—25 cases (14%); medications—23 cases (13%); and exercise—12 cases (7%). Allergic reactions to food were found to be the most common cause of anaphylactic reactions outside of the hospital, being observed more frequently than reactions to bee sting and drugs combined. Extrapolating from the Sorsensen data, this finding would suggest that approximately 2500 food-induced anaphylactic reactions occur in the United States each year, with about 125 deaths. Peanuts and nuts were

the most common foods causing serious anaphylactic reactions. Bock surveyed 73 emergency departments in Colorado over a 2-year period and identified 25 cases of severe anaphylactic reactions to food, including one death (8). From these data, Bock concluded that at least 950 cases of severe food-induced anaphylaxis occur in the United States annually. The author cautioned that his survey underestimated the problem, however, as patients had been referred to him who were not included in the survey, and the proportion of reactions was higher in the rural emergency departments serving smaller populations than in the busier metropolitan departments. A 5-year survey of anaphylactic reactions treated at the Children's Hospital of Philadelphia also showed that food allergy was the most common cause of anaphylaxis outside of the hospital (Dibs SD, Baker MD; presented at the Ambulatory Pediatrics Association, San Diego, CA, 1995).

The first of several reports on fatal food-induced anaphylaxis was published in 1988 by Yunginger and colleagues, who reported seven cases of fatal anaphylaxis evaluated during a 16-month period (9). In all but possibly one case, the victims unknowingly ingested a food that provoked a previous allergic reaction. Similarly, six fatal and seven near-fatal food-induced anaphylactic reactions in children (aged 2 to 17 years) were accumulated from three metropolitan areas over a 14-month period (10). Common risk factors were noted in these cases: all patients had asthma (although it was generally well controlled); all patients were unaware that they were ingesting the food allergen; all patients had experienced previous allergic reactions to the incriminated food (although in most cases symptoms had been much milder); and all patients had immediate symptoms, with approximately half experiencing a quiescent period prior to a major respiratory collapse. In both series, no patient who died received adrenaline immediately; three patients with near-fatal reactions did, however, receive adrenaline within 15 minutes of developing symptoms but still went on to develop respiratory collapse and hypotension requiring mechanical ventilation and vasopressor support for 12 hours to 3 weeks. Interestingly, patients investigated with life-threatening food-induced anaphylaxis had no significant increase in serum tryptase, raising questions about the exact mechanism of food-induced anaphylaxis (10).

Table 15.1
Three-Year Retrospective Survey of Anaphylaxis Occurring Outside of the Hospital Treated by the Mayo Clinic Emergency Department (7)

Presumed Etiology of Anaphylaxis	Number	Percentage
Food	59	33%
Idiopathic	34	19%
Hymenoptera	25	14%
Medications	23	13%
Exercise	12	7%
Other	8	4%
False diagnosis	18	10%

Foods Implicated in 18 Patients Who Were Skin-Tested

Peanut	4
Cereals	6
Egg	2
Nuts	9
Milk	2

The incidence of food-dependent exercise-induced anaphylaxis appears to be increasing, possibly due to the increased popularity of exercising over the past decade. Two forms of food-dependent exercise-induced anaphylaxis have been described: reactions following the ingestion of specific foods (e.g., celery, shellfish, wheat) (11–15) and, more rarely, reactions following the ingestion of any food (16). Anaphylaxis occurs when a patient exercises within 2 to 4 hours of ingesting a food, although the patient can otherwise ingest the food without any apparent reaction and can exercise without any apparent reaction as long as the specific food (or any food, in the case of nonspecific reactors) has not been ingested within the past several hours. The disorder is twice as common in females, and more than 60% of cases occur in individuals less than 30 years of age. In a recent survey of 199 individuals experiencing exercise-induced anaphylaxis, ingestion of food within 2 hours of exercise was suspected to be a factor in the development of attacks in 54% of the cases (17). Symptoms generally begin with a sensation of generalized pruritus that progresses to urticaria and erythema, respiratory obstruction, and cardiovascular collapse. Patients with specific food-dependent exercise-induced anaphylaxis generally have positive prick skin tests to the food that provokes symptoms; occasionally, they may have a history of reacting to the food at a younger age. As discussed below, specific management of this disorder involves identifying the food(s) that cause the reaction (i.e., DBPCFC with exercise).

Several factors appear to predispose an individual to food-induced anaphylaxis, including a personal history of atopy, family history of atopy, age, and dietary exposure. Atopic patients with asthma have an apparent increased risk of developing more severe food allergic reactions (10, 18, 19). In the reports of Yunginger *et al.* (9) and Sampson *et al.* (10), the majority of individuals were highly atopic, and all had histories of asthma. Although atopy reportedly does not predispose individuals to an increased risk of anaphylaxis (20), it does tend to predispose patients to more severe reactions. Individuals inherit the ability to produce antigen-specific IgE to food proteins, although no conclusive evidence exists that hypersensitivity to a specific food is inherited.

Age may play a role in predisposing an individual

to food-induced anaphylaxis. The incidence of food allergy appears greatest in the first 2 years of life and decreases with age. Consequently, foods introduced during the first year (e.g., cow's milk, egg, soy, wheat, and, in the United States, peanut (in the form of peanut butter) are more apt to induce hypersensitization. Allergic reactions to milk, egg, soybean, and wheat are generally "outgrown" (21, 22). The age of onset of milk allergy is usually in the first year of life, with about 85% of infants "outgrowing" their sensitivity by the third year of life (23, 24). In contrast, food sensitivity to peanuts, tree nuts, fish, and shellfish often persist into adulthood (18, 25). Only rarely will a patient develop clinical tolerance to peanuts and tree nuts.

Dietary exposure can influence the occurrence of food-induced anaphylaxis in several ways. Different populations and nationalities may consume more of certain foods, and the increased exposure may result in increased prevalence of that specific food allergy. In the United States, peanut is one of the most common food allergies (26, 27), in part because Americans ingest several tons of peanuts daily (25) (FDA 1986). By contrast, in Scandinavia, where fish consumption is high, a greater incidence of allergic reactions to codfish is observed (FDA 1986). Rice and buckwheat allergy are quite rare in the United States, unlike in Japan, where these foods are eaten in large quantities.

Etiology

FOODS

A large variety of foods have been reported to have precipitated an anaphylactic reaction. The list of foods that potentially may induce an anaphylactic reaction is unlimited, and, in theory, any food protein is capable of causing an anaphylactic reaction. As indicated in Table 15.2, certain foods tend to be cited most frequently as the cause of anaphylaxis, including peanuts (and to a lesser extent, other legumes such as soybeans, pinto beans, peas, green beans, and garbanzo beans), fish (e.g., cod, whitefish), shellfish (shrimp, lobster, crab, scallops, oyster), tree nuts (hazelnuts, walnuts, cashew, almonds, pistachio), cow's milk, egg, fruits (banana, kiwi), seeds (cotton-

Table 15.2
Foods Most Frequently Implicated
in Food-Induced Anaphylaxis

Peanut
Tree nuts: hazelnuts (filberts), walnuts, cashews, pistachios, Brazil
    nuts
Fish: less often tuna
Shellfish: shrimp, crab, lobster, oyster, scallop
Cow's milk: goat's milk
Hen's egg
Seeds: cottonseed, sesame seed, pine nuts, sunflower seed
Beans: soybeans, green peas, pinto beans, garbanzo beans, green
    beans
Fruit: banana, kiwi
Cereal grains: wheat, barley, oat, buckwheat
Potato

seed, sunflower seed), and cereals or grains (wheat, rice, rye, millet, buckwheat).

Recent reports appear to indicate that certain foods are more likely to induce an anaphylactic reaction. These foods include peanuts and tree nuts (7, 9, 10), fish (27), and shellfish (27). Individuals typically do not "outgrow" these food sensitivities, unlike sensitivities to foods such as milk, eggs, and soybeans. The potency of particular foods in inducing an anaphylactic reaction appears to vary and also depends upon the sensitivity of the individual. In general, for some foods such as peanuts, microgram quantities may be sufficient to induce a reaction. In oral food challenge studies where food-allergic patients are tested on a regular basis (e.g., annually) over a period of years, patients who eventually become tolerant to a food often appear to tolerate more of the antigen in successive years. For example, the initial challenge may be positive after 500 mg of the food; in the subsequent challenge 1 year later, the patient may tolerate 5 g of the food. The next challenge in the following year may reveal that the patient is no longer sensitive to that food.

In theory, prior exposure and sensitization to food allergens must precede the initial anaphylactic reaction. Numerous reports of an anaphylactic reaction occurring after the first known exposure to a food substance have surfaced, however. Several possibilities may account for this apparent paradox: infants are typically sensitized to foods passed in maternal breast milk during lactation; sensitization may occur following an unknown exposure to a food antigen (e.g., milk formula given during the night in the newborn nursery, food given by another care-giver such as a babysitter or grandparent, or food hidden in another product); and sensitization may occur because of cross-sensitization to a similar allergen [e.g., kiwi or banana allergy in a latex-sensitive individual (28)]. Data also suggest that sensitization may occur in utero (29).

FOOD ADDITIVES

Although food additives are often suspected of provoking anaphylactic reactions, sulfites and papain are the only food additives for which significant evidence of precipitation of an anaphylactic reaction exists. One of the initial reports detailed an atopic, nonasthmatic patient who experienced an anaphylactic reaction after consuming a restaurant meal that contained significant sodium bisulfite (30). Specific IgE to sodium bisulfite was demonstrated by skin testing and transfer of passive cutaneous anaphylaxis, and an oral food challenge produced itching of the ears and eyes, nausea, warmness, cough, tightness in the throat, and erythema of the shoulders. These symptoms resolved following treatment with epinephrine. Other scattered case reports in the literature confirm sulfite-induced anaphylaxis (31–33).

One patient reportedly experienced anaphylaxis following the ingestion of a beefsteak that had been treated with papain as a meat tenderizer (34). In prick skin testing, the patient was found to have specific IgE to papain; the patient also experienced a positive oral challenge to papain with palatal itching and throat tightness. One study suggested that MSG could provoke asthma and anaphylaxis in some patients, but this theory remains somewhat controversial (35).

Clinical Features

The hallmark of a food-induced anaphylactic reaction is the onset of symptoms within seconds to minutes following the ingestion of the food allergen. The time course of the appearance and perception of symptoms and signs differ among individuals. Almost invariably, some symptoms begin within the first 60 minutes following the exposure. Generally the later the onset of anaphylactic signs and symptoms, the less severe the reaction. Approximately 25% to 30% of patients will experience a biphasic reaction (10), in which classic symptoms develop initially, the patient appears to be recovering (and may become asymptomatic), and then significant, often catastrophic symptoms recur. The intervening quiescent period may last as long as 1 to 3 hours. In the report by Sampson and colleagues, three of seven patients with near-fatal anaphylaxis experienced protracted anaphylaxis, with symptoms lasting from 1 day to 3 weeks (10). Most reports suggest that the earlier epinephrine is administered in the course of anaphylaxis, the better the chance of a favorable prognosis, although this therapy does not necessarily affect the prevalence of biphasic or protracted symptoms. In addition, in very rare cases patients have received a single injection of epinephrine almost immediately but still progressed to fatal anaphylaxis. Even with appropriate treatment in a medical facility, rarely is it possible to reverse an anaphylactic reaction once it has begun.

The symptoms of anaphylaxis generally affect the gastrointestinal, respiratory, cutaneous, and cardiovascular systems. Symptoms may also affect other organ systems, albeit much less commonly. The sequence of symptom presentation and severity will vary from one individual to the next. In addition, a patient who experiences anaphylaxis to more than one type of food may experience a different sequence of symptoms with each food. While many patients will develop similar allergic symptoms on subsequent occasions following the ingestion of a food allergen, patients with asthma and peanut and/or nut allergy appear to follow a less predictable course. In many cases, peanut-allergic children who reacted with minimal cutaneous and gastrointestinal symptoms as young children later developed asthma and then experienced a catastrophic anaphylactic event after ingesting peanut in their teenage years.

The first symptoms experienced often involve the oropharynx, and may include edema and pruritus of the lips, oral mucosa, palate, and pharynx. Young children may scratch at their tongues, palates, anterior necks, or external auditory canals (presumably because of referred pruritus of the posterior pharynx).

Evidence of laryngeal edema may include a "dry staccato" cough, dysphonia, and dysphagia. Gastrointestinal symptoms include nausea, vomiting, crampy abdominal pain, and diarrhea. Emesis generally contains large amounts of "stringy" mucus. Respiratory symptoms may comprise a deep repetitive cough, stridor, dyspnea, and wheezing. Cutaneous symptoms of anaphylaxis may include flushing, urticaria, angioedema, and an erythematous macular rash. The development of cardiovascular symptoms, along with airway obstruction, create the greatest concern in anaphylactic reactions. Cardiovascular symptoms may include syncope, a feeling of faintness, and chest pain. Hypotension or shock may result from vascular collapse, cardiac arrhythmia, or asphyxia. Anaphylaxis may be complicated by myocardial ischemia.

Other signs and symptoms reported frequently in anaphylaxis include periocular and nasal pruritus, sneezing, diaphoresis, disorientation, fecal or urinary urgency or incontinence, and uterine cramping. In addition, patients often report a "sense of doom." In some instances, the initial manifestation of anaphylaxis may involve the loss of consciousness. Death may ensue in minutes, but has also been reported to occur days to weeks after anaphylaxis (36). Late deaths generally represent manifestations of organ damage experienced early in the course of anaphylaxis.

Several factors appear to increase the risk of more severe anaphylactic reactions. Patients taking beta-adrenergic antagonists or calcium-channel blockers may be resistant to standard therapeutic regimens and, therefore, at increased risk for severe anaphylaxis (37). Patients with asthma appear to be at increased risk for severe symptoms, as noted in two of the recent reports concerning fatal and near-fatal food anaphylactic reactions (9, 10). Similar findings have been reported in patients with insect sting allergy (38) and in patients experiencing anaphylaxis as a result of immunotherapy (39). These patients developed significant, acute bronchospasm along with other symptoms of anaphylaxis.

In a review of 43 fatal cases of anaphylaxis—approximately 80% of which were due to injections of medications—Delage and Irey (40) noted that symptoms developed within 20 minutes in 86% of cases and that death ensued within 30 minutes in

Table 15.3
Presenting Symptoms in 43 Fatal Cases of Anaphylaxis

Symptoms	Number	Percentage
Respiratory	16	37%
Circulatory collapse	14	33%
Seizures	11	26%
Cyanosis	11	26%
Nausea and vomiting	6	23%
Dizziness and weakness	6	14%
Skin eruption	3	7%

From Delage and Irey (40).

Table 15.4
Clinical Signs and Symptoms of Anaphylaxis

Respiratory (major shock organ)
Laryngeal: pruritus and sensation of tightness in the throat, dysphagia, dysphonia and hoarseness, dry "staccato" cough, and sensation of itching in the external auditory canals
Lung: shortness of breath, dyspnea, chest tightness, "deep" cough, and wheezing
Nose: pruritus, congestion, rhinorrhea, and sneezing

Cardiovascular
Feeling of faintness, syncope, chest pain, arrhythmia, and hypotension

Skin
Flushing, pruritus, urticaria, angioedema, morbilliform rash, and pilor erecti

Gastrointestinal
Nausea, abdominal pain (colic), vomiting (large amounts of "stringy" mucus), and diarrhea

Oral
Pruritus of lips, tongue, and palate, and edema of lips and tongue

Other
Periorbital pruritus, erythema and edema, conjunctival erythema, and tearing; uterine contractions in women; and aura of "doom"

33% of individuals, within 1 hour in 51%, and within 5 hours in 19% of cases (Table 15.3). Respiratory distress and circulatory collapse were the presenting symptoms in 37% and 33% of patients, respectively, and skin symptoms constituted the presenting symptom in only 7% of cases. Pathologic findings identified pulmonary congestion in 90% of patients, pulmonary edema in 50%, intra-alveolar hemorrhage in 45%, tracheobronchial secretions in 45%, and laryngeal edema in 38% of cases (marked laryngeal edema was observed in only 10% of cases). In six cases of fatal food-induced anaphylaxis (10), initial symptoms developed within 3 to 30 minutes and severe respiratory symptoms within 20 to 150 minutes. Symptoms involved the lower respiratory tract in six of six children, the gastrointestinal tract in five of six patients, and the skin in only one of six children. **Anaphylaxis should never be ruled out on the basis of absent skin symptoms.** In evaluation of Hymenoptera-allergic patients undergoing venom immunotherapy, intentional bee stings resulted in 14 systemic reactions (36). Three patients experienced severe bronchospasm and hypotension that initially appeared refractory to epinephrine and large volumes of fluid; none developed any skin symptoms.

Diagnosis

Because of its abrupt and dramatic nature, the diagnosis of systemic anaphylaxis is generally readily apparent (Table 15.4). In many cases in which a food is implicated, the inciting food is obvious from the temporal relationship between the ingestion and the onset of symptoms. The initial step in determining the cause of an episode of anaphylaxis involves taking a very careful history, especially when the cause of the episode is not straightforward. Specific questions to address include the type and quantity of food eaten, the last time that the food was ingested, the time frame between ingestion and the development of symptoms, the nature of the food (cooked or uncooked), other times when similar symptoms occurred (and if the food in question was eaten on those occasions), and the involvement of any other precipitating factors (e.g., exercise).

Basically, any food may precipitate an anaphylactic reaction, but a few specific foods appear to be implicated most often in the etiology of food-induced anaphylactic reactions: peanuts, tree nuts, fish, and shellfish. In cases where the etiology of the anaphylactic reaction is not readily apparent, a dietary history should review all ingredients of the suspected meal, including any concealed ingredients or food additives. The food provoking the reaction may be merely a contaminant (knowingly or unknowingly) in the meal.

For example, peanuts or peanut butter are frequently added to cookies, candies, pastries, or sauces such as chili, spaghetti, and barbecue sauces. Chinese restaurants frequently use peanut butter to hold together the overlapping ends of egg rolls, employ pressed or "extruded" peanut oil in their cooking, and reuse the same wok to cook a variety of different meals, resulting in residual contaminant carryover.

Another infrequent (but not rare) cause of food contamination occurs during the manufacturing process. Such contamination may occur with scraps of candy that are "reworked" into the next batch of candy or where production switches from one product to the next in a processing plant. As an example, a reaction to almond butter by a peanut-allergic patient started an investigation that determined that 10% of the almond butter produced in one plant was contaminated with peanut butter (FDA 1986) after a production changeover from peanut butter to almond butter. Other examples include popsicles run on the same line as creamsicles, fruit juices packaged in individual cartons where milk products have previously been packaged, and milk-free desserts packaged in dairy plants (41).

Food items with "natural flavoring" designated on the label may contain an unsuspected allergen (e.g., casein in canned tuna fish, hot dogs, or bologna, and soy in a variety of baked goods). In addition, some foods do not indicate the presence of certain proteins when they represent less than 2% of total protein (e.g., some crackers contain milk protein, and some cookies contain egg).

Food allergy can develop at any age, although it appears more commonly in the first 3 years of life. Not uncommonly a patient may tolerate a food (i.e., shrimp) for his or her entire life and then experience a major allergic reaction after ingesting the food at some point in mid-adulthood. Such patients may experience no forewarning of the impending episode, but on detailed questioning will not infrequently describe some previous minor symptoms, such as oral pruritus or nausea and cramping. Cooking or processing of some foods may potentially remove, diminish, or even enhance their allergenicity as well.

Some clinical conditions may be confused with food anaphylaxis, such as scombroid poisoning, factitious allergic emergency, and vasovagal collapse. In the absence of urticaria and angioedema, one must consider arrhythmia, myocardial infarction, hereditary angioedema, aspiration of a bolus of food, pulmonary embolism, and seizure disorders as causes of the episode.

With the presence of laryngeal edema, especially when accompanied by abdominal pain, the diagnosis of hereditary angioedema must be considered. In general, this disorder has a slower onset, does not include urticaria, and often presents with a family history of similar reactions. Systemic mastocytosis results in flushing, tachycardia, pruritus, headache, abdominal pain, diarrhea, and syncope. A factitious allergic emergency may occur when patients knowingly and secretively ingest a food substance to which they are known to be allergic (42).

In vasovagal syncope, the patient may collapse after an injection or a painful or disturbing situation. The patient typically has a pale appearance and complains of nausea prior to the syncopal episode, but does not complain of pruritus or become cyanotic. Respiratory difficulty does not occur, and symptoms are almost immediately relieved by recumbency. Profuse diaphoresis, slow pulse, and maintenance of blood pressure generally complete the syndrome. Hyperventilation may cause breathlessness and collapse. Other signs and symptoms of anaphylaxis generally do not appear, except for peripheral and perioral tingling sensations. Blood pressure and pulse generally remain normal.

Laboratory Evaluation

The laboratory evaluation of patients with an anaphylactic reaction should be directed at identifying specific IgE antibodies to the food in question. IgE antibody can be recognized in vivo by prick or puncture skin testing. Although not absolutely proven in patients with anaphylaxis, a negative prick/puncture skin test serves as an excellent predictor for a negative IgE-mediated food reaction to the suspected food. In contrast, a positive prick skin test does not necessarily indicate that the food is the inciting agent. Nevertheless, in patients with classic histories of anaphylaxis following ingestion of an isolated food and a positive prick/puncture skin test to that food, this laboratory test appears to provide a good positive predictor of allergic reactivity.

Skin testing has some limitations that need to be recognized. Some researchers speculate that skin testing shortly after the occurrence of anaphylaxis may fail to yield a positive response because of temporary anergy. Although not demonstrated in food allergy, this phenomenon has been demonstrated in Hymenoptera sensitivity following an insect sting (43). Possible causes of false-negative prick skin tests include improper skin test technique, concomitant use of antihistamines, or use of food extracts with reduced or inadequate allergenic potential. With some foods, processing of the food for commercial extracts may diminish antigenicity (44), especially in some fruits and vegetables. If a food is strongly suspected to have precipitated an anaphylactic reaction even though the prick skin test is negative, the patient should be tested with the natural food utilizing the "prick + prick" method to ensure an absence of detectable IgE antibody (45). Some caution should be exercised when performing this procedure as the amount of antigen on the prick device will not be controlled. Appropriate negative controls should be performed as well.

Appropriate skin testing should be undertaken in each patient, although in vitro measurement of food-specific IgE may be evaluated initially. Many patients with anaphylaxis require limited prick skin testing to confirm the etiology of the anaphylactic reaction. In cases of idiopathic anaphylaxis, more extensive prick skin testing may help in diagnosis (31). The clinician must decide how many skin tests are practical and justified, taking into account the anticipated low yield of positive results in idiopathic anaphylaxis and the value of discovering an etiology in this serious disorder.

Intradermal skin tests are sometimes performed following negative prick/puncture skin tests, although a positive intradermal test following a negative prick/puncture test has dubious diagnostic significance, and probably no clinical benefit (36). Anaphylactic reactions have been documented following intradermal skin tests to foods (39), so extra caution should be exercised with any intradermal tests. **Under no circumstances should an intradermal skin test be performed prior to performing a prick/puncture test.** In cases where extreme hypersensitivity is suspected, alternative approaches may be warranted, including further dilution of the food extract prior to prick skin testing or use of a food-specific in vitro test (e.g., radioallergosorbent test; RAST). Overall, RAST is considered less sensitive and specific than the prick skin test. In high-quality laboratories, a 3+ to 4+ RAST (on a 1+ to 4+ RAST scale) probably has a positive predictive accuracy similar to that of a prick skin test that is 3 mm greater than the negative control (46).

Massive activation of mast cells during anaphylaxis results in a dramatic rise in plasma histamine and, somewhat later, a rise in plasma or serum tryptase (47–49). Plasma histamine rises during the first several minutes of a reaction and generally remains elevated for a brief period of time. It requires special collection techniques and will degrade unless the plasma sample is frozen immediately. Consequently, measurement of plasma histamine to document anaphylaxis is impractical except in research situations. Whether measurement of urinary methyl-histamine will prove useful in the documentation of anaphylaxis remains to be demonstrated. Serum tryptase rises over the first hour and may remain elevated for many hours. It remains fairly stable at room temperature and can be obtained from post-mortem specimens. Tryptase has been shown to be markedly elevated in most cases of bee sting or drug-induced anaphylaxis (48, 49), but is often not elevated in food-induced anaphylaxis (10). The reason for this discrepancy is not clear, but suggests that other cells—such as basophils or monocytes/macrophages—may have greater importance in food-induced anaphylaxis.

Double-blind, placebo-controlled food challenges (DBPCFC) are contraindicated in patients with an unequivocal history of anaphylaxis following the isolated ingestion of a food to which they have significant IgE antibodies. If several foods were ingested and the patient has positive skin tests to several foods, however, the responsible food must first be identified. Patients have reportedly experienced repeated anaphylactic reactions because physicians incorrectly assumed that they had identified the responsible food (10). Young children who experience anaphylactic reactions to foods other than peanuts, tree nuts, fish, and shellfish may eventually outgrow their clinical reactivity. Thus, an oral challenge may be warranted following an extended period of food elimination with no history of reactions to accidental ingestions.

Treatment

Treatment of food-induced anaphylaxis may be subdivided into acute and long-term management. While physicians spend hours preparing for management of an acute attack, long-term measures ultimately provide the best quality of life for the food-allergic patient.

ACUTE MANAGEMENT

Acute management strategies are outlined in Table 15.5. Fatalities may occur if treatment of a food-induced anaphylactic reaction is not immediate (9, 10). Data from the review of fatal beesting-induced anaphylactic reactions indicate that the longer that

---

Table 15.5
Acute Management of Anaphylaxis

Rapid assessment of:
Extent and severity of symptoms
Adequacy of oxygenation, cardiac output, and tissue perfusion
Potential confounding medications
Suspected cause of the reaction

Initial therapy:
Epinephrine: 0.01 mg/kg/dose up to 0.3–0.5 mg S.C. or I.M. up to 3 times every 20 minutes
Oxygen: 40% to 100% by mask
Intravenous fluids: 30 mL/kg of crystalloid up to 2 liters over the first hour (or more depending upon blood pressure and response to medications)

Secondary medications:
Nebulized albuterol: may be continuous
Antihistamines: H_1 antagonist (diphenhydramine—1 mg/kg up to 75 mg for 6 hours)
H_2 antagonist (cimetidine—4 mg/kg up to 300 mg for 6–8 hours)
Corticosteroids: solumedrol—1–2 mg/kg/dose for 8 hours
Dopamine: for hypotension refractory to epinephrine; IV drip: 2–20 μg/kg/min
Norepinephrine: for hypotension refractory to epinephrine
Glucagon: for hypotension refractory to epinephrine and norepinephrine; especially patients on beta blockers

---

initial therapy is delayed, the greater the incidence of complications and fatalities (36). Initial treatment must be preceded by a rapid assessment that determines the following: the extent and severity of the reaction; the adequacy of oxygenation, cardiac output, and tissue perfusion; any potential confounding medications (e.g., beta blockers); and the suspected cause of the reaction (5). Initial therapy should be directed at maintaining an effective airway and circulatory system. Epinephrine (adrenaline) is the drug of choice in the treatment of anaphylaxis. The first step in the management of anaphylaxis involves the subcutaneous or intramuscular injection of 0.01 mL/kg of aqueous epinephrine 1 : 1000 (maximal dose is 0.3 to 0.5 mL, or 0.3 to 0.5 mg). Intravenous administration of epinephrine may cause fatal arrhythmias or myocardial infarction, particularly in adults, and should be reserved for refractory hypotension requiring cardiopulmonary resuscitation. In patients with pulmonary symptoms, supplemental oxygen should be administered.

The importance of epinephrine in the treatment of anaphylaxis is most evident in the cases of fatal and near-fatal food-induced anaphylaxis. In general, patients who die from the anaphylactic reaction have received no epinephrine (or an inadequate dose) during their acute reaction (9, 10, 36). In contrast, patients who survive a near-fatal anaphylactic reaction generally receive epinephrine early in the course of their reaction, and many receive repeated doses of epinephrine.

To insure that patients receive epinephrine as early as possible, they, their family members, and other care providers should be instructed in the self-administration (or administration) of epinephrine. Preloaded syringes with epinephrine should be provided to any patients at risk for food-induced anaphylaxis (i.e., patients with a history of a previous anaphylactic reaction and patients with asthma and food allergy, especially if they are allergic to peanuts, nuts, fish, or shellfish). In the United States, premeasured doses of epinephrine at this time can be obtained in two forms: Epi-Pen, which is distributed by Center Laboratories (Port Washington, New York) and Ana-Kit or Ana-Guard, both of which are distributed by Miles Inc., Allergy Products (West Haven, Connecticut). The Epi-Pen is a disposable drug delivery system with a spring-activated concealed needle intended for a single intramuscular injection. It can be obtained in two sizes: the Epi-Pen—0.3 mg for adults and the Epi-Pen Jr.—0.15 mg for children weighing less than 22 to 25 kg. The device is pressed firmly into the thigh muscle (or trigger-activated with the newer version of the Epi-Pen) and held in place for several seconds to allow injection of the medication. Although residual epinephrine remains in the device after its use, no more epinephrine is accessible once the needle has been exposed. Because the Epi-Pen can deliver only a single dose, two Epi-Pens may be prescribed for patients who have experienced a previous anaphylactic reaction or who are at high risk and do not have ready access to a medical center. The Ana-Guard and Ana-Kit each contain a special calibrated syringe that allows separate delivery of two doses. Prior to injecting the medication, the plunger is turned clockwise 90°. Pushing the plunger to the first stop delivers 0.3 mg of epinephrine either S.C. or I.M. Lesser amounts of adrenaline can be injected by discarding a specified portion of the medication as the syringes include 0.1 mL (mg) calibration marks. Whichever device is prescribed, it is imperative that the patient and/or family members practice with appropriate training devices to ensure that they can use the device proficiently in case of an emergency. Patients should be notified that these preloaded devices have a 1-year shelf life and, therefore, should be renewed each year.

Sustained-release preparations of epinephrine are not appropriate treatment for acute anaphylaxis. Inhaled epinephrine (either nebulized or via metered-dose inhaler; e.g., Primatine Mist in the United States) has been recommended by the European Academy of Allergy and Clinical Immunology (50). A minimum of 20 puffs inhaled correctly can produce blood levels similar to an injection of 0.3 to 0.5 mg of epinephrine in adults, and 10 to 15 puffs in a child can deliver the equivalent of 0.15 mg injected subcutaneously (51–53). Lesser doses may reverse laryngeal edema or persistent bronchospasm.

Once epinephrine has been administered, other therapeutic modalities may produce additional benefits. Studies have suggested that the combination of an H_1 antihistamine (i.e., diphenhydramine at 1 mg/kg up to 75 mg) administered either intramuscularly or intravenously and an H_2 antihistamine (i.e., cimetidine at 4 mg/kg up to 300 mg) administered intravenously may be more effective than either agent administered alone (54). Both histamine antagonists should be infused slowly if given intravenously as rapid infusion of diphenhydramine is associated with arrhythmias and cimetidine with falls in blood pressure.

The role of corticosteroids in the treatment of anaphylaxis remains unclear. Most authorities recommend giving prednisone (1 mg/kg orally) for mild to moderate episodes of anaphylaxis and solumedrol (1 to 2 mg/kg intravenously) for severe anaphylaxis in an attempt to modulate the late-phase response. Patients who have been receiving glucocorticosteroid therapy for other reasons should be assumed to have hypothalamic-pituitary-adrenal-axis suppression and should be administered stress doses of hydrocortisone intravenously during resuscitation.

If wheezing is prominent, an aerosolized β-adrenergic agent (i.e., albuterol) is recommended intermittently or continuously, depending upon the patient's symptoms and the availability of cardiac monitoring. Intravenous aminophylline may also be useful for recalcitrant respiratory symptoms. Aerosolized epinephrine may help prevent life-threatening upper airway edema, although a tracheotomy may be required to prevent fatal laryngeal obstruction in approximately 10% of cases (40).

Hypotension, which results from a shift in fluid from the intravascular to extravascular space, may be severe and refractory to epinephrine and antihistamines. Depending upon the blood pressure, large volumes of crystalloid (e.g., lactated Ringer's solution or normal saline) infused rapidly are frequently required to reverse the hypotensive state. An alternative to crystalloid solution is hydroxyethyl starch, a colloid. Children may need as much as 30 mL/kg of crystalloid over the first hour (55) and adults up to 2 liters (56) over the first hour to control hypotension. Patients taking beta blockers may require much larger volumes (e.g., 5 to 7 liters) of fluid before pressure stabilizes (56). Although epinephrine and fluids represent the mainstay of hypotension treatment, other vasopressor drugs may be used as well. Dopamine administered at a rate of 2 to 20 μg/kg/minute while carefully monitoring the blood pressure may be lifesaving. In addition, 1 to 5 mg of glucagon given as a bolus, followed by an infusion of 5 to 15 μg/minute titrated against clinical response, may be helpful in refractory cases or in patients taking beta blockers. The best treatment of patients experiencing anaphylaxis while taking beta-adrenergic blocking drugs remains a matter of some concern. If combined β_1- and β_2-receptor blockers (e.g., propranolol) are used, epinephrine may be administered for its alpha-adrenergic activity and isoproterenol in an attempt to overcome the beta blockade. Because patients may experience a biphasic response, all patients should be monitored for a minimum of 4 hours—longer in cases of more severe anaphylaxis.

Although it remains a controversial strategy, some authorities suggest the use of activated charcoal to prevent further absorption of food allergens from the gut. Others suggest that some attempt should be made to evacuate the stomach, if vomiting has not already occurred. Some investigators advocate the use of gastric lavage when large amounts of the allergen have been ingested. Whether these measures will prove beneficial in ameliorating food-induced anaphylaxis remains to be demonstrated.

Patients who are at risk for food-induced anaphylaxis should have medical information concerning their condition available on them at all times (e.g., a Medic Alert bracelet). This information may be lifesaving as it will expedite the diagnosis and appropriate treatment of a patient experiencing an anaphylactic reaction.

LONG-TERM MANAGEMENT

The life-threatening nature of anaphylaxis makes prevention the cornerstone of therapy (Table 15.6). If the causative food allergen is not clearly delineated, an evaluation to determine the etiology should be promptly initiated to prevent a lethal reoccurrence. The central focus of prevention of food-induced anaphylaxis requires the appropriate identification and complete dietary avoidance of the specific food allergen. Certain factors place some individuals at increased risk for more severe anaphylactic reactions (Table 15.7): (1) history of a previous anaphylactic reaction; (2) history of asthma, especially if it is poorly controlled; (3) allergy to peanuts, nuts, fish,

Table 15.6
Long-term Management of Food-Induced Anaphylaxis

Identify positively the food that provoked the anaphylactic reaction
Educate the patient, his or her family, and/or care providers on how to avoid all exposure to the food allergen
Provide patient at risk with self-injectable epinephrine and thoroughly teach him or her when and how to use this medication (i.e., practice with Epi-Pen trainer)
Provide patient with liquid antihistamine (diphenhydramine or hydroxyzine) and teach them when and how to use this medication
Establish a formal *emergency plan* in case of a reaction:
    Proper use of "emergency medications"
    Transportation to nearest emergency facility (capable of resuscitation and endotracheal tube placement)

and shellfish; (4) use of beta blockers or ACE inhibitors; and (5) possibly female gender. An educational process is imperative to ensure that the patient and family understand how to avoid all forms of the food allergen and the potential severity of a reaction if the food is inadvertently ingested. The *Food Allergy Network* is a nonprofit organization in Fairfax, Virginia, United States (telephone: 701-691-3179 or 800-929-4040; fax: 701-691-2713) that provide patients with information about food allergen avoidance and that offers several programs for schools and parents of children with food allergies and anaphylaxis.

Patients experiencing a previous food allergic reaction often subsequently demonstrate some instinctive avoidance measure. This condition may be typified by extreme dislike for the taste or even smell of the offending food. The sensitized person must take a very proactive role to completely avoid a food that has previously caused an anaphylactic reaction. Many patients may even require total removal of the food from the household. Educational measures must be directed at the patient, his or her family, and school personnel, other caretakers, or fellow workers so that they understand the potential severity and

Table 15.7
Factors That Suggest Increased Risk for Severe Anaphylaxis

History of a previous severe anaphylactic reaction
Patient with asthma, especially if poorly controlled
Allergy to peanuts, nuts, fish, and/or shellfish
Patients on beta blockers or ACE inhibitors
Female gender (possibly)

scope of the problem. If a patient ingests a food prepared outside the home, they must always be very cautious and should not hesitate to ask very specific and detailed questions concerning ingredients of foods they are planning to eat. Unfortunately, it is not uncommon for patients dining in restaurants to ingest a food that they were assured did not exist in the meal.

Although changes in food labeling laws in the United States have simplified somewhat the reading of labels for food-allergic individuals, several problems still remain. These problems fall into one of five categories: (1) misleading labels (e.g., "non-dairy" creamers usually contain some milk protein); (2) ingredient switches (e.g., a name brand food may alter the ingredients with no significant change on the label); (3) a "natural flavoring" designation that allows a product to contain a small amount of other food proteins for flavoring purposes without identifying that protein (e.g., casein in canned tuna fish); (4) legal labeling loopholes that allow proteins representing less than 2% of total protein to be included in a product without designating its presence; and (5) inadvertent contamination that may occur when more than one product is manufactured on a line and residual protein from the previous run adulterates the subsequent run (e.g., non-dairy ice cream desserts). It is still imperative that patients and their families be taught the many "words" that indicate the presence of a particular food protein as an ingredient of a food product and that they try to be aware of products where certain food proteins may unexpectedly occur.

Prognosis

For many young children diagnosed with anaphylaxis to foods such as milk, egg, wheat, and soybeans, the clinical sensitivity may eventually be outgrown after several years. Children who develop their food sensitivity after 3 years of age, however, are less likely to lose their food reactions over a period of several years. Allergies to foods such as peanuts, tree nuts, fish, and seafood are generally not outgrown no matter at what age they develop. Individuals with

such allergies appear likely to retain their sensitivity for a lifetime. Consequently, several groups are evaluating new strategies to "desensitize" patients to these foods.

REFERENCES

1. Sheffer A. Anaphylaxis. J Allergy Clin Immunol 1985;75:227–233.
2. Portier P, Richet C. De l'action anaphylatique de certains venins. C R Soc Biol (Paris) 1902;54:170–172.
3. Anderson J, Sogn D, eds. Adverse reactions to foods. Bethesda, MD: National Institute of Allergy and Infectious Disease, NIH Public. #84-2442 ed., 1984.
4. Goldbert T, Pattereon R, Pruzansky J. Systemic allergic reactions to ingested antigens. J Allergy 1969;44:96–107.
5. Bochner B, Lichtenstein L. Anaphylaxis. N Engl J Med 1991;324:1785–1790.
6. Sorensen H, Nielsen B, Nielsen J. Anaphylactic shock occurring outside hospitals. Allergy 1989;44:288–290.
7. Yocum MW, Khan DA. Assessment of patients who have experienced anaphylaxis: a 3-year survey. Mayo Clin Proc 1994;69:16–23.
8. Bock S. The incidence of severe adverse reactions to food in Colorado. J Allergy Clin Immunol 1992;90:683–685.
9. Yunginger JW, Sweeney KG, Sturner WQ, Giannandra LA, Teigland JD, Bray M, et al. Fatal food-induced anaphylaxis. JAMA 1988;260:1450–1452.
10. Sampson HA, Mendelson LM, Rosen JP. Fatal and near-fatal anaphylactic reactions to food in children and adolescents. N Engl J Med 1992;327:380–384.
11. Kidd J, Cohen S, Sosman A, Fink J. Food-dependent exercise-induced anaphylaxis. J Allergy Clin Immunol 1983;71:407–411.
12. Dohi M, Suko M, Sugiyama H, Yamashita N, Tadokoro K, Juji F, et al. Food-dependent, exercise-induced anaphylaxis: a study on 11 Japanese cases. J Allergy Clin Immunol 1991;87:34–40.
13. Romano A, Fonso M, Giuffreda F, Quaratino D, Papa G, Palmieri V, et al. Diagnostic work-up for food-dependent, exercise-induced anaphylaxis. Allergy 1995;50:817–824.
14. Maulitz R, Pratt D, Schocket A. Exercise-induced anaphylactic reaction to shellfish. J Allergy Clin Immunol 1979;63:433–434.
15. Kushimito H, Aoki T. Masked type I wheat allergy—relation to exercise-induced anaphylaxis. Arch Dermatol 1985;121:355–360.
16. Novey H, Fairshter R, Sainess K, Simon R, Curd J. Postprandial exercise-induced anaphylaxis. J Allergy Clin Immunol 1983;71:498–504.
17. Horan R, Sheffer A. Food-dependent exercise-induced anaphylaxis. Immunol Allergy Clin North Am 1991;11:757.
18. Atkins FM, Steinberg SS, Metcalfe DD. Evaluation of immediate adverse reactions to foods in adult patients. I. Correlation of demographic, laboratory, and prick skin test data with response to controlled oral food challenges. J Allergy Clin Immunol 1985;75:348–355.
19. DeMartino M, Novembre E, Gozza G, DeMarco A, Bonazza P, Verucci A. Sensitivity to tomato and peanut allergens in children monosensitized to grass pollen. Allergy 1988;43:206–213.

20. Settipane G, Klein D, Boyd G. Relationship of atopy and anaphylactic sensitization: a bee sting allergy model. Clin Allergy 1978;8:259–264.
21. Bock SA. The natural history of food sensitivity. J Allergy Clin Immunol 1982;69:173–177.
22. Sampson HA, Scanlon SM. Natural history of food hypersensitivity in children with atopic dermatitis. J Pediatr 1989;115:23–27.
23. Goldman AS, Anderson DW, Sellers WA, Saperstein A, Kniker WT, Halpern SR. Milk allergy. I. Oral challenge with milk and isolated milk proteins in allergic children. Pediatrics 1963;32:425–443.
24. Host A. Cow's milk protein allergy and intolerance in infancy. Pediatr Allergy Immunol 1994;5:5–36.
25. Bock SA, Atkins FM. The natural history of peanut allergy. J Allergy Clin Immunol 1989;83:900–904.
26. Sampson HA. Peanut anaphylaxis. J Allergy Clin Immunol 1990;86:1–3.
27. Settipane G. Anaphylactic deaths in asthmatic patients. Allergy Proc 1989;10:271–274.
28. Moneret-Vautrin D, Beaudouin E, Widmer S, Mouton C, Kanny G, Prestat F, et al. Prospective study of risk factors in natural rubber latex hypersensitivity. J Allergy Clin Immunol 1993;92:668–677.
29. Warner J, Miles E, Jones A, Quint D, Colwell B, Warner J. Is deficiency of interferon gamma production by allergen triggered cord blood cells a predictor of atopic disease? Clin Exp Allergy 1994;24:423–430.
30. Prenner B, Stevens J. Anaphylaxis after ingestion of sodium bisulfite. Ann Allergy 1976;37:180–182.
31. Stricker W, Anorve-Lopez E, Reed C. Food skin testing in patients with idiopathic anaphylaxis. J Allergy Clin Immunol 1986;77:516–519.
32. Twarog F, Leung D. Anaphylaxis to a component of isoetharine (sodium bisulfite). J Am Med Assoc 1982;248:2031.
33. Clayton D, Busse W. Anaphylaxis to wine. Clin Allergy 1980;10:341–343.
34. Mansfield L, Bowers C. Systemic reaction to papain in a nonoccupational setting. J Allergy Clin Immunol 1983;71:371–374.
35. Allen D, Delohery J, Baker G. Monosodium l-glutamate-induced asthma. J Allergy Clin Immunol 1987;80:530–537.
36. Barnard J. Studies of 400 Hymenoptera sting deaths in the United States. J Allergy Clin Immunol 1973;52:259.
37. Kivity S, Yarchovsky J. Relapsing anaphylaxis to bee sting in a patient treated with β-blocker and Ca blocker. J Allergy Clin Immunol 1990;85:669–670.
38. Settipane G, Chafee R, Klein DE, Boud G, Sturam J, Freye H. Anaphylactic reactions to Hymenoptera stings in asthmatic patients. Clin Allergy 1980;10:659–665.
39. Lockey R, Benedict L, Turkeltaub P, Bukantz S. Fatalities form immunotherapy and skin testing. J Allergy Clin Immunol 1987;79:660–667.
40. Delage C, Irey N. Anaphylactic deaths: a clinicopathologic study of 43 cases. J Forensic Sci 1972;17:525–540.
41. Gern J, Yang E, Evrard H, Sampson H. Allergic reactions to milk-contaminated "non-dairy" products. N Engl J Med 1991;324:976–979.
42. Weiszer I. Allergic emergencies. In: Patterson R, ed. Allergy diseases—diagnosis and management. Philadelphia: JB Lippincott, 1985, 418–439.
43. Settipane G, Chafee F. Natural history of allergy of Hymenoptera. Clin Allergy 1979;9:385–390.
44. Ortolani C, Ispano M, Pastorello EA, Ansaloni R, Magri GC. Comparison of results of skin prick tests (with fresh foods and commercial food extracts) and RAST in 100 patients with oral allergy syndrome. J Allergy Clin Immunol 1989;83:683–690.
45. Rosen J, Selcow J, Mendelson L, Grodofsky M, Factor J, Sampson H. Skin testing with natural foods in patients suspected of having food allergies . . . is it necessary? J Allergy Clin Immunol 1994;93:1068–1070.
46. Sampson HA. Comparative study of commercial food antigen extracts for the diagnosis of food hypersensitivity. J Allergy Clin Immunol 1988;82:718–726.
47. Sampson HA, Jolie PL. Increased plasma histamine concentrations after food challenges in children with atopic dermatitis. N Engl J Med 1984;311:372–376.
48. Schwartz L, Yunginger J, Miller J, et al. The time course of appearance and disappearance of human mast cell tryptase in the circulation after anaphylaxis. J Clin Invest 1989;83:1551–1555.
49. Schwartz L, Metcalfe D, Miller J, et al. Tryptase levels as an indicator of mast cell activation in systemic anaphylaxis and mastocytosis. N Engl J Med 1987;316:1622–1626.
50. Muller U, Mosbech H, Aberer W, Dreborg S, Ewan P, Kunkel G, et al. EAACI position statement: adrenaline for emergency kits. Allergy 1995;50:783–787.
51. Heilborn H, Hjemdahl P, Daleskog M, Adamsson U. Comparison of subcutaneous injection and high-dose inhalation of epinephrine. J Allergy Clin Immunol 1986;78:1174–1179.
52. Warren J, Doble N, Dalton N, Ewan P. Systemic absorption of inhaled epinephrine. Clin Pharmacol Ther 1986;40:673–678.
53. Heilborn H, Hjemdahl P, Daleskog M, Adamsson U. Comparison of subcutaneous injection and high-dose inhalation of epinephrine—implication for self-treatment to prevent anaphylaxis. J Allergy Clin Immunol 1986;78:1174–1179.
54. Kambam J, Merrill W, Smith B. Histamine-2 receptor blocker in the treatment of protamine-related anaphylactoid reactions: two case reports. An J Anaesth 1989;36:463–465.
55. Saryan J, O'Loughlin J. Anaphylaxis in children. Pediatr Ann 1992;21:590–598.
56. Eon B, Papazian L, Gouin F. Management of anaphylaxis and anaphylactoid reactions during anesthesia. Humana Press 1991;9:415–429.

16

INFANTILE COLIC AND FOOD HYPERSENSITIVITY

David J. Hill
Clifford S. Hosking

*F*ussing and crying, especially in the evening, are normal developmental phenomena in infants in the first 3 months of life (1). Unexplained paroxysms of irritability, fussing, or crying that persist for more than 3 hours per day, for more than 3 days in one week (2), are claimed to represent a separate clinical condition termed infantile colic (3). During such episodes the legs may be drawn up to the abdomen and the infant may become flushed. Abdominal distention and increased passage of flatus are often noted.

Table 16.1 shows the varying incidences of colic reported from different countries (4). Most infants in these studies suffered from "severe colic," even though no criteria have yet defined mild, moderate, or severe colic. Moreover, the term "colic" implies a mechanism responsible for the distress displayed by these infants. Such a mechanism has never been demonstrated. For this reason many recent workers have referred to these infants as suffering from crying, fussing, or distressed behavior.

In the following discussion the term "colic" will be used interchangeably with each of these terms, although it is to be emphasized that use of this term in no way implies the cause of the infant distress.

Broadly, pediatricians managing infantile colic take one of two approaches:

- Assumption that colic is an extreme form of "normal" crying behavior. The abdominal distention and excess flatus are attributed to air swallowing. Colic is managed with a behavioral approach.

- Assumption that colic is a distinct entity from normal crying behavior and results from an adverse reaction to foods.

This review will discuss:

1. Evidence that infants with colic differ significantly in their pattern of distressed behavior from non-colic infants.
2. The incidence of colic in children with food allergy.
3. The incidence of food allergy in children presenting with colic.
4. The outcome of trials focusing on the dietary management of colic.
5. The outcome of recent studies involving behavior modification in colic.

Some of the contents of this chapter were presented at a Conference on Intestinal Immunology and Food Allergy in 1993 and published as part of the proceedings of that meeting (5).

Evidence That Infants with Colic Differ Significantly in Their Pattern of Distressed Behavior from Non-Colic Infants

Brazelton (1) used parental recording in cry charts to document the natural history of distressed behavior in infancy. Figure 16.1 summarizes the pattern of

Table 16.1
Prevalence of Infantile Colic

Author	Country	Year	Prevalence
Wessel	United States	1954	24%
Illingworth	England	1957	20%
Jakobsson	Sweden	1979	20%
Boulton	Australia	1979	41%
Thomas	Australia	1981	35%
Carey	United States	1984	10%
Hide	England	1982	16%
Lothe	Sweden	1989	17.4%

distressed or fussing behavior in a group of 80 non-colic infants studied in the first 12 weeks of life. Brazelton showed how distressed behavior frequently deteriorated until the children were about 6 weeks of age and then gradually improved. Both he and Wessel (2) described the predominance of fussing behavior during the late afternoon and evening period, although Wessel noted that distress was not confined to this period in one-third of infants. As discussed below, the authors' studies suggest that this pattern of distress may be influenced by whether the infant is breast- or formula-fed.

Brazelton contrasted the pattern of distressed behavior in non-colic normal infants with that of a group of colic infants. He found that the colic infant's distress was more marked, peaked later than the normal age of 6 weeks, and persisted to the 12-week follow-up (1).

Wessel's and Brazelton's distress diaries were not validated against objective methods for measuring crying, however. Barr et al. developed a 24-hour crying chart validated against objective measurements of infant distress (6). This group compared information recorded by parents on specifically designed crying data sheets with data recorded on voice activated audio taped (VAR) of negative vocalizations (i.e., crying) over a 24-hour period. Their study of 10 infants showed a moderate correlation between VAR "negative" vocalization clusters and (1) the frequency of diary-recorded episodes of crying or fussing behavior (R = +0.64; p = 0.03) and (2) the duration of crying (R = +0.67; p = 0.02).

Elimination of one "outlier" considerably strengthened the correlation between the VAR objective recorded data and episodes of crying/fussing behavior (R = +0.85) and the duration of crying (R = +0.90). Using these validated cry charts, Hunziker et al. (7) confirmed the natural history of

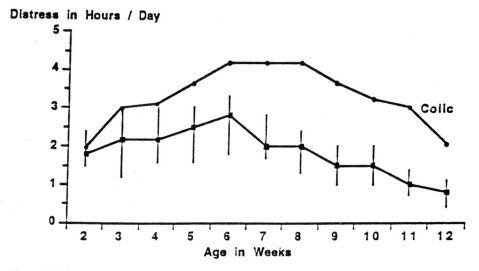

Figure 16.1

Total crying time of 80 non-colic infants and 6 colic infants in the first 12 weeks of life. From Brazelton (1).

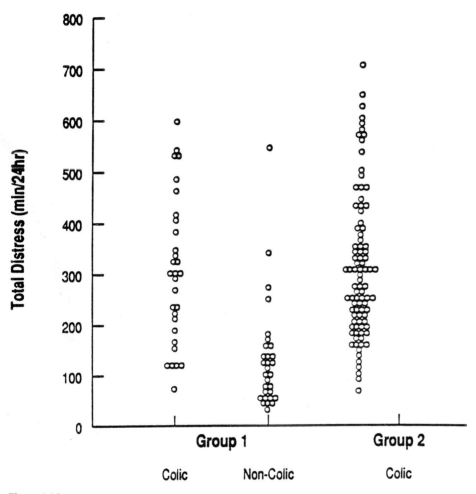

Figure 16.2

Duration of total distress (the sum of cry and fuss time) recorded over 24 hours in 30 colic and 30 non-colic infants (Group 1). The colic group showed significantly more total distress (median 300 minutes) than the non-colic group (median 105 minutes) ($p < 0.001$). The median total distress score of a second group of 90 colic infants (Group 2) was 280 minutes.

distressed behavior previously described by Brazelton (1).

Recent studies from the authors' center have compared the pattern and duration of distressed behavior in a group of 30 colic and non-colic infants (8). Figure 16.2 shows the higher levels of distressed behavior in the colic infants as compared with that in the non-colic infants. The findings were confirmed in a separate group of 90 colicky infants. The evaluation of distressed behavior on an hour-by-hour basis

confirmed the predominance of nocturnal symptoms, but like Hide and Guyer (9) the authors found colic and distressed behavior frequently occurred in colicky infants during other time periods (Fig. 16.3). At all time periods, the colic infants were more distressed than the non-colic infants. Table 16.2 shows the duration of distress broken down into 6 hourly periods.

In the authors' colic patients, the levels of distress at different time points during 24 hours were com-

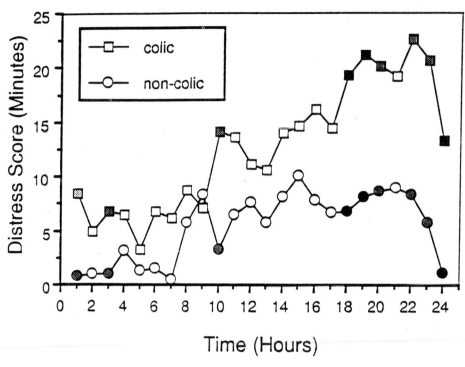

Figure 16.3

One-hour distress scores (minutes). One hourly mean duration of total distress. Sum of cry and fuss time, recorded over 24 hours. Colic infants showed significantly more distress (p < 0.01) than non-colic infants at periods marked -o- finishing at 6 P.M., 7 P.M., and 12 midnight; periods marked -o- indicate differences in colic and non-colic behavior at p < 0.01–0.05 level.

pared between formula-fed and breast-fed infants. While the total distress was similar over the 24 hours, formula-fed infants showed more distress before 12 noon than breast-fed infants (p = 0.05), whereas breast-fed infants were more distressed after noon (p = 0.03). When results were analyzed on an hourly basis, formula-fed infants showed significantly more distress at 3 A.M. (p = 0.04), 9 A.M. (p = 0.02), and 10 A.M. (p = 0.01). Thus, if dietary protein intolerance contributes to distress behavior, formula feeding with high-dose antigen exposure is more likely to elicit a rapid-onset distress response than prolonged low-dose antigen exposure through breast milk.

These data suggest the distressed behavior of colic infants may not simply represent an exaggeration of the normal distressed pattern of non-colic infants. Hunziker's studies, which reported that "sup-

plemental carrying" reduced distressed behavior in "non-colic" (7) but not colic infants at 6 weeks of age (10), is consistent with this hypothesis.

The Incidence of Colic in Children with Proven Food Allergy

Studies from our group have used cow's milk allergy (CMA) as a model of food allergy. Descriptions of the effects of cow's milk challenge in young children suspected of having CMA demonstrate the diverse manifestations of this disorder (11). Associated markers of immune hypersensitivity mechanisms have also been reported (12–15). In a sequential group of 100 patients with challenge-proven CMA (median age

Table 16.2
Comparison of Total Distress Between Colic and Non-Colic Infants*

Time Periods	Colic (*n* = 30) Median (minutes)	95% CI	Non-Colic (*n* = 30) Median (minutes)	95% CI	P-value
Midnight–6 A.M.	10.0	(0.0, 25.0)	2.5	(0.0, 5.0)	0.038
6 A.M.–noon	55.0	(30.0, 75.0)	25.0	(15.0, 37.7)	0.045
Noon–6 P.M.	75.0	(60.0, 100.4)	30.0	(20.0, 35.0)	0.001
6 P.M.–midnight	105.0	(80.0, 146.6)	30.0	(10.0, 57.7)	0.001

*Comparison of total distress (i.e., cry + fuss), in minutes, between colic and non-colic infants at 6-hourly time periods over 24 hours. P-value of Mann-Whitney test based on medians.

16.2 months), 44% displayed irritable and colicky behavior during the cow's milk challenge procedure (11).

A clustering algorithm (K-means) identified three groups of patients with common clinical features (11). Predominant clinical findings in each of the three groups along with relevant immunological markers are shown in Tables 16.3 and 16.4. Children who developed immediate reactions (i.e., Group 1), reacted with small volumes of cow's milk within 1 hour of commencing the cow's milk challenge procedure. In contrast, the children in Group 2 (intermediate reactors) usually tolerated 60 to 200 mL of cow's milk before symptoms of vomiting and diarrhea developed over several hours. The third group of patients usually tolerated near-normal volumes of cow's milk for 24 to 72 hours before symptoms of CMA commenced.

From these data, each of the patient groups showed statistically significant differences in incidence of challenge-induced skin eruptions, vomiting, diarrhea, and respiratory symptoms. By contrast, the incidence of distressed behavior (i.e., colic elicited by cow's milk challenge) was the same in the three patient groups. As shown in Table 16.3, each of the clinical groups exhibits different immunological features. Thus, colic is not associated with any one immunological marker of CMA in that the children with IgE immediate-type hypersensitivity (Group 1), non-IgE-associated enteropathy (Group 2), or delayed onset T-cell associated disease (Group 3) all showed colic features.

One other point to emerge from these studies was that children with hypersensitivity to cow's milk frequently demonstrated similar reactions to other foods, including eggs, nuts, wheat, and soy, casein,

Table 16.3
Effect of Milk Challenge in CMA

	Group 1	Group 2	Group 3	P-value
Patients	27	53	20	
Angioedema/urticaria	21[ab]	6[a]	2[b]	a = < 0.001 b = > 0.001
Eczema	3	2[a]	7[a]	a = 0.001
Morbilli	1	4	0	
Vomiting	9[ab]	32[ac]	0[bc]	a = 0.02 b = 0.003 c = < 0.001
Diarrhea	4[ab]	32[a]	12[b]	a = < 0.001 b = 0.001
Colic/irritable	10	24	10	
Cough/wheeze	8[a]	2[ab]	10[b]	a = 0.002 b = < 0.001
Stridor	2	0	0	
Rhinitis	2	4	6	

Frequency of symptoms induced by formal milk challenge in Groups 1, 2, and 3. Level of difference indicated if P < 0.05 by chi-squared analysis and Fisher's exact test. No significant difference was observed in frequency of morbilliform eruptions, colic, stridor, or rhinitis.

Table 16.4
Immune Features of Children with
Challenge-Proven CMA

	Group 1	Group 2	Group 3
Clinical	Skin	Gastrointestinal	Mixed
Immunoglobulin	IgE↑	IgA↓	IgM↑
SPT/RAST	+++	±	+
Anti-milk IgG	↓	↓	↓
LIF	±	NK	++
GIFN	±	NK	+
Rotavirus	+	++	NK

and whey hydrolysate preparations (16). Recently, the authors' group has shown in double-blind, placebo-controlled challenge studies that even these hypoallergenic formulas may elicit distress symptoms (17).

Thus, children with true CMA often show colic and distressed behavior as one manifestation of the disease. It remains less clear how many children with "colic, putatively due to cow's milk allergy" fail to display other manifestations of CMA.

The Incidence of Food Allergy in Children Presenting with Colic

Iacono *et al.* put 70 cow's milk formula-fed infants with severe colic on a soy milk formula (18). After one week, the parents of 50 of the infants reported improvement of colic that relapsed within 24 hours after cow's milk was reintroduced into their diet. Within 3 weeks 8 of 50 infants developed soy allergy, and at the age of 9 months 18 of 50 patients developed other symptoms of CMA at challenge. Only 1 of 20 of the patients whose colic did not respond initially to soy milk developed other features of CMA (p < 0.02).

Lothe *et al.* noted a similar phenomenon (19). Of 43 infants with colic who responded to exclusion of cow's milk, 18% developed other features of CMA by the age of 6 months, and 13% retained these features to at least 12 months of age.

While the severity of colic at presentation in these infants may have possibly overshadowed other minor features of CMA, it is more likely that colic

represented one early manifestation of true food protein hypersensitivity.

Sleep disturbance is a major feature of infants presenting with colic. In a report of 146 children referred for sleep disturbance, Kahn (20) identified 15 (median age 13 months) in whom sleep disturbance resolved within 5 weeks of commencing a cow's milk-free diet. In a subsequent double-blind, placebo-controlled challenge, this sleep disturbance recurred within 4 days of the reintroduction of cow's milk. The effect of milk exclusion and reintroduction was monitored via polysomnographs to document arousal and sleep disturbance patterns and evaluated by measurement of skin water evaporation during nonrapid eye movement sleep.

Gastroesophageal reflux and other cardiorespiratory dysrhythmias as a source of the distressed sleep pattern were excluded.

This study did not determine how many children developed symptoms other than sleep disturbance and distressed behavior following reintroduction of cow's milk, but more than half showed features of eczema, vomiting, and diarrhea before receiving the cow's milk-free diet.

The Outcome of Trials of Dietary Management of Colic

Following a preliminary study (21), Jakobsson *et al.* noted that one-third of breast-fed colic infants developed remission and then relapse of colic when mothers excluded and subsequently reintroduced cow milk (22). Evans *et al.* (23), however, were unable to confirm these findings but associated increased colic with increased variety of foods in the maternal diet. Maternal ingestion of cow's milk, egg, chocolate, fruit, and nuts were implicated in producing symptoms. Lothe *et al.* reported that 11 of 60 colic infants on cow's milk formula responded to soy formula; another 32 infants improved following administration of a casein hydrolysate formula (19). These preliminary studies have since been criticized because some of the populations were selected (22), the numbers were too small to identify a real effect (23), the protocol was not truly double-blind (19), and objective data of crying or fussing behavior were not obtained (19, 21–23).

Other investigations of the role of diet in colic have addressed some of these shortcomings. Lothe *et al.* (24) implemented a 5-day cow's milk-free diet using casein hydrolysate. A marked diminution of distressed symptoms occurred in 24 of 27 colicky infants. In these infants, the total crying time decreased from 5.6 hours to 0.7 hour (p < 0.001). The 24 responding infants then entered into a randomized double-blind, crossover trial of a whey protein formula. The active or placebo challenge was conducted on a single day with an intervening 3-day washout period. Crying and disturbed sleep were more prevalent in the whey feeding phase (whey 3.2 +/− 2.4 hours versus placebo 1.0 +/− 1.6 hours) (p < 0.01). Of the 24 infants challenged, 18 (i.e., two-thirds of the original study population) demonstrated increased distress on challenge with milk protein.

In a crossover design of 17 colicky infants, Forsyth (25) ensured that the smell of formula would not lead to unblinding of the study. Casein hydrolysate, or casein hydrolysate and cow's milk formula were fed alternately for four periods, each of which lasted 4 days. Significant decreases in distressed behavior were noted in the first two formula-change periods only. Over the four formula challenge periods, only 2 (11.8%) of the infants showed a reproducible effect of formula change on colic behavior. Previously, Lothe (19) had suggested that approximately 25% of infants with colic responded to dietary change.

The conclusions of Forsyth's study have been questioned because of the small numbers of patients studied and the accuracy of diary recording over 16 days; in addition, critics have noted that the volume of milk protein administered in challenge was only half that normally given to infants of this age. Furthermore, the effect of returning these infants to normal volumes of cow's milk formula upon completion of the study was not recorded. Forsyth concluded that diet was likely to be only one factor in the causation of colic (25). He particularly drew attention to the feelings of helplessness, frustration, and decreased confidence in parenting ability that parents of colic patients suffer.

Results of these studies are summarized in Table 16.5.

Table 16.5
Studies Supporting the Role of Diet as a Cause of Infantile Colic

Author	Study Details	Outcome
Jakobsson (22)	Breast $n = 10$	Conditional probability (p = 0.95) whey protein implicated in colic
Evans (23)	Breast $n = 20$	Range of maternal diet significant (p < 0.05)
Lothe (24)	Formula $n = 24$	Casein hydrolysate 1.0 hours versus whey protein 3.2 hours (p < 0.001)
Forsyth (25)	Formula $n = 17$	Cow's milk distress > casein hydrolysate distress (p < 0.01)

The Outcome of Recent Studies of Behavior Modification in Colic

In a series of studies, Taubman demonstrated the effectiveness of parental counseling in the management of distressed infants (26). In the first phase of a study of 21 colic infants, he found that parental counseling reduced distressed behavior to a similar extent as introduction of a cow's milk-free diet. In the second phase of his study, however, patients who had received only dietary treatment in the first phase returned to their prestudy diet while their parents received counseling. The distressed behavior of these infants with diet-responsive colic further decreased with parental counseling. Taubman concluded that, in many infants suffering from colic, the crying results from parental misinterpretation of infant cries and is not caused primarily by milk protein allergy. The relatively small number of patients in this study and the difficulty of blinding counseling procedures bring the validity and generalizability of Taubman's findings into question. Nevertheless, they do emphasize the importance of parental counseling in the management of infantile colic.

Hunziger *et al.* (7) also implied that distressed behavior in infancy may reflect parental misinterpretation of normal crying behavior. Following their observations that normal infants showed less crying behavior when regularly nurtured by supplemental carrying, Barr *et al.* studied the effect of supplemental carrying on 66 colic infants (10). Overall, the "treatment" group carried their infants 6.1 hours per day (2.2 hours more than the control group) throughout the intervention period. At 6 weeks of age, when a significant effect of treatment was expected, none could be shown. Hunziger's group concluded that this difference in response to carrying may be due to an underlying pathological process such as protein hypersensitivity or irritable bowel.

Recent studies by Rautava *et al.* (27) suggest an important role for maternal distress during pregnancy and childbirth and unsatisfactory sexual relationships, but not for socio-demographic factors, in the etiology of colic in Finnish infants. Wolke *et al.* (28) examined the effect of different behavior strategies in 92 mother/colicky infant pairs. After 3 months, all of the infants' distress had improved. Infants whose mothers received advice on behavior modification improved distress by 51%, however, compared with those whose mothers received empathic support (37%) and the control group (35%). Interestingly, all but 3 of the 92 infants in this study were ingesting hypoallergenic formula during the study period. Thus, although behavior modification clearly improved distress in this cohort of colic infants, the role of hypoallergenic formula in influencing the outcome of the study was not examined.

The results of these studies are summarized in Table 16.6.

The Melbourne Colic Study

The role of diet was examined in a recent investigation of 115 colic infants who were reportedly distressed for more than 3 hours per day, for more than 3 days per week, for more than 3 weeks (29). Infants were referred from community-based pediatric facilities and were studied over a 1-week period. All mothers of breast-fed infants were placed on an artificial color-free, preservative-free, additive-free diet program. In addition, those assigned the active low-allergen diet excluded all milk, egg, wheat, and nuts. Formula-fed infants were assigned a casein hydrolysate preparation (low-allergen diet) or cow's milk-based formula. In the double-blind, placebo-controlled study, the response to diet was assessed by comparing the level of distress behavior at the outset and at the end of the 1-week diet treatment. Parents recorded distress levels on the previously validated infant distress charts described above.

If successful outcome was defined as "a reduction in distress of 25% or more," after adjusting for age and feed mode, infants on active diet had a significantly higher rate of improvement than those on the control diet (odds ratio 2.32; 95% confidence interval, 1.07–5.0) (p = 0.03). In addition, the results were assessed by comparing the distress ratio of day 8 to day 1 for infants assigned the active diet compared with those assigned the control diet. Distress was

Table 16.6
Studies Investigating Disturbed Family Interaction as a Cause of Colic

Author	Study Details	Outcome: Change in Distress (hours per 24-hour period)
Hunziker (7)[a]	Carrying n = 49	1.2
	Control n = 50	2.2 (p < 0.001)
Barr (10)	Carrying n = 31	3.3
	Control n = 35	3.4 (p > 0.05)
Taubman (26)	Counseling n = 10	3.2 versus 1.06 (p = 0.001)
	Diet n = 10	3.2 versus 2.03 (p = 0.01)
Wolke (28)	Empathy n = 27	6.3 versus 3.7 (p < 0.001)
	Behavior modification n = 21	5.8 versus 2.8 (p < 0.001) [b]
	Control n = 44	5.7 versus 3.7 (p < 0.001)

[a] Study of non-colic infants.
[b] Behavior modification superior to empathy and control (p < 0.02).

reduced by 39% (95% CI, 26–50) in infants on the active diet compared with 16% (95% CI, 0–30) for those on the control diet. After again adjusting for age and feed mode, these differences proved statistically significant (p = 0.012). This finding translates into a median reduction in distress scores for infants on the active diet of 117 minutes compared with 46 minutes for those on the control diet.

These results were achieved by studying a cohort of infants whose contact was restricted to the study period. Subjects entered the study irrespective of previous use of anti-colic medications, dietary manipulation, or presence of psychosocial factors likely to contribute to colic. The findings may have general applicability because infants were referred by community-based pediatricians, family practitioners, and child health practitioners. They had distress times comparable to infants in other investigations of diet and behavior intervention strategies in colic. The apparent benefits of diet in this study must be tempered by the following limitations associated with the study, however.

First, a high drop-out rate was noted, with 36 infants not completing the full study. No difference was observed in the active or control diet assigned to patients, nor did socio-economic factors differ between the drop-outs and those who completed the study. Second, in determining sample size, based on the data available, the incidence of spontaneous improvement in colic was underestimated by as much as 30% in the different groups. This condition meant that only one group of patients (breast-fed infants older than 6 weeks) included a sufficient number of patients to adequately test the effect of diet in different subgroups.

One striking feature that emerged from the study was the difference in the effect of the two diet programs on breast-fed infants less than 6 weeks of age. In this age group, only infants on the active diet *decreased* their distress, whereas those on the control diet *increased* distress during the study period. The breast-fed infants younger than 6 weeks of age on the active diet decreased distress by 24% (73 min/24 hours), whereas those on the control diet increased distress by 34% (67 min/24 hours). This difference in the response to diet was statistically significant

(p = 0.006). When these data were examined according to whether the infants reduced distress by 25% or more, 6 out of 12 assigned the active diet reduced distress according to this parameter, whereas none of the 10 on the control diet achieved this reduction (p = 0.015).

The findings of this study suggest that diet is one factor that contributes to colic in infants but it was unclear whether this effect was global or whether only a subpopulation of distressed infants are responsive. The results suggest that, in particular, breast-fed infants younger than 6 weeks of age may benefit from this intervention; in older infants, the incidence of spontaneous remission of colic is such that a large number of patients need to be studied to detect an effect of diet change. These findings suggest that some infants have colic because of transient protein intolerance that improves beginning at about 6 weeks of age.

In the authors' study, the degree of dietary restriction on breast-feeding mothers was severe. If this approach is to be followed for more than 1 week, nutritional support for breast-feeding mothers is essential.

Conclusion

Colic is a clinical syndrome that can be defined and quantified. General consensus has emerged about its etiology but it is likely to be multifactorial. The two major schools of thought attribute colic to either a disturbance in the parent–child interaction (behavioral) or a food protein hypersensitivity reaction (allergy). The following observations may help to reconcile the apparent differences between these conflicting views.

First, Barr *et al.* (10) observed that colicky infants younger than 6 weeks respond poorly to a form of behavior modification shown to benefit normal crying infants (6). Second, Forsyth (25) noted that the response to diet-change in formula-fed infants with colic is transient. Our group's study (17) has demonstrated that breast-fed infants of less than 6 weeks of age with colic respond particularly well to a hypoallergenic diet. Finally, Wolke *et al.* noted that older infants with excessive crying who were ingesting hypoallergenic formula diets responded to behavior modification (28).

Thus, we hypothesize that in colic infants, transient food protein intolerance in the first weeks of life leads to distress that may then persist due to behavior patterning and disturbed parent–infant interactions.

REFERENCES

1. Brazelton TB. Crying in infancy. Pediatrics 1960;26:579–588.
2. Wessel MA, Cobb SC, Jackson EB, et al. Paroxysmal fussing in infancy: sometimes called "colic." Pediatrics 1954;14:421–434.
3. Illingworth RS. Three months of colic. Arch Dis Child 1954;29:165–174.
4. Lothe L. Studies on infantile colic. Thesis; University of Lund, Malmo, 1989.
5. Hill DJ, Hosking CS. Role of adverse food reactions in infantile colic. In: De Weck AL, Sampson HA, eds. Intestinal Immunology and Food Allergy. Nestle Nutrition Workshop Series, vol. 34, New York: Raven Press, 1995, 131–139.
6. Barr RG, Kramer MS, Boisjoly C, et al. Parental diary of infants cry and fuss behaviour. Arch Dis Child 1988;63:380–387.
7. Hunziker VA, Barr RG. Increased carrying reduces infant crying: a randomized control trial. Pediatrics 1986;5:641–647.
8. Hill DJ, Menahem S, Hudson I, Sheffield LJ, Shelton MJ, Oberklaid F, Hosking CS. Charting infant distress—an aid to defining colic. J Pediatr 1992;121:755–758.
9. Hide DW, Guyer BM. The prevalence of infant colic. Arch Dis Child 1982;57:559–560.
10. Barr RG, McMullan SJ, Speiss H, et al. Carrying as colic "therapy": a randomized control trial. Pediatrics 1986;87:623–630.
11. Hill DJ, Firer MA, Shelton MJ, Hosking CS. Manifestations of milk allergy in infancy: clinical and immunological findings. J Pediatr 1986;109:270–276.
12. Firer MA, Hosking CS, Hill DJ. Humoral immune response to cow's milk in children with cow's milk allergy. Int Arch Allergy Appl Immunol 1987;84:173–177.
13. Hill DJ, Ball G, Hosking CS. Clinical manifestations of cow's milk allergy in childhood. I. Association with in vitro cellular immune responses. Clin Allergy 1988;18:469–479.
14. Hill DJ, Duke AM, Hosking CS, et al. Clinical manifestations of cow's milk allergy in childhood: II. The diagnostic value of skin tests and RAST. Clin Allergy 1988;5:481–490.
15. Hill DJ, Ball G, Hosking CS, Wood PR. Gamma-interferon production in cow milk allergy. Allergy 1993;48:75–80.
16. Bishop JM, Hill DJ, Hosking CS. Natural history of cow milk allergy—clinical outcome. J Pediatr 1990;116:862–867.
17. Hill DJ, Cameron DJS, Francis DEM, Gonzalez A, Hosking CS. Challenge confirmation of late onset reactions to extensively hydrolysed formula in infants with multiple food protein intolerance. J Allergy Clin Immunol. 1995; 96:386–394.
18. Iacono G, Carroccio A, Montalto G, et al. Severe infantile colic and food intolerance; a long term prospective study. J Pediatr Gastroenterol Nutr 1991;12:332–335.
19. Lothe L, Lindberg T, Jakobsson I. Cow's milk formula as a cause of infantile colic: a double-blind study. Pediatrics 1982;70:7–10.
20. Kahn A, Mozin MJ, Rebuffat E, et al. Milk intolerance in children with persistent sleeplessness; a prospective double-blind crossover evaluation. Pediatrics 1989;84:595–603.
21. Jakobsson I, Lindberg T. Cow's milk proteins cause infantile colic in breast fed infants. Lancet 1978;2:437–439.
22. Jakobsson I, Lindberg T. Cow's milk proteins cause infantile colic in breast-fed infants: a double-blind crossover study. Pediatrics 1983;71:268–271.
23. Evans RW, Fergusson DM, Allardyce RA, Taylor B. Maternal diet and infantile colic in breast-fed infants. Lancet 1981;1:1340–1342.
24. Lothe L, Lindberg T. Cow's milk whey protein elicits symptoms of infantile colic in colicky formula-fed infants: a double-blind crossover study. Pediatrics 1989;83:262–266.
25. Forsyth BW. Colic and the effect of change in formulas: a double-blind multiple-crossover study. J Pediatr 1989;115:521–526.
26. Taubman B. Parental counselling compared with elimination of cow's milk or soy milk protein for the treatment of infantile colic: a randomised trial. Pediatrics 1988;81:756–761.
27. Rautava P, Helenius H, Lehtonen L. Psycho-social predisposing factors for infantile colic. Brit Med J 1993;307:600–604.
28. Wolke D, Gray P, Meyer R. Excess infant crying: a control study of mothers helping mothers. Pediatrics 1994;94:322–332.
29. Hill DJ, Hudson IL, Sheffield LJ, Shelton MJ, Hosking CS. A low allergen diet is a significant intervention in infantile colic: results of a community-based study. J Allergy Clin Immunol 1995; 96:886–892.

17

EOSINOPHILIC GASTROENTERITIS

Kyung-Up Min

*E*osinophilic gastroenteritis (EG) is characterized by peripheral eosinophilia, eosinophilic infiltration of the bowel wall, and gastrointestinal symptoms. The variable terminology describing this disease has included pyloric hypertrophy with eosinophilic infiltration, gastric lesion of Löffler's syndrome, gastric granuloma with eosinophilic infiltration, eosinophilic granuloma, infiltrative eosinophilic gastritis, and eosinophilic (allergic) gastroenteritis (1). The sites of involvement include the esophagus, stomach, small intestine, colon, and rarely extraintestinal organs. Approximately one-half of the cases have allergic features and may be related to food allergy.

Epidemiology

Eosinophilic gastroenteritis is uncommon, but cases have been recognized in North and South America, Europe, Australia, the Pacific, South Africa, and the Middle East. Although more than 150 case reports have appeared in the literature (2), the true prevalence of EG is not known. The peak age of onset is in the third decade, and although EG occurs mainly in infants, children, and young adults, no age is immune to it (3, 4). Males are affected slightly more than females. The disease is sporadic in distribution, but a case of familial EG has been reported (5).

Etiology

The cause of EG is unknown, although an allergic or immunologic reaction to food antigen seems likely in some cases (6). A mast-cell-mediated mechanism dependent on immunoglobulin E (IgE) has been advocated for the immunologic basis of this disorder. Atopic diseases, such as childhood food sensitivities, eczema, allergic rhinitis, bronchial asthma, and a therapeutic response to steroids are common in patients with EG (7). Moreover, many patients have eosinophilia in the peripheral blood, elevated serum IgE concentrations, and positive radioallergosorbent tests (RAST) for specific IgE antibodies to food antigen (3, 8). Sometimes, these results correlate with positive skin tests and symptomatic response to these food substances (9, 10). Mononuclear cells containing IgE have been identified in the lamina propria of the intestine, and the number of IgE-containing cells and eosinophils has been reported to decrease after an elimination diet, which was accompanied by clinical improvement (11).

Because the lymphokines IL-4, IL-5, and γ-interferon regulate IgE synthesis and eosinophilopoiesis in vitro, Jaffe *et al.* recently examined whether an imbalance occurs in their production in allergic eosinophilic gastroenteritis. Three adult patients with allergic eosinophilic gastroenteritis were studied (12). Flow cytometric studies of peripheral blood mononuclear cells did not reveal evidence of T-cell activation or disturbance of T-cell numbers or subsets. T cells were capable of normal mitogenic activation in vitro. With mitogenic stimulation, IL-4 and IL-5 production were markedly elevated. Most IL-4 and IL-5 production was by CD4+ T cells. Synthesis of IL-5 by CD4+ T lymphocytes in three patients and CD8+ T lymphocytes in two patients occurred in the absence of mitogen. Mitogen-stimulated GM-CSF and γ-interferon synthesis by CD4+ T cells was normal. γ-Interferon mRNA was not detected by reverse transcription/polymerase chain reaction in biopsies from patients with allergic eosinophilic gastroenteritis but was present in controls. These lymphokine abnormalities were consistent with the elevated IgE and eosinophilia seen in allergic eosinophilic gastroenteritis.

Participation of an allergic mechanism has been demonstrated in cow's milk allergy of childhood. A milk challenge resulted in an infiltration of eosinophils, an increase of IgE-positive plasma cells, and mast cell degranulation in the small-intestinal mucosa (13). Eosinophils infiltrating the bowel mucosa were both activated and degranulated, and in this way may have induced tissue damage by releasing the eosinophil cationic protein (ECP) and major basic protein (MBP) (5). Ultrastructural study of mucosal eosinophils obtained from damaged duodenum showed that the electron core density of eosinophil granules was inverted or disappeared and tubulovesicular structures appeared. The major basic protein was detected diffusely in the matrix of eosinophil granules, supporting a role for major basic protein in tissue damage in EG (14). Indeed, many pediatric cases of intolerance to food protein, such as milk protein or soy protein, have been classified as allergic gastroenteropathy when convincing evidence of an allergic mechanism existed and when the clinical findings were those of EG (15). In these cases, the children frequently improved following elimination of the incriminated food antigen (16). The basis of allergic pathogenesis remains to be elucidated.

All patients with EG, however, are not atopic, and all cases cannot be explained by food allergy (17). Only one-half of patients have findings consistent with atopy. Many patients show no personal or family history of allergy, no adverse reactions to food, no positive skin tests for food allergens, and no elevation in serum IgE. Even in patients with suspected food allergies, sequential withdrawal of various food substances may fail to result in amelioration of symptoms, and a poor correlation may appear between the results of skin tests to specific food antigens and the results of an elimination diet. In addition, there are patients who show no abnormality following extensive immunologic studies, including serum immunoglobulins, complement levels, lymphocyte quantitation, and lymphocyte responses to nonspecific mitogens (8).

An Arthus-type hypersensitivity reaction has also been suggested as responsible for attracting eosinophils to the site of antigen–antibody complex deposition. An antigen in food could react with specific antibody in the gut wall. The activation of the complement pathway would then draw eosinophils to the site of complex formation (18). At present little evidence exists to support this possibility.

A number of other etiologic processes, including viral infections, parasitic infestations, and malignancies, have been considered as an explanation for EG in patients without obvious food allergies. Viral infections have been proposed because of the observation that EG may follow viral gastroenteritis. A history of flu-like symptoms, laboratory data including viral cultures and serologies, gastric histology showing inclusion bodies, and spontaneous remissions in a few weeks are consistent with this hypothesis. Several patients have had evidence of infection with cytomegalovirus or parainfluenza virus (19). Interestingly, it has been reported that certain viral infections may provoke allergic reactions by preferentially depressing IgE T suppressor cells (20), thereby allowing T helper cells to stimulate IgE production. Moreover, the increased absorption of antigen through mucosa damaged by a viral infection may stimulate immune responses.

Parasite infestation in tissues is often associated with peripheral eosinophilia and eosinophilic infiltrations. Eosinophilic gastroenteritis due to *Schistosoma* (21) and the herring parasite *Eustoma rotundatum* (22) have been reported. This possibility can be eliminated in most cases, however.

The association of massive eosinophilia with nonhematopoietic malignancy is described (23). EG has been reported in a patient with ovarian malignancy with regression of eosinophilic gastritis after resection of this tumor (24). Other diseases associated with EG include scleroderma, polymyositis, dermatomyositis (25), polyarteritis nodosa (26), dermatitis herpetiformis, and gluten-sensitive enteropathy (27). The mechanisms behind such associations are poorly understood, but the gastrointestinal disease may foretell the development of these diseases, sometimes by several years.

Classification

Rational classification of a disease is best developed out of an understanding of its etiology and pathogenesis. Lacking a precise knowledge of these aspects in EG, any attempt to classify this disorder cannot be conclusive (28). That being said, three types of diffuse eosinophilic gastroenteritis have been proposed, linking the clinical manifestations and depth of the maximal disease process (29). In this classification scheme, type I disease is predominantly mucosal and characterized by fecal blood loss, iron-deficiency anemia, protein-losing enteropathy, and malabsorption. Type II disease is predominantly a muscle layer disease with obstructive symptoms due to thickening and rigidity of the gut. Type III disease is predominantly a subserosal disease with eosinophilic ascites. More than one site may be involved in a given patient.

Most of the earlier recorded cases involved patients first treated as surgical emergencies with symptoms of intestinal obstruction, or type II disease. With increasing awareness of the condition and its recognition by other means such as radiology, peroral small-bowel biopsy, and endoscopy, more cases with mucosal involvement have been found. The subserosal type, which accounts for approximately 10% of the reported cases, is the least frequent type of the three (30). Colonic or esophageal involvement, isolated or combined, is also being recognized with increasing frequency, suggesting that the designation of this disease as gastroenteritis is too limiting.

The term "allergic gastroenteropathy" has been used for a childhood disease with mucosal abnormalities and a clinical diagnosis of allergy. Considerable clinical and histologic overlap is noted between reported cases of allergic gastroenteropathy with malabsorption and the mucosal type of EG, perhaps justifying their inclusion in a single category of disease (15). The childhood disease, food protein-sensitive enteropathy, appears to be closely related to EG (16). It has clinical findings similar to EG but is transient, begins in the first year of life, remits on withdrawal of the food from the diet, and seems not uniformly associated with IgE-mediated immediate hypersensitivity. The precise relationship between these clinically similar diseases remains undefined.

Pathology

MACROSCOPIC FINDINGS

Eosinophilic gastroenteritis most commonly involves the stomach and the small bowel, with esophageal (31) and colonic involvement rarely encountered. Typically, the gastric antrum is affected. The duodenum and, to a lesser extent, the jejunum tend to be affected in association with the stomach rather than alone (32). The affected portion of bowel is thickened and swollen with varying degrees of induration, edema, hyperemia, and nodularity, sometimes obstructing the lumen. The rugal folds of the stomach or intestinal valves of the small intestine are enlarged. Multiple small, discrete mucosal ulcerations may occur (7). The serosa appears reddened with yellow or grayish patches.

Regional lymphadenopathy is sometimes quite marked. Ascites may be present. The appendix may be involved, in which case EG may present as acute appendicitis (33). Involvement of other organs such as the liver, spleen, gallbladder, pancreas, and urinary bladder has been described, but is rare (34, 35).

MICROSCOPIC FINDINGS

The two striking microscopic features of EG are dense eosinophilic infiltration and edema (4) (Fig. 17.1). The degree of eosinophilic infiltration is extremely variable, even within the same specimen. The lamina propria or submucosa is usually infiltrated to a maximum degree. A tendency to perivascular aggregation of the eosinophils has been observed. In some instances, large numbers of eosinophils are observed in the subserosal layer or in the muscle coat with separation of the muscle bundles. The extent of the tissue eosinophilia does not have a constant relationship to the number of eosinophils in the peripheral blood (4). Muscular hypertrophy has been noted, with necrosis of muscle fibers and vessels, and a giant cell reaction in the stomach. The sinusoids of enlarged regional lymph nodes are engorged with eosinophils.

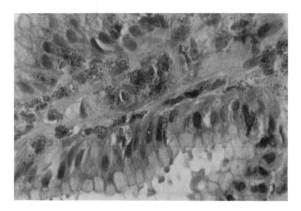

Figure 17.1

Small-bowel biopsy specimen. The lamina propria is densely infiltrated with eosinophilic leukocytes, which contain many eosinophilic granules. The villous architecture is preserved. (Hematoxylin and eosin stain, ×400.)

Clinical Manifestations

The clinical manifestations of EG depend on the area of maximal gastrointestinal involvement and the depth of the maximal disease process (Table 17.1).

Table 17.1
Clinical Manifestations of Eosinophilic Gastroenteritis Related to the Depth of the Maximal Disease Process

Type	Predominant Involvement	Manifestations
I	Mucosal	Abdominal pain Nausea Vomiting Iron-deficiency anemia Diarrhea Growth retardation Weight loss Fecal blood loss
II	Muscular	Abdominal pain Nausea Vomiting Weight loss Early satiety
III	Subserosal	Abdominal pain Nausea Vomiting Diarrhea Ascites

In patients with mucosal involvement, postprandial nausea, vomiting, cramping, periumbilical pain, and loose, watery diarrhea are common. Weight loss due to malabsorption may progress to cachexia. Generalized edema secondary to protein-losing enteropathy may occur (19). Pallor is due to iron-deficiency anemia, usually resulting from fecal blood loss. Growth retardation may be profound in children.

In patients with predominantly muscle layer involvement, manifestations of intermittent gastric or small-bowel obstruction are seen (6, 36). Epigastric pain, nausea, vomiting, and weight loss are frequent. Nocturnal regurgitation, heartburn, hematemesis, or melena may be encountered. Duodenal involvement may result in biliary obstruction (37).

The chief manifestation of EG in patients with predominant subserosal involvement is ascites (30). Abdominal distention, abdominal pain, and diarrhea are the usual symptoms. Nausea and vomiting may accompany these problems. Eosinophilic pleural effusions may also be noted. It is not unusual to find multiple-layer involvement, even though it is not clinically apparent. Small-bowel perforations involving the entire thickness of the bowel wall have been seen (38).

The patients with colonic or rectal involvement may experience recurrent cramping lower abdominal pain, weight loss, and frequent liquid, blood-streaked stools (39–41). Eosphageal involvement in EG may manifest in intermittent dysphagia, epigastric pain, or vomiting (42). When the appendix is infiltrated with eosinophils, the clinical signs and symptoms may be indistinguishable from those of acute suppurative appendicitis (33). The clinical course of EG may be that of chronic or recurrent acute episodes of gastrointestinal symptoms. Occasionally the condition is self-limiting.

Laboratory Findings

The most characteristic laboratory finding of EG is a prominent eosinophilia (up to 80%) in the peripheral blood (43). The eosinophils are mature and show no abnormality in morphology. The bone marrow may be infiltrated with eosinophils but reveals no evidence of a blood dyscrasia. The total white blood cell count is frequently elevated. In contrast, the erythrocyte sedimentation rate may be normal.

There may also be varying degrees of iron-deficiency anemia, depending on the site, extent, and duration of bowel involvement. Stools are usually positive for occult blood, and may contain gross blood. Charcot-Leyden crystals, presumably from extruded mucosal eosinophils, may be found on microscopic examination of the stool. When present the ascites is invariably an exudate and contains many eosinophils. Abnormal D-xylose absorption tests indicative of mucosal disease may be evident. Hypoalbuminemia secondary to protein-losing enteropathy or malabsorption is occasionally seen in these patients (44, 45). Some patients have elevated serum IgE levels that rise with exposure to specific foods (10). Specific IgE and positive skin reactions to multiple food antigens may be detected.

Radiologic Findings

There is no pathognomonic radiologic finding in EG. In mucosal disease, the stomach exhibits mucosal thickening similar to hypertrophic gastritis or Ménétrier's disease. With further thickening of the folds, a polypoid gastritis or a discrete polyp may be observed, sometimes simulating lymphosarcoma (46). The changes in the small bowel may be striking with patchy thickening and distortion of the folds, spasm, irritability, and increased secretions, more prominent in the jejunum (47). The thickened folds may produce a nodular configuration along the contour of the bowel.

In the muscular type, changes in the stomach are usually limited to the antrum, producing a radiologic appearance of hypertrophic pyloric stenosis. The triangular cleft noted on the greater curvature of the prepyloric segment in hypertrophic pyloric stenosis is not observed, however. When muscular thickening is diffuse, an appearance simulating scirrhous carcinoma may be produced. Segments of small intestine may show a pipe-stem appearance with no mucosal folds. If EG involves only the subserosa, radiologic findings will be those of ascites.

Colonic changes include mild mucosal irregularity, narrowing, thumb-printing, or spasm, and may simulate inflammatory bowel disease. In esophageal involvement, the radiologic findings are mucosal irregularities or narrowing of the lumen. The motility is disturbed, with incomplete relaxation of the lower sphincter, mimicking achalasia.

Diagnosis

The diagnosis of EG is not difficult if the histology of the bowel wall reveals heavy eosinophilic infiltration in a patient with peripheral eosinophilia and characteristic clinical symptoms. The pertinent clinical setting for an IgE-mediated pathogenesis includes a personal and family history of atopic disease, and characteristic gastrointestinal symptoms. Iron-deficiency anemia, hypoproteinemia, and an increased IgE level may be present. The erythrocyte sedimentation rate is almost normal. Food-specific IgE antibodies may be detected in the serum, and the patient may show positive skin tests to multiple food antigens. Symptoms may be related to exposure to specific foods (10). Challenge with a suspected food may severely exacerbate symptoms and should not routinely be performed, although food challenge may aid in diagnosis under carefully controlled conditions.

The histologic diagnosis may be made by mucosal biopsy in patients with mucosal disease. Patients with infiltration of deeper layers may require full-thickness biopsies (41). Alterations of the gastric antrum are more constant and profound, suggesting that biopsy specimens from this site are the most sensitive and discriminating for diagnosis, even when gastric involvement is not suspected clinically (48). The intestinal lesions are often patchy, and multiple biopsies may be required.

DIFFERENTIAL DIAGNOSIS

Many disorders may mimic the findings of EG. Eosinophilic infiltrations of the gut are often seen in eosinophilic granuloma, polyarteritis nodosa, intestinal parasite infestation, lymphoma, intestinal carcinoma (24), peptic ulcer disease, and hypereosinophilic syndrome (29). However, peripheral eosinophilia is not a consistent feature of eosinophilic granuloma, lymphoma, intestinal carcinoma, or peptic ulcer disease. Moreover, increased erythrocyte sedimentation rates are common in polyarteritis nodosa and lymphoma, unlike the usually normal erythrocyte sedimentation rate in EG.

In infants with small-bowel involvement, celiac disease, intestinal lymphangiectasia, cystic fibrosis, and immune deficiency should be differentiated. In those with large-bowel involvement, the findings are of a colitis. Such features may simulate ulcerative colitis or Crohn's disease.

Treatment

The ideal treatment of EG is to identify and remove the causative antigen if it exists. In pediatric cases, food antigens are the most commonly incriminated cause of EG. Milk, soy, egg, and wheat flour are frequently at fault. Administration of an elemental, hypoallergic diet may result in a rapid clinical recovery (31). Replacement of cow's milk with soy formula is successful in the treatment of children allergic to cow's milk protein (49, 50), but there is a tendency to develop sensitivity to soy protein when it is fed during an active disease process. So it may be necessary to rest the inflamed bowel by total parenteral nutrition for a time before shifting to another diet. During this time the damaged bowel wall can recover mucosal integrity.

In adults, the causative agents are usually not as evident. A trial elimination diet is justified in patients with an atopic diathesis, although it is not usually successful. Substances known or suspected by the patient to exacerbate symptoms should be rigidly excluded. In the absence of a clinically suspected food sensitivity, trial elimination diets can be based on results of skin testing and RAST (18). Some patients with food hypersensitivity may have anaphylactic episodes following exposure to certain foods. These patients must be identified and instructed to avoid these incriminated foods and should be prepared to self-administer adrenalin if a systemic reaction occurs following inadvertent exposure.

Steroids are successfully used in patients with EG who fail to respond to elimination diets. The dosages initially employed range from 20 to 40 mg of prednisone daily. The response is usually prompt. Occasion-

ally, patients require continuous administration of a low dose of steroids every other day to control symptoms. Cromolyn sodium (26, 48) and ketotifen (51) have been used in some patients, but with no consistent effect.

Surgery should be reserved for patients with obstructive symptoms, bowel perforation, or uncertain diagnosis. It is possible that bowel obstruction can be managed with steroids if detected early (52). A few patients have shown a persistent remission of EG after surgical excision of the involved bowel segment (38).

Prognosis

The long-term prognosis for young patients with EG is good. Pediatric patients with EG usually respond to an elimination diet when the disease is related to food sensitivity. Frequently, the sensitivity to foods resolves spontaneously by 2 to 3 years of age. Some children have recurrent symptoms after a short period of improvement with an elimination diet. Adult patients may experience chronic recurrent disease (53). The recurrent symptoms can be managed by dietary manipulation and steroid therapy. Fatal cases are rare, and are usually due to bowel perforation or other associated diseases (54–56). Patients with EG have no known increased risk of gastrointestinal malignancies.

REFERENCES

1. Edelman MJ, March TL. Eosinophilic gastroenteritis. Am J Roentgen 1964;91:773–778.
2. Blackshaw AJ, Levison DA. Eosinophilic infiltrates of the gastrointestinal tract. J Clin Pathol 1986;39:1–7.
3. Trounce JQ, Tanner MS. Eosinophilic gastroenteritis. Arch Dis Child 1985;60:1186–1188.
4. Johnstone JM, Morson BS. Eosinophilic gastroenteritis. Histopathology 1978;2:335–348.
5. Keshavarzian A, Saverymuttu SH, Tai PC, Thompson M, Barter S, Spry CJF, Chadwick VS. Activated eosinophils in familial eosinophilic gastroenteritis. Gastroenterology 1985;88:1041–1049.
6. Caldwell JH, Mekhjian HS, Hurtubise PE, Beman FM. Eosinophilic gastroenteritis with obstruction: immunological studies of seven patients. Gastroenterology 1978;74:825–829.
7. Lucak BG, Sansaricq CS, Snyderman SE, Greco MA, Fazzini EP, Bazaz GR. Disseminated ulcerations in allergic eosinophilic gastroenteritis. Am J Gastroenterol 1982;77:248–252.

8. Elkon KB, Sher R, Seftel HC. Immunological studies of eosinophilic gastro-enteritis and treatment with disodium cromoglycate and beclomethasone dipropionate. S Afr Med J 1977;52:838–841.

9. Caldwell JH, Sharma HM, Hurtubise PE, Colwell DL. Eosinophilic gastroenteritis in extreme allergy: immunopathological comparison with nonallergic gastrointestinal disease. Gastroenterology 1979;77:560–564.

10. Caldwell JH, Tennenbaum JI, Bronstein HA. Serum IgE in eosinophilic gastroenteritis: response to intestinal challenge in two cases. N Engl J Med 1975;292:1388–1390.

11. Jenkins HR, Pincott JR, Soothill JF, Milla PJ, Harries JT. Food allergy: the major cause of infantile colitis. Arch Dis Child 1984;59:326–329.

12. Jaffe JS, James SP, Mullins GE, Braun-Elwert L, Lubensky I, Metcalfe DD. Evidence for an abnormal profile of interleukin-4, IL-5, and γ-interferon in peripheral blood T cells from patients with allergic eosinophilic gastroenteritis. J Clin Immunol 1994;14:299–309.

13. Oyaizu N, Uemura Y, Izumi H, Morii S, Nishi M, Hioki K. Eosinophilic gastroenteritis: immunochemical evidence for IgE mast cell-mediated allergy. Acta Pathol Jpn 1985;35:759–766.

14. Torpier G, Colombel JF, Mathieu-Chandelier C, et al. Eosinophilic gastroenteritis: ultrastructural evidence for a selective release of eosinophil major basic protein. Clin Exp Immunol 1988;74:404–408.

15. Goldman H, Proujansky R. Allergic proctitis and gastroenteritis in children: clinical and mucosal biopsy features in 53 cases. Am J Surg Pathol 1986;10:75–86.

16. Katz AJ, Twarog FJ, Zeiger RS, Falchuk ZM. Milk-sensitive and eosinophilic gastroenteropathy: similar clinical features with contrasting mechanisms and clinical course. J Allergy Clin Immunol 1984;74:72–78.

17. Leinbach GE, Rubin CE. Eosinophilic gastroenteritis: a simple reaction to food allergens? Gastroenterology 1970;59:874–889.

18. Cello JP. Eosinophilic gastroenteritis: a complex disease entity. Am J Med 1979;67:1097–1104.

19. Stillman AE, Sieber O, Manthei U, Pinnas J. Transient protein-losing enteropathy and enlarged gastric rugae in childhood. Am J Dis Child 1981;135:29–33.

20. Frick OL, German DF, Mills J. Development of allergy in children. 1. Association with virus infections. J Allergy Clin Immunol 1979;63:228–241.

21. Hesdorffer CS, Ziady F. Eosinophilic gastroenteritis—a complication of schistosomiasis and peripheral eosinophilia? A case report and review of the pathogenesis. S Afr Med J 1982;61:591–593.

22. Ashby BS, Appleton PJ, Dawson I. Eosinophilic granuloma of gastro-intestinal tract caused by herring parasite Eustoma rotundatum. Br Med J 1964;1:1141–1145.

23. Tsutsumi Y, Ohshita T, Yokoyama T. A case of gastric carcinoma with massive eosinophilia. Acta Pathol Jpn 1984;31:117–122.

24. Reshef R, Manaster J, Ezekiel E, Suprun H, Manor E. Malignant tumor masquerading as eosinophilic gastroenteritis. Isr J Med Sci 1987;23:281–283.

25. DeSchryver-Kecskemeti K, Clouse RE. A previously unrecognized subgroup of "eosinophilic gastroenteritis": association with connective tissue diseases. Am J Surg Pathol 1984;8:171–180.

26. Heatley RV, Harris A, Atkinson M. Treatment of a patient with clinical features of both eosinophilic gastroenteritis and polyarteritis nodosa with oral sodium cromoglycate. Dig Dis Sci 1980;25:470–472.

27. Bennet RA, Whitelock T III, Kelly JL Jr. Eosinophilic gastroenteritis, gluten enteropathy, and dermatitis herpetiformis. Am J Dig Dis 1974;19:1154–1161.

28. Ureles AL, Alschibaja T, Lodico D, Stabins SJ. Idiopathic eosinophilic infiltration of the gastrointestinal tract, diffuse and circumscribed: a proposed classification and review of the literature with two additional cases. Am J Med 1961;30:899–909.

29. Klein NC, Hargrove RL, Sleisenger MH, Jeffries GH. Eosinophilic gastroenteritis. Medicine (Baltimore) 1970;49:299–319.

30. Harmon WA, Helman CA. Eosinophilic gastroenteritis and ascites. J Clin Gastroenterol 1981;3:371–373.

31. Kelly KJ, Lazenby AJ, Rowe PC, Yardley JH, Perman JA, Sampson HA. Eosinophilic esophagitis attributed to gastroesophageal reflux: improvement with an amino acid-based formula. Gastroenterology 1995;109:1503–1512.

32. Zora JA, O'Connell EJ, Sachs MI, Hoffman AD. Eosinophilic gastroenteritis: a case report and review of the literature. Ann Allergy 1984;53:45–47.

33. Zona JZ, Belin RP, Burke JA. Eosinophilic infiltration of the gastrointestinal tract in children. Am J Dis Child 1976;130:1136–1139.

34. Everett GD, Mitros FA. Eosinophilic gastroenteritis with hepatic eosinophilic granulomas: report of a case with 30-year follow-up. Am J Gastroenterol 1980;74:519–521.

35. Robert F, Omura E, Durant JR. Mucosal eosinophilic gastroenteritis with systemic involvement. Am J Med 1977;62:139–143.

36. Steele RJC, Wright RG, Gilmore HM. Eosinophilic gastroenteritis presenting as acute intestinal obstruction. Scott Med J 1983;28:183–184.

37. Rumans MC, Lieberman DA. Eosinophilic gastroenteritis presenting with biliary and duodenal obstruction. Am J Gastroenterol 1987;82:775–778.

38. Lysey J, Eid A. Eosinophilic gastroenteritis with small bowel perforation. J Clin Gastroenterol 1986;8:694–695.

39. Chisholm JC, Martin HI. Eosinophilic gastroenteritis with rectal involvement: case report and a review of literature. J Natl Med Assoc 1981;73:749–753.

40. Partyka EK, Sanowski RA, Kozarek RA. Colonoscopic features of eosinophilic gastroenteritis. Dis Colon Rectum 1980;23:353–359.

41. Haberkern CM, Christie DL, Haas JE. Eosinophilic gastroenteritis presenting as ileocolitis. Gastroenterology 1978;74:896–899.

42. Matzinger MA, Daneman A. Esophageal involvement in eosinophilic gastroenteritis. Pediatr Radiol 1983;13:35–38.

43. Burhenne HJ, Carbone JV. Eosinophilic (allergic) gastroenteritis. Am J Roentgenol Radium Ther Nucl Med 1966;96:332–338.

44. Kaplan SM, Goldstein F, Kowlessar OD. Eosinophilic gastroenteritis: report of a case with malabsorption and protein-losing enteropathy. Gastroenterology 1970;58:540–545.

45. Greenberger NJ, Tennenbaum JI, Ruppert RD. Protein-losing enteropathy associated with gastrointestinal allergy. Am J Med 1967;43:777–784.

46. Marshak RH, Lindner A, Maklansky D, Gelb A. Eosinophilic gastroenteritis. JAMA 1981;245:1677–1680.

47. Goldberg HI, O'Kieffe D, Jenis EH, Boyce HW. Diffuse eosinophilic gastroenteritis. Am J Roentgenol Radium Ther Nucl Med 1973;119:342–351.

48. Katz AJ, Goldman H, Grand RJ. Gastric mucosal biopsy in eosinophilic (allergic) gastroenteritis. Gastroenterology 1977;73:705–709.

49. Stringel G, Mercer S, Sharpe D, Shipman R, Jimenez C. Eosinophilic gastroenteritis. Can J Surg 1984;27:182–183.

50. Kravis LP, South MA, Rosenlund ML. Eosinophilic gastroenteritis in the pediatric patient. Clin Pediatr 1982;21:713–717.

51. Slichtman DM, Lentz J, Stringer D, Sherman P. Eosinophilic gastroenteritis presenting in an adolescent with isolated colonic involvement. Gut 1986;27:1219–1222.

52. Howlett SA, Nelson FW, Spivey JC, Kramer DC, Cerda JJ Eosinophilic gastroenteritis. South Med J 1976;69:427–429.

53. Carmichael JL, Mauldin JL, Sullivan MB. Eosinophilic gastroenteritis. South Med J 1982;75:742–744.

54. Felt-Bersma RJF, Meuwissen SGM, von Velzen D. Perforation of the small intestine due to eosinophilic gastroenteritis. Am J Gastroenterol 1984;79:442–445.

55. Konrad EA, Meister P. Fatal eosinophilic gastroenterocolitis in a two-year-old child. Virchows Arch [A] 1979;382:347–353.

56. Tytgat GN, Grijm R, Dekker W, den Hartog NA. Fatal eosinophilic enteritis. Gastroenterology 1976;71:479–484.

18

FOOD PROTEIN-INDUCED COLITIS AND GASTROENTEROPATHY IN INFANTS AND CHILDREN

Alan M. Lake

Introduction

The gastrointestinal tract serves as the portal of entry for a nearly infinite array of dietary and microbial antigens. Two major factors determine the ability of a dietary protein to induce disease. The first involves the integrity of the enteric immune system featuring secretory antibodies (IgA and IgM), systemic antibodies (IgG, IgM, and IgE), and cellular immune systems. The second factor is the permeability of the gastrointestinal mucosa. Increased permeability is present in the newborn, especially with prematurity, the acute and recovery phases of viral enteritis, during malnutrition, and with any chronic inflammatory disease of the mucosa. The infant, facing new antigens with increased mucosal permeability and an immature secretory antibody response, is at greatest risk. While breast feeding adds significant immune benefit, maternal dietary antigens can be transported into the infant intestine.

Dietary proteins are introduced in a somewhat orderly fashion throughout early infancy. Not surprisingly, the earliest antigens introduced are those most commonly implicated in disease: cow's milk, soybean, wheat, and egg. In other cultures, other antigens play equally prominent roles—such as rice in Japan and fish in Scandinavia. While mechanisms of disease have been defined in animal systems (1), the relative roles of genetic predisposition, age at antigen exposure, and degree of intestinal permeability have yet to be determined in childhood.

Table 18.1 summarizes the four major clinical conditions induced in childhood by dietary food proteins that are reviewed in this chapter. The table presents the typical age of onset and anticipated duration of sensitivity. The proteins most commonly implicated and major clinical features are also listed to enable comparisons among the condition. In addition to these syndromes, this chapter will examine the potential role for dietary protein to induce idiopathic inflammatory bowel disease in childhood.

As the review of these four conditions will reveal, classic type I immediate hypersensitivity plays a minimal role. Indeed, with the exception of a mild association of eczema in some children with enteropathy and enterocolitis, systemic features of an IgE-mediated nature are essentially absent. Furthermore, none of the four major conditions appears to predispose a child to either chronic injury or subsequent allergy. A case can, therefore, be made that local enteric inflammatory disease, while perhaps severe in early infancy, could be yet another level of protection of the child from food allergy in these situations.

Food-Induced Enterocolitis Syndrome

In 1940, Rubin reported an infant with rectal bleeding responsive to elimination of cow's milk from the diet (2). By 1967, Grybowski had demonstrated inflammatory colitis induced by cow's milk in eight infants (3). The clinical presentation and course of enterocolitis have evolved from a number of subsequent reports (3–10).

Presentation can be as early as the first day of life after the first formula feeding, or as late as 9

Table 18.1
Food Protein-Induced Enteric Syndromes

	Food-Induced Enterocolitis Syndrome	Benign Eosinophilic Proctitis	Food-Induced Enteropathy/ Malabsorption	Iron Deficiency
Age at onset	1 day–9 months	4 days–4 months	2–18 months	2–20 months
Duration	9–18 months	6–9 months	18–36 months	14–36 months
Proteins implicated	Cow's milk	Breast milk	Cow's milk	Cow's milk
	Soy	Cow's milk	Soy, egg	
	Chicken	Soy	Gluten, rice, Chicken, fish	
Features				
FTT	Moderate	No	Moderate	Minimal
Emesis	Prominent	No	Intermittent	No
Edema	Acute, severe	Rare	Moderate	Mild
Diarrhea	Severe	Minimal	Moderate	Minimal
Bloody stools	Severe	Moderate	Minimal	No
Villus injury	Moderate	No	Moderate	Mild

FTT = failure to thrive.

months with the transition from formula to cow's milk. Thus, both heat-labile and heat-stable proteins could be implicated. The usual presentation takes place from 3 days to 3 months of age with protracted, often blood-streaked diarrhea, emesis, and a reduced rate of growth. Modest dehydration usually mandates hospitalization and exclusion of sepsis or necrotizing enterocolitis. Transient methemoglobinemia and metabolic acidosis may be observed (11), as well as peripheral eosinophilia and eczema. While the fecal polymorphonuclear leukocytes (PMN) suggest colitis, the features of reduced D-xylose absorption, anemia, lactose malabsorption, and hypoproteinemia implicate small-bowel injury (3–5, 7, 10).

Proctoscopic examination reveals diffuse colitis, with biopsy specimens confirming chronic inflammation (Fig. 18.1). Crypt abscess formation may be prominent. Small-bowel biopsies reveal edema, acute inflammation, and mild villus injury.

While acute colitic manifestations are prominent many infants with this condition also present with erosive gastritis and reflux esophagitis (12–17). In addition, hematemesis, protein-losing enteropathy with Menetrier's histology, anemia, and eventual failure to thrive may be noted. Endoscopic features include focal erosive gastritis and esophagitis. Histologic features include prominent eosinophilia and mild to moderate villus atrophy. The histologic overlap with eosinophilic gastroenteritis is great, with clinical distinction based on early age and prominence of associated colitis. The degree of malnutrition correlates with the duration of disease.

At the time of presentation, the majority of affected infants have received several infant formula preparations. As a result, the specific offending protein may not be immediately obvious. As noted, most such infants will require hospitalization and a brief interval of intravenous hydration. Gradual institution of a hydrolyzed casein formula will generally be tolerated within 5 to 7 days, precluding the need for prolonged parenteral nutrition. Nonetheless, intractable diarrhea has been encountered.

To confirm the offending protein, Powell developed a standardized challenge protocol (5). After stabilization and clinical recovery lasting at least 2 weeks, the challenge is undertaken with the suspected protein (0.6 g/kg of body weight) administered in a single feeding. To date, cow's milk, soy protein, chicken (8), and rice (18) have been implicated as antigens. Because the enteric reaction can prove acute and severe (including shock), the challenge is best undertaken in a hospital. A positive response develops in less than 12 hours and consists of peripheral blood leukocytosis (an increase in polymorphonuclear leukocytes of more than 3500 cells/mm^3 at 6 to 8 hours), fecal heme, and fecal leukocytes. Emesis, transient

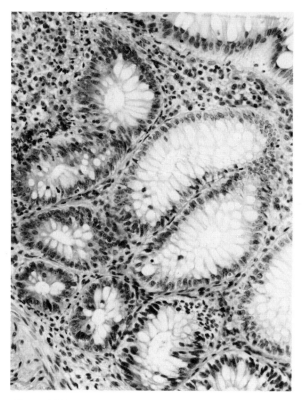

Figure 18.1

Colonic biopsy specimen (280×) from a 6-week-old male with soy protein-induced enterocolitis. There is a diffuse inflammatory cell infiltrate with prominent plasma cells. Distortion of crypt architecture and increase crypt mitotic activity are noted.

disaccharide intolerance, and a mild increase in serum B-I-C globulin may be noted as well. Eosinophils may appear in the stool.

Infants with cow's milk or soy enterocolitis will generally grow and thrive on a hydrolyzed casein formula. No advantage has been ascribed to the use of goat's milk, beef-based, lamb-based, or whey hydrolysate formulas (19–23). The rare child with persistent colitis or anaphylactic response to casein hydrolysate formula (24, 25) will require transient use of an amino-acid-based formula. These formulas are continued until the child reaches at least 1 year of age. After 18 months, gradual resumption of the offending protein is usually well tolerated, although rare exceptions are reported, especially in children

with persistent eosinophilia (26). Colonic stricture has been described as a long-term complication of dietary protein-induced enterocolitis (6).

Although the acute nature of the injury potentially implicates anaphylaxis, the immunologic mechanism for the development of enterocolitis remains unknown. Serum antibody, skin test, and complement data gathered to date are inconclusive. Specific protein-induced alteration in lymphocyte stimulation has been reported (9), but the significance of this observation has not been determined, as lymphocytes from most normal individuals also respond to food antigens.

Benign Eosinophilic Proctitis (Food-Induced Proctocolitis)

The syndrome of proctitis from dietary protein was first described in 1982 in six infants (27). In striking contrast to the well-described infants with enterocolitis, these infants were breast-fed and, aside from the blood-streaked stools, appeared clinically healthy. Over the ensuing years, the clinical and histologic features of this condition have been defined in reviews from Goldman (28), Katz (29), Winter (30), Odze (31), and Machida (32). At the time of diagnosis, more than 50% of reported infants were exclusively breast-feeding.

Infants typically present in the first four months of life, usually at 1 to 3 weeks of age with blood-streaked normal to moderately loose stools. Breast-fed infants affected by this condition are often older. No anatomic fissure or vascular malformation is found, and cultures of the stool test negative for pathogens. In addition to the gross bleeding, a smear of the fecal mucus usually features increased leukocytes. Systemic features such as growth failure, emesis, edema, fever, or dehydration are lacking. Blood loss, while modest, will eventually produce anemia (27, 33, 34). When systematically investigated, both peripheral blood eosinophilia and mild hypoalbuminemia may be seen (32). The average duration of symptoms before diagnosis was 25 days (31).

Endoscopic evaluation yields a wide variety of mucosal alterations, from focal aphthoid ulceration to patchy erythema and friability, to linear erosions, to diffuse colitis (27, 30–32, 35). While rectal involvement is universal, the patchy distribution of inflammation precludes reliable diagnosis by a single-blind rectal biopsy (28, 29, 31). Extension of disease more than 15 cm from the rectum is unusual.

In contrast to the variability in gross endoscopic features, a surprisingly uniform biopsy histology has been noted (30 32). A modest acute inflammation occurs, with striking eosinophilic infiltration of the epithelium, lamina propria, and muscularis. The numbers of eosinophils consistently exceed 10 to 20 per high-power field. In infants less than 3 months of age or with less than 1 month of symptoms, histologic features of chronic colitis are absent (27) and crypt architecture is well maintained (31). While discrete granulomas are not reported, giant cells are occasionally seen (36).

By definition, resolution of the visible rectal bleeding occurs within 72 to 96 hours of elimination of the offending protein from the diet. Formula-fed infants are given hypoallergenic hydrolyzed protein formulas (19). Only rarely do patients remain symptomatic on casein hydrolysate (32). Repeated dietary protein challenge is unnecessary to establish the diagnosis (28).

Breast-fed infants usually respond to strict maternal dietary restriction. In the author's experience with 70 breast-fed infants with eosinophilic proctitis, 44 had clinical resolution with maternal elimination of cow's milk protein from the diet. Other implicated proteins have included egg (14 patients), corn (4 patients), soy (2 patients), and chocolate (but not cow's milk) (2 patients). Strict attention must be paid to food labels as very small inadvertent exposures can produce a flare of symptoms. Only two mothers had to eliminate more than one protein—both cases involved infants sensitive to both milk and egg. In six breast-fed infants, symptoms resolved on a casein hydrolyzed formula but recurred whenever nursing was resumed despite diligent maternal efforts at dietary elimination. Three of these infants continued to nurse, with gradual resolution of symptoms over the subsequent 6 to 10 weeks. All became mildly anemic, but none progressed to more dramatic colitis nor did they exhibit reduced rates of growth.

Hydrolyzed formula is generally continued until 6 to 9 months, with 25% of involved infants becoming tolerant of the previously offending protein by 6 months and 95% tolerant by 9 months. As the symptoms appear more benign than those seen in infants with dietary food protein-induced enterocolitis, the introduction of formula is usually carried out at home with a gradual advance from 1 oz. per day up to full feedings over 2 weeks. Normal exposures to cereal, fruit, or vegetables may continue. Long-term follow-up of the infants with benign eosinophilic proctitis up to 10 years reveals no apparent increased risk for allergic disease or chronic inflammatory bowel disease.

Why or how oral protein induces disease that remains restricted to the rectum and distal colon is unknown. Because breast milk contains only trace amounts of antigenic protein (37, 38), the dose of antigen is clearly very small. An IgE-mediated process is implicated only in the very rare infant with an anaphylactic response (39). As symptoms can be induced within a few hours of exposure, an immune-complex-mediated process may possibly be involved. The striking degree of eosinophilia cannot be ignored, especially given that the eosinophil is now considered a pro-inflammatory cell (32, 40).

Many of the infants with proctitis and rectal bleeding present with colonoscopic (35) and/or histologic (32) features of lymphoid nodular hyperplasia of the colon. Mucosal nodularity with overlying erosions and friability is noted as well. While eosinophilic infiltration is inconsistently associated with these infants, they usually respond to dietary protein intervention. Persistent symptomatic lymphoid nodular hyperplasia of the colon suggests a humoral immune dysfunction.

Enteropathy (Food-Induced Enteropathy/Malabsorption Syndrome)

The ability of infant feedings based on cow's milk to produce a malabsorption syndrome with diarrhea, emesis, and impaired growth was first reported in 1903 by Schlossmann (41). By 1963, Lamy and associates had histologically confirmed that cow's milk could induce small-bowel injury (42). In 1965, Davidson induced an enteropathy with β-lactoglobulin, a major cow's milk protein (43). The first large series, reported by Kuitunen and associates in 1975 (44), emphasized the enteropathy's overlapping features with gluten-induced celiac disease. In the past two decades, studies have confirmed enteropathy with cow's milk, soybean, and gluten proteins (44–47). Additional case reports have confirmed enteropathy induced by egg, chicken, rice, and fish in children with coexistent cow's milk enteropathy (48–50).

The majority of affected infants develop symptoms in the first 9 months of life that may endure to the age of 18 months. Thus, such infants are a little older and not usually as acutely ill as those with the enterocolitis syndrome. A predisposing family history of cow's milk allergy is no more prevalent than in the normal population (46). In Kuitunen's series, eczema was occasionally reported (44). The gradual evolution of the enteropathy may mean that symptoms are first noted in the form of complications of malabsorption rather than acute diarrhea.

In many infants, the onset of symptoms mimics acute enteritis with transient emesis and anorexia complicated by protracted diarrhea. Indeed, the acute small-bowel injury of a viral enteritis has been postulated to predispose the child to subsequent protein-induced enteropathy (51–53). In other circumstances, acute injury from cow's milk is postulated to predispose to subsequent injury from soy protein (54) and even gluten (55). The clinical features of soy protein enteropathy are essentially identical to those noted with injury induced by cow's milk. Any infant who develops acute illness with emesis following the exposure to soy-based formula must also be considered to have possible fructose intolerance from the sucrose sugar commonly employed in soy formula.

The laboratory features at presentation resemble those of small-bowel villus injury, often complicated by increased enteric protein loss. Colitic features such as bloody stools and fecal leukocytes are distinctly absent. The frequency of anemia (40%) exceeds the frequency of documented blood in the stool (5%), suggesting that malabsorption of iron or folate is a major contributing factor to this condition. Although reductions in albumin are most commonly measured, the increased enteric loss of protein occurs independently of molecular weight. Consequently, fecal α_1-antitrypsin, for example, may serve as a marker of protein-losing enteropathy. The absorption of the pentose sugar D-xylose is reduced in the majority of patients reported, reflecting the reduced villus surface area (56, 57). Disaccharide intolerance can be confirmed in the majority of symptomatic infants with monosaccharide intolerance, a rare complication (58, 59). Radiography reveals that the features mimic those of chronic edema of the small-bowel wall, with thickening of the valvulae conniventes and ileal narrowing (60).

Food protein enteropathy is diagnosed via confirmation of villus injury on small-bowel biopsy. Although the degree of villus injury can be either severe or flat, the majority of biopsy specimens from untreated infants reveal a patchy, subtotal villus injury (47, 61–63) (Fig. 18.2). Intraepithelial lymphocytes are often prominent (64), while mucosal infiltration with eosinophils is inconsistent (65, 66). Mucosal lipid content may be increased (67), but scanning electron microscopy reveals a reduced glycocalyx (69), suggesting impaired crypt epithelial hypertrophy in response to villus injury. The histologic features of soybean-induced enteropathy are similar to those noted for cow's milk (45, 53, 54, 70, 71). Immunohistochemical studies of the mucosal biopsies in untreated and challenge-positive infants demonstrate nonspecific increases in mucosal IgA, IgG, and IgM (72) with inconsistent increases in IgE (72, 73).

Using the challenge model from gluten-sensitive enteropathy to document post-challenge small-bowel injury in enteropathy induced by cow's milk or soy protein has led to conflicting data (74, 75). Because the sensitivity to protein can resolve spontaneously by the age of 9 to 12 months, delays in challenge may lead to tolerance of the protein both clinically and histologically. In patients who remain clinically sensitive, biopsy specimens obtained 24 hours after challenge reveal no characteristic alterations (75), a finding that argues against an acute anaphylactic or IgE-mediated injury. With current technology, therefore, routine challenge for biopsy is rarely indicated. In summary, in contrast to children with gluten-sensitive enteropathy, infants with cow's milk or soy protein enteropathy have an earlier age of onset, a transient age-dependent sensitivity, and an enteropa-

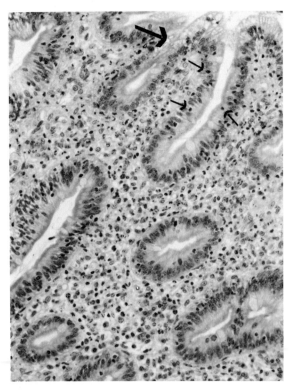

Figure 18.2

Small-bowel biopsy specimen (280×) from a 6-month-old female with cow's milk protein-induced enteropathy. The villi are blunted *(large arrow)* but not flattened. The inflammatory cell infiltrate is diffuse and nonspecific. Increased intrepithelial lymphocytes are prominent *(small arrows)*.

thy that is both patchy in distribution and subtotal in terms of degree of villus injury.

Management consists of identification of the offending protein and its total elimination from the diet. As the vast majority of affected infants are less than 1 year of age, casein hydrolysate formulas constitute the foundation of nutritional therapy. Human breast milk potentially has value, although appropriate pooled sources are extremely limited. Goat's milk is generally avoided because of its lactose content, shortage of folic acid, and equal antigenicity (19).

On many occasions, the parents have switched to soybean-based formula early in the symptomatic course of cow's milk enteropathy. These formulas offer the advantages of relatively low cost, ready availability, and frequent success in post-enteritis lactose intolerance. In early infancy, however, soy protein is equally as antigenic as cow's milk protein (76). As some infants with cow's milk enteropathy have been subsequently sensitized to soybean formulas, casein hydrolysate formulas are suggested until 1 year of age (19). After 1 year of age, most affected children can tolerate gradual reintroduction of cow's milk, and tolerance is the rule after 3 years of age.

In two large studies of long-term follow-up of infants with documented cow's milk enteropathy, no evidence has appeared to suggest the development of significant IgE anti-cow's milk antibody (77, 78). On the other hand, a significant elevation of IgG anti-cow's milk antibody is frequently noted, although this feature is common in many intestinal inflammatory states in childhood (79).

Iron-Deficiency Anemia (Wilson-Heiner-Lahey Syndrome)

In 1962, Wilson, Heiner, and Lahey described a group of infants with cow's milk protein-induced occult rectal bleeding with universal symptoms of anemia, and frequent hypoproteinemia and respiratory signs (80). In these infants, the hypoproteinemia was subsequently confirmed to result from increased enteric protein leakage (81). The classic malabsorptive features of the enteropathy syndrome are not seen with this condition, and growth and development are usually normal. Symptoms occur between 2 months and 20 months of age, frequently following the transition from breast milk or formula to cow's milk. The syndrome has not been reported with soy or wheat proteins.

In a large prospective study from Scandinavia, the frequency of cow's milk-induced anemia and hypoproteinemia is approximately 1 in 7000 infants (82). When infants from 4 months to 12 months of age are fed whole cow's milk, 27% of the infants develop iron depletion. The major contributing factor to this anemia was reduced iron absorption, however—not increased fecal heme losses (83).

The tolerance of cow's milk formulas and intolerance of cow's milk itself suggests that the etiologic cow's milk protein is heat-labile, and that it is rendered inactive by the additional heating employed in preparing cow's milk formula. Indeed, Fomon and associates demonstrated that more than 40% of infants fed pasteurized cow's milk at 6 months would have occult fecal blood loss as opposed to less than 10% of infants fed the same milk after additional heat treatment, and 0% of the infants left on a cow's milk formula (84).

Small-bowel biopsy data for this syndrome are sparse and often distorted by the observation that iron deficiency alone can produce a nonspecific villus injury responsive to iron therapy independent of eliminating cow's milk from the diet (82, 85). Biopsies performed to date reveal a less "immunologic" appearance than with the enteropathy syndrome, with few intraepithelial lymphocytes, minimal cytotoxicity, and no significant increase in local antibody synthesis (85).

Anemia can also represent the chief feature in infancy of cow's milk protein-induced gastroduodenitis (12, 15, 17, 86, 87) or esophagitis (88). A large overlap exists, of course, with infants having eosinophilic antral gastritis (89, 90).

The respiratory symptoms in infants with anemia induced by cow's milk may be attributable to an associated pulmonary hemosiderosis (91, 92). Iron-laden macrophages are recovered from bronchial and gastric aspirates. Biopsy specimens of the lung reveal deposition of IgG, IgA, and C'3, with no evidence of increased local IgE (93). Thus, a local immune-complex-induced injury is presumed to be at fault. Unlike intestinal features, which rarely persist after 3 years, pulmonary symptoms may recur for several years following subsequent cow's milk exposure (93).

Inflammatory Bowel Disease

The etiology of chronic inflammatory bowel diseases, ulcerative colitis, and regional enteritis (Crohn's disease) remains unknown. A role for dietary proteins has been postulated for nearly half a century, but supporting evidence remains scant. A few adults with colitis have experienced a remission following elimi-

nation of cow's milk from the diet (94). Elevations of IgE anti-cow's milk antibody are occasionally reported (95), although skin test data have proved inconclusive. Histologically, biopsy specimens of acute colitis demonstrate enhanced local IgE (as well as other antibody) synthesis (97). Furthermore, mast cell degranulation represents a prominent feature in regional enteritis (97). In adults, both an allergic proctitis (98) and hypereosinophilic colitis (99) are observed. Hypereosinophilic colitis has been reported in a 7-year-old with bloody diarrhea, hepatosplenomegaly, and hypoalbuminemia (100).

Similarities in the clinical presentation and histopathology create a potential overlap of cow's milk-induced enterocolitis and ulcerative colitis in infants and toddlers. Presentation of inflammatory bowel disease (IBD) prior to the age of 2 years occurs in 5% to 8% of children diagnosed with IBD (101). Among these patients, the reported etiologic relationship to cow's milk varies from 25% (102) to 100% (7).

After the age of 2 years, the colitis rarely responds to cow's milk elimination or challenge. Regional enteritis is less likely to be confused with dietary protein enterocolitis, owing to the frequency of stricture (103) and the histologic feature of granuloma formation. In infancy, the extraintestinal manifestations of IBD such as uveitis, arthritis, or erythema nodosum rarely appear.

Conclusion

A number of food protein-induced intestinal syndromes in infants and children have been reviewed. The characteristic features of each usually allow a high degree of confidence in the distinction between syndromes. Most are age-specific, with an excellent long-term prognosis.

One risk associated with these conditions is the abuse of excessively restricted diets, which may limit normal growth in children presumptively diagnosed with "food allergy" (104, 105). Fortunately, alternative formula feedings are readily available for use in infancy. Factitious food allergy in which multiple food restrictions contributed to failure to thrive was encountered in 5% of patients referred to a large allergy program (106). For older children who require prolonged use of an elimination diet, a nutritional review of the diet and appropriate counseling of the child and family should be conducted.

REFERENCES

1. Lake AM. Experimental models for the study of gastrointestinal food allergy. Ann Allergy 1983;51:226–228.
2. Rubin MI. Allergic intestinal bleeding in the newborn: a syndrome. Am J Med Sci 1940;200:385–390.
3. Gryboski JD. Gastrointestinal milk allergy in infants. Pediatrics 1967;40:354–362.
4. Halpin TC, Byrne WJ, Ament ME. Colitis, persistent diarrhea, and soy protein intolerance. J Pediatr 1977;91:404–407.
5. Powell GK. Milk- and soy-induced enterocolitis of infancy. J Pediatr 1978;93:553–560.
6. Schwarzenberg SJ, Whittington PF. Colonic stricture complicating formula protein intolerance enterocolitis. J Pediatr Gastroenterol Nutr 1983;2:190–192.
7. Jenkins HR, Pincott JR, Soothill JF, Milla PJ, Harries JT. Food allergy: the major cause of infantile colitis. Arch Dis Child 1984;59:326–329.
8. Vandenplas Y, Edelman R, Sacré L. Chicken induced anaphylactic reaction and colitis. J Pediatr Gastroenterol Nutr 1994;19:240–241.
9. Van Sickle GJ, Powell GK, McDonald PJ, Goldblum RM. Milk and soy-protein-induced enterocolitis: evidence for lymphocyte sensitization to specific food proteins. Gastroenterology 1985;88:1915–1921.
10. Goldman H, Provjansky R. Allergic proctitis and gastroenteritis in children. Am J Surg Pathol 1986;10:75–86.
11. Murray KF, Christie DL. Dietary protein intolerance in infants with transient methemoglobinemia and diarrhea. J Pediatr 1993;122:90–92.
12. Coello-Ranurez P, Larrosa-Haro A. Gastrointestinal occult hemorrhage and gastroduodenitis in cow's milk protein intolerance. J Pediatr Gastroenterol Nutr 1984;3:215–218.
13. Forget P, Arenda JW. Cow's milk protein allergy and gastroesophageal reflux. Eur J Pediatr 1985;144:298–300.
14. Kokkonen J, Simila S, Herva R. Impaired gastric function in children with cow's milk intolerance. Eur J Pediatr 1979;132:1–7.
15. El-Mouzan MI, Al-Quorain AA, Anim JJ. Cow's milk induced erosive gastritis in an infant. J Ped Gastroenterol Nutr 1990;10:111–113.
16. Fishbein M, Kirschner BS, Gonzales-Villina R, Ben-Ami T, Lee PC, Weisenberg E, Schmidt-Sommerfield E. Menetrier's disease associated with formula protein allergy and small bowel intestinal injury in an infant. Gastroenterology 1992;103:1664–1668.
17. Heldenberg D, Abudy Z, Keren S, Auslaender L. Cow's milk-induced hematemesis in an infant. J Pediatr Gastroenterol Nutr 1993;17:451–452.
18. Borchers SD, Li BUK, Friedman RA, McClung HJ. Rice-induced anaphylactic reaction. J Pediatr Gastroenterol Nutr 1992;15:321–324.
19. Kleinman KRE, Bahna S, Powell GF, Sampson HA. Use of infant formulas in infants with cow's milk allergy: a review of recommendations. Pediatr Allergy Immunol 1991;2:146–155.
20. Sampson HA, Bernhisel-Broadbent J, Young E, Scanlon S. Safety of casein hydrolysate formula in children with cow's milk allergy. J Pediatr 1991;118:520–525.
21. Wahn U, Wahl R, Rugo E. Comparison of the residual allergenic activity of six different hydrolyzed protein formulas. J Pediatr 1992;121:S80–S84.
22. Merritt RJ, Carter M, Haight M, Eisenberg LD. Whey protein hydrolysate formula for infants with gastrointestinal intolerance to cow's milk and soy protein in infant formulas. J Pediatr Gastroenterol Nutr 1990;11:78–81.
23. Ellis MII, Short JA, Heiner DC. Anaphylaxis after ingestion of a recently introduced hydrolyzed whey protein formula. J Pediatr 1991;118:74–77.
24. Saylor JD, Bahna SL. Anaphylaxis to casein hydrolysate formula. J Pediatr 1991;118:71–73.
25. Lifschitz C, Hawkins HK, Guerra C, Byrd M. Anaphylactic shock due to cow's milk protein hypersensitivity in a breast fed infant. J Pediatr Gastroenterol Nutr 1988;7:141–144.
26. Ament ME. Malabsorption syndromes in infancy and childhood. Part 1. J Pediatr 1972;81:685–697.
27. Lake AM, Whittington PF, Hamilton SR. Dietary protein-induced colitis in breast fed infants. J Pediatr 1982;101:906–910.
28. Goldman H, Proujanski R. Allergic proctitis and gastroenteritis in children. Am J Surg Pathol 1986;10:75–86.
29. Katz AJ, Twarog FJ, Zeiger RS, Falchuk ZM. Milk-sensitive and eosinophilic gastroenteropathy; similar clinical features with contrasting mechanisms and clinical course. J Allergy Clin Immunol 1984;74:72–78.
30. Winter HS, Antonioli DA, Fukagawa N. Allergy related proctocolitis in infants: diagnostic usefulness of rectal biopsy. Mod Pathol 1990;3:5–10.
31. Odze RD, Bines J, Leichtner AM, Goldman H, Antonioli D. Allergic proctocolitis in infants: a prospective clinicopathologic biopsy study. Human Pathol 1993;24:668–674.
32. Machida HM, Smith AGC, Gall DG, Travenen C, Scott RB. Allergic colitis in infancy: clinical and pathologic aspects. J Pediatr Gastroenterol Nutr 1994;19:22–26.
33. Wilson NW, Self TW, Hamburger RW. Severe cow's milk induced colitis in an exclusively breast-fed neonate. Clinical Pediatr 1990;29:77–80.
34. Perisic VN, Filipovic D, Kokai G. Allergic colitis and rectal bleeding in an exclusively breast-fed neonatal. Acta Pediatr Scand 1988;77:163–164.
35. Dupont C, Badoual J, Lehuyer B, LeBourgens C, Banbet JP, Voyer M. Rectosigmoidoscopic findings during isolated rectal bleeding in the neonate. J Pediatr Gastroenterol Nutr 1987;6:257–264.
36. Raafat F, Castro R, Booth IW. Eosinophilic proctitis with giant cells: a manifestation of cow's milk protein intolerance. J Pediatr Gastroenterol Nutr 1990;11:128–132.
37. Gerrard JW. Allergy in breast-fed babies to ingredients in breast milk. Ann Allergy 1979;42:69–71.
38. Lovegrove JA, Osman DL, Morgan JB, Hampton SM. Transfer of cow's milk β-lactoglobulin to human serum after a milk load-a-pilot study. Gut 1993;34:203–207.
39. Lifschitz CH, Hawkins HK, Guerra C, Byrd N. Anaphylactic shock due to cow's milk protein hypersensitivity in a breast-fed infant. J Pediatr Gastroenterol Nutr 1988;7:141–144.
40. Lake AM. The polymorph in red is no lady. J Pediatr Gastroenterol Nutr 1994;19:4–6.
41. Schlossmann NA. Uber die giftwirkung des artfremden eiwe-

isses in der milch auf den organismus des sauglings. Arch Kinderheilkunde 1905;41:99–103.

42. Lamy M, Nezelof C, Jos J, Frezel J, Rey J. La biopsie de la muqueuse intestinale chez l'enfant. Premiers resultats d'une etude des syndromes de malabsorption. Presse Med 1963;71:1267–1270.

43. Davidson M, Burnstine RC, Kugler MM, Bauer CH. Malabsorption defect induced by ingestion of beta-lactoglobulin. J Pediatr 1965;66:545–554.

44. Kuitunen P, Visakorpi JK, Savilahti E, Pelkonen P. Malabsorption syndrome with cow's milk intolerance: clinical findings and course in 54 cases. Arch Dis Child 1975;50:351–356.

45. Ament ME, Rubin EC. Soy protein. Another cause of the flat intestinal lesion. Gastroenterology 1972;62:227–234.

46. Walker-Smith JA. Food sensitive enteropathies. Clin Gastroenterol 1986;15:55–69.

47. Iyngkaran N, Yadav M, Boey CG, Lam KL. Severity and extent of upper small bowel mucosal damage in cow's milk protein-sensitive enteropathy. J Pediatr Gastroenterol Nutr 1988;7:667–674.

48. Ford RPK, Fergusson DM. Egg and cow milk allergy in children. Arch Dis Child 1980;55:608–610.

49. Iyngkaran N, Abidin Z, Meng LL, Yadav M. Egg-protein-induced villous atrophy. J Pediatr Gastroenterol Nutr 1982;1:29–33.

50. Vitoria JC, Camarero C, Sojo A, Ruiz A, Rodriguez-Soriano T. Enteropathy related to fish, rice, and children. Arch Dis Child 1982;57:44–48.

51. Iyngkaran N, Robinson MJ, Prathap K, Sumithran E, Yadav M. Cow's milk protein-sensitive enteropathy. Arch Dis Child 1978;53:20–26.

52. Walker-Smith JA. Cow's milk intolerance as a cause of post-enteritis diarrhea. J Pediatr Gastroenterol Nutr 1982;1:163–166.

53. Iyngkaran N, Yadav M, Looi LM, et al. Effect of soy protein on the small bowel mucosa of young infants recovering from acute gastroenteritis. J Pediatr Gastroenterol Nutr 1988;7:68–75.

54. Whitington PF, Gibson R. Soy protein intolerance: four patients with concomitant cow's milk intolerance. Pediatrics 1977;59:730–732.

55. Gryboski JD, Katz J, Reynolds D, Herskovic T. Gluton intolerance following cow's milk sensitivity: two cases with coproantibodies to milk and wheat protein. Ann Allergy 1968;26:33–36.

56. Ford RPK, Barnes GL, Hill DJ. Gastrointestinal hypersensitivity to cow's milk protein: the diagnostic value of gut function tests. Aust Paediatr J 1986;22:37–42.

57. Iyngkaran N, Abidin Z. One hour D-xylose in the diagnosis of cow's milk protein sensitive enteropathy. Arch Dis Child 1982;57:40–43.

58. Iyngkaran N, Abidin Z, Davis K, et al. Acquired carbohydrate intolerance and cow milk protein-sensitivity enteropathy in young infants. J Pediatr 1979;95:373–378.

59. Poley JR, Bhatia M, Welsh JD. Disaccharidase deficiency in infants with cow's milk intolerance. Digestion 1978;17:97–107.

60. Richards DG, Somers S, Issenman RM, Stevenson GW. Cow's milk protein/soy protein allergy. Radiology 1988;167:721–723.

61. Kuitunen P, Rapola J, Savilahti E, Visakorpi JK. Response of the jejunal mucosa to cow's milk in the malabsorption syndrome with cow's milk intolerance. Acta Pediatr Scand 1973;62:585–595.

62. Fontaine JL, Navarro J. Small intestinal biopsy in cow's milk protein allergy in infancy. Arch Dis Child 1975;50:357–362.

63. Shiner M, Ballard J, Brook CGD, Herman S. Intestinal biopsy in the diagnosis of cow's milk protein intolerance without acute symptoms. Lancet 1975;2:1060–1063.

64. Kuitunen P, Kosnai I, Savilahti E. Morphometric study of the jejunal mucosa in various childhood enteropathies with special reference to intraepithelial lymphocytes. J Pediatr Gastroenterol Nutr 1982;1:525–531.

65. Withrington R, Challacombe DN. Eosinophil counts in duodenal tissue in cow's milk allergy. Lancet 1979;1:675–677.

66. Kosnai I, Kuitunen P, Savilahti E, Sipponen P. Mast cells and eosinophils in jejunal mucosa of patients with intestinal cow's milk allergy and celiac disease of childhood. J Pediatr Gastroenterol Nutr 1984;3:368–372.

67. Variend S, Placzek M, Raafat F, Walker-Smith JA. Small intestinal mucosal fat in childhood enteropathies. J Clin Pathol 1984;37:373–377.

68. Poley JR. Loss of the glycocalyx of enterocytes in small intestine: a feature detected by scanning electron microscopy in children with gastrointestinal intolerance to dietary protein. J Pediatr Gastroenterol Nutr 1988;7:386–394.

69. Maluenda C, Phillips AD, Bridden A, Walker-Smith JA. Quantitative analysis of small intestinal mucosa in cow's milk sensitive enteropathy. J Pediatr Gastroenterol Nutr 1984;3:349–356.

70. Poley JR, Klein AW. Scanning electron microscopy of soy protein-induced damage of small bowel mucosa in infants. J Pediatr Gastroenterol Nutr 1983;2:271–287.

71. Perkkio M, Savilahti E, Kuitunen P. Morphometric and immunochemical study of jejunal biopsies from children with intestinal soy allergy. Eur J Pediatr 1981;137:63–69.

72. Stern M, Dietrich R, Muller J. Small intestinal mucosa in coeliac disease and cow's milk protein intolerance: morphometric and immunofluorescent studies. Eur J Pediatr 1982;139:101–105.

73. Rosenkrans PCM, Meijer CJLM, Cornelise CJ, van der Wal AM, Lindeman J. Use of morphometry and immunohistochemistry of small intestinal biopsy specimens in the diagnosis of food allergy. J Clin Pathol 1980;33:125–130.

74. De Sousa JS, de Silva A, Pereira V, Soares J, Romalho PM. Cow's milk protein-sensitive enteropathy: number and timing of biopsies for diagnosis. J Pediatr Gastroenterol Nutr 1986;5:207–209.

75. Berg NO, Jakobsson I, Lindberg T. Do pre- and post-challenge biopsies help to diagnose cow's milk protein intolerance. Acta Pediatr Scand 1979;68:657–661.

76. Eastham EJ, Lichauco T, Grady M, Walker WA. Antigenicity of infant formulas: role of immature intestine on protein permeability. J Pediatr 1978;93:561–564.

77. Danneus A, Johansson SGO. A follow-up study of infants with adverse reactions to cow's milk. Acta Pediatr Scand 1979;68:337–341.

78. Hill DJ, Finer MA, Ball G, Hosking CS. Recovery from milk allergy in early childhood: antibody studies. J Pediatr 1989;114:761–766.

79. Eastham EJ, Walker WA. Adverse effects of milk formula ingestion on the gastrointestinal tract: an update. Gastroenterology 1979;76:365–374.

80. Wilson JF, Heiner DC, Lahey ME. Evidence of gastrointestinal dysfunction in infants with iron deficiency anemia: a preliminary report. J Pediatr 1962;60:787–789.

81. Woodruff CW, Clark JL. The role of fresh cow's milk in iron deficiency. I. Albumin turnover in infants with iron deficiency anemia. Am J Dis Child 1972;24:18–23.

82. Lundstrom U, Perkkio M, Savilahti E, Siimes M. Iron deficiency anemia with hypoproteinemia. Arch Dis Child 1983;58:438–441.

83. Fuchs G, DeWeir M, Hutchinson S, Sundeen M, Schwartz S, Suskind R. Gastrointestinal blood loss in older infants: impact of cow milk versus formula. J Pediatr Gastroenterol Nutr 1993;16:4–9.

84. Fomon SJ, Ziegler EE, Nelson SE, Edwards BB. Cow milk feeding in infancy: gastrointestinal blood loss and iron nutritional status. J Pediatr 1981;98:540–542.

85. Savilahti E, Verkassalo M. Intestinal cow's milk allergy: pathogenesis and clinical presentation. Clin Rev Allergy 1984;2:7–23.

86. Coello-Ramirez P, Larrosa-Haro A. Gastrointestinal occult hemorrhage and gastroduodenitis in cow's milk protein intolerance. J Pediatr Gastroenterol Nutr 1984;3:215–218.

87. Kokkonen J, Simila S. Cow's milk intolerance with melena. Eur J Pediatr 1980;135:189–194.

88. Forget P, Arends JW. Cow's milk protein allergy and gastroesophageal reflux. Eur J Pediatr 1985;144:298–300.

89. Katz AJ, Twarog FJ, Zeiger RS, Falchuk ZM. Milk-sensitive and eosinophilic gastroenteropathy: similar clinical features with contrasting mechanisms and clinical course. J Allergy Clin Immunol 1984;74:72–78.

90. Snyder JD, Rosenblum N, Wershil B, Goldman H, Winter HS. Pyloric stenosis and eosinophilic gastroenteritis in infants. J Pediatr Gastroenterol Nutr 1987;6:543–547.

91. Heiner DC, Sears JW. Chronic respiratory disease associated with multiple circulating precipitins to cow's milk. Am J Dis Child 1960;100:500–502.

92. Boat TF, Polmar SH, Whitman V, et al. Hyperreactivity to cow milk in young children with pulmonary hemosiderosis and cor pulmonale secondary to nasopharyngeal obstruction. J Pediatr 1975;87:23–29.

93. Lee SK, Kniker WT, Cook CD, Heiner DC. Cow's milk induced pulmonary disease in children. Adv Pediatr 1978;25:39–57.

94. Truelove SC. Ulcerative colitis provoked by milk. Br Med J 1961;1:154–156.

95. Jewell DR, Truelove SC. Reaginic hypersensitivity in ulcerative colitis. Gut 1973;13:903–906.

96. O'Donoghue DP, Kumar P. Rectal IgE cells in inflammatory bowel disease. Gut 1979;20:149–153.

97. Dvorak AM, Monahan RA, Osage JE, et al. Mast cell degranulation in Crohn's disease. Lancet 1978;1:498–499.

98. Rosenkrans PCM, Meijer CJLM, Van der Wal AM, Lindeman J. Allergic proctitis, a clinical and immunopathological entity. Gut 1980;21:1017–1023.

99. Spry CJF, Davies J, Tai PC, Olsen EGJ, Oakley CM, Goodwin JF. Clinical features of fifteen patients with the hypereosinophilic syndrome. Q J Med 1983;52:1–22.

100. Falade AG, Darbyshire PJ, Raafat F, Booth IW. Hypereosinophilic syndrome in childhood appearing as inflammatory bowel disease. J Pediatr Gastroenterol Nutr 1991;12:276–279.

101. Gryboski JD, Hillemeier AC. Inflammatory bowel disease in children. Med Clin North Am 1980;1185–1207.

102. Enzer NB, Hijmans JC. Ulcerative colitis beginning in infancy. J Pediatr 1963;63:437–440.

103. Miller RC, Larson E. Regional enteritis in early infancy. Am J Dis Child 1971;122:301–311.

104. Lloyd-Still JD. Chronic diarrhea of childhood and the misuse of elimination diets. J Pediatr 1979;95:10–13.

105. David TJ, Waddington E, Stanton RHJ. Nutritional hazards of elimination diets in children with atopic eczema. Arch Dis Child 1984;59:323–325.

106. Roesler TA, Barry PC, Bock SA. Factitious food allergy and failure to thrive. Arch Pediatr Adolesc Med 1994;148:1150–1155.

19

GLUTEN-SENSITIVE ENTEROPATHY (CELIAC DISEASE)

Anne Ferguson

Wheat and Gluten Intolerance

Many diseases and symptoms exist within the broad diagnostic category of adverse clinical reactions to ingested food or drink (1). Celiac disease (currently defined as a permanent gluten-sensitive enteropathy) is one of the best characterized of these conditions. Diagnostic criteria, which are based on the effects of dietary manipulation on small-bowel mucosal histopathology, are entirely objective.

Not all wheat—or even gluten—intolerance is due to celiac disease, however. Wheat gluten in a meal impairs the absorption of starch (2), and large but palatable doses (100–150 g) of gluten daily can lead to fat malabsorption (3). An elimination diet that excludes wheat is said to cure the symptoms of some patients with the irritable bowel syndrome (4), and non-celiac gluten-sensitive diarrhea, with normal jejunal biopsy architecture, has been described as well (5).

Wheat or gluten sensitivity may also be expressed as enteropathy—that is, as measurable changes in the histopathology of the jejunum associated with the presence of dietary gluten. In celiac disease, this form of intolerance is permanent, whereas gluten is only one of many foods that can produce transient enteropathy in infants. A condition of "latent" gluten-sensitive enteropathy clearly exists in which the person has a normal jejunal biopsy while taking a normal, gluten-containing diet, but celiac-like pathology is found (6–8) at other times (e.g., after gluten-loading for a few weeks). This area is the subject of active research, discussed at length elsewhere (9, 10), but its relevance in general clinical practice remains to be established.

Historical Background and Definition

The first important clinical description of the disease was published in 1888, when Samuel Gee wrote of the celiac affection (11). In the early 1950s, when the successful treatment of celiac disease with a gluten-free diet was recognized and later published (12), the cause of the malabsorption spurred great controversy. In 1948, John Paulley had suggested at a London meeting of the Royal Society of Tropical Medicine and Hygiene that "the absorptive defect is due to a non-specific jejunitis" (cited in 13). Shortly thereafter, he presented supportive evidence from full-thickness intestinal biopsies taken at laparotomy in three cases of idiopathic steatorrhea (13). The definitive paper describing the pathology of the small bowel in this disease (having been delayed by being rejected both by *Gastroenterology* and *Lancet*) was finally published in the *British Medical Journal* in 1954 (14).

Evolution of a Working Definition of Celiac Disease

Until the 1950s, the diagnosis of celiac disease (idiopathic steatorrhea, nontropical sprue) was entirely based on the presence of clinical features of malabsorption and the absence of infection. During the 1950s, it was recognized that both clinical remission and reduction in fecal fat excretion occurred after treatment with a gluten-free diet. Techniques for peroral small-bowel biopsy were widely introduced in the 1960s, and patients with malabsorption were found to have either an absolutely normal or a characteristically flat jejunal biopsy, with partial or subtotal villus atrophy. Later, increased understanding of intestinal epithelial cell kinetics and of gut mucosal immunology directed attention to the hyperplasia of the crypts of Lieberkuhn that accompanies the villus changes, to cytological details of the enterocytes, and to the lymphoid cells of the mucosa. For the provisional diagnosis of celiac disease, patients present with short or absent villi, crypt hyperplasia, cuboidal surface enterocytes with a clearly abnormal brush border, intense lymphoid cell infiltrate in the lamina propria, and a high density of surface intraepithelial lymphocytes (IEL).

In pediatric practice, abnormal small-bowel morphology with villus atrophy occurs not infrequently—for example, in giardiasis—as does immunodeficiency with infection. Also, infants exhibit many transient food-sensitive enteropathies, including cow's milk protein intolerance and enteropathy due to soy, chicken, and egg. Transient wheat-sensitive enteropathy has also been described.

To avoid diagnostic confusion, the European Society of Paediatric Gastroenterology and Nutrition proposed strict diagnostic criteria for celiac disease (ESPGAN criteria) (15) "(i) malabsorption syndrome, with a flat jejunal biopsy, which (ii) recovers to normal on a gluten-free diet, and (iii) relapses on subsequent gluten reintroduction (gluten challenge)." Many thousands of children were subjected to this protocol during the 1970s and 1980s. When the first two criteria have been met, gluten challenge produces positive results in between 95% and 99% of cases. In the majority of children, histopathological relapse occurs within 3 to 6 months of gluten reintroduction, but in some cases may go undetected for several years. For example, of 67 children who had presented under the age of 2 years with symptoms and classical small-bowel histology of celiac disease, and then improved on a gluten-free diet, 64 relapsed within 2 years based on gluten challenge results.

ESPGAN criteria have since been revised and simplified (16). In everyday clinical practice it is still essential to obtain biopsy confirmation in every patient before starting dietary treatment. This result, with a follow-up biopsy demonstrating mucosal recovery after gluten withdrawal, is usually sufficient to confirm the diagnosis.

Simple pathological reporting based on pattern recognition is less valuable than a careful and thorough description of the structural and cellular details of the different compartments within the mucosa: crypt/villus architecture, surface and crypt epithelium, and lymphoid cell types and numbers in the various microenvironments (Table 19.1). Features such as a normal intraepithelial lymphocyte count (17) can distinguish the post-enteritis syndrome or idiopathic chronic intractable diarrhea in infancy from celiac disease and related enteropathies. In difficult diagnostic situations, immunohistochemical methods can be used to assess whether T-cell activation has occurred (18).

GLUTEN CHALLENGE

In certain groups of patients, gluten challenge remains essential (19). These populations include the following:

1. Patients in whom a gluten-free diet has been started without an initial diagnostic biopsy.
2. Patients in whom the original biopsy is technically poor or in whom the histopathology is not classically that of celiac disease.
3. Patients in whom infection or immunodeficiency was present at the time of the original diagnostic biopsy.
4. Patients with a strong personal or family history of atopic disease.

Table 19.1
Factors That an Ideal Description of a Small-Bowel Mucosal Biopsy Should Address

Sizes of villi and crypts
Crypt mitoses (appropriate to villus size)
Enterocytes
Brush border
Other epithelial cells
Intraepithelial lymphoid cells (surface, crypt)
Lamina propria cells (density, types)
Matrix abnormalities (e.g., collagen)
Infectious agents
Tumor cells
Erosions, ulcers, granulomas, etc.
Polymorphs (epithelial, lamina propria, crypt abscesses)

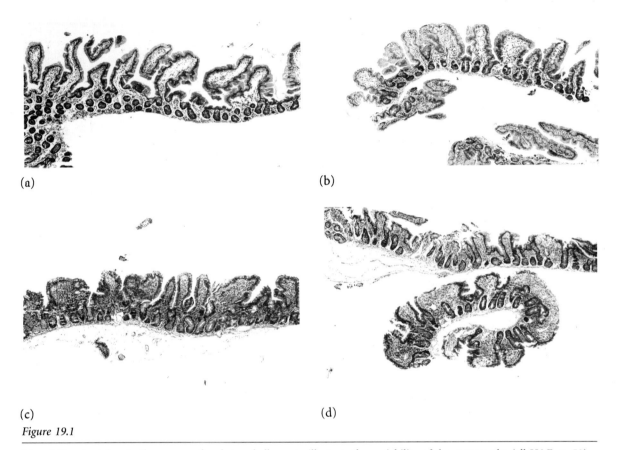

(a)

(b)

(c)

(d)

Figure 19.1

Jejunal biopsies taken in the course of a gluten challenge to illustrate the variability of the enteropathy (all H&E $\times$ 50). (a) Prechallenge biopsy—normal. (b) After 3 months, gluten challenge at 20 g gluten powder daily. Biopsy contains a couple of broad villi but is considered within normal limits. (c, d) Three of multiple jejunal biopsies taken after 1 year of continuing gluten ingestion. Crypt hyperplasia is evident in all biopsies, although the degree of villus abnormality is variable.

If gluten challenge is performed only in patients in whom a jejunal biopsy is normal at the time of gluten reintroduction, symptoms are extremely rare and never serious.

Several different techniques and protocols can be used for the challenge. We either continue to prescribe a gluten-free diet and add 20 g daily of gluten powder, or advise the patient to take a normal diet and assess accurately the amount of gluten being eaten—between 15 and 20 g daily. Usually, the histopathological changes associated with dietary manipulation are so striking that subjective comparison by an experienced pathologist is sufficient to confirm improvement or worsening of the pathology (Fig. 19.1). On the other hand, it may be necessary to use ob-

jective techniques to assess changes in the jejunal mucosa. Figures 19.2–19.4 illustrate some of the improvements seen after 3 to 6 months of a gluten-free diet in celiac patients; after gluten challenge, abnormalities can be clearly recognized and measured (19).

Variation in Celiac Disease Incidence with Time and Place

Acceptable data on the epidemiology of celiac disease require pathological confirmation of the diagnosis in all cases. Even in populations with a similar genetic

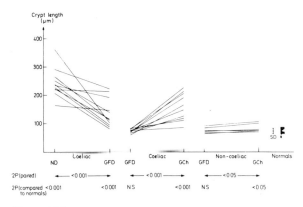

Figure 19.2

Effects of gluten-free and gluten-containing diets on lengths of jejunal crypts. ND, normal diet (gluten-containing); GFD, gluten-free diet (3 to 6 months); GCH, gluten challenge (approximately 20 g gluten daily for 3 to 6 months) (19).

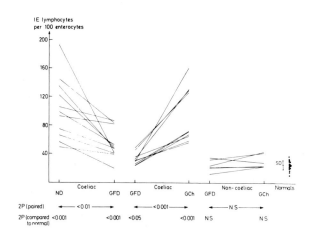

Figure 19.3

Effects of gluten-free and gluten-containing diets on jejunal IEL counts. ND, normal diet (gluten-containing); GFD, gluten-free diet (3 to 6 months); GCH, gluten challenge (approximately 20 g gluten daily for 3 to 6 months) (19).

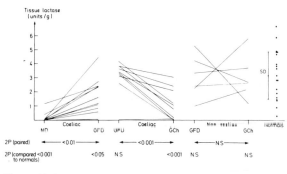

Figure 19.4

Effects of gluten-free and gluten-containing diets on jejunal lactase activity. ND, normal diet (gluten-containing); GFD, gluten-free diet (3 to 6 months); GCH, gluten challenge (approximately 20 g gluten daily for 3 to 6 months) (19).

background, the incidence varies very considerably, indicating that some environmental trigger plays a key role in addition to the importance of possessing certain gene or genes conferring predisposition. The best examples are the rarity of celiac disease in the United States, even in families of Scottish and Irish background; in addition, 1 in 300 children born in some parts of Sweden develop celiac disease early in life compared with an incidence of one in several thousand in nearby Denmark. Celiac disease rarely if ever occurs in persons of Chinese or African descent, although many well-documented cases have involved Asians from the Indian subcontinent.

Estimates of the incidence of celiac disease at various periods in the last 30 years and in different parts of Europe range widely, from 1 in 300 to around 1 in 10,000. The author has recently completed a study of histologically confirmed celiac disease in Edinburgh and the Lothians (20), from which a number of interesting points have emerged. A total of 704 celiacs were registered, of whom 469 were alive and residing in Lothian in 1979. Integration of this information with population statistics gives a prevalence of 61 per 100,000. The male-to-female ratio was 1 : 1.6, and striking variation was found in incidence of births of celiacs (this variation being mainly related to changes in the numbers of females in different age groups). Peaks of births of celiacs oc-

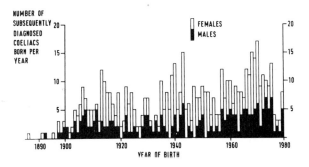

Figure 19.5

Patterns of births of individuals subsequently diagnosed as having celiac disease, in Lothian region. Data from Logan *et al.* (20).

curred around 1915–1920, 1940–1945, and 1969–1970 (Figs. 19.5 and 19.6).

The decline in the incidence of celiac disease since 1970 has also been observed mainly in Northern and Central European countries, but not in Southern Europe (21). The reasons for these striking differences are unknown but may be related to changes in infant feeding practices. If our hypothesis (described at the end of this chapter) is correct—that celiac disease is due to an abnormal cell-mediated immune reaction

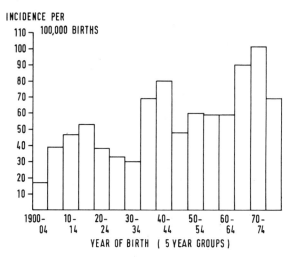

Figure 19.6

Incidence of celiac disease in Lothian region. Data from Logan *et al.* (20).

to gluten—then the variations in incidence must be due to modulation of the induction of the individual's immune responses in some way. Candidate mechanisms include both environmental and social factors—nature, quantity and age of introduction of dietary gluten, patterns of infection and immunization in the first year of life, or breast feeding and weaning habits.

Clinical Heterogeneity

Because the standard diagnostic test is based entirely on small-bowel biopsy pathology, specific clinical features are not included in the definition. Indeed, patients subsequently diagnosed as celiac may have presented with any of a wide range of clinical manifestations.

SILENT AND ACTIVE CELIAC DISEASE

In some individuals, celiac disease is **clinically silent**—that is, patients are asymptomatic healthy people in whom jejunal biopsy has been performed as part of a family study, in screening of blood donors, or in the clinical investigation of an unrelated disorder. In patients with **active celiac disease,** unequivocal nutrient deficiencies or gastrointestinal symptoms such as abdominal distention and diarrhea are present. Today, a full-blown malabsorption syndrome is rarely seen.

PRESENTATIONS IN CHILDREN

The textbook description of a celiac child is of a grumpy, rickety, anemic, growth-retarded toddler with diarrhea, a pot belly, and muscle wasting. In many children, however, the effects of malabsorption are much less severe and only a single symptom or sign may be present—for example, growth retardation, iron-deficiency anemia, or mild rickets. On the other hand, if gluten has been included in the diet from infancy, an accelerated form of the disease may occur, with abdominal distention, vomiting, and constipation, suggestive of intestinal obstruction.

The clinical pattern of celiac disease in a particular country shows some correlation with incidence rate (22). For example, in Naples, Italy, where incidence continues to be high, most cases have presented by the age of 2 years; clinical features typically include anorexia, abdominal distention, diarrhea, growth failure, and occasionally vomiting. In contrast, in Tampere, Finland, no cases of celiac disease have been diagnosed in the first year of life for the last 18 years. The average age at diagnosis is 5 years, and only 50% of the children present with diarrhea. In a group of 96 cases recently described, 11 exhibited isolated growth failure, seven had anemia alone, six had delayed puberty, five had arthritis, and five had diabetes (the last two groups of patients were diagnosed only because disease associations with celiac diseases drew the attention of Finnish pediatricians).

PRESENTATIONS IN ADULTS

In adult life, the condition may present as anemia, metabolic bone disease, diarrhea, or weight loss. Recent series have drawn attention to the numbers presenting with trivial, often unrelated, illness. In our study in Scotland (23), only 1 in 6 celiac patients had malabsorption syndrome; presentation as a result of symptoms from anemia, osteomalacia, or hypocalcemia occurred virtually only in women; only 41 of 102 patients had diarrhea, a further 5 had abdominal pain, dyspepsia or dysphagia, and the remaining 56 patients had no gastrointestinal symptoms. In a similar study of English celiacs, Swinson and Levi (24) found that only 26% of their patients with celiac disease had classic symptoms of steatorrhea, osteomalacia, or anemia. In 44% of 88 cases, the disease was suspected only because of an unexplained abnormality on a full blood count, which in half of the patients appeared as red-cell macrocytosis without anemia.

Many cases of celiac disease emerge as a result of investigation of weight loss alone, of minor abnormalities found on routine blood tests, or in the thorough work-up of patients with diseases known to be associated with celiac disease, such as hyposplenism, recurrent aphthous ulceration, jejunal ulceration, abdominal lymphoma, and old rickets. As an example of the wide clinical spectrum associated with celiac disease, we have reported a patient with morbid obesity despite the presence of jejunal villous atrophy (25).

In adults, probably the greatest influence on the symptoms of a cohort of patients diagnosed in a particular center is the level of awareness of clinicians. For example, in a comparison of the presentation of patients diagnosed as celiac disease in Edinburgh teaching hospitals in the early 1960s and the late 1970s, striking differences were noted in the symptoms of the patients and in the laboratory features of malabsorption (Table 19.2). If celiac disease is included in the differential diagnosis only when patients have classic malabsorption syndrome, many cases will remain undetected. The continuing underdiagnosis of this condition is suggested by the considerable geographic variation in England and Wales in membership of the Coeliac Society, and by the correlation between membership of the Coeliac Society and sales of jejunal biopsy capsules in different Health Regions (p < 0.02) (24).

Indications for Small-Bowel Biopsy

The clinical decision to perform a small-bowel biopsy should take into account the wide range of presenting symptoms of celiac disease listed above. The importance of this consideration is only increasing with changes in clinical practice and biopsy techniques, and case mix.

Small-bowel biopsy should be included in the routine investigation of patients with many different presentations (Table 19.3). A well-orientated biopsy of either the second part of the duodenum (taken at endoscopy) or a peroral capsule biopsy of jejunum

Table 19.2
Features of Celiac Disease at Presentation

	1960–1964	1975–1979
Male to female ratio	19:19	27:75
Malabsorption syndrome	64%	13%
Single-nutrient deficiencies	18%	15%
Diarrhea	18%	27%
Trivial indications	45%	?
Hemoglobin low	79%	43%
Albumin low	68%	20%
Calcium low	31%	13%
Total cases	38	102

Data from Logan et al. (23).

Table 19.3
Indications for Jejunal Biopsy

1. *Classic presentations of celiac disease*
   Malabsorption syndrome
   Iron deficiency anemia, if no evidence of blood loss
   Folate deficiency
   Steatorrhea
   High-volume diarrhea
   Metabolic bone disease (old rickets)
   Unexplained weight loss/growth delay
   Other vitamin or mineral deficiencies
   History of celiac disease in childhood

2. *Diseases diagnosed that are known to be associated*
   with celiac disease
   Abdominal lymphoma
   Small-bowel adenocarcinoma
   Dermatitis herpetiformis
   Benign small-bowel ulcers/strictures
   Hyposplenic blood film with no splenectomy
   IgA deficiency
   Collagenous and lymphocytic colitis
   Many other rarer conditions

3. *Consider coexisting celiac disease in some of the following cases*
   Crohn's disease
   Ulcerative colitis
   Autoimmune liver disease
   Cystic fibrosis
   Severe aphthous ulceration
   Insulin-dependent diabetes mellitus

4. *Reassurance/screening*
   Healthy family members of celiacs
   Some patients with multiple symptoms
   Food sensitivity

should be examined by an experienced pathologist as discussed above.

Many factors should be borne in mind in the interpretation of biopsy appearances; some of these issues are considered below.

AMOUNT OF GLUTEN IN THE DIET

In the patient with untreated celiac disease, the amount of gluten ingested daily can influence the severity of enteropathy. For example, a diabetic taking limited carbohydrate or a relative of a celiac (who may live in a household in which family meals include many gluten-free products) may have relatively low-grade pathological changes. Clinicians should provide pathologists with information on dietary gluten if it is likely to vary substantially from the "normal" diet

status of the population. In the United Kingdom, for example, most people take between 10 and 30 g gluten daily.

DRUGS

Immunosuppressive, cytotoxic, and anti-inflammatory drugs prescribed for other indications may produce improvement of some features of the enteropathy. Effects of drugs such as corticosteroids, azathioprine, and cyclosporine may make it almost impossible for the pathologist to recognize unusual intestinal pathology as attributed to celiac disease.

ENDOSCOPIC DUODENAL BIOPSIES AND THE CONFUSION WITH PEPTIC DUODENITIS

In patients who have duodenal ulcer or severe peptic duodenitis, biopsies from macroscopically affected areas of the first part of the duodenum may be distinctly abnormal with short villi, long crypts, and increased infiltration with inflammatory cells. Such biopsies usually include polymorphs, however. Even in peptic disease, biopsies from the second part of the duodenum, when assessed by careful morphometry, may appear entirely normal. If endoscopic biopsies are being taken to assess the presence or absence of celiac disease, the endoscopist should take biopsies with large-bite forceps, from visually normal areas of the second part of the duodenum. The visual appearances should then be drawn to the attention of the pathologist who will interpret the slides. In our experience, a few polymorphs (unusual features of the lesion of celiac disease in the jejunum) may be present in duodenal biopsies from celiacs, which can sometimes cause confusion. In fact, with most of the present generation of endoscopes, the surface and the presence (or absence) of a villus architecture can usually be determined.

PRIMARY AND ACQUIRED IMMUNODEFICIENCY

The occasional celiac patient who also has hypogammaglobulinemia is likely to have very few infiltrating plasma cells in the lamina propria; these cells will be of the IgM isotype.

So-called "villus atrophy" is a feature of small-bowel pathology in many patients with HIV infections and diarrhea. Crypt hyperplasia is not as prominent a feature as occurs in celiacs, however, and, in most patients, crypts in the gut lesions of patients with AIDS are short. Furthermore, IEL counts appear normal in the epithelium covering the short villi in HIV.

Non-Invasive Alternatives to Small-Bowel Biopsy

As yet, none of the currently available immunological or absorptive tests can substitute for proper examination of a small-bowel mucosal biopsy. If celiac disease is seriously being considered as a diagnosis, a negative result in a screening test cannot substitute for biopsy examination. In any event, patients with malabsorption or nutrient deficiencies may have some other small-bowel disease that requires mucosal biopsy for diagnosis, such as transient food-sensitive enteropathy, giardiasis, HIV or enteropathy, or disaccharidase deficiency. Nevertheless, a number of useful laboratory tests are now available for screening programs, as ancillary aids to differential diagnosis, and as non-invasive measures to monitor the clinical response of a patient to a gluten-free diet.

ANTI-GLIADIN ANTIBODIES

The best-studied immunological tests are serum IgG and IgA class antibodies to gliadin (antigliadin antibody, or AGA) (26). IgG AGA is usually positive in untreated celiac disease but often negative in other gastrointestinal diseases and even in a proportion of healthy individuals; the presence of serum IgA AGA is more likely to indicate celiac disease. This test is positive in the majority of untreated celiac children but only in 70% of untreated celiac adults. Approximately 1 in 50 celiacs is IgA-deficient.

ANTI-ENDOMYSIUM ANTIBODIES

The presence of anti-reticulin antibody in celiac disease has been recognized for many years. The technical variant of this study, based on the use of monkey esophagus or human umbilical cord as substrate in an immunofluorescence test, has revealed that IgA endomysium antibody (AEA) is present in a much higher proportion of untreated celiacs than is IgA AGA (27, 28). Patients in whom celiac disease occurs in association with IgA deficiency will have negative results, however, and the majority of studies report 5% to 15% of IgA AEA-negative, untreated celiac patients despite classic severe enteropathy.

INTESTINAL PERMEABILITY TESTS

Various tests of intestinal permeability are valuable aids to diagnosis, particularly for follow-up of celiac patients (30–32). These permeability tests are sensitive but not entirely specific, as abnormal results may occur in other small-bowel diseases, including Crohn's disease, and also with NSAID therapy.

Management

A strict gluten-free diet, excluding wheat, oats, rye, and barley, for life is the cornerstone of management of celiac disease. Rice and maize are not toxic to celiacs, and can be useful as alternatives to protein-free, wheat-derived flours. Unfortunately, patient compliance on such long-term treatment is not always ideal. Patient support groups, such as the Coeliac Society in the United Kingdom, play an important role in treatment, offering practical advice on gluten-free products and recipes. Explicit food labeling is invaluable to celiacs, particularly for convenience foods. In some countries, suitable baby and some other foods are marked with a "gluten-free" symbol.

The effects of treatment should be monitored by simple clinical assessment (e.g., cessation of diarrhea) and, at 3 to 6 months, by repeated jejunal biopsy. The small-bowel mucosa may not become completely normal in adults, and improvement may continue for 2 or more years.

General nutritional treatments should also be used as required, such as hematinics, vitamins, and mineral supplements. These substances can be discontinued when the biopsy returns to normal.

In patients who do not respond to a gluten-free diet, the physician should first determine whether the patient is complying with the dietary regime. A complicating lymphoma, ulcerative jejunitis, and pancreatic insufficiency should then be excluded. Other conditions such as inflammatory bowel disease and collagenous colitis may coexist.

Nevertheless, a small number of *celiac* patients, despite not having the above complications, fail to respond to a gluten-free diet. Strictly speaking, their diagnosis is not celiac disease but non-celiac enteropathy. Corticosteroids can produce considerable clinical improvement in such patients, and it may also be valuable to try elemental diet therapy for 4 to 6 weeks.

Disease Associations and Complications

Many diseases have been found with a higher-than-normal frequency in a series of celiac patients (Table 19.4), and several good clinical reviews of this subject exist (e.g., 33–36). In particular, a cluster of autoimmune diseases is linked with the HLA A1,B8 DR3/7 phenotype. Diabetes in a celiac can produce considerable management difficulties, pernicious anemia requires parenteral vitamin B_{12} treatment indefinitely, autoimmune Addison's disease may be missed in a patient who requires steroids for relief of symptoms attributed to celiac disease, and in thyrotoxicosis, diarrhea and weight loss continue despite gluten-free diet therapy.

Other unexplained immune associations include IgA deficiency, in itself relatively harmless, and splenic atrophy. In addition, bizarre neurological disease may coexist with celiac disease.

Benign ulcerative jejunitis, a relatively rare complication (37), is considered by some to be a forerunner of lymphoma (38). This hypothesis is difficult to disprove, but we have observed several patients who remain well years after surgery of strictures, although other similar patients have later progressed to lymphoma. The ulcers may bleed, perforate, or cause small-bowel obstruction. Because abdominal pain is

Table 19.4
Celiac Disease and Related Disorders

Definite
Diabetes mellitus
Thyrotoxicosis
Hypothyroidism
IgA deficiency
Sarcoidosis
Vasculitis
Dermatitis herpetiformis
Encephalopathy and cerebellar atrophy
Myasthenia
Peripheral neuropathy
Malignant lymphomas
Small-intestinal adenocarcinomas
Esophageal and pharyngeal squamous carcinoma

Probable
Addison's disease
Rheumatoid arthritis
Sjögren's syndrome
Bird fancier's lung
Farmer's lung
Pernicious anemia
Exocrine pancreatic insufficiency
Inflammatory bowel disease
Primary biliary cirrhosis
Collagenous colitis

Adapted from Mulder and Tytgat (34).

not a feature of uncomplicated celiac disease, this symptom should be investigated by barium radiology of the small bowel. Treatment of ulcerative jejunitis remains unsatisfactory: many patients require laparotomy with resection of affected segments of the small intestine, while those patients who do not require surgery may respond to corticosteroids.

Dermatitis herpetiformis (DH) is characterized by a symmetrical pruritic skin rash with subepidermal blisters and granular subepidermal deposits of IgA in remote, uninvolved skin (39). Most DH patients have abnormal small-intestinal biopsy pathology that is histologically indistinguishable from that of celiac disease and returns to normal after dietary exclusion of gluten (40–42). An interpretation of these observations is that most patients with DH also have celiac disease, but a minority prove completely tolerant of gluten. Alternatively, intestinal gluten sensitivity may exist in all cases with a variable requirement of dietary gluten for its clinical expression (i.e., a latent enteropathy exists in the minority) (43).

Malignancy and Celiac Disease

Lymphoma-complicating celiac disease was first reported in 1962 (44); since that time, it has become clear that patients with celiac disease have a 50- to a 100-fold greater risk of developing malignant lymphoma than the general population. An apparent excess of non-lymphomatous malignancies in celiacs was also recognized in the 1960s (45).

Some years ago, gastroenterologists and pathologists in the United Kingdom collected and published details of a large number of celiac patients who also suffered from malignant disease (46). From these data, tumor types were identified that were present in significant excess in celiacs when compared with U.K. cancer statistics for the general population. The key findings are given in Tables 19.5 and 19.6. In the 235 patients studied, 259 histologically confirmed malignancies were reported: 133 (51.4%) were malignant lymphomas, 62 were gastrointestinal tract non-lymphomatous tumors, 61 were other tumors, and 3 were unclassifiable.

Malignant lymphoma in association with celiac disease had been described initially as Hodgkin's disease or reticulum cell sarcoma. Later, the term "malig-

Table 19.6
Classification of 133 Lymphomas Occurring in Celiac Patients

Morphological Classification	Number of Cases
Well-differentiated lymphocytic	2
Undifferentiated large cell	9
Histiocytic*	107
Mycosis fungoides	1
Unclassified	14

*Now called EATCL. Adapted from Swinson *et al.* (46).

nant histiocytosis of the intestine" (MHI) was used. Current evidence, however, suggests that the tumor is a T-cell lymphoma (47), and the nomenclature suggested by this finding, "enteropathy-associated T-cell lymphoma" (EATCL), will be used in this chapter. The recent U.K. study has provided valuable information on the incidence, prognosis, and clinical features of patients with EATCL.

Disputes have arisen over whether patients presenting with a flat mucosa and lymphoma actually have celiac disease or whether the changes in mucosal architecture are caused by abnormally activated malignant cells or their secreted products. After all, substantial evidence suggests that cytokines secreted

Table 19.5
Non-lymphomatous Malignancies in Celiac Disease

Site	Observed	Expected	Significance (p)
Mouth	3	1.55	ns
Pharynx	4	0.69	<0.001 (excess)
Esophagus	10	2.04	<0.001 (excess)
Stomach	7	7.01	ns
Small intestine	19	0.23	<0.001 (excess)
Colon	6	7.77	ns
Rectum	7	5.38	ns
Other gastrointestinal	4	4.51	ns
Lung	9	21.79	<0.001 (deficit)
Breast	4	15.95	<0.001 (deficit)
Skin	6	11.80	ns
Bladder	5	4.83	ns
Prostate	0	2.79	ns
Cervix	0	3.58	ns
Ovary	4	3.07	ns
Uterus	0	2.89	ns
CNS	4	2.10	ns
Larynx	2	1.18	ns
Testis	6	1.75	<0.001 (excess)
Other	16	15.07	ns

Adapted from Swinson *et al.* (46).

by gut mucosal T cells can produce celiac-like changes in intestinal mucosal architecture (49, 50). For several reasons, which we have reviewed elsewhere (48), we hold the view that celiac disease is the primary condition involved.

The majority of lymphomas in celiac patients are intestinal, occurring not only in the jejunum, but in any part of the small intestine. Ulcers, strictures, or nodules of tumor may occur, and occasionally only microscopic foci are noted. In the majority of cases, widespread dissemination is observed at the time of diagnosis, particularly to mesenteric lymph nodes, liver, spleen, and bone marrow.

Lymphoma may present as either a clinical deterioration in a celiac patient previously well controlled on a gluten-free diet or de novo, with the diagnosis of celiac disease and lymphoma being made simultaneously. Most patients present with malaise, anorexia, weight loss, and diarrhea, often accompanied by abdominal pain. Physical signs included fever, lymphadenopathy, skin rash, hepatomegaly, and a palpable abdominal mass. Approximately 50% of patients require laparotomy for complications of hemorrhage, perforation, or obstruction. In the U.K. study, the diagnosis was made at autopsy in 20% of patients.

Even in cases of early diagnosis, the prognosis remains poor. In the recent U.K. study, the overall survival rate following diagnosis was 43% at 6 months, 36% at 1 year, and 10% at 5 years. No clear guidelines for treatment have been formulated. Given that most tumors are widely disseminated at presentation, chemotherapy would logically be preferred but no regimes for this rare disease have yet been subjected to formal clinical trial.

Apart from lymphoma, patients with celiac disease face increased risk of developing esophageal and pharyngeal squamous carcinomas and small-intestinal adenocarcinoma. In the U.K. study, the relative risk of developing small-intestinal adenocarcinoma was 82.6; nevertheless, the risk to the individual patient is extremely low, with the expected incidence among patients with celiac disease of approximately 50 per 100,000 per year. Similarly, routine screening of celiacs for pharyngo-esophageal tumors would appear unnecessary although any relevant symptoms such as dysphagia must be taken seriously.

The clinical and pathological features of non-lymphoid malignancies are similar in both celiac and non-celiac patients. The only difference arises in that the majority of small intestinal adenocarcinomas in celiac patients occurred in the duodenum and jejunum, whereas the duodenum, jejunum, and ileum are affected equally in the general population.

A report from Birmingham (51) has recently provided evidence that dietary compliance reduces the risks of lymphoma and other malignancies in celiac disease. Previous studies had had too short an observation period, inadequate patient numbers, and problems in the recognition of gluten-sensitivity that prevented collection of such data. The English report follows up on 210 celiac patients who had been initially reviewed in 1974. At that time, no evidence of a protective effect from a gluten-free diet was known. The patients have been kept under surveillance, and at the end of 1985 only 4 could not be traced, giving a 98% follow-up, for a minimum of 13 years or until death. The latest analysis shows that, for celiac patients who have taken a gluten-free diet for 5 years or more, the risk of developing a malignancy was similar to (not statistically different from) that of the general population. Patients whose dietary compliance was poor or who ate a normal diet had an excess of cancers of the mouth, pharynx, and esophagus and of lymphoma. This compelling evidence supports the prescription of a lifelong gluten-free diet in celiac disease.

Pathogenesis of Gluten-Sensitive Enteropathy

Although theories of peptidase deficiency and lectin-like gluten related toxicity are not completely eliminated from consideration, it seems likely that food protein sensitive enteropathies—including celiac disease—have an immunological basis (52).

DELAYED-TYPE HYPERSENSITIVITY

Strong circumstantial evidence supports the concept of immune activation of T cells in the celiac lesion. Lamina propria CD4+ T cells in celiac mucosa express CD25 antigen (which identifies the α chain of the IL-2 receptor), and this production is linked to gluten exposure (53). Human crypt epithelium does not normally express HLA-DR antigens, and the crypt cell HLA-DR expression in celiac disease, which is gluten-dependent (54), provides further evidence that activation of T effector cells in the mucosa occurs.

Most, but not all, of the features of the celiac lesion can be reproduced in model systems of T-cell activation, such as graft-versus-host reaction in the mouse (49)—crypt hyperplasia, shortening of villi, high density of IEL infiltrate in the villus epithelium, IEL mitosis, and HLA class II expression by crypt cells. Different cell activation and cytokine signals may underlie these components—gamma-interferon and IL-2–influencing crypt cells, TNF associated with villus flattening, and cytotoxic cells or other cytokines involved in the rare, severe hypoplastic lesion. Some immune features that occur in celiac disease, however, probably have a different pathogenesis. The author has examined this issue in a group of non-celiacs, who were selected to have a high frequency of immune abnormalities on careful testing. Expression of HLA-DR on crypt cells was significantly associated with high total IEL count and high CD3+ IEL count, but not with high $\gamma\delta$ IEL count, overexpression of IgM, gut permeability, or serum anti-gliadin antibodies (55).

COMPLEMENT

The striking damage to surface enterocytes that occurs in celiac disease is not a feature in models of delayed-type hypersensitivity, and cannot be attributed merely to direct gluten toxicity. The cells at the surface of a "flat" biopsy taken after an overnight fast will have moved out of the crypts onto the surface during the preceding 8 to 12 hours and, therefore, have not been exposed to gluten. Good evidence exists for a role of complement in the celiac lesion (56), and IgM/IgG immune complex/complement-mediated damage probably coexists with DTH in untreated patients. The latter characteristic may be the major factor responsible for reduced enterocyte height and derangement of entocyte brush border.

GLIADIN-TOXIC SEQUENCE OR GENETICALLY DETERMINED IMMUNE RECOGNITION?

Today, the methods of structural biochemistry and molecular medicine can be used to describe the precise structure of individual gliadin molecules and to prepare, by synthesis rather than by degradation, gliadin peptides for immunogenicity testing. By applying the approaches used for other proteins, it will be possible to examine the precise interactions, at the molecular level, between gliadin antigens and antibodies or T-cell receptors. A great deal of research remains to be done on the immunogenicity of gliadins, particularly to establish whether this development is influenced by the individual's genetic make-up. Central to this line of work is the fact that T and B cells recognize different regions of antigens. Many investigators have tried and failed to produce clones of gluten-reactive T cells, but success in this endeavor was only recently reported from Norway (57). Interestingly, the clones produced were HLA-DQ restricted, rather than reacting to DR associated with gluten, which might be the way antigen would be presented by the gut epithelium (the crypt cells overexpress DR but not DQ in celiacs).

As both T cells and antibodies in the fully expressed enteropathy may contribute to immunogenicity, it will be important that workers continue to pursue the regulation of B-cell as well as T-cell function in these new and exciting lines of research.

INDUCTION OF IMMUNITY OR TOLERANCE TO FED ANTIGEN

Fundamental information on human immune responses to dietary antigens, in normal individuals as well as in celiacs, remains scanty. As a result, **induction** and **expression** must be considered separately.

Much work has been performed in rodents showing that feeding of protein antigens, including gliadin, induces the specific immune response of **oral tolerance.** This response comprises a powerful and prolonged suppression and down-regulation of the capacity of the animal to mount active antibody- and

T-cell-mediated immune responses to the antigen concerned.

It is accepted that celiacs have an abnormal state of sensitization to gluten. Proper analysis of the pathogenesis involved requires knowing the precise immune status of normal individuals in this respect. Are they actively tolerant or merely not sensitized? No such data are available for humans, but comparative studies of immune responsiveness of genetically identical mice from gluten-free and gluten-containing diet colonies have clearly shown that mice eating a normal diet are tolerant (58).

CMI IN THE GUT MUCOSA: DO THE GENETIC FACTORS INFLUENCE INDUCTION OR EXPRESSION?

The author's studies with mice showed that immunological sensitization to gliadin does not trigger the development of a T-cell-mediated lesion of the intestine when the diet contains gluten (59). Additional cofactors were required, which could then act via enhanced antigen presentation, recruitment of specific T cells in the mucosa, up-regulation of the expression of class II antigens, or failure of suppression.

A gene that modulates the expression of mucosal DTH, whether HLA- or non-HLA-associated, represents a possible second factor. In other words, the genetic factor in celiac disease could act not only via induction of abnormal immunity, but also by influencing the severity of pathological effects of expression of CMI in the intestine.

Hypothesis: The Pathogenesis of Celiac Disease

Integration of knowledge about oral tolerance combined with recent changes in our perspectives of gluten sensitivity suggests the following hypothetical sequence as the pathogenesis of gluten-sensitive enteropathy (35):

1. Oral tolerance for T-cell-mediated immunity fails to develop, either globally (many antigens) or as confined to gluten.

2. The genetically predisposed individual becomes vulnerable to being actively immunized to the food antigen (gluten) if a particular combination of diet, gut permeability, mucosal, and systemic immunomodulatory signals coincide. The frequency with which this immunization occurs in non-tolerant individuals, and at what age, depends on many intrinsic and environmental factors.

3. When active T-cell sensitization has occurred and the diet contains gluten, relatively subtle effects on the gut mucosa (low-grade pathology, such as high IEL count with normal villi) occur, but only in a proportion of those patients at risk.

4(a). A critical combination of antigen dose and activated mucosal T effector cells eventually occurs, which precipitates the evolution of severe enteropathy and malabsorption.

4(b). Simultaneously with stage 4(a), a wide range of immune effector cells are recruited. Other dietary antigens—and possibly autoantigens—become involved, perpetuating and worsening the enteropathy, and explaining why tissue damage persists for weeks or months after strict dietary exclusion of gluten.

This scheme can accommodate the important advances in celiac disease research made in recent years. The genetic predisposition may act at several steps—via immune response genes, immune recognition of gluten peptides, or the regulation of expression of T-cell-mediated enteropathy. The important phenomenon of latent celiac disease spans stages 2 and 3, depending on whether subtle immune abnormalities (e.g., high count of IEL, high $\gamma\delta$ IEL counts, overexpression of mucosal IgM) appear. Our work, and that of Marsh, on the evolution of enteropathy from high IEL count to the flat lesion, links stages 3 and 4.

Differences in the proportion of "at risk" patients who progress to the next step (i.e., $1 \rightarrow 2$, $2 \rightarrow 3$, $3 \rightarrow 4$) will explain striking differences in disease frequency in groups that share the same genetic make-up (e.g., Swedes and Danes; British infants in the late 1960s; healthy and affected relatives of celiacs).

REFERENCES

1. A joint report of the Royal College of Physicians and the British Nutrition Foundation. Food intolerance and food aversion. J R Coll Physicians Lond 1984;18;83–123

2. Anderson IH, Levine AS, Levitt MD. Incomplete absorption of the carbohydrate in all-purpose wheat flour. N Engl J Med 1981;304:891–892.

3. Levine RA, Briggs GW, Harding RS, Nolte LB. Prolonged gluten administration in normal subjects. N Engl J Med 1966; 274:1109–1114.

4. Alun Jones V, McLaughlan P, Shorthouse M, Workman E, Hunter JO. Food intolerance: a major factor in the pathogenesis of irritable bowel syndrome. Lancet 1982;ii:1115–1117.

5. Cooper BT, Holmes GKT, Ferguson R, Thompson RA, Allan RN, Cooke WT. Gluten-sensitive diarrhea without evidence of celiac disease. Gastroenterology 1980;79:801–806.

6. Weinstein WM. Latent celiac sprue. Gastroenterology 1974; 66:489–493.

7. Doherty M, Barry RE. Gluten-induced mucosal changes in subjects without overt small-bowel disease. Lancet 1981;i:517–520.

8. Ferguson A, Blackwell JN, Barnetson RStC. Effects of additional dietary gluten on the small intestinal mucosa of volunteers and of patients with dermatitis herpetiformis. Scand J Gastroenterol 1987;22:543–549.

9. Arranz E, Ferguson A. Intestinal antibody pattern of coeliac disease: occurrence in patients with normal jejunal biopsy histology. Gastroenterology 1993;104:1263–1272.

10. Arranz E, Ferguson A. Small bowel crypt HLA-DR expression: Association with high count of intra-epithelial lymphocytes, but not with γδ intra-epithelial lymphocyte counts or intestinal antibody patterns. Gut (submitted).

11. Gee S. On the coeliac affection. Saint Bartholomew's Hospital Reports 1888; xxiv:17–20.

12. Dicke WK, Weijers HA, Van de Kamer JH. Coeliac disease. II. The presence in wheat of a factor having a deleterious effect in cases of coeliac disease. Acta Pediatr 1953;42:43–52.

13. Paulley JW. In discussion. Trans Roy Soc Trop Med Hyg 1952c;46:594.

14. Paulley JW. Observation on the aetiology of idiopathic steatorrhoea. Br Med J 1954;ii:1318–1321.

15. Meeuwisse G. Diagnostic criteria in coeliac disease. Acta Paediat Scand 1970;59:461–464.

16. Walker-Smith JA, Guandalini S, Schmitz J, Schmerling DH, Visakorpi JK. Revised criteria for diagnosis of coeliac disease. Arch Dis Child 1990;65:909–911.

17. Ferguson A, McClure JP, Townley RRW. Intraepithelial lymphocyte counts in small intestinal biopsies from children with diarrhoea. Acta Paediatr Scand 1976;65:541–546.

18. Cuenod B, Brousse N, Goulet O, et al. Classification of intractable diarrhea in infancy using clinical and immunohistological criteria. Gastroenterology 1990;99:1037–1043.

19. Ziegler K, Ferguson A. Coeliac disease. In: Batt RM, Lawrence TLJ, eds. Function and dysfunction of the small intestine. Liverpool University Press, 1984, 149–166.

20. Logan RFA, Rifkind EA, Busuttil A, Gilmour HM, Ferguson A. Prevalence and "incidence" of celiac disease in Edinburgh and the Lothian Region of Scotland. Gastroenterology 1986;90:334–342.

21. Greco L, Maki M, Di Donato F, Visakorpi JK. Epidemiology of coeliac disease in Europe and the Mediterranean area. In: Auricchio S, Visakorpi JK, eds. Common food intolerances 1: epidemiology of coeliac disease. Dyn Nutr Res. Basel: Karger, 1992, 25–44.

22. Maki M, Holm K, Ascher H, Greco L, Factors affecting clinical presentation of coeliac disease: Role of type and amount of gluten-containing cereals in the diet. In: Auricchio S, Visakorpi JK, eds. Common food intolerances 1: epidemiology of coeliac disease. Dyn Nutr Res. Basel: Karger, 1992, 76–82.

23. Logan RFA, Tucker G, Rifkind EA, Heading RC, Ferguson A. Changes in clinical features of coeliac disease in adults in Edinburgh and the Lothians 1960–1979. Br Med J 1983; 286:95–97.

24. Swinson CM, Levi AJ. Is coeliac disease underdiagnosed? Br Med J 1980;281:1258–1260.

25. Logan RFA, Ferguson A. Jejunal villous atrophy with morbid obesity: death after jejunoileal bypass. Gut 1982;23:999–1004.

26. Troncone R, Ferguson A. Anti-gliadin antibodies. J Pediatr Gastroenterol Nutr 1991;12:150–158.

27. Burgin-Wolff A, Gaze H, Hadziselimovic F, et al. Antigliadin and antiendomysium antibody determination for coeliac disease. Arch Dis Child 1991;66:941–947.

28. Ferreira M, Lloyd Davies S, Butler M, Scott D, Clark M, Kumar P. Endomysial antibody: is it the best screening test for coeliac disease. Gut 1992;33:1633–1637.

29. Ladinser B, Rossipal E, Pittschieler K. Endomysium antibodies in coeliac disease: an improved method.. Gut 1994;35:776–778.

30. Menzies IS, Pounder R, Heyer S, et al. Abnormal intestinal permeability to sugars in villous atrophy. Lancet 1979;2:1107–1109.

31. Hamilton I, Cobden I, Rothwell J, Axon ATR. Intestinal permeability in coeliac disease. The response to gluten withdrawal and single dose gluten challenge. Gut 1982;23:202–210.

32. Strobel S, Brydon WG, Ferguson A. Cellobiose/mannitol sugar permeability test complements biopsy histopathology in clinical investigation of the jejunum. Gut 1984;25:1241–1246.

33. Losowsky MS. The protean clinical manifestations of coeliac disease. In: Advanced medicine. Tunbridge Wells: Pitman, 1984, 48–60.

34. Mulder CJJ, Tytgat GNJ. Coeliac disease and related disorders. Neth J Med 1987;31:286–299.

35. Ferguson A. Coeliac disease research and clinical practice—maintaining momentum into the twenty-first century. In: Howdle. Coeliac disease, Bailliere's clinical gastroenterology; Bailliere Tindall, London, 1995;9:2:395–412.

36. Holmes GKT. Long-term health risks for unrecognized coeliac patients. In: Auricchio S, Visakorpi JK, eds. Common food intolerances 1: epidemiology of coeliac disease. Dyn Nutr Res. Basel: Karger, 1992, 105–118.

37. Robertson DAF, Dixon MF, Scott BB, et al. Small intestinal ulceration: diagnostic difficulties in relation to coeliac disease. Gut 1983;24:565–574.

38. Isaacson PG, Wright DH. Malignant histiocytosis of the intestine: its relationship to malabsorption and ulcerative jejunitis. Human Pathol 1978;9:661–677.

39. Fry L, Seah PP. Dermatitis herpetiformis: an evaluation of diagnostic criteria. Br J Dermatol 1974;90:137–146.

40. Marks J, Schuster S, Warson AJ. Small bowel changes in dermatitis herpetiformis. Lancet 1966;2:1280–1282.

41. Gawkrodger DJ, Blackwell JN, Gilmour HM, Rifkind EA, Heading RC, Barnetson RStC. Dermatitis herpetiformis: diagnosis, diet and demography. Gut 1984;25:151–157.

42. Gawkrodger DJ, McDonald C, O'Mahony S, Ferguson A. Small intestinal function and dietary status in dermatitis herpetiformis. Gut 1991;32:377–382.

43. O'Mahony S, Vestey JP, Ferguson A. Similarities in intestinal humoral immunity in dermatitis herpetiformis without enteropathy and in coeliac disease. Lancet 1990;335:1487–1490.

44. Gough KR, Read AE, Naish JM. Intestinal reticulosis as a complication of idiopathic steatorrhoea. Gut 1962;3:232–239.

45. Brzechwa-Ajdukiewicz A, McCarthy CF, Austad W, et al. Carcinoma, villous atrophy and steatorrhoea. Gut 1966;7:572–577.

46. Swinson CM, Slavin G, Coles FC, Booth CC. Coeliac disease and malignancy. Lancet 1983;1:111–115.

47. Isaacson PG, O'Connor NTJ, Spencer J, et al. Malignant histiocytosis: a T cell lymphoma. Lancet 1985;2:688–691.

48. O'Mahony S, Ferguson A. Celiac disease. In: Eastwood G, ed. Premalignant conditions of the gastrointestinal tract. New York: Elsevier, 1991, 167–183.

49. Ferguson A. Models of immunologically driven small intestinal damage. In: Marsh MN, ed. Immunopathology of the small intestine. Chichester: John Wiley, 1987, 225–252.

50. Troncone R, Ziegler K, Strobel S, Ferguson A. Gliadin, intestinal hypersensitivity, and food protein-sensitive enteropathy. In: Cunningham-Rundles S, ed. Nutrient modulation of the immune response. New York: Marcel Dekker, 1993, 319–337.

51. Holmes GKT, Prior P, Lane MR, Pope D, Allan RN. Malignancy in coeliac disease—effect of a gluten free diet. Gut 1989;30:3:333–338.

52. Marsh MN. Gluten, major histocompatibility complex and the small intestine. Gastroenterology 1992;102:330–354.

53. Halstensen TS, Brandtzaeg P. Activated T lymphocytes in the celiac lesion: non-proliferative activation (CD25) of CD4+ α/β cells in the lamina propria but proliferation (Ki-67) of α/β and γ/δ cells in the epithelium. Eur J Immunol 1993;23:505–510.

54. Fais S, Mauri L, Pallone F, et al. Gliadin induced changes in the expression of MHC-class II antigens by human small intestinal epithelium. Organ culture studies with coeliac disease mucosa. Gut 1992;33:472–475.

55. Ferguson A, Arranz E, Kingstone K. Clinical and pathological spectrum of celiac disease. In: Malignancy and chronic inflammation in the gastrointestinal tract—new concepts. Proceedings of Falk Symposium held in Berlin, Germany, November 1994, Eds EO Riecken, M Zeitz, A Stallmach, W Helse. 1995;51–63.

56. Haltensen TS, Hvatum M, Scott H, Fausa O, Brandtzaeg P. Association of subepithelial deposition of activated complement and immunoglobulin G and M response to gluten in celiac disease. Gastroenterology 1992;102:751–759.

57. Lundin KEA, Scott H, Hansen T, et al. Gliadin-specific, HLA (—1*0501, β1*0201) restricted T cells isolated from the small intestinal mucosa of celiac disease patients. J Exp Med 1993;178:187–196.

58. Troncone R, Ferguson A. Gliadin presented via the gut induces oral tolerance in mice. Clin Exp Immunol 1988;72:284–287.

59. Troncone R, Ferguson A. Animal model of gluten induced enteropathy in mice. Gut 1991;32:871–875.

20

EXERCISE- AND PRESSURE-INDUCED SYNDROMES

Stephen A. Tilles
Alan L. Schocket

*T*he association of physical urticaria syndromes with the ingestion of foods or other substances has only recently been described. The relationship remains relatively controversial, although the body of evidence that supports its existence is growing. The concept implies that two or more subthreshold stimuli that would not cause mediator release when encountered individually, will produce the release of allergic mediators when combined in a temporal relationship. Such a combination of factors might include foods against which a patient has developed specific antibodies and a physical stimulus such as exercise or pressure. The clinical manifestation of the cellular reaction is a syndrome ranging in severity from itching and hives to anaphylactic shock. Although the mechanism appears logical, it has neither been proved nor strictly complies with the classic concept of allergic sensitivity—that is, that exposure to a single antigen such as a specific food to which the individual has previously been sensitized directly induces a clinical allergic reaction. The two physical urticaria syndromes in which the ingestion of food represents an important but "subthreshold" precipitating factor are exercise-induced anaphylaxis and delayed pressure urticaria (DPU).

Exercise-Induced Anaphylaxis and Urticaria

The clinical syndrome of exercise-induced anaphylaxis and urticaria has been well described in several comprehensive reviews (1–7). It is characterized by the onset, during or shortly after exercise, of symptoms and signs including cutaneous erythema, itching, and urticaria, which may progress to vascular collapse or upper respiratory obstruction. Other symptoms may include headaches, angioedema, choking, wheezing, and nausea. Attacks may be precipitated by various types of exercise, including running, walking, tennis, dancing, and sports such as basketball. The association of this syndrome with an underlying atopic history is not consistent, although atopy is clearly more common than in the general population (1). In some studies of patients with this syndrome, the reactions have been reproduced in the laboratory (8). Elevated histamine levels are associated with the development of symptoms (2–4, 6), and skin biopsies performed with symptoms during challenge testing confirm mast cell degranulation (9).

As described by Maulitz and associates (10), the first case of exercise-induced anaphylaxis associated with food ingestion involved a runner who developed anaphylactic reactions when running within 8 to 12 hours after ingestion of shellfish. The patient ran on a regular basis, averaging 50 to 130 km per week, usually without problems. Over a 3-year period prior to diagnosis of the condition, the patient sustained approximately 10 bouts of transient facial flushing and edema, with diffuse urticaria and intense pruritus occurring during or immediately after exercise. Two of the exercise-induced reactions resulted in almost complete upper airway obstruction requiring emergency therapy with epinephrine and antihistamines. The patient had no initial suspicion of allergic sensitivity to, or clinical reactions following, shellfish ingestion, but eventually made the association between his reactions and the prior ingestion of shellfish. During further evaluation, he had positive immediate reactions with epicutaneous skin testing to clams, oysters, shrimp, and crab (all at a weight–volume ratio of 1 : 2 0), peanuts, trees, grass, and weeds. Once the diagnosis was made and the causative foods identified, avoidance of ingestion of these foods for at least 12 hours prior to exercise resulted in almost complete elimination of any further reactions.

Following Maulitz's original case, Kidd and colleagues reported a series of four cases of exercise-induced anaphylaxis temporally related to the ingestion of food (11). The reactions occurring during or immediately after exercise were similar to those in Maulitz's report and included urticaria, abdominal cramps, wheezing, dyspnea, angioedema, and pruritus. All of the attacks began with generalized tingling, itching, and warmth. In three patients, celery was implicated as the offending food; in the other patient, any food ingested within 2 hours prior to exercise induced the reaction. In one patient, the reaction was precipitated by the ingestion of food after exercise. Of the three patients whose reactions were precipitated by specific foods, all had positive skin tests to celery as well as other antigens. Food skin tests were negative in the patient who developed reactions after eating any food prior to exercise. It is interesting to note that all three patients had problems with celery, a member of the dill family (along with carrots). Two patients had skin reactivity to dill and carrot but did not exhibit clinical sensitivity after eating these foods. This report suggests that celery may possess a unique antigen that predisposes to anaphylactic sensitivity. The authors emphasized that care must be taken to ensure that the food antigen used for skin tests is potent. Fresh celery used as a "puddle test" may be required to detect sensitivity.

In a case reported by Novey and colleagues (12), a patient developed anaphylaxis during exercise followed by meals; as with the one patient described in the previous study, no specific foods were implicated. Subsequent articles describing exercise-induced anaphylaxis in other patients have again implicated celery (13) and shellfish (14, 15), as well as wheat (15–17), lentils (19), peaches (20), apple (21), grapes (18), eggs (15), hazelnut (22), and a cheese sandwich (8).

The diagnosis of an underlying food sensitivity in patients with exercise-induced anaphylaxis may at times prove difficult. The history, as noted in the initial case report (10), represents the most important diagnostic tool. The best clue comes from the presence of intermittent or sporadic reactions superimposed on the baseline of consistent, uneventful exercise. While a specific food is sometimes implicated as a necessary coprecipitating factor, most cases of exercise-induced anaphylaxis are labeled "idiopathic." The time lag between ingestion and reaction may extend to 12 hours, however, so that identifying a specific food trigger by history is often extremely difficult. Skin testing is useful, as all cases of exercise-induced anaphylaxis with a specific food as a coprecipitating factor have positive skin tests to the implicated food. Allergens not present on routine skin test batteries may also act as specific coprecipitating factors. Therefore, some patients in the "idiopathic" category may possibly be reacting to unidentified ingestants.

Some types of exercise-induced anaphylaxis may represent variants of cholinergic urticaria. Cholinergic urticaria patients are typically not atopic and symptoms are usually not dramatic, although anaphylaxis has been documented (2, 4). The classic symptom triggers involve application of generalized heat, including exercise, anxiety, and hot showers. As described by Kaplan and associates (4), symptoms in cholinergic urticaria patients with anaphylaxis occur consistently with exercising to a certain work level. In some cases, careful desensitization protocols using regular graded exercise in conjunction with antihistamine therapy have been useful prophylactically.

In contrast to cholinergic urticaria with anaphylaxis, exercise-induced anaphylaxis symptoms cannot usually be predicted. If a required specific ingestant is identified, avoidance of exposure to this ingestant for at least 8 to 12 hours prior to exercise will usually prevent an urticarial or anaphylactic reaction during exercise. In those patients who fall in the "idiopathic" category, however, management becomes more difficult. Exercise after a fast—especially first thing in the morning or on an empty stomach—is recommended. In addition, antihistamines, taken either regularly or one-half hour before exercise, may help blunt the attack. No data, however, exist to support this therapy or to suggest that it can eliminate or prevent episodes. Patients with a history of life-threatening reactions should avoid exercising alone and should carry self-injectable epinephrine (e.g., Epi-Pen). Emergency treatment at the time of the reaction may be lifesaving, although no confirmed deaths have been attributed to exercise-induced anaphylaxis.

Delayed Pressure Urticaria

Another syndrome in which an association has been made between the ingestion of food and the development or exacerbation of a physically induced urticarial reaction is delayed pressure urticaria (DPU) (23–30). This unusual disease, which is probably more prevalent than previously appreciated, is characterized by the delayed onset of deep cutaneous swellings in areas exposed to pressure of various intensities. The onset of the lesion usually occurs 4 to 8 hours following application of pressure from various stimuli (e.g., prolonged walking for the feet, carrying a golf bag for the shoulder, or hammering nails for the hands). The lesions usually peak 6 to 9 hours after pressure and may last as long as 36 hours. In 30% to 90% of patients, DPU is associated with "common" chronic urticaria (27, 28, 30). A significant number of patients develop "flu-like" symptoms of malaise and fever in association with the skin lesions. An elevated erythrocyte sedimentation rate and mild leukocytosis may be seen in almost half of DPU patients. These prolonged systemic symptoms have been interpreted by some observers as evidence for pro-inflammatory cytokine release. Usually the delayed pressure symptoms parallel the activity of chronic urticaria. The disease has been noted to persist for 30 years (27). In many cases, the condition creates a significant functional disability, especially in individuals whose occupations require heavy physical labor such as carpenters, construction workers, and auto mechanics.

Delayed pressure urticaria is best diagnosed by a good history. Without previous awareness of the nature of this disease, many patients have been diagnosed as having refractory angioedema in association with their chronic urticaria. The diagnosis can be confirmed using several tests (25–29). The most common and reliable test involves a 15 lb weight split into two sandbags connected by a strap; this device is then suspended over the shoulder for a period of 15 minutes (27). The shoulder is examined 4 to 8 hours after the challenge for the development of a deep, frequently painful, erythematous swelling. Most cases give a positive test the first time, but in patients with a good history and a negative initial test, a follow-up test after several days may have positive results. The test is often negative when the disease is quiescent or in remission.

The pathogenesis of DPU remains unclear. It was thought initially to be a manifestation of an Arthus phenomenon, but biopsy failed to reveal either immunoglobulin or complement in the vessel walls (25). Lesions can be induced by the injection of the mast cell degranulator compound 48/80 into the skin, suggesting that the induction of the lesion relates to release of mast cell mediators (31). Increased histamine levels have been shown in skin blisters above the lesions (29). Biopsy specimens reveal mild mononuclear perivascular infiltrates with some eosinophils and a small number of polymorphonuclear leukocytes (32). The presence of fibrin deposition and edema among the collagen fibers at the pressure challenge site suggest a similarity between the lesions of DPU and those generated by the cutaneous late-phase reaction seen after allergen injection (33). The relation of lesion production to kallikrein generation, leukotriene production (29), and even cytokine release (34) has been hypothesized but, to date, not confirmed.

The pressure-induced lesions of most patients with DPU respond poorly to milder drugs commonly used in the treatment of chronic urticaria and angioedema. The delayed pressure component almost uniformly fails to respond to conventional H_1 antihistamines alone or a combination of H_1 and H_2 antihistamines (25–27, 30). The urticarial lesions usually respond to this therapy, however, leaving unresolved the problem of the delayed pressure swellings, which often are suspected to be refractory angioedema. A partial response to nonsteroidal anti-inflammatory agents has been reported in some patients (27), but has not been confirmed in other studies (30). A clinical response was reported with cetirazine (35, 36), a newer-generation antihistamine with some anti-inflammatory properties. The only medications that consistently relieve the delayed pressure symptoms are corticosteroids (25–27, 30). Some patients require relatively high doses of these agents and prolonged therapy to remain functional and able to work.

Consequently, if an underlying "allergic" aggravating factor could be identified whose removal would improve or resolve this potentially debilitating disease, an investigation would be worthwhile.

In an article by Davis and coworkers, specific food ingestion was identified as an exacerbating factor in some patients with DPU (37). In this preliminary report, six selected patients with challenge-proved DPU were studied. All required daily prednisone for symptomatic control. The patients were either fasted, receiving only water, or given a diet of unflavored Vivonex for a minimum of 48 hours. Five of the six patients were clear of both spontaneous urticarial lesions and pressure-induced symptoms after 24 to 48 hours of fasting. Although a control group of patients with chronic urticaria was treated in the same way, none responded to the fast.

The patients were tested to a panel of foods using both skin tests and RAST. Interestingly, several patients developed delayed cutaneous responses to food. Most of these delayed responses followed an immediate cutaneous reaction by an average of 6 hours after testing, similar to late cutaneous reactions. A significant number of the delayed reactions, however, were not preceded by an immediate cutaneous response. In addition, all of the RAST results were negative. All five patients who improved with the fast had positive or delayed reactions to at least one food in the skin tests. Challenge with those foods elicited a reaction in all patients within 2 to 24 hours after food ingestion.

Although this study was not blinded, several of its findings are quite interesting. First, some selected patients apparently have a specific food that may contribute to DPU symptoms. The mechanism by which this contribution occurs, however, remains unclear. In some patients, late cutaneous reactions (after 6 hours) followed a positive immediate cutaneous reaction to food skin testing, while other subjects experienced only late cutaneous reactions. None of the patients, however, had immunoglobulin E (IgE) antibodies to foods demonstrable by RAST. Elimination diets excluding the identified offending foods resulted in not only improvement of chronic urticaria but also loss of the positive delayed pressure response to provocative testing. Those patients who responded to the dietary elimination of the offending foods were

eventually either withdrawn from corticosteroid or required significantly lower doses for control of their disease. It is unclear from this article what percentage of patients with DPU have a food sensitivity as an underlying aggravating factor or when the evaluation for this condition should be undertaken.

A subsequent report described two patients with DPU in whom lesions could be elicited when they had eaten normal food but not when they had been on an elimination diet for at least 5 days (38). In those patients, DPU was a reproducible phenomenon. Response to skin testing was not described, however.

In studies conducted by Czarnetski and colleagues (28, 39), patients with positive cutaneous responses to foods failed to respond to elimination diets. In one report, the group presented 13 patients with DPU (39). All of the subjects received prick skin tests to a large battery of common allergens, including food extracts. Seven of these patients had positive early cutaneous reactions (after 15 minutes) and six developed positive late cutaneous reactions (after 6 hours). Two patients had only early cutaneous reactions, and four experienced only late cutaneous reactions to food antigens. None of the patients, however, showed any improvement on diets that eliminated those food antigens to which they reacted with a late cutaneous reaction. It is not clear whether any of the patients fasted for any prolonged period of time to exclude other allergens that were not part of the skin test battery.

Thus, although a role for food ingestion in the causation of DPU has been suggested, it has not yet been well documented or proved. Nevertheless, given the high morbidity of DPU in some patients, including the potential requirement for long-term systemic corticosteroid therapy, it is a worthwhile effort to exclude ingestants as aggravating factors in almost any patient with significant or debilitating DPU.

Pathophysiology

Clinical syndromes relating physical urticarias such as delayed pressure urticaria and exercise-induced anaphylaxis to food ingestion have been described in the literature; nevertheless, their existence remains controversial. In large part, this controversy stems from the relative lack of well-controlled studies confirming food ingestion as a causal factor in these syndromes. In addition, the pathophysiologic mechanisms underlying the role of food ingestion in these diseases are not yet well defined. From the nature of these syndromes, one could infer that they are caused by two or more subthreshold stimuli that individually are inadequate to produce mediator release from mast cells or basophils, but when combined in a temporal relationship will produce mast cell or basophil degranulation, resulting in a clinically apparent event.

The clinical precedent creates a compelling argument. In a review article (40), Wong and colleagues described several studies in which patients developed dermographism when treated with certain medications. They also described patients with exercise-induced dermographism and cold-precipitated dermographism. The cutaneous passive transfer of the dermographic response with serum—in some cases IgE—has been described as well (41–43). Further studies by Moore-Robinson and Warin noted a worsening of cold urticaria after exercise (44). A report by Doeglas noted a high incidence of aspirin sensitivity in patients with both chronic urticaria and physical urticarias, including cholinergic and pressure-induced urticaria (45). In a later paper, however, Moore-Robinson and Warin failed to identify any ability of aspirin to exacerbate physical challenges in their patients with dermographism, cold urticaria, and cholinergic urticaria (46). At a cellular level, Murdoch and associates demonstrated that certain dyes (azo and non-azo) and other additives, including butylated hydroxyanisole (BHA), butylated hydroxytoluene (BHT), sodium benzoate, and aspirin at pharmacologic levels, released histamine from leukocytes of both normal subjects and patients with urticaria and increased the spontaneous release from patients with urticaria (47). These studies suggest that certain factors are potentially able to release mediators and may also lower thresholds for the release of mediators from mast cells or basophils without directly causing them to degranulate.

In the clinical situation, the major questions revolve around the factors that alter mast cell releasability and those that are present in the individual patient. Many naturally occurring endogenous peptides have been shown to be capable of releasing histamine from mast cells both in vivo and in vitro (48). These peptides include substance P (49), vasoactive intestinal peptide, or VIP (50), calcitonin gene-related peptide (50), gastrin (51), pentagastrin (51), and endorphins (48), to name but a few members of a growing list. Release of these peptides occurs via various stimuli, including digestion, anxiety, pain, exercise, and local irritation. Any of these factors could be involved in physical urticarias and other allergic syndromes, including chronic urticaria, asthma, allergic rhinitis, and anaphylaxis. A study by Wallengren and colleagues highlighted this mechanism by demonstrating increased levels of certain peptides in skin blisters from patients with urticaria and dermographia as compared with normal subjects (50). Three studies on patients with exercise-induced anaphylaxis and urticaria have demonstrated a decreased cutaneous mast cell releasability threshold during a reaction (52–54). Two of these investigations (52, 53) used compound 48/80 (a nonspecific mast cell degranulator); the other (54) used codeine (a mast cell degranulator sometimes used as a positive control in skin tests). Exercise-induced anaphylaxis patients exhibited greater skin test reactivity to these agents post-exercise, while control patients' skin test reactivity did not change (54).

The mechanisms creating the role played by food sensitivities in exercise-induced anaphylaxis and urticaria, although not proved, appear plausible; the pathophysiology of delayed pressure urticaria related to food sensitivity, however, is much less clear. Histopathologically, the lesions of DPU resemble the late cutaneous IgE response (33) and are reproducible in affected patients by the injection of compound 48/80 (31). The factors that alter mast cell releasability and predispose to a late-phase type of cutaneous reaction in patients with DPU have not been definitively identified (55, 56). In the study described above relating food sensitivity to the clinical syndrome of DPU, specific IgE to the implicated food could not be demonstrated by RAST (37). Furthermore, in some patients the development of a late cutaneous reaction to certain foods was not preceded by an immediate wheal-and-flare reaction as seen in the IgE-mediated late-phase cutaneous reactions. A later study noted similar skin test phenomenon in these patients (39). In the DPU patients described, elimination of the foods causing positive skin tests did not ameliorate the clinical syndrome. Thus, although certain patients appear to have DPU from food sensitivity, IgE antibodies to foods are not demonstrable. Other factors such as IgG4 may play important roles but have not been studied in this disease.

Conclusion

Increasing evidence suggests that in some physical urticaria syndromes—specifically, exercise-induced anaphylaxis and urticaria and delayed pressure urticaria—the presence of a food sensitivity or allergy and the subsequent ingestion of the specific food can either induce or exacerbate the clinical disease. Although this relationship remains controversial, the hypothesis is quite provocative. It suggests that the commonly accepted mechanism of direct mediator release from mast cells and basophils, induced by the binding of a food antigen to specific IgE on their surfaces, is not the only form of food allergy. Another, more subtle mechanism may be at work by which an IgE antigen–antibody complex formation alters the threshold of releasability on the surface of the mast cell. Complexes are most likely insufficiently dense to alter the cell membrane enough to initiate the cascade of mediator release. The density, however, may be adequate to permit mast cell degranulation by other factors, especially physical stimuli or endogenous substances such as peptides or hormones, which would ordinarily be inadequate to cause this release. This mechanism may potentially explain some of the well-known variability and irreproducibility of clinical reactions and challenge testing to foods seen in some patients with otherwise credible histories.

REFERENCES

1. Shefer AL, Austen KR. Exercise induced anaphylaxis. J Allergy Clin Immunol 1980;66:106–111.
2. Lewis J, Lieberman P, Treadwell G, Erffmeyer J. Exercise-induced urticaria, angioedema, and anaphylactoid episodes. J Allergy Clin Immunol 1981;68:432–437.
3. Sheffer AL, Soter NA, McFadden ER, Austen KR. Exercise-induced anaphylaxis: a distinct form of physical allergy. J Allergy Clin Immunol 1983;71:311–316.
4. Kaplan AP, Natbony SF, Tawil AP, Fruchter L, Foster M.

5. Songsiridej V, Busse WW. Exercise-induced anaphylaxis. Clin Allergy 1983;13:317–321.
6. Casale TB, Kehey TM, Kaliner M. Exercise-induced anaphylactic syndromes: insights into diagnostic and pathophysiologic features. JAMA 1986;255:2049–2053.
7. Tilles S, Schocket A, Milgrom H. Exercise-induced anaphylaxis related to specific foods. J Pediatrics 1995 (in press).
8. Tilles SA, Schocket AL. Exercise-induced anaphylaxis. Pact Allergy Immunol 1994;9:64–67.
9. Sheffer AL, Tong AK, Murphy GF, et al. Exercise-induced anaphylaxis: a serious form of physical allergy asssociated with mast cell degranulation. J Allergy Clin Immunol 1985;75:479–484.
10. Maulitz RM, Pratt DS, Schocket AL. Exercise-induced anaphylactic reaction to shellfish. J Allergy Clin Immunol 1979;63:433–434.
11. Kidd JM, Cohen SH, Sosman AJ, Fink JN. Food-dependent exercise induced anaphylaxis. J Allergy Clin Immunol 1983;71:407–411.
12. Novey HS, Fairshter RD, Salness K, Simon RA, Curd JG. Postprandial exercise-induced anaphylaxis. J Allergy Clin Immunol 1983;71:498–504.
13. Silverstein SR, Frommer DA, Dobozin B, Rosen P. Celery-dependent exercise-induced anaphylaxis. J Emerg Med 1986;4:195–199.
14. McNeil D, Strauss RH. Exercise-induced anaphylaxis related to food intake. Ann Allergy 1988;61:440–442.
15. Fukutomi O, Kondo N, Agata H, et al. Abnormal responses of the autonomic nervous system in food-dependent exercise-induced anaphylaxis. Ann Allergy 1992;68:438–445.
16. Kushimoto H, Aoki T. Masked type I wheat allergy. Arch Dermatol 1985;121:355–360.
17. Dohi M, Suko M, Sugiyama H, et al. Food-dependent exercise-induced anaphylaxis: a study on eleven Japanese cases. J Allergy Clin Immunol 1992;87:34–40.
18. Okazaki M, Kitani H, Mifune T, et al. Food-dependent exercise-induced anaphylaxis. Intern Med 1992;31:1052–1055.
19. Sabbah A, Drouet M. Anaphylaxie induite par l'exercice et liee a l'allertie alimentaire. Presse Med 1984:2390–2391.
20. Buchbinder EM, Bloch KJ, Moss J, Guiney TE. Food-dependent exercise-induced anaphylaxis. JAMA 1983;250:2973–2974.
21. Anibarro B, Dominguez C, Diaz JM, Martin MF, Garcia-Ara MC, Boyano MT, Ojeda JA. Apple-dependent exercise-induced anaphylaxis. Allergy 1994;49:482.
22. Munoz MF, Lopez CJM, Villas F, Contreras JF, Diaz JM, Ojeda JA. Exercise-induced anaphylactic reaction to hazelnut. Allergy 1994;49:314–316.
23. Kalz M, Bower C, Prichard H. Delayed and persistent dermographia. Arch Dermatol Syph 1950;61:772–780.
24. Baughman RD, Jillson OF. Seven specific types of urticaria: with special reference to delayed persistent dermographism. Ann Allergy 1963;21:248–255.
25. Ryan TJ, Shim-Young N, Turk JL. Delayed pressure urticaria. Br J Dermatol 1968;80:485–490.
26. Warin R, Champion RH. Urticaria. London: WB Saunders, 1974.
27. Sussman GL, Harvey RP, Schocket AL. Delayed pressure urticaria. J Allergy Clin Immunol 1982;70:337–342.
28. Czarnetzki B. Urticaria. Berlin: Springer-Verlag, 1986.
29. Czarnetzki B, Meentken J, Rosenbach T, Pokropp A. Clinical,

pharmacological and immunological aspects of delayed pressure urticaria. Br J Dermatol 1984;111:315–323.

30. Dover JS, Black AK, Ward AM, Greaves MW. Delayed pressure urticaria: clinical features, laboratory investigations, and response therapy of 44 patients. J Am Acad Dermatol 1988;18:1289–1298.

31. Davis K, Mekori Y, Kohler P, Schocket A. Late cutaneous reactions in patients with delayed pressure urticaria. J Allergy Clin Immunol 1984;73:810–812.

32. Czarnetzki B, Meentken J, Kolde G, Brocker E. Morphology of the cellular infiltrate in delayed pressure urticaria. J Am Acad Dermatol 1985;12:253–259.

33. Mekori Y, Dobozin B, Schocket A, Kohler P, Clark R. Delayed pressure urticaria histologically resembles cutaneous late-phase reactions. Arch Dermatol 1988;124:230–235.

34. Shelley W, Shelley E. Delayed pressure urticaria syndrome: a clinical expression of interleukin 1. Acta Derm Venereol (Stockh) 1987;67:438–441.

35. Kontou-Fili K, Maniatakou G, Paleologos G, Aroni K. Cetirizine inhibits delayed pressure urticaria (part 2): skin biopsy findings. Ann Allergy 1990;65:520–522.

36. Kontou-Fili K, Maniatakou G, Demaka P, Gonianakis M, Paleologos G. Therapeutic effects of cetirizine in delayed pressure urticaria (part 1): effects on weight tests and skin window cytology. Ann Allergy 1990;65:517–519.

37. Davis K, Mekori Y, Kohler P, Schocket A. Possible role of diet in delayed pressure urticaria—preliminary report. J Allergy Clin Immunol 1986;77:566–569.

38. Rajka G, Mork NJ. Clinical observations of the mechanisms of delayed pressure urticaria. In: Champion RH, Greaves MW, Black AK, Pye RJ, eds. The urticarias. New York: Churchill Livingstone, 1985, 191–193.

39. Czarnetzki B, Cap H, Forck G. Late cutaneous reactions to common allergens in patients with delayed pressure urticaria. Br J Dermatol 1987;117:695–701.

40. Wong RC, Fairley JA, Ellis CN. Dermographism: a review. J Am Acad Dermatol 1984;11:643–652.

41. Smith JA, Mansfield LE, Fokakis A, Nelson HS. Dermographia caused by Ige mediated penicillin allergy. Ann Allergy 1983;51:30–32.

42. Murphy GM, Zollman PE, Greaves MW, Winkelmann RK. Symptomatic dermographism (factitious urticaria)—passive

transfer experiments from human to monkey. Br J Dermatol 1987;116:801–804.

43. Mikhailov P, Berova N, Andreev VC. Physical urticaria and sport. Cutis 1977;20:381–390.

44. Moore-Robinson M, Warin R. Some clinical aspects of cholinergic urticaria. Br J Dermatol 1968;80:794–799.

45. Doeglas H. Reactions to aspirin and food additives in patients with chronic urticaria, including the physical urticarias. Br J Dermatol 1975;93:135–144.

46. Moore-Robinson M, Warin R. Effect of salicylates in urticaria. Br Med J 1967;4:262–264.

47. Murdoch RD, Pollock I, Young E. Effects of food additives on leukocyte histamine release in normal and urticaria subjects. J R Coll Physicians Lond 1987;21:251–256.

48. Foreman JC, Piotrowski W. Peptides and histamine release. J Allergy Clin Immunol 1984;74:127–131.

49. Miadonna A, Tedeschi A, Leggieri E, et al. Activity of substance P on human skin and nasal airways. Ann Allergy 1988;61:220–223.

50. Wallengren J, Moller H, Ekman R. Occurrence of substance P, vasoactive intestinal peptide, and calcitonin gene-related peptide in dermographism and cold urticaria. Arch Dermatol Res 1987;279:512–515.

51. Tharp MD, Thirlby R, Sullivan TJ. Gastrin induces histamine release from human cutaneous mast cells. J Allergy Clin Immunol 1984;74:159–165.

52. Errington G, Mekori Y, Silvers W, Schocket A. Altered mast cell threshold in exercise-induced anaphylaxis. J Allergy Clin Immunol 1985;75:193 (abstr).

53. Kivity S, Ephraim S, Greif J, Topilsky M, Mekori Y. The effect of food and exercise on the skin response to compound 48/80 in patients with food associated exercise-induced urticaria-angioedema. J Allergy Clin Immunol 1988;81:1155–1158.

54. Lin RY, Barnard M. Skin testing with food, codeine, and histamine in exercise-induced anaphylaxis. Ann Allergy 1993;70:475–478.

55. Estes SA, Yung CW. Delayed pressure urticaria: an investigation of some parameters of lesion induction. J Am Acad Dermatol 1981;5:25–31.

56. Keahey TM, Indrisano J, Lavker RM, Kaliner MA. Delayed vibratory angioedema: insights into pathophysiologic mechanisms. J Allergy Clin Immunol 1987;80:831–838.

21

OCCUPATIONAL REACTIONS TO FOOD ALLERGENS

Carol E. O'Neil
Samuel B. Lehrer

*I*n the United States alone, more than 21 million people are employed in some aspect of the food industry. Of these people, 2.1 million work in the farm sector and the remainder work in processing, manufacturing, transportation, or eating establishments (Table 21.1) (1). As a result of their employment, such individuals are exposed to a wide variety of substances, many of which are known to induce allergic diseases. Most sensitizing materials are food-derived protein allergens, including green coffee beans, flour, and shellfish. In addition, nonfood agents can induce allergic disease—for example, honey bees, grain storage mites, antibiotics, thermophilic actinomycetes, and even rubber boots. Exposure routes (inhalation and contact) vary depending on agents and industries, but are the same as for other environmental allergens (2). Allergic diseases associated with workplace exposures include occupational asthma (OA), hypersensitivity pneumonitis (HP) (extrinsic allergic alveolitis), and dermatitis.

Definitions

Occupational asthma is a reversible airway obstruction induced by inhaled agents encountered in the workplace. Asthma occurring at the workplace is not necessarily "occupational asthma," and it is important, for medicolegal reasons, to draw this distinction. Many persons have a preexisting hypersensitivity to common allergens, such as dust or molds, and may develop symptoms if exposed to these materials in the course of their employment.

Hypersensitivity pneumonitis is a disease spectrum characterized by a diffuse, predominantly mononuclear inflammation of the lung parenchyma, particularly of the interstitium and alveoli. In some instances, HP advances such that granulomas and fibrosis occur. This disease is associated with intense and often prolonged exposure to organic dusts. Although it is almost exclusively an occupational disease, individuals can also be exposed to sensitizing agents via heating, humidification, or air-conditioning systems.

Traditionally, the term "contact dermatitis" has been used to describe any rash resulting from a substance touching the skin. Three major forms of contact dermatitis occur: irritant, allergic contact, and photoallergic. Irritant dermatitis is not an allergic process, and thus does not require previous sensitization. Allergic contact dermatitis (Fig. 21.1) is characterized by an eczematous skin reaction appearing 48 hours after exposure to antigen. The result of a cell-mediated immune response, it occurs following an acquired sensitivity to a given substance. Some materials can induce both irritant and allergic dermatitis. Photo contact dermatitis is also a T-cell-mediated eczematous disease; concomitant exposure to an etiologic agent and ultraviolet irradiation are, however, required to elicit a reaction. Contact urticaria, an occupational skin disease encountered in the food industries, is usually associated with the immediate release of mast cell mediators. Careful examination

Table 21.1
Employment of Individuals Working in the Food and
Fiber Sector, 1992

Employment	Number Working (in millions)
Food and Fiber Total	28.2*
Farm sector	2.0
Non-farm sector	20.8
Food processing	1.5
Manufacturing	3.0
Transportation, trade, retailing	7.8
Eating establishments	5.2
Other	3.4

* 18% of total work force.
(Adapted from national data book and guide to sources. Statistical abstract of the United States, 114th ed. Washington, D.C.: U.S. Department of Commerce, Bureau of the Census, 1994, Table 1077.)

of the affected area reveals a transient wheal-and-flare response, rather than dermatitis.

Prevalence and Incidence

To determine prevalence or incidence of occupational diseases with any certainty is difficult, particularly in the food industries. Both employees and physicians tend to underreport health problems, and epidemiologic data on agriculture workers and food handlers remain scanty.

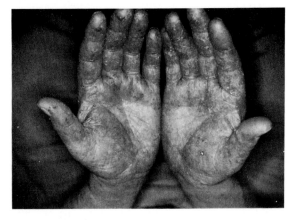

Figure 21.1

Allergic contact dermatitis of the hands caused by shrimp. Reprinted, with permission, from Fisher AA. Allergic contact urticaria of the hands due to seafood in food handlers. Cutis 1988;42:388–389.

The overall prevalence of asthma in the general population probably lies between 2% and 6% (3), with approximately 2% to 15% of all cases of adult asthma attributable to occupational exposure (4, 5). In those food-related industries in which prevalence of OA are available, rates do not significantly differ from those found in nonfood industries. For example, OA occurs in 3% (6) to 10% (7) of workers exposed to green coffee beans, 15% of snow crab processing workers (8), and 10% to 30% of bakers (9). By comparison, 5% of individuals exposed to toluene diisocyanate (TDI) (10) or Western red cedar (11) develop asthma; approximately 70% of individuals exposed to complex salts of platinum (12) or river flies (13) become sensitized.

The incidence of HP is difficult to determine because of the disease's generally low occurrence, problems with differential diagnosis, and the lack of prospective epidemiologic studies. Incidence also depends on exposure levels of the offending antigen and varies widely in different industries or even in areas of the same plant. Climatic factors may also contribute to variations in incidence. For example, in farmer's lung, the incidence ranges from 2.3% to 8.6%, with farmers living in regions with high rainfall being more susceptible to disease (14, 15).

Most epidemiologic studies of dermatologic reactions in food-industry workers have included only subjects already diagnosed with occupational skin disease. Consequently, although types of skin reactions can be distinguished and many of the important etiologic agents can be identified, the true prevalence of disease remains difficult to determine. In a study of 1052 workers in the Finnish food industry, 17% were identified as having a skin disease (16). In that study, 8.5% of 541 female workers had occupational eczema, most commonly caused by fish, meat, and vegetables. In a 5-year retrospective study, 3662 consecutive patients, including 180 food handlers, were patch-tested (17). In 91 of 180 subjects (50.5%), dermatitis resulted from an occupational exposure. Patch tests were positive in 59 of 180 patients (32.7%), and 25 of 180 (13.8%) had dermatitis resulting from exposure to meats or vegetables. Hjorth and Roed-Petersen evaluated 33 cases of occupational dermatitis occurring in restaurant kitchen workers (18). Metals, onions, and garlic were implicated most frequently in contact dermatitis; fish and shellfish were the major agents responsible for provoking contact urticaria. The same food allergens were also identified as the most important in a study of caterers (19).

Several studies have been performed in workers exposed to celery. In one investigation, 163 of 203 celery harvesters (54%) developed phototoxic dermatitis after handling of celery infected with the fungus *Sclerotinia sclerotiorum* (20). Another study demonstrated that 68.8% of workers developed dermatitis when exposed to this fungus (21). Healthy celery can also induce phytophotodermatitis in exposed workers (22). For 30 of 127 grocery store workers (23.6%), disease developed after they handled celery containing high concentrations of furocoumarins.

Host Factors

Physicochemical properties of occupational agents, as well as dose, duration and route of exposure, allergenic potency, and industrial hygiene and engineering practices influence their potential to induce allergic disease. As only a small proportion of exposed workers develop occupational reactions, however, host factors clearly play an important role in disease development. These factors may include atopy, human leukocyte antigen (HLA) type, cigarette smoking, and preexisting nonspecific bronchial hyperreactivity (NSBH).

ATOPY

Atopic individuals have a personal or family history of hayfever, asthma, or eczema and exhibit a greater tendency to develop sensitivity to environment agents than do normal subjects. Atopic individuals frequently show elevated total immunoglobulin E (IgE) levels. Nevertheless, history alone is not sufficient for the diagnosis of atopy, as identical symptoms can arise from allergic and nonallergic mechanisms. A wheal-and-flare skin reactivity is often used along with history to establish a diagnosis.

Occupational asthma is frequently associated with increased production of specific IgE antibodies. Even so, atopy per se is not always associated with an increased incidence of disease. Atopy appears to be an important factor in workers sensitized to papain (23), flour (9), and green coffee beans (6). In some instances where the incidence of OA might be expected to be influenced by a worker's atopic status, such as in snow crab processing workers (8) or grain handlers (24), no relationship between atopy and development of disease has been discerned. It is possible, however, that affected workers have left the workplace, creating a "healthy worker population." Unlike with OA, atopic individuals appear less likely to develop HP than nonatopic individuals.

The role of atopy has not been clearly defined in the pathophysiology of occupational dermatoses. In general, atopic dermatitis and urticaria appear more likely to occur in atopic subjects. Evaluation of 33 patients with a variety of occupational skin diseases resulting from exposure to foods demonstrated, however, that only 7 had a personal or family history of atopy (18).

HLA TYPE

Almost no information has been gathered on tissue type and its relationship to the development of OA, particularly OA resulting from exposure to allergens in the food industry. A relationship may exist between HP and HLA type, as suggested by an apparent familial (25) or ethnic occurrence of HP, and by several laboratory studies (26, 27). Results from other investigations have failed to confirm this association (28, 29). Some evidence suggests an increased prevalence of HLA-A3 and HLA-A9 in patients with atopic dermatitis (30), but this hypothesis has not been evaluated in subjects exposed to food allergens.

SMOKING

The role of cigarette smoke in development, exacerbation, or pathogenesis of OA is not clear. Exposure to cigarette smoke increases bronchial epithelial permeability (31), which might potentially allow inhaled antigens increased access to immunocompetent cells and evoke an immune response. A potential relationship between asthma, cigarette smoke, and dust, aerosol, or vapor exposure appears intriguing, but epidemiologic studies in this area are limited. Smokers exposed occupationally to green coffee bean or castor bean dust appear to be at higher risk for the development of occupationally induced allergies than similarly exposed nonsmokers (32). Furthermore, a significantly higher proportion of smokers appear among "sensitized" than "nonsensitized" coffee factory workers, and sensitization appears to progress more rapidly in smokers (33). In grain handlers, symptoms of allergy occurred with similar frequency in atopic and nonatopic individuals, but appeared to be more highly correlated with smoking status than with the presence of positive skin tests (34). Pulmonary effects of smoking and grain dust exposure are additive (35). These findings underscore the importance of imposing controls for smoking during data analysis.

Smokers appear less likely to develop HP than nonsmokers (36–38). Reasons for this discrepancy are not immediately obvious, but cigarette smoke can reportedly affect distribution patterns of particles (39), hasten clearance of particles from the lungs (40), and hinder deposition of some inhaled particles (41). These observations may help to explain the epidemiologic findings.

AIRWAY HYPERREACTIVITY

Occupational asthma, like allergic asthma, is usually associated with NSBH, as demonstrated by provocative challenge testing with histamine or methacholine. It is not clear whether NSBH is a preexisting risk factor or if it develops concomitantly with asthma. Because asthma is not a feature of HP, NSBH is not usually associated with this disease.

Agents Associated with Allergic Occupational Diseases of Food Workers

Hundreds of agents are known to cause occupational asthma. Most of these substances are chemicals, pharmaceuticals, wood dust, and metals (42, 43); in addition, more than 50 agents encountered in food or food-related industries are known to induce OA. In some industries, such as coffee factories, OA is a well-recognized problem; in other types of work-places, only individual case reports have been reported.

Table 21.2
Materials Used in Food or Food-Related Industries That Are Known to Induce Occupational Asthma or Rhinitis

Agents	Occupational Exposure	References
Animal Products		
Sea animals		
Prawn	Seafood processing	44, 45
Crab	Seafood processing	46
Crab, king	Seafood processing	47
Crab, snow	Seafood processing	8, 48
Lobster	Seafood processing	49
Oyster	Culture oyster workers	49, 50
Clams	Seafood processing	51
Shrimpmeal	Aquaculture	52
Fishmeal	Factory workers	53
Fish flour	Factory workers	54
Mother of pearl	Button factory workers	55
Sea squirt	Oyster shuckers	56, 57
Seashells	Shell grinders	58
Trout		59
Farm products		
Cows	Dairy farmers	60–62
Milk	Factory workers	63
Hogs	Hog farmers	64, 65
Swine food	Hog workers	66
Poultry	Poultry workers	67
Pheasants, quail, doves	Breeders	68
Eggs	Egg processors, bakery workers	69–72
Egg lysozyme		73

Table 21.2
(Continued)

Agents	Occupational Exposure	References
Insects		
Poultry mites	Poultry workers	74, 75
(*Ornithonyssus sylviarum*)		
Grain storage mites	Grain workers	76–78
(*Glycyphagus destructor*)		
Honey bees	Beekeepers, honey processors	79–81
Bee-moth	Fish-bait breeders	82
Rice flower beatle	Rice flower workers	83
Enzymes		
Pepsin	Pharmaceutical workers	84
Trypsin	Pharmaceutical workers	85
Pancreatic enzymes	Pharmaceutical workers	86, 87
Miscellaneous		
Spiramycin	Chick breeders	88
Pyrolysis products of polyvinyl chloride or label adhesives	Meat wrappers	89–95
Plant/Fungi		
Grains/flours		
Flour (wheat, rye)	Bakers, millers	96–98
Buckwheat	Food workers	99, 100
Carob bean flour	Food workers	101
Rice	Rice millers	102–103
Soybeans	Agricultural workers	104
Soybean lecithin		105
Grain dust	Grain handlers	106–109
Spices/herbs		
Garlic	Factory workers, farmers	110–113
Coriander, mace, ginger, paprika	Factory workers	114, 115
Cinnamon	Spice workers	116
Paprika plants	Greenhouse workers	117
Vegetables		
Green beans	Homemaker	118
Okra		119
Enzymes		
Bromelain	Factory workers	120–122
Papain	Factory workers	123–126
Miscellaneous		
Coffee	Coffee factory workers	6, 127
Castor	Factory workers, dock workers	128
Tea	Tea factory workers, tea garden workers	129–131
Herbal tea	Herbal tea workers	132
Pollen	Sugarbeet workers	133
	Sunflower workers	134
	Grape growers	135
Pectin		136, 137
Alkaline hydrolysis derivative of bluten	Bakers	138
Alternaria/Aspergillus	Poultry vendors	139
Colophony	Poultry vendors	140
Hops	Brewery chemists	141
Devil's tongue	Food workers	142
(*Amorphophallus konjac*)		
Mushrooms	Soup manufacturers	143
	Growers	144
Fungal amylase	Bakers	145, 146
Verticillium albo-atrum	Greenhouse workers	147

Agents encountered in food industries that are known to induce OA are listed in Table 21.2. It is not possible to discuss each agent, or even each group of agents, in detail in this chapter; instead specific examples will be given when appropriate.

Organic dust derived from bacteria, fungi, protozoa, plant and animal products, and simple chemicals can induce hypersensitivity pneumonitis. A list of agents encountered in food industries that are known to induce HP are given in Table 21.3. Many of these

materials are of fungal origin. Coffee dust has been omitted from this list because the single case of "coffee worker's lung" (180) was subsequently redescribed as cryptogenic fibrosing alveolitis associated with rheumatoid arthritis (181).

A wide variety of foods, additives, and flavorings, as well as materials used in food preparation, are known to induce several types of occupational skin disease. Table 21.4 lists etiologic agents, along with diagnoses. Some materials, such as seafood and garlic,

Table 21.3
Etiology of Hypersensitivity Pneumonitis Occurring in Food and Food-Related Industries

Agent	Source	Disorders	References
Thermophilic Actinomycetes			
Faenia rectivirgula	Moldy hay	Farmer's lung	148
(*Micropolyspora faeni*)	Moldy compost	Mushroom worker's lung	149
Thermoatinomyces sacchari	Moldy sugar cane	Bagassosis	150
T. vulgaris	Moldy compost	Mushroom worker's lung	151
	Moldy hay	Farmer's lung	152
T. viridis	Vineyards	Vineyard sprayer's lung	153
Fungus			
Aspergillus clavatus	Moldy barley/malt	Malt worker's lung	154–156
A. clavatus	Moldy cheese	Cheese worker's lung	157
A. flavus	Moldy corn	Farmer's lung	158
A. fumigatus	Vegetable compost		159
A. oryzae	Soy sauce brewer		160
Cladosporium	Moldy hay	Farmer's lung	152
Mucor stolonifer	Moldy paprika pods	Paprika slicer's disease	161
Penicillium sp.	Moldy hay	Farmer's lung	152
P. caseii	Cheese	Cheese worker's lung	162, 163
P. roqueforti	Cheese	Cheese worker's lung	164
Botrytis cinerea	Moldy grapes	Wine-grower's lung	165
Insects			
Grain weevil (*Sitophilus grainarius*)	Infested wheat	Miller's lung	166, 167
Cheese mites (*Acarus siro*)	Cheese	Cheese worker's lung	168
Animal Products			
Duck proteins	Feathers	Duckfever	169
Chicken proteins	Chicken products	Feather plucker's disease	170, 171
	Hen litter		172
Turkey proteins	Turkey products	Turkey handler's disease	173
Goose proteins	Feathers		169
Bird proteins	Fishermen		174
Fish meal	Fishmeal workers		175
Plant Products			
Mushrooms	Spores	Mushroom worker's disease	176
Miscellaneous			
Erwina herbicoa (*Enterobacter agglomerans*)	Contaminated grain	Grain worker's lung	177
Tea plants		Tea grower's lung	178
Oyster shells	Oyster shell dust		179

Table 21.4
Dermatitis in Food Processing and Food Service Workers

Industry	Exposure	Diagnosis	References
Agriculture			
Milk controllers, milk recorders, milkers	Bronopol, Kathon CG	Dermatitis	182, 183
Milk testers	Chrome, dichromate		184, 185
Milk analyzers	Dichromate	Allergic contact dermatitis	186
Ewe milker		Dermatitis	187
Celery harvesters	Celery fungus (*Sclerotinia sclerotiorum*)	Phototoxic dermatitis	20, 21
Apple packers	Apples sprayed with ethoxyquin	Allergic contact dermatitis	188
Orange pickers	Omite-CR	Dermatitis	189
Grocery Workers	Celery (furocoumarins)		22, 190
Food Preparation			
Fish factory workers	Fish, mustard	Dermatitis, contact urticaria	191
Cooks	Mustard, rape	Eczema	192
Cooks	Garlic/onions	Eczema	193
Cooks	Paprika, curry	Contact dermatitis	194
Salad makers	Mustard	Dermatitis	195
Food workers	Cashew nuts (cardol)	Dermatitis	196
Sandwich makers	Codfish, plaice, chicken, onion, garlic	Dermatitis	18
Food workers	Lettuce	Dermatitis	197
Food workers	Lettuce, chicory, endive	Contact dermatitis	198
Bakers	Sodium metabisulfite	Dermatitis	200
	Persulfate		201
	Cinnamon		202
	Sorbic acid		203
	Propyl gallate	Allergic contact dermatitis	204
	Dodecyl gallate	Eczema	205
	Propyl gallate	Eczema	206
	Chromium	Eczema	207
	Flour mite	Dermatitis	207
	Sugar mite	Dermatitis	208
	Karaya gum	Dermatitis	209
	Flour	Contact urticaria	207
Butchers/Poultry Processors			
Butchers	Rubber boots	Allergic contact dermatitis	210
Butchers	Knife handle	Dermatitis	211, 212
Butchers	Povidone-iodine	Allergic contact dermatitis	213
Slaughtermen	Blood (cow and pig)	Contact urticaria	214
Slaughterhouseman	Gut casings	Eczema	215
Butchers	Calf's liver	Urticaria	216
Butchers	Pig's gut	Urticaria	217
Butchers	Beef	Urticaria	218
Poultry workers	Various	Irritant allergic dermatitis, eczema	219
Chicken vaccinators	Antibiotics	Contact dermatitis	220
Seafood			
Fishmarket workers	Shrimp	Allergic contact urticaria	221
Caterers	Shrimp	Contact urticaria	222
Seafood processors	Prawns	Asthma, dermatitis	45
Oyster shuckers	Oysters	Dermatitis	223
Mussel processors	Mussels	Dermatitis	224
Food handlers	Fish and shellfish	Contact dermatitis	18
Food handlers	Cuttlefish		225

Table 21.4
(Continued)

Industry	Exposure	Diagnosis	References
Seafood (*cont.*)			
Fishermen	Fish	Skin diseases	226
Fish workers	Fish	Contact urticaria	227
Cooks	Fish	Contact urticaria	228
Fishermen	Fish	Dermatoses	229
Caterers	Fish	Dermatitis	19
Trawlermen	Bryozoa	Dermatitis, eczema	230
			231
Fishermen	Rubber boots	Dermatitis	232
Fishnet repairers	Fishnets	Dermatitis	233
Miscellaneous			
Snackbar meat products	Penicillin residues	Dermatitis	234
Spice workers	Turmeric	Allergic contact dermatitis	235
Spice workers	Cinnamon, cinnamic aldehyde		236
Margarine manufacturers	Octyl gallate	Eczema	237
Margarine workers		Dermatitis	238
Peanut butter manufacturers	Octyl gallate	Dermatitis	239
Food workers	Sesame oil	Contact sensitivity	240
Food workers	Artichokes	Eczema	241
Confectioners	Cardamom	Allergic contact dermatitis	242
Cookie workers	"Thin mint" cookies	Eczema	243
Beekeepers	Propolis	Dermatitis	244, 245
Beekeepers	Beeswax (poplar resin)	Dermatitis	246
Coconut climber	Coconut trees/coconuts	Dermatitis	247
Bartender	Citrus peel, geraniol citral	Allergic contact dermatitis	248

commonly induce dermatitis, whereas others, including nonfood items such as betadine, are seldom reported to cause occupational skin disease.

Occupational Asthma

The characteristic bronchospasm observed in OA may result from irritative, pharmacologic, or type I, IgE-mediated mechanisms (249). Complex organic mixtures, such as grain dust, have numerous biological actions, which may or may not be pathogenic. Other agents induce OA by as-yet-undefined mechanisms.

IRRITATIVE RESPONSES

Irritative responses, which do not require prior sensitization, can result from high-level exposure to any dust, aerosol, or vapor. They are particularly associated with exposure to several organic dusts. For example, green coffee beans are known to induce IgE-mediated OA in susceptible individuals. Because roasting destroys or denatures the allergen (250, 251), workers exposed to only roasted beans do not develop IgE-mediated disease. On the other hand, some individuals exposed occupationally to roasted coffee report irritation or burning of the skin, eyes, nose, or throat, and nasal bleeding (33, 252). Cinnamon workers (116) and chili grinders (253) also experience what are presumed to be irritant responses.

PHARMACOLOGIC MECHANISM

The classic example of acute asthma caused by a pharmacologic mechanism occurs in farm workers exposed to organophosphate insecticides (254). These chemicals irreversibly inactivate cholinesterase, which causes an accumulation of acetylcholine, with subsequent bronchospasm.

IMMUNE MECHANISMS

Many agents encountered in the workplace are antigenic or allergenic and elicit type I, IgE-mediated reactions in sensitized individuals. As with other agents inducing IgE-mediated OA, only a small proportion of exposed workers develop disease. A latent period, ranging from several weeks to years, precedes onset of symptoms. Several specific examples resulting from exposure to allergens found in food industries are reviewed below.

Coffee Worker's Asthma

For centuries, the growing, production, and importing and exporting of coffee have represented important components of world trade. In 1982, 150 coffee companies employed 11,800 persons in the United States alone. Exposure to allergens from green coffee (or castor) beans has been shown to induce OA (6, 255–257), which is IgE-mediated (127, 258–260). In one study, all individuals diagnosed as having OA by provocative inhalation challenge had positive results to a skin and radioallergosorbent test (RAST) (127). In workers who did not have asthma per se, but who reported respiratory symptoms, 69% had positive skin tests to coffee extracts, as compared with 14% of those without symptoms (7). Jones and associates (6) demonstrated that although 17% to 18% of workers with respiratory symptoms produced positive skin tests, only 3% to 5% had OA. The decreased prevalence of skin reactivity and OA in the latter population of coffee workers may reflect the more sophisticated industrial hygiene practices in today's automated coffee plants.

A link appears to exist between the atopic state and disease induced by green coffee bean dust. Seventy-four percent of individuals with work-related symptoms and specific skin reactivity were atopic, as compared with 40% of those reporting neither symptoms nor skin reactivity (7). Another study of 50 selected workers showed that 40% of sensitized individuals—but only 10% of nonsensitized individuals—were atopic (33). The prevalence rates of coffee-related symptoms in individuals with asthma or bronchitis were 85% and 90%, respectively, suggesting that an irritative mechanism induced or exacerbated symptoms in these individuals (7).

Cereal-Grain-Induced Lung Diseases

Occupational exposure to cereal grains affects both grain handlers and bakers. In Canada, an estimated 175,000 farmers handle grain; an additional 30,000 workers are employed in grain elevators. Equivalent numbers of individuals are exposed to grain or grain dust in the United States, Australia, the former Soviet Union, and Argentina (261). It has been known for centuries that exposure to grain dust can induce respiratory diseases (262); these conditions have been subsequently described as chronic obstructive pulmonary disease (263, 264), "grain fever" (265, 266), and OA (267, 268). A variety of mechanisms—both allergic and nonallergic—have been postulated to generate grain-dust-induced bronchospasm. A correlation between positive skin reactions to grain dust extracts and decline in lung function has been shown by some investigators (267), although others found no such relationship (268, 269). Grain dust can activate complement by both the classic and alternative pathways (270) and can release mast cell mediators from human lung fragments (271). Identification of the etiologic agent has proved extremely difficult, as the dust is a complex mixture consisting of a variety of cereal grains and their disintegration products, pollens, fungi, insects, mites, pigeon and rodent excrement, silicon dioxide, and pesticides (272).

By contrast, the pathophysiology of asthma in bakers is more clearly understood. It is IgE-mediated (96, 98, 273, 274), and wheat and rye flour have been implicated as etiologic agents (98, 275–277). Furthermore, most cereal grains, including wheat, rye, triticale, barley, and oat, share common allergenic determinants (96, 278). Sensitization to wheat flour is correlated with atopy, NSBH, duration of exposure (279), and dust levels (273). Although few studies have examined the prevalence of OA in established bakers, the prevalence of flour allergy in bakers or millers is estimated to vary from 10% to 30%. The results of one study evaluating development of skin reactivity suggested that duration of exposure is an important factor. Bakery apprentices in West Berlin were skin-tested, and a progressive increase was noted in individuals whose skin tests were positive—8% to 30%—over a 5-year period (9). These figures correspond with the number of established bakers reporting allergic symptoms (258). In the former West Germany, approximately 300 bakers per year claim occupational disease and one-fourth of them receive compensation for their illness.

Beekeeper or Honey Processor's Respiratory Disease

More than 1600 commercial beekeepers—that is, individuals who keep more than 300 colonies—operate in the United States. Approximately 30 companies process honey on a year-round basis for interstate shipment. In addition, thousands of hobbyists keep bees for production of honey. Workers in these industries are exposed to several potential allergens, most notably honey bee venom and fragmented bees. Although allergic reactions have been associated with exposure to either or both allergens, OA appears to be more closely associated with inhalation of fragmented bees. No systemic epidemiologic studies have been conducted among beekeepers or honey processors, and industry-wide prevalences of sensitization to these allergens are unknown. According to one report, 3 of 17 workers (17.6%) in a honey processing plant experienced adverse symptoms following seasonal exposure to honey bees (79). Skin test and RAST demonstrated the presence of honey bee whole-body-specific IgE antibodies in symptomatic workers; RAST inhibition was used to demonstrate that bee body parts and venom were distinct components (80). Individuals may also be sensitive to both allergens. In another study, 14 of 19 atopic beekeepers or their family members (73.7%) gave clinical histories that suggested whole-body sensitivity (81).

Exposure to honey per se is seldom implicated in adverse allergic reactions, occupational or otherwise. In individuals exposed occupationally to bees or pollens, incidents of apparent honey allergy have been reported (134, 251). Pollen grains, which contaminated the honey, were the etiologic agent.

Hypersensitivity Pneumonitis

Type III or type IV hypersensitivity reactions are thought to occur in subjects with HP. The presence of IgG-precipitating antibodies in symptomatic individuals is highly suggestive of a type III reaction, although the role of precipitins in disease pathogenesis is disputed (282). Data suggesting a cell-mediated type IV response also confuse the issue (178). Mushroom worker's lung represents a good example of this disease.

MUSHROOM WORKER'S LUNG

During 1986 and 1987, more than 615 million pounds of mushrooms (with a cash value of $539 million) were produced by 476 growers in the United States. Hypersensitivity pneumonitis among mushroom workers was first reported in 1959 (151), and the term "mushroom worker's lung" was coined in 1967 (149). As with most allergic respiratory diseases in food-related industries, no systematic studies of this disease have been conducted, and information is derived from isolated cases and small "outbreaks" (Table 21.5).

Mushroom worker's lung is caused by a variety of antigens associated with the cultivation of mushrooms—notably microorganisms and mushroom spores (Table 21.5). Specific exposures depend on where an individual works in the operation, harvest conditions, and which mushroom species are involved. Most cultivated mushrooms are grown in compost. During fermentation of compost, temperatures as high as 60 °C are generated and growth of thermophilic organisms flourishes. Meanwhile, a growth medium is inoculated with mushroom spores; after growth begins, this material is transferred onto grain. The combination, called spawn, is mixed with fermented compost prior to seeding mushroom beds. High levels of thermophilic actinomycetes are liberated during the mixing process, with actinomycete spore levels of $7.4 \times 10^8/m^3$ having been detected (298). Thermophilic organisms are the traditional source of "mushroom worker's lung antigen." Species may potentially include *Thermomonospora* sp., *Streptomyces* sp., *Thermoactinomyces vulgaris*, and *Faenia rectivirgula* (298). *Fungi imperfecti*, including *Aspergillus fumigatus* and *Penicillium notatum*, also occur in mushroom houses; although they have been associated with respiratory symptoms, conclusive immunologic evidence of their involvement in disease pathogenesis is lacking.

Mushroom spores can also cause HP in sensitive individuals. Although most commercial mushrooms

Table 21.5
Reported Cases of Mushroom Worker's Lung

Number of Patients	Geographic Location	Antibodies	Reference
16	U.S.A.	*T. vulgaris*	151
4	U.K.	*Faenia rectivirgula*	149
2	U.K.	Mushroom compost	283
2	Canada		284
1	Canada	Compost (prior to spawn)	285
6	U.K.	Compost, spores (*Pleurotus ostreatus*)	286
NS	Germany	"Spore-rich part of fungus"	287
NS			288
17	U.K.	A variety of thermophilic actinomycetes, but not *F. rectivirgula* or *T. vulgaris*; *Aspergillus fumigatus*	289
	France		290
NS	Germany	*P. ostreatus*, "spore-rich part of fungus"	291
8			292
1	U.S.A.		293
1	U.S.A.	*T. vulgaris, F. rectivirgula, Cephalosporium acremonium, Pullalaria pullulons, Psalliota campestris*	294
3	France		295
4	U.K.		296
4	U.S.A.		297

NS = not stated.

(*Agaricus* sp.) are harvested prior to sporulation, workers can be exposed to high spore levels if picking occurs after this stage, or if other, more exotic mushrooms, such as oyster (*Pleurotus ostreatus*) and shiitake (*Lentinus edodes*), which sporulate continuously, are cultivated. Spore loads greater than $10^6/m^3$ have been detected in shiitake growing facilities (299).

Occupational asthma has been shown to occur in both mushroom growers (144) and soup processors (143). In growers, the etiologic agent is spores, while the antigen is dried mushroom powder in soup processors. Asthma resulting from exposure to mushrooms is distinct from HP and occurs in different individuals.

Occupational Dermatitis

In addition to OA, bakers can suffer from a variety of skin diseases associated with occupational exposure to dough, flour, additives, and flavorings (Table 21.6). Most reactions are irritant, rather than allergic, and result from continuous exposure to wet, sticky dough, sweetening agents, or flavorings. Irritant responses can be distinguished from allergic reactions by patch testing with putative agents. In addition, atopic dermatitis is frequently seen as the result of exposure to a variety of antigens (Table 21.6). Flour itself can induce contact urticaria, and flour contaminants—for example, mites—can induce occupational dermatoses in sensitive workers.

Table 21.6
Additives Encountered by Bakers That Can Cause Skin Disease

Irritants	Allergens
Emulsifiers	Benzoyl peroxide
Acetic acid	Potassium bromate
Lactic acid	Cinnamon oil
Calcium acetate/sulfate	Limonen, oil of
Yeast	Balsam of Peru
Potassium iodide/bromate	*p*-Amino-azo-benzene
Potassium bicarbonate	Eugenol
Bleaching agents	Vanilla
Ascorbinic acid	Sorbic acid
	Karaya gum
	Ammonium persulfate
	Sodium metabisulfite

Relationship of Sensitization Routes: Inhalation at the Workplace Versus Ingestion at Home

The relationship between sensitization by inhalation and symptomatology following inhalation or ingestion of the same or a related antigen is intriguing. Exposure to food allergens typically occurs only via ingestion. Having subjects sensitized to traditional food allergens by inhalation presents an opportunity to compare elements of the two exposure routes. Most food-related occupational allergens have not been shown to induce symptoms following ingestion by workers sensitized by inhalation. In some individuals, certain allergens (e.g., garlic) can elicit symptoms following inhalation and ingestion. A spice factory worker who developed asthma following inhalation of garlic dust noted the immediate onset of wheezing after eating garlic-containing foods (110). A provocative challenge with garlic aerosol produced an immediate 35% reduction in forced expiratory volume in 1 second (FEV_1). An oral challenge with 1600 mg of garlic (in capsules) induced apprehension, flushing, and nausea within 10 minutes. Diarrhea, increased pulse rate, and a 21% reduction in FEV_1 appeared within 2 hours. In contrast to the immediate response to inhalation challenge and natural ingestion of garlic-containing foods, maximal symptoms were noted 2 hours after laboratory challenge, suggesting that inhalation of garlic vapors or absorption through the oral mucosa was necessary to produce an immediate response. Buckwheat (300), pineapple protease (122), snow crab (48), and honey/pollens (134, 281) have also been shown to produce allergic reactions following inhalation and ingestion by sensitive subjects.

Some individuals sensitized by inhalation to one occupational agent report symptoms following ingestion of a related antigen. A bird breeder developed OA following exposure to birds concomitant with an exquisite gastrointestinal sensitivity to ingested chicken eggs. Her primary sensitization involved bird serum antigens, which cross-reacted with ingested egg yolk proteins (68). Butcher and colleagues (301) described an individual who developed and lost sensitivity to TDI vapor and ingested radishes, which contain isothiocyanates. The latter case is of particular interest, because, unlike vapors, the vast majority of particulates and aerosols that are nominally inhaled are actually swallowed.

Diagnosis

HISTORY

Individuals with suspected OA usually experience episodic dyspnea, chest tightness, or wheezing. When a subject with suspected OA is evaluated, the diagnosis of asthma must be confirmed via physical examination and objective evidence of reversible airway disease. It is also vital to obtain a complete history, including an occupational history. The history should identify whether symptoms began a short time after a job or workplace change, if new materials or processes were introduced into the workplace, if agents with known asthma-inducing potential are used in the workplace, and if other workers exhibit similar symptoms. Usually, a latent period occurs between first exposure and development of symptoms; the length of this latency can range from weeks to more than 20 years. In individuals with OA, symptoms must be temporally correlated with workplace exposure. In immediate-type asthma, this relationship is usually apparent. In subjects with late, dual, or recurrent nocturnal asthma (described below), a workplace connection may be less obvious.

Hypersensitivity pneumonitis can manifest in two forms (157, 178, 302). Intermittent exposure usually produces acute disease characterized by dyspnea, chills, fever, cough, and malaise beginning 4 to 6 hours after exposure (303, 304). Symptoms usually subside 18 to 24 hours after cessation of exposure; they may, however, recur with subsequent exposure. Repeated episodes may lead to weight loss. When exposure is continuous but less intense, chills and fever may be absent; cough, exertional dyspnea, fatigue, and weight loss are common, however. As no laboratory tests are available for diagnosis of HP, physical examination and history have paramount importance.

In the acute form of HP, physical examination reveals fine bilateral crackles. Occasionally, rhonchi or wheezes can be detected, although asthma rarely constitutes a part of this disease syndrome. Peripheral blood leukocytosis, with or without eosinophilia, also occurs (305). Chest radiographs are usually consistent with a diffuse interstitial or alveolar filling process; occasionally findings suggest pulmonary edema. If episodes are infrequent, radiographs may be normal. As with OA, history is extremely important and disease must be temporally correlated with exposure.

In evaluating patients with occupational skin disease, physical examination is also important. The appearance helps to determine whether the dermatitis is endogenous (constitutional), contact, or a combination of the two. Atopic dermatitis is characterized by large areas of pruritic, confluent papules and prominent lichenification. Distribution may suggest a probable cause. Approximately 90% of occupational dermatitis involves the hands—usually the backs and palmar surface of the wrist (2). When occupational disease is suspected, matching the location of the dermatitis and the exposure source becomes necessary. Actual or simulated workplace practices may aid in accomplishing this task.

LABORATORY TESTS

Knowledge of the etiologic agent is important to understanding pathogenetic mechanisms. Identification of the agent may ultimately lead to changes in the workplace environment and decreased incidence of disease. When the putative agent is antigenic, laboratory tests may help establish a diagnosis of OA. Some of these tests can be performed at the workplace, but others must be conducted in a laboratory.

Skin prick tests with common environmental antigens, including pollens, molds, and dusts, are used to identify atopic individuals. In addition, skin testing with specific occupational allergens may assist in establishing a diagnosis of OA or monitoring workplace populations; positive skin tests are not themselves diagnostic, however. Antigens encountered in food industries are very suitable for this type of testing. As with all skin testing, care must be exercised, particularly with allergens of extreme potency, such as bromelain, which may induce systemic reactions (120).

Specific IgE levels can be assessed using RAST. Like skin prick tests, RAST can be used to evaluate both individuals and populations. Although it is less sensitive than skin tests, RAST is more convenient for the testing of industrial populations. Serum can be collected during the worker's regular plant physical, so that the employee does not have to be removed from the production line for testing, and a physician's presence is not required. RAST can also be used for retrospective studies (306).

RAST inhibition is used to confirm the specificity of the RAST. Such testing can also be used to evaluate cross-reactivity among allergens (127), to identify allergens in areas where workers are exposed to multiple or complex agents, and to carry out environmental monitoring (79).

Double gel diffusion is frequently used to document exposure to relevant antigens in subjects with suspected HP. Many individuals with this disease have antibodies directed against the offending antigen. For example, as many as 90% of individuals with farmer's lung have serum precipitins; on the other hand, a significant percentage of farmers exposed to moldy hay who have no history of disease also have serum precipitins (307, 308). Thus, the presence of such antibodies merely confirms exposure and cannot be used to make a definitive diagnosis.

The patch test represents the only practical assay for demonstrating allergic contact dermatitis (309). In the classic patch test, the putative agent is applied to a piece of cloth or paper that is then placed on intact skin and covered with an impermeable substance. The patch is affixed to the skin with tape. After 24 or 48 hours, the patch is removed and the underlying skin examined. No standard method of testing for contact urticaria has been developed. Many materials produce urticaria following contact with intact skin; clinically relevant allergens can be demonstrated only after application to dermatitic skin or by skin prick test. Regardless of the technique used, tests are read at 20 to 30 minutes. As some agents, including balsam of Peru, can induce positive results by nonimmunologic mechanisms, appropriate controls must be included in the test.

RESPIRATORY REACTIONS IN WORKERS EXPOSED TO FOOD ANTIGENS

Respiratory response patterns seen in individuals with OA or HP resulting from exposure to food antigens do not differ from those observed in subjects with allergic lung disease due to exposure to common environmental or other occupational antigens. Three types of airway responses are noted in asthma: immediate, late, and dual. Figure 21.2 illustrates these responses in sensitized seafood workers. In an immediate response, a decline in expiratory flow rates (usually expressed as a decline in FEV_1) occurs within minutes of exposure, reaches a peak within 30 minutes, and resolves, frequently spontaneously, within 2 hours. Late reactions are not manifested clinically for several hours (2–10 hours); they reach their peak several hours thereafter and can last 36 hours or more. One type of late-phase reaction, recurrent nocturnal asthma, recurs at approximately the same time on successive nights following a single exposure; this response has been described in subjects exposed to the grain mite *(Glycyphagus destructor)* (310). Some individuals experience a dual response (combined immediate and late). If exposure dose is controlled, as could occur in a laboratory challenge, dose dependency can sometimes be demonstrated.

Individuals with acute forms of HP may undergo a restrictive effect, with a decline in forced vital capacity (FVC), diffusion capacity, and compliance (Fig. 21.3). This response usually occurs 4 to 6 hours after challenge and is characterized clinically by chills, fever, dyspnea, and crepitant rales on auscultation. Some individuals with HP may also experience an immediate response characterized by a decline in FVC and expiratory flow rates. These events are followed by the more characteristic delayed response (157).

Challenge Testing

NONSPECIFIC BRONCHIAL HYPERREACTIVITY

Nonspecific bronchial hyperreactivity is usually assessed by provocative challenge with methacholine or histamine; methods have been described previously

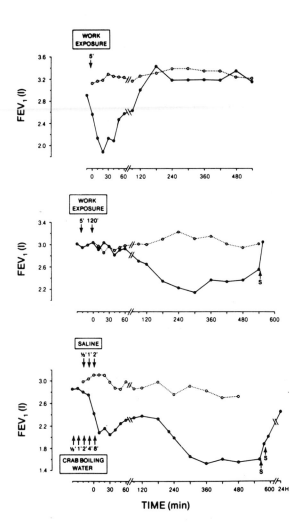

Figure 21.2

Examples of the three patterns of asthmatic responses (immediate, late or nonimmediate, and dual) are illustrated at the top, middle, and bottom, respectively. Open circles are values obtained on control days; solid circles, on exposure days. The examples in the top and middle graphs illustrate challenges performed in the work environment, whereas the challenge illustrated in the bottom graph was carried out under laboratory conditions by nebulization of saline (open circles) and crab-boiling water extract (solid circles). Salbutamol (albuterol) inhalation. Reprinted, with permission, from Cartier A, Malo J-L, Forest P, *et al.* Occupational asthma in snow crab processing workers. J Allergy Clin Immunol 1984;74:261–269.

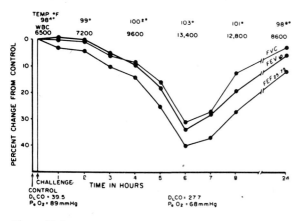

Figure 21.3

Typical clinical and physiologic response to inhalation challenge with *Micropolyspora faeni* in a patient with farmer's lung disease. FEF_{25-75}, forced expiratory flow at 25% to 75% FVC; D_LCO, pulmonary diffusing capacity. Reprinted, with permission, from Schlueter DP. Infiltrative lung disease hypersensitivity pneumonitis. J Allergy Clin Immunol 1982;70:50–55.

(311, 312). These tests confirm the diagnosis of asthma, but cannot determine the putative agent or the pathogenic mechanisms. The majority of individuals with OA appear to have NSBH, although this result is not a universal finding (134). The relationship between development of OA and methacholine sensitivity is not clear. Late asthmatic reactions to occupational agents are associated with transient increases in airway hyperresponsiveness (313, 314). The increase in NSBH following a late or dual asthmatic reaction suggests that it may result from an inflammatory response—a finding that is true of all such reactions and is not limited to exposure to occupational agents (315).

It is not clear whether NSBH predisposes an individual to develop OA. It appears, however, that NSBH may develop concomitantly with asthma, as individuals with no history of disease prior to entering the workplace may develop and continue to demonstrate bronchial reactivity in the absence of exposure (316). Prospective studies are needed to assess more fully the relationship between NSBH and specific occupational sensitization.

SPECIFIC CHALLENGE

Traditionally, challenges with food allergens are performed by ingestion. To simulate industrial exposures, on the other hand, inhalation challenges must be performed. Provocative inhalation challenge can be conducted at the workplace or in a controlled laboratory environment. In a simple workplace "challenge," spirometry is performed before and after the work shift. This type of testing simply demonstrates a decline in lung function over the work period. Although spirometry cannot identify putative agents or even a definite temporal relationship with a workplace exposure, it can give important information concerning lung function of exposed populations. This type of testing has been used successfully in tea (130), herb tea (132), and grain workers (317, 318), as well as meat wrappers (93).

In the more traditional workplace challenge, subjects use a portable peak-flow meter to make recordings at preestablished time intervals, both at work and at home. Workplace readings are compared with those obtained during time away from work. A temporal relationship between decline in peak flow and work suggests the presence of a work-related obstructive airway disease (Fig. 21.4). Workplace challenges have been used successfully in both the seafood (8) and egg processing industries (70).

This type of testing has several advantages: (1) risk is minimal, as the individual has presumably encountered this level of exposure previously; (2) cost is low; and (3) hospital admission is unnecessary. Disadvantages include the following: (1) the lack of close supervision means that, although overt fraud is uncommon, test results may reflect submaximal effort; (2) tests cannot be "blinded"; (3) it is difficult to perform adequate controls; (4) workers find it demanding to perform these tests; and (5) the tests usually cannot identify the causative agent definitively.

Laboratory challenge is the method of choice for diagnosis of OA and identification of the etiologic agent (319). This type of testing is indicated when evaluations involve materials not previously known to induce asthma or when precise identification of the etiologic agent is necessary, as when litigation may follow. No other test provides such definitive

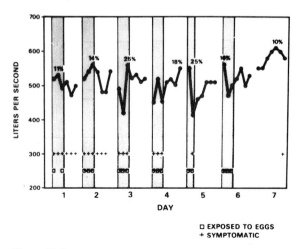

Figure 21.4

Changes in peak-flow measurements during a workplace challenge in subjects reactive to eggs. Reprinted, with permission, from Smith AB, Bernstein DI, Aw T-C, *et al.* Occupational asthma from inhaled egg protein. Am J Ind Med 1987;12:205–218.

results; specificity and sensitivity of provocative challenge can reach 100%. Other tests are less time-consuming, potentially hazardous, and costly, however.

Treatment

The best "treatment" for allergic occupational disease is prevention. In some industries, reduction of exposure levels may reduce the incidence of respiratory symptoms among workers. Even in industries in which threshold limit values have been established, however, levels of exposure that induce hypersensitivity reactions are not known. Once an individual has experienced such reactions, asthmatic responses will occur at minute exposure levels, usually less than any industrial plant can maintain.

Preemployment screening and periodic health monitoring have been suggested as ways to prevent development of allergic respiratory disease. Questions arise over which tests are appropriate. In industries in which atopy is suggested as a predisposing factor for the development of asthma, exclusion of atopic

individuals from the workplace has been demonstrated not to eliminate the problem (320). Skin prick testing with specific allergens may prove useful for monitoring, although positive responses do not necessarily correlate with disease.

Preemployment methacholine testing has also been proposed. Mounting evidence suggests, however, that NSBH develops concomitantly in many individuals who develop OA.

Once an occupational respiratory disease has been diagnosed, the individual should be removed permanently from further exposure. For OA, even brief, intermittent exposure following sensitization can increase the severity of disease (300, 321). Moreover, continued exposure after onset of symptoms may adversely affect prognosis (322).

In rare cases when the worker cannot be removed from the offending environment, prophylactic bronchodilator or cromolyn therapy may be attempted. The efficacy of these treatments applied on a regular basis in the workplace is not known. No data have been gathered that suggest that drug treatment can prevent development of chronic OA. For HP, corticosteroids represent the treatment of choice if avoidance cannot be immediately effected. Protective devices, including dust masks or respirators, can also minimize exposure, but frequently prove ineffective because of poor fit or lack of compliance.

More extreme treatment measures, such as immunotherapy, have been attempted on a limited scale. In a double-blind immunotherapy trial with partially purified green coffee bean extract, Osterman found that responses of skin and challenge testing diminished during treatment (33). Immunotherapy is contraindicated as a treatment for HP because of the possibility of immune-complex-mediated damage to the vascular system (157).

As with respiratory disease, drug treatment of occupational dermatoses produces only temporary benefit unless the individual receives no further exposure. This isolation can be difficult to achieve in an occupational setting if suitable alternative employment for the affected individual cannot be found. Furthermore, in industry, replacement of materials that are allergenic with other appropriate ones may not be feasible. Protective measures that reduce skin contact, such as rubber gloves, may be used if avoidance is impossible. It should not be automatically assumed that such devices are impervious to all materials; however, and latex gloves themselves have been demonstrated to induce allergic reactions in sensitive subjects (323–326).

Prognosis

To date, follow-up studies on individuals with OA who are employed in food industries have been limited to snow crab workers (322). The average period of follow-up was 13.4 ± 6.0 months. Subjects with OA continued to have bronchospasm and increased NSBH following cessation of exposure. When compared with subjects in a non-food-related industry, like those exposed to Western red cedar, workers with crab-induced asthma demonstrated a significant improvement in NSBH following cessation of exposure. The small sample size should be borne in mind, however, before any definitive conclusions are drawn.

Factors influencing prognosis in subjects with OA have not been clearly identified. Nevertheless, they probably include the duration of symptoms before diagnosis, the type of airway response (immediate versus late or dual), lower initial values for pulmonary function tests, and the degree of NSBH (322, 327).

One important question is whether an individual with OA who no longer demonstrates specific antigen reactivity can be reintroduced into the workplace. One snow crab processing worker who continued to suffer from symptoms of asthma 1 year following removal from the workplace had a negative provocative challenge, and was subsequently reintroduced into a crab processing area. Her respiratory symptoms worsened, and upon a later rechallenge with crab, she experienced an asthmatic exacerbation (322). Although this example was the only one that we could find in a food-related industry, similar results have been reported in the chemical industry (328). Together these data support the hypothesis that any individual with OA should be removed permanently from the workplace.

The prognosis for individuals with HP depends primarily on the amount of damage at the time of diagnosis and the ability of the individual to avoid contact with the etiologic agent. Avoidance of the allergen can prove particularly difficult in the case of small, family-run farms. In the acute form of the disease, clinical abnormalities reverse themselves, and, as long as no further exposure occurs, the subjects remain symptom-free. Individuals with chronic disease who have severe pulmonary function abnormalities do not have reversible disease (157).

The majority of individuals with contact dermatitis have an excellent prognosis, provided that exposure to the allergen is eliminated. If an employee cannot change jobs, dermatitis can become chronic. Chronic dermatitis can also occur in some subjects despite the apparent elimination of allergen exposure. This condition is particularly troublesome in industrial settings and may reflect complex exposures or mixed disease—endogenous or irritant dermatitis, or psoriasis.

Conclusion

Exposure to a wide variety of food-derived and food-associated materials encountered in the workplace is associated with development of occupational asthma, hypersensitivity pneumonitis, or dermatitis in sensitized individuals. The number of causative agents will undoubtedly continue to rise as new agents are introduced into the workplace and as physician awareness of these conditions continues to grow. Very little is known about the prevalence and incidence, importance of host factors, preemployment screening, treatment, or prognosis of the occupational diseases resulting from exposure to these antigens. As the number of individuals employed in the food industry grows, the need for this type of information will increase significantly.

Acknowledgments

The authors acknowledge Drs. Robert M. Adams and Maria Christina Soto-Aquilar's review of the manuscript and the word processing of Mrs. Anita Kivell.

Support by the National Institute of Allergy and Infectious Disease (grant AI-19266) and by a grant from the National Fisheries Institute is gratefully acknowledged.

REFERENCES

1. National data book and guide to sources. Statistical abstract of the United States, 108th ed. Washington, D.C.: U.S. Department of Commerce, Bureau of the Census, 1988, 607.
2. Emmett EA. Occupational skin diseases. J Allergy Clin Immunol 1983;72:649–656.
3. Butcher BT, Hendrick DJ. Occupational asthma. Clin Chest Med 1983;4:43–53.
4. Kobayashi S. Different aspects of occupational asthma in Japan. In: Frazier CA, ed. Occupational asthma. New York: Van Nostrand Reinhold, 1980, 229–244.
5. Gervais P, Rosenberg N. Occupational respiratory allergy: epidemiologic and medicolegal aspects. In: Reed CE, ed. Proceedings of the XII International Congress of Allergology and Clinical Immunology. St. Louis: CV Mosby, 1986, 480–485.
6. Jones RN, Hughes JM, Lehrer SB, et al. Lung function consequences of exposure and hypersensitivity in workers who process green coffee beans. Am Rev Respir Dis 1982;125:199–202.
7. Kaye M, Freedman SO. Allergy to raw coffee—an occupational disease. Can Med Assoc J 1961;84:469–471.
8. Cartier A, Malo J-L, Forest F, et al. Occupational asthma in snow-crab processing workers. J Allergy Clin Immunol 1984;74:261–269.
9. Herxheimer H. The skin sensitivity to flour of baker's apprentices: a final report of long term investigation. Acta Allergologica 1967;28:42–49.
10. NIOSH criteria for a recommended standard. Occupational exposure to diisocyanate. NIOSH publication 78-215. Washington, D.C.: U.S. Department of Health, Education and Welfare, 1978.
11. Chan-Yeung M. Occupational asthma. Clin Rev Allergy 1986;4:251–266.
12. Parrot JL, Hebert R, Saindelle A, Ruff A. Platinum and platinosis. Allergy and histamine release due to some platinum salts. Arch Environ Health 1969;19:685–691.
13. Figley KD. Mayfly (Ephemerida) hypersensitivity. J Allergy 1940;11:376–387.
14. Grant INB, Blyt W, Wardrop VE, Gordon RM. Prevalence of farmer's lung in Scotland: a pilot survey. Br Med J 1972;1:530–534.
15. Madsen D, Klock LE, Wenzel FJ, Robbins JL, Schmidt CD. The prevalence of farmer's lung in an agricultural population. Am Rev Respir Dis 1976;113:171–174.
16. Peltonen L, Wickstrom G, Vaahtoranta M. Occupational dermatoses in the food industry. Dermatosen 1985;33:166–169.
17. Veien N, Hattel T, Justesen O, Norholm A. Causes of eczema in the food industry. Dermatosen 1983;31:84–86.
18. Hjorth N, Roed-Petersen J. Occupational protein contact dermatitis in food handlers. Contact Dermatitis 1976;2:28–42.
19. Cronin E. Dermatitis of the hands in caterers. Contact Dermatitis 1987;17:265–269.
20. Birmingham DJ, Key MM, Tubich GE, Perone VB. Phototoxic bullae among celery harvesters. Arch Dermatol 1961;83:73–87.
21. Austad J, Kavli G. Phototoxic dermatitis caused by celery infected by Sclerotinia sclerotiorum. Contact Dermatitis 1983;9:448–451.
22. Berkley SF, Hightower AW, Beier RC, et al. Dermatitis in grocery workers associated with high natural concentrations of furocoumarins in celery. Ann Intern Med 1986;105:351–355.
23. Novey HS, Keenan WJ, Fairshter RD, Wells ID, Wilson AF, Culver BD. Pulmonary disease in workers exposed to papain: clinico-physiological and immunological studies. Clin Allergy 1980;10:721–731.
24. Mink JT, Gerrard JW, Cockcroft DW, Cotton DJ, Dosman JA. Increased bronchial reactivity to inhaled histamine in nonsmoking grain workers with normal lung functions. Chest 1980;77:28–31.
25. Brummund W, Kurup VP, Resnick A, Milson TJ Jr, Fink JN. Immunologic response to Faenia rectivirgula (Micropolyspora faeni) in a dairy farm family. J Allergy Clin Immunol 1988;82:190–195.
26. Allen DH, Basten A, Woolcock AJ. HLA and bird breeder's hypersensitivity pneumonitis. Monogr Allergy 1977;11:45.
27. Flaherty DK, Iha T, Chmelik F. HLA-8 in farmer's lung disease. Lancet 1975;2:507.
28. Rittner C, Sennekamp J, Vogel F. HLA-B8 in pigeon fancier's lung. Lancet 1975;2:1303.
29. Rodey EF, Fink J, Koethe S, et al. A study of HLA-A, B, C, and DR specificities in pigeon breeder's disease. Am Rev Respir Dis 1979;119:755–759.
30. Rasmussen JE, Provost TT. Atopic dermatitis. In: Middleton E Jr, Reed CE, Ellis EF, eds. Allergy, principles and practice, 2nd ed. St. Louis: CV Mosby, 1983, 1297–1312.
31. Hulbert WC, Walker DC, Jackson A, Hogg JC. Airway permeability to horseradish peroxidase in guinea pigs: the repair phase after injury by cigarette smoke. Am Rev Respir Dis 1981;123:320–326.
32. Zetterstrom O, Osterman K, Machado L, Johanson SGO. Another smoking hazard: raised serum IgE concentration and increased risk of occupational allergy. Br Med J 1981;283:1–7.
33. Osterman K. Coffee worker's allergy. A clinical and immunological study. PhD dissertation, Uppsala University, 1984, 48.
34. Patel KR, Symington IS, Pollack R, Shaw A. A pulmonary survey of grain handlers in the west of Scotland. Clin Allergy 1981;11:121–129.
35. Cotton DJ, Graham BL, Li KY, Froh F, Barnett CD, Dosman JA. Effects of respiratory symptoms and lung function. J Occup Med 1983;25:131–141.
36. Belin L. Clinical and immunological data on "wood trimmer's disease" in Sweden. Eur J Respir Dis 1980;61(suppl 17):169–176.
37. Warren SPW. Extrinsic allergic alveolitis: a disease commoner in non-smokers. Thorax 1977;32:567.
38. Hapke EJ, Seal RME, Thomas GO, Hayes M, Meek JC. Farmer's lung: a clinical, radiographic, functional and serological correlation of acute and chronic stages. Thorax 1968;23:451–468.
39. Parkes WR. Occupational lung disorders, 2nd ed. London: Butterworths, 1982.
40. Albert RE, Peterson HT Jr, Bohning DE, Lippman M. Short-term effects of cigarette smoking on bronchial clearance in humans. Arch Environ Health 1975;30:361–367.
41. Gough J. Emphysema in relation to occupation. Ind Med Surg 1960;29:283–285.

42. Chan-Yeung M, Lan S. Occupational asthma. Am Rev Respir Dis 1986;133:686–703.
43. O'Neil CE, Salvaggio JE. The pathogenesis of occupational asthma. In: Kay AB, ed. Ballieres clinical immunology and allergy. The allergic basis of asthma, vol. 2. Philadelphia: WB Saunders, 1988, 143–175.
44. Gaddie J, Legge J, Friend JAR, Reid TMS. Pulmonary hypersensitivity in prawn workers. Lancet 1980;2:1350–1353.
45. McSharry C, Wilkinson PC. Serum IgG and IgE antibody against aerosolized antigens from *Nephrops norwegicus* among seafood process workers. Adv Exp Med Biol 1987;216A:865–868.
46. Asthma-like illness among crab-processing workers—Alaska. MMWR 1982;31:95–96.
47. Orford R, Wilson JT. Epidemiologic and immunologic studies in processors of the King crab. Am J Ind Med 1985;7:155–169.
48. Cartier A, Malo J-L, Ghezzo H, McCants M, Lehrer SB. IgE sensitization in snow crab-processing workers. J Allergy Clin Immunol 1986;78:344–348.
49. Patel PC, Cockcroft DW. Occupational asthma caused by exposure to cooking lobster in the work environment: a case report. Ann Allergy 1992;68:360–361.
50. Nakashima T. Studies on bronchial asthma observed in cultured oyster workers. Hiroshima J Med Sci 1969;18:141–184.
51. Wada S, Nishimoto Y, Nakashima T, Shigenobu T, Onari K. Clinical observation of bronchial asthma in workers who culture oysters. Hiroshima J Med Sci 1967;16:255–266.
52. Carino M, Elia G, Molinini R, Nuzzaco A, Ambrosi L. Shrimp-meal asthma in the aquaculture industry. Med Lav 1985;76:471–475.
53. Droszcz W, Kowalski J, Piotrowska B, Pawlowicz A, Piebruszewzka E. Allergy to fish meal in fish meal factory workers. Int Arch Occup Environ Health 1981;49:13–19.
54. Zuskin E, Kanceljak B, Schacter EN, Witek TJ, Maayani S, Goswami S, Marom Z, Rienzi N. Immunological and respiratory changes in animal food processing workers. Am J Ind Med 1992;21:177–191.
55. Tas J. Respiratory allergy caused by mother of pearl. Isr J Med Sci 1972;81:630.
56. Jyo T, Komoto K, Tsubai S, Katsutani T, Otsuka T, Oka S. Sea squirt asthma—occupational asthma induced by inhalation of antigenic substances contained in sea squirt body fluid. Allergy Immunol 1974/1975;20/21:435–448.
57. Jyo T, Katsutani T, Otsuka T. Studies on sea squirt asthma. Sea squirt asthma in workers engaged in pearl cultivations. Arerugi 1967;16:668–672.
58. Kim WH, Lee SK, Lee HC, et al. Shell-grinder's asthma. Yonsei Med J 1982;23:123–130.
59. Sherson D, Hansen I, Sigsgaard T. Occupationally related respiratory symptoms in trout-processing workers. Allergy 1989;44:336–341.
60. Rautalahti M, Terho EO, Vohlomen I, Husman K. Atopic sensitization of dairy farmers to work-related and common allergens. Eur J Respir Dis 1987;71(suppl 152):155–164.
61. Terho EO, Husman K, Vohlonen I, Rautalahti M, Tukiainen H. Allergy to storage mites or cow dander as a cause of rhinitis among Finnish dairy farmers. Allergy 1985;40:23–26.
62. Virtanen T, Vilhunen P, Husman K, Manyjarvi R. Sensitization of dairy farmers to bovine antigens and effects of exposure on specific IgG and IgE titers. Int Arch Allergy Appl Immunol 1988;87:171–177.
63. Bernaola G, Echechipia S, Urrutia I, Fernandez E, Audicana M, Fernandez de Corres L. Occupational asthma and rhino-conjunctivitis from inhalation of dried cow's milk caused by sensitization of alpha-lactalbumin. Allergy 1994;49:189–191.
64. Harries MG, Cromwell O. Occupational asthma caused by allergy to pig's urine. Br Med J 1982;284:867.
65. Matson SC, Swanson MC, Reed CE, Yuninger JW. IgE and IgG-immune mechanisms do not mediate occupation-related respiratory or systemic symptoms in hog farmers. J Allergy Clin Immunol 1983;72:299–304.
66. Zuskin E, Kanceljak B, Schacter EN, Mustajbegovic J, Goswami S, Maayani S, Marom Z, Rienzi N. Immunological and respiratory findings in swine farmers. Environ Res 1991;56:120–130.
67. Bar-Sela S, Teichtahl H, Lutsky I. Occupational asthma in poultry workers. J Allergy Clin Immunol 1984;73:271–275.
68. Hoffman DR, Guenther DM. Occupational allergy to avian proteins presenting as allergy to ingestion of egg yolk. J Allergy Clin Immunol 1988;81:484–488.
69. Bernstein DI, Smith AB, Moller DR, et al. Clinical and immunologic studies among egg-processing workers with occupational asthma. J Allergy Clin Immunol 1987;80:791–797.
70. Smith AB, Bernstein DI, Aw T-C, et al. Occupational asthma from inhaled egg protein. Am J Ind Med 1987;12:205–218.
71. Edwards JH, McConnochie K, Trotman DM, Collins D, Saunders MJ, Latham SM. Allergy to inhaled egg material. Clin Allergy 1983;13:427–432.
72. Smith AB, Bernstein DI, London MA, Gallagher J, Ornella GA, Gelletly SK, Wallingford K, Newman MA. Evaluation of occupational asthma from airborne egg protein exposure in multiple settings. Chest 1990;98:398–404.
73. Bernstein JA, Kraut A, Bernstein DI, Warrington R, Bolin T, Warren CP, Bernstein IL. Occupational asthma induced by inhaled egg lysozyme. Chest 1993;103:532–535.
74. Lutsky I, Teichtahl H, Bar-Sela S. Occupational asthma due to poultry mites. J Allergy Clin Immunol 1984;73:56–60.
75. Lutsky I, Bar-Sela S. Northern fowl mite (*Ornithonyssus sylviarum*) in occupational asthma of poultry workers (letter). Lancet 1982;2:874–875.
76. Cuthbert OD, Brostoff J, Wraith DG, Brighton WD. "Barn allergy": asthma and rhinitis due to storage mites. Clin Allergy 1979;9:229–236.
77. Ingram CG, Jeffrey IG, Symington IS, Cuthbert OD. Bronchial provocation studies in farmers allergic to storage mites. Lancet 1979;2:1330–1332.
78. Cuthbert OD, Jeffrey IG, McNeil HB, Wood J, Topping MD. Barn allergy among Scottish farmers. Clin Allergy 1984;14:197–206.
79. Ostrom NK, Swanson MC, Agarwal MK, Yuninger JW. Occupational allergy to honeybee-bodydust in a honey-processing plant. J Allergy Clin Immunol 1986;77:736–740.
80. Reisman RE, Hale R, Wypych JL. Allergy to honey-bee body components: distinction from bee venom sensitivity. J Allergy Clin Immunol 1983;71:18–20.
81. Yuninger JW, Jones RT, Leiferman KM, Paull BR, Welsh PW, Gleich GJ. Immunological and biochemical studies in bee-keepers and their family members. J Allergy Clin Immunol 1978;61:93–101.
82. Randolph H. Allergic response to dust of insect origin. JAMA 1934;103:560–562.
83. Schultze-Werninghaus G, Zachgo W, Rotermund H, Wiewrodt R, Merget R, Wahl R, Burow G, zur Strassen R. *Tribolium*

confusum (confused flour beetle, rice flour beetle)—an occupational allergen in bakers: demonstration of IgE antibodies. Int Arch Allergy Appl Immunol 1991;94:371–372.

84. Cartier A, Malo J-L, Pineau L, Dolovich J. Occupational asthma due to pepsin. J Allergy Clin Immunol 1984;73:574–577.

85. Colten HR, Polakoff PL, Weinstein SE, Strieder DJ. Immediate hypersensitivity to hog trypsin resulting from industrial exposure. N Engl J Med 1975;292:1050–1053.

86. Pilat L, Teculescu D. Bronchial asthma and allergic rhinitis associated with inhalation of pancreatic extracts (letter). Am Rev Respir Dis 1975;112:275.

87. Hill D. Pancreatic extract lung sensitivity. Med J Aust 1975;2:553–555.

88. Paggiaro PL, Loi AM, Toma G. Bronchial asthma and dermatitis due to spiramycin in a chick breeder. Clin Allergy 1979;9:571–574.

89. Andrasch RH, Bardana EJ Jr, Koster F, Pirofsky B. Clinical and bronchial provocation studies in patients with meatwrapper's asthma. J Allergy Clin Immunol 1976;158:291–298.

90. Polakoff PI, Lapp NL, Reger R. Polyvinyl chloride pyrolysis products: a potential cause of respiratory impairment. Arch Environ Health 1975;30:269–271.

91. Pauli G, Bessot JC, Kopferschmitt MC, *et al*. Meat wrapper's asthma: identification of the causal agent. Clin Allergy 1980;10:263–269.

92. Butler J, Culver BH, Robertson HT. Meat-wrapper's asthma. Chest 1980;80(suppl):71–73.

93. Eisen EA, Wegman DH, Smith TJ. Across-shift changes in the pulmonary function of meat wrappers and other workers in the retail food industry. Scand J Work Environ Health 1985;11:21–26.

94. Aelony Y. "Meat-wrapper's asthma" (letter). JAMA 1976;236:21–26.

95. Andrasch RH, Bardana EJ. Thermoactivated price-label fume intolerance. A cause of meat-wrapper's asthma. JAMA 1976;235:937.

96. Block G, Tse KS, Kijek K, Chan H, Chan-Yeung M. Baker's asthma: clinical and immunologic studies. Clin Allergy 1983;13:359–370.

97. Wilbur RD, Ward GW. Immunological studies in a case of baker's asthma. J Allergy Clin Immunol 1976;58:366–372.

98. Hendrick DJ, Davies RJ, Pepys J. Baker's asthma. Clin Allergy 1976;6:241–250.

99. Gohte CJ, Wieslander G, Ancher K, Forsbeck M. Buckwheat allergy: health food, an inhalation health risk. Allergy 1983;38:155–159.

100. Valdivieso R, Moneo I, Pola J, Munoz T, Zapata C, Hinojosa M, Losada E. Occupational asthma and contact urticaria caused by buckwheat flour. Ann Allergy 1989;63:149–152.

101. van der Brempt X, Ledent C, Mairesse M. Rhinitis and asthma caused by exposure to carob bean flour. J Allergy Clin Immunol 1992;90(pt 1):1008–1010.

102. Lim HH, Domala Z, Joginder S, Lee SH, Lin CS, Abu Baker CM. Rice miller's syndrome: a preliminary report. Br J Ind Med 1984;41:445–459.

103. World Health Organization. Recommended health-based occupational exposure limits for selected vegetable dusts. Technical report series 684. Geneva: WHO, 1983.

104. Bush RK, Cohen M. Immediate and late onset asthma from occupational exposure to soybean dust. Clin Allergy 1977;7:369–373.

105. Lavaud F, Perdu D, Prevost A, Vallerand H, Cossart C, Passemard F. Baker's asthma related to soybean-lecithin-induced asthma in bakers. Allergy 1994;49:159–162.

106. Tse KS, Warren P, Janusz M, McCarthy DS, Cherniack RM. Respiratory abnormalities in workers exposed to grain dust. Arch Environ Health 1973;27:74–77.

107. Cockcroft AE, McDermott M, Edwards JH, McCarthy P. Grain exposure—symptoms and lung function. Eur J Respir Dis 1983;64:189–196.

108. Darke CS, Knowelden J, Lacey J, Ward AM. Respiratory disease of workers harvesting grain. Thorax 1976;31:294–302.

109. doPico GA, Reddan W, Flaherty D, *et al*. Respiratory abnormalities among grain handlers. Am Rev Respir Dis 1977;115:915–927.

110. Lybarger JA, Gallagher JS, Pulver DW, Litwin A, Brooks S, Bernstein IL. Occupational asthma induced by inhalation and ingestion of garlic. J Allergy Clin Immunol 1982;69:448–454.

111. Falleroni AE, Zeiss CR, Levitz D. Occupational asthma secondary to inhalation of garlic dust. J Allergy Clin Immunol 1981;68:156–160.

112. Henson GE. Garlic: an occupational factor in the etiology of bronchial asthma. J Fla Med Assoc 1940;27:86.

113. Couturier P, Bousquet J. Occupational allergy secondary to inhalation of garlic dust. J Allergy Clin Immunol 1982;70:145.

114. van Toorenenberger AW, Dieges PH. Immunoglobulin E antibodies against coriander and other spices. J Allergy Clin Immunol 1985;76:477–481.

115. Zuskin E, Kanceljak B, Skuric Z, Pokrajac D, Schacter EN, Witek TJ, Maayani S. Immunological findings in spice-factory workers. Environ Res 1988;47:95–108.

116. Uragoda C. Asthma and other symptoms in cinnamon workers. Br J Ind Med 1984;41:224–227.

117. van Toorenenberger AW, Dieges PH. Occupational allergy in horticulture: demonstration of immediate-type allergic reactivity in freesia and paprika plants. Int Arch Allergy Appl Immunol 1984;75:44–47.

118. Igea JM, Fernandez M, Quirce S, de la Hoz B, Gomez MLD. Green bean hypersensitivity: an occupational allergy in a homemaker. J Allergy Clin Immunol 1994;94:33–35.

119. Ueda A, Manda F, Aoyama K, Ueda T, Obama K, Li Q, Tochigi T. Immediate-type allergy related to okra (*Hibiscus esculentus* Linn) picking and packing. Environ Res 1993;62:189–199.

120. Gailhofer G, Wilers-Truschnig M, Smolle J, Ludvan M. Asthma caused by bromelain: an occupational allergy. Clin Allergy 1988;18:445–450.

121. Galleguillos F, Rodriguez JC. Asthma caused by bromelain inhalation. Clin Allergy 1978;8:21–24.

122. Baur X, Fruhmann G. Allergic reactions, including asthma to the pineapple protease bromelain following occupational exposure. Clin Allergy 1979;9:443–450.

123. Baur X, Fruhmann G. Papain-induced asthma: diagnosis by skin test, RAST and bronchial provocation test. Clin Allergy 1979;9:75–81.

124. Baur X, Konig G, Bencze K, Fruhmann G. Clinical symptoms and results of skin test, RAST and bronchial provocation test in thirty-three papain workers: evidence for strong immunogenic potency and clinically relevant proteolytic effects of airborne papain. Clin Allergy 1982;12:9–17.

125. Milne J, Brand S. Occupational asthma after inhalation of

dust of the proteolytic enzyme, papain. Br J Ind Med 1975;32:302–307.

126. Flindt ML. Respiratory hazards from papain. Lancet 1978;1:430–432.

127. Karr RM, Lehrer SB, Butcher BT, Salvaggio JE. Coffee worker's asthma: a clinical appraisal using the radioallergosorbent test. J Allergy Clin Immunol 1978;62:143–148.

128. Patussi V, De Zotti R, Riva G, Fiorito A, Larese F. Allergic manifestations due to castor beans: an undue risk for the dock workers handling green coffee beans. Med Lav 1990;81:301–307.

129. Uragoda CG. Tea maker's asthma. Br J Ind Med 1970;27:181–182.

130. Zuskin E, Skuric Z. Respiratory function in tea workers. Br J Ind Med 1984;41:88–93.

131. MacKay DM. Disease patterns in tea garden workers in Bangladesh. J Occup Med 1975;19:469–472.

132. Castellan RM, Boehlecke BA, Petersen MR, Thedell TD, Merchant JA. Pulmonary function and symptoms in herbal tea workers. Chest 1981;79:81S–85S.

133. Dulton LO. Beet pollen and beet sugar seed dust causing hayfever and asthma. J Allergy 1938;9:607–609.

134. Bousquet J, Dhivert H, Clauzel A-M, Hewitt B, Michel F-B. Occupational allergy to sunflower pollen. J Allergy Clin Immunol 1985;75:70–74.

135. Tsukioka K, Hirono S, Ishikawa K. A case of occupational grape pollinosis. Arerugi Jpn J Allergol 1984;33:247–250.

136. Cohen AJ, Forse MS, Tarlo SM. Occupational asthma caused by pectin inhalation during the manufacture of jam. Chest 1993;103:309–311.

137. Kraut A, Peng Z, Becker AB, Warren CP. Christmas candy maker's asthma. IgG4-mediated pectin allergy. Chest 1992;102:1605–1607.

138. Lachance P, Cartier A, Dolovich J, Malo J-L. Occupational asthma from reactivity to an alkaline hydrolysis derivative of gluten. J Allergy Clin Immunol 1988;81:385–390.

139. Klaustermeyer WB, Bardana EJ, Hale FC. Pulmonary hypersensitivity to Alternaria and Aspergillus in baker's asthma. Clin Allergy 1977;7:227–233.

140. So SY, Lam WK, Yu D. Colophony-induced asthma in a poultry vender. Clin Allergy 1981;11:395–399.

141. Newmark FM. Hops allergy and terpene sensitivity: an occupational disease. Ann Allergy 1978;41:311–312.

142. Kobayashi S. Occupational asthma due to inhalation of pharmacologic dusts and other chemical agents with some reference to other occupational asthma in Japan. In: Yamamura Y, Frick O, Hariuchi Y, et al., eds. Allergology. Amsterdam: excerpta medica, 1974, 124–132.

143. Symington IS, Kerr JW, McLean DA. Type I allergy in mushroom soup processors. Clin Allergy 1981;11:43–47.

144. Shichijo K, Kondo T, Yamada M, Aoki M, Shimoyama K, Taya T. A case of bronchial asthma caused by spore of Lentinus edodes (Berk) Sing. Jpn J Allergy 1969;18:35–39.

145. Flindt MLH. Allergy to alpha-amylase and papain. Lancet 1979;1:1407–1408.

146. Blanco Carmona JG, Juste Picon S, Garces Sotillos M. Occupational asthma in bakeries caused by sensitization to alpha-amylase. Allergy 1991;46:274–276.

147. Davies PDO, Jacobs R, Mullins J, Davies BH. Occupational asthma in tomato growers following an outbreak of the fungus Verticillium albo-atrum in the crop. J Soc Occup Med 1988;38:13–17.

148. Cross T, Maciver A, Lacey L. The thermophilic actinomycetes in mouldy hay: Micropolyspora faeni sp. J Gen Microbiol 1968;50:351–359.

149. Sakula A. Mushroom worker's lung. Br Med J 1967;3:708–710.

150. Seabury J, Salvaggio J, Buechner H, Kundur VG. Bagassosis. III. Isolation of thermophilic and mesophilic actino-mycetes and fungi from moldy bagasse. Proc Soc Exp Biol Med 1969;129:351–360.

151. Bringhurst LS, Byrne RN, Gershon-Cohen J. Respiratory disease of mushroom workers. JAMA 1959;171:15–18.

152. Belin L. Health problems caused by actinomycetes and moulds in the industrial environment. Allergy 1985;40(suppl):24–29.

153. Salvaggio JE. Diagnosis and management of hypersensitivity pneumonitis. Hosp Prac November 1980:93–103.

154. Channell S, Blyth W, Lloyd M, et al. Allergic alveolitis in maltworkers. A clinical, mycological and immunological study. QJ Med 1969;38:351–376.

155. Grant IW, Blackadder ES, Greenberg M, Blyth W. Extrinsic allergic alveolitis in Scottish maltworkers. Br Med J 1976;1:490–493.

156. Riddle HFV, Channell S, Blyth W, et al. Allergic alveolitis in a malt-worker. Thorax 1968;23:271–280.

157. Fink J. Hypersensitivity pneumonitis. J Allergy Clin Immunol 1984;74:1–9.

158. Patterson R, Sommers H, Fink JN. Farmer's lung following inhalation of Aspergillus flavus growing in mouldy corn. Clin Allergy 1974;4:79–86.

159. Vincken W, Roels P. Hypersensitivity pneumonitis due to Aspergillus fumigatus in compost. Thorax 1984;39:74–75.

160. Tsuchiya Y, Shimokata K, Ohara H, Nishiwaki K, Kino T. Hypersensitivity pneumonitis in a soy sauce brewer caused by Aspergillus oryzae. J Allergy Clin Immunol 1992;89:1061–1062.

161. Hunter D. The diseases of occupations. London: The English Universities Press, 1959, 942.

162. De Weck AL, Gutersohn J, Butikofer E. La maladie des laveurs de fromage ("Kasewascherkrankheit") une forme particuliere du syndrome du poumon du fermier. Schweiz Med Wochenchr 1969;99:872–876.

163. Minning H, De Weck AL. Die "Kasewascher-krankheit." Immunologische epidemiologische studien. Schweiz Med Wochenschr 1972;102:1205–1212.

164. Campbell JA, Kryda MJ, Treuhaft MW, Marx JJ Jr, Roberts RC. Cheese worker's hypersensitivity pneumonitis. Am Rev Respir Dis 1983;127:495–496.

165. Popp W, Ritschka L, Zwick H, Rauscher H. "Beerenausleselunge" oder Winzerlunge-eine exogen-allergische alveolitis ausgelost durch Botrytis cinerea-Sporen. Prax Klin Pneumol 1987;41:165–169.

166. Lunn JA. Millworker's asthma: allergic response to the grain weevil (Sitophilus granarius). Br J Ind Med 1966;23:149–152.

167. Lunn JA, Hughes DTD. Pulmonary hypersensitivity to the grain weevil. Br J Ind Med 1967;24:158.

168. Pepys J. Occupational allergic lung disease caused by organic agents. J Allergy Clin Immunol 1986;78:1058–1062.

169. Plessner MM. Une maladiedes trieurs de plumes: la fieve de canard. Arch Mal Prof 1960;21:67–69.

170. Warren CPW, Tse KS. Extrinsic allergic alveolitis owing to hypersensitivity to chickens—significance of sputum precipitins. Am Rev Respir Dis 1974;109:672–677.

171. Elman AJ, Tebo T, Fink JN, Barboriak JJ. Reactions of poultry farmers against chicken antigens. Arch Environ Health 1968;17:98–100.

172. Korn DS, Florman AL, Gribetz I. Recurrent pneumonitis with hypersensitivity pneumonitis to hen litter. JAMA 1968;205:114–115.

173. Boyer RS, Klock LE, Schmidt CD, et al. Hypersensitivity lung disease in the turkey raising industry. Am Rev Respir Dis 1974;109:630–635.

174. Luksza AR, Bennett P, Earis JE. Bird fancier's lung: hazard of the fishing industry. Br Med J (Clin Res Ed) 1985;291:1766.

175. Avila R. Extrinsic allergic alveolitis in workers exposed to fish meal and poultry. Clin Allergy 1971;1:343–346.

176. Cox A, Folgering HTM, van Griensven LJLD. Extrinsic allergic alveolitis caused by spores of the oyster mushroom Pleurotus ostreatus. Eur Respir J 1988;1:466–468.

177. Dutkiewicz J, Kus L, Dutkiewicz E, Warren CPW. Hypersensitivity pneumonitis in grain farmers due to sensitization to Erwinia herbicola. Ann Allergy 1985;54:65–68.

178. Hammar S. Hypersensitivity pneumonitis. In: Rosen PP, Fechner RE, eds. Pathology annual: 1988, part 1. Norwalk, CT: Appleton and Lange, 1988, 195–215.

179. Weiss W, Bauer X. Antigens of powdered pearl-oyster shell causing hypersensitivity pneumonitis. Chest 1987;91:146–168.

180. Van Toorn DW. Coffee worker's lung. A new example of extrinsic allergic alveolitis. Thorax 1970;25:339–405.

181. Van den Bosch JM, Van Toorn DW, Wegenaar SS. Coffee worker's lung: reconsideration of a case report. Thorax 1983;38:720.

182. Grattan GEH, Harman RRM, Tan RSH. Milk recorder dermatitis. Contact Dermatitis 1986;14:217–220.

183. Grattan GEH, Harman RRM. Bronopol eczema in a milk controller. Br J Dermatol 1985;113:43.

184. Rogers S, Burrows D. Contact dermatitis to chrome in milk testers. Contact Dermatitis 1975;1:387.

185. Rudski E, Czerwinska-Dihnz I. Sensitivity to dichromate in a milk analysis laboratory. Contact Dermatitis 1977;3:107–108.

186. Huriez C, Martin P, Lefebvre M. Sensitivity to dichromate in a milk analysis laboratory. Contact Dermatitis 1975;1:247–248.

187. Quirce S, Olaguibel JM, Muro MD, Tabar AI. Occupational dermatitis in a ewe milker. Contact Dermatitis 1992;27:56.

188. Wood WS, Fulton R. Allergic contact dermatitis from ethoxyquin in apple packers. Contact Dermatitis Newsletter 1972;11:295.

189. Saunders LD, Ames RG, Knaak JB, Jackson RJ. Outbreak of Omite-CR-induced dermatitis among orange pickers in Tulare County, California. J Occup Med 1987;29:409–413.

190. Seligman PJ, Mathias CG, O'Malley MA, et al. Phytophotodermatitis from celery among grocery store workers. Arch Dermatol 1987;123:1478–1482.

191. Kavli G, Moseng D. Contact urticaria from mustard in fishstick production. Contact Dermatitis 1987;17:153–155.

192. Meding B. Immediate hypersensitivity to mustard and rape. Contact Dermatitis 1985;13:121–122.

193. Van Ketel WG, de Haan P. Occupational eczema from onion and garlic. Contact Dermatitis 1978;4:53–54.

194. Hafner J, Riess CE, Wuthrich B. Protein contact dermatitis from paprika and curry in a cook. Contact Dermatitis 1992;26:51–52.

195. Dannaker CJ, White IR. Cutaneous allergy to mustard in a salad maker. Contact Dermatitis 1987;16:212–214.

196. Marks JG Jr, DeMelfi T, McCarthy MA, et al. Dermatitis from cashew nuts. J Am Acad Dermatol 1984;10:627–631.

197. Binkel HJ, Bayleat RM. Occupational dermatitis due to lettuce. JAMA 1932;98:137–138.

198. Friis B, Njorth N, Vail JT Jr, Mitchell JC. Occupational contact dermatitis from Cichorium (chicory, endive) and Lactuca (lettuce). Contact Dermatitis 1975;1:311–313.

199. Aberer W. Occupational dermatitis from organically grown parsnip (Pastinaca sativa L.). Contact Dermatitis 1992;26:62.

200. Apetato M, Marques MSJ. Contact dermatitis caused by sodium metabisulfite. Contact Dermatitis 1986;14:194.

201. White IR, Catchpole HE, Rycroft RJG. Rashes amongst persulphate workers. Contact Dermatitis 1982;8:168–172.

202. Malten KE. Four bakers showing positive patch tests to a number of fragrance materials, which can also be used as flavors. Acta Derm Venereol (Stockh) 1979;59:117–121.

203. Fisher AA. Cutaneous reactions to sorbic acid and potassium sorbate. Cutis 1980;25:350, 352, 423.

204. Bojs G, Nicklasson B, Svenson A. Allergic contact dermatitis to propyl gallate. Contact Dermatitis 1987;17:294–298.

205. Brun R. Kontaktekzem auf Laurylgallat und p-hyroxy-benzolsaureester. Berufsdermatosen 1964;12:281–284.

206. Heine A, Fox G. Backerekzema durch Chromverbindung in Mechlen. Dermatosen 1980;28:113–115.

207. Fisher AA. Hand dermatitis—"a baker's dozen." Cutis 1982;29:214–221.

208. Baker EW, Wharton GW. Acarology. New York: Macmillan, 1952, 327.

209. Figley KD. Karaya gum hypersensitivity. JAMA 1940;114:747–748.

210. Ho VC, Mitchell JC. Allergic contact dermatitis from rubber boots. Contact Dermatitis 1985;12:110–111.

211. Fancalanci S, Giorgini S, Gola M, Sertoli A. Occupational dermatitis in a butcher. Contact Dermatitis 1984;11:320.

212. Cronin E, Calnan CD. Rosewood knife handle. Contact Dermatitis 1975;1:121.

213. Lachapelle JM. Occupational allergic contact dermatitis to providine-iodine. Contact Dermatitis 1984;11:189–190.

214. Goransson K. Occupational contact urticaria to fresh cow and pig blood in slaughtermen. Contact Dermatitis 1981;7:281–282.

215. Hjorth N. Gut eczema in slaughterhouse workers. Contact Dermatitis 1978;4:49–52.

216. Fisher AA, Stengel F. Allergic occupational hand dermatitis due to calf's liver. An urticarial "immediate" type hypersensitivity. Cutis 1977;19:561–565.

217. Moseng D. Urticaria from pig's gut. Contact Dermatitis 1982;8:134–144.

218. Jovanovic M, Oliwiecki S, Beck MH. Occupational contact urticaria from beef associated with hand eczema. Contact Dermatitis 1992;27:188–189.

219. Marks JG, Rainey CM, Rainey MA, Andreozzi RJ. Dermatoses among poultry workers. "Chicken poison disease." J Am Acad Dermatol 1983;9:852–857.

220. Vilaplana J, Romaguera C, Grimalt F. Contact dermatitis from lincomycin and spectinomycin in chicken vaccinators. Contact Dermatitis 1991;24:225–226.

221. Fisher AA. Allergic contact urticaria of the hands due to seafood in food handlers. Cutis 1988;42:388–389.

222. Maibach AI. Regional variation in elicitation of contact urticaria syndrome: shrimp. Contact Dermatitis 1986;15:100.
223. Yamura T, Kurose H. Oyster-shucker's dermatitis. Arerugi 1966;15:813.
224. Zhoutyi VR, Borzov MV. Dermatitis in workers processing mussels. Vestn Dermatol Venerol 1973;47:71–73.
225. Burches E, Morales C, Pelaez A. Contact dermatitis from cuttlefish. Contact Dermatitis 1992;26:277.
226. Rasheia-Kotel'ba B, Khoetska A, Karas Z, Preisler A. Skin diseases in fisherman. Vestn Dermatol Venerol 1979;5:46–47.
227. Beck HI, Nissen BK. Contact urticaria to commercial fish in atopic persons. Acta Derm Venereol (Stockh) 1983;63:257–260.
228. Goransson K. Contact urticaria to fish. Contact Dermatitis 1981;7:282–283.
229. Sabatini C. Fisherman's dermatoses. Folia Med (Napoli) 1969;52:109–117.
230. Newhouse ML. Dogger bank itch among Lowestoft trawlermen. Proc R Soc Med 1966;59:1119–1120.
231. Audebert C, Lamoureux P. Professional eczema of trawlermen by contact with bryozoaires in the "baie de scine": (first French cases 1975–1977). Ann Dermatol Venereol 1978;105:187–192.
232. Ross JB. Rubber boot dermatitis in Newfoundland: a survey of 30 patients. Can Med Assoc J 1969;100:13–19.
233. Rasheia-Kotel'ba B, Chojecka A, Flieger M, Karas Z. Occupational dermatitis and skin changes in workers manufacturing and repairing fishing nets. Przegl Dermatol 1979;66:367–374.
234. de Boer EM, van Ketel WG. Occupational dermatitis caused by snackbar meat products. Contact Dermatitis 1984;11:322.
235. Goh CL, Ng SK. Allergic contact dermatitis to *Curcuma longa* (turmeric). Contact Dermatitis 1987;17:186.
236. Meding B. Skin symptoms in a spice factory. Contact Dermatitis 1993;29:202–205.
237. Burckhardt W, Fierz U. Antioxydantien in der Margarine als Ursache von Gewerbeekzemen. Dermatologica 1964;129:431–432.
238. Rudzki E, Baranowska A. Reactions to gallic acid esters. Contact Dermatitis 1975;1:393.
239. van Ketel WG. Dermatitis from octyl gallate in peanut butter. Contact Dermatitis 1978;4:60–61.
240. Kubo Y, Nonaka S, Yoshida H. Contact sensitivity to unsaponifiable substances in sesame oil. Contact Dermatitis 1986;15:215–217.
241. Gougerot S. Occupational eczema due to artichokes. Bull Soc Franc Dermat Syph 1936;43:1463–1467.
242. Mobacken H, Fregert S. Allergic contact dermatitis from cardamom. Contact Dermatitis 1975;1:175–176.
243. Spencer LV, Fowler JF Jr. "Thin-mint" cookie dermatitis. Contact Dermatitis 1988;18:185–186.
244. Bunney MH. Contact dermatitis in beekeepers due to propolis (bee glue). Br J Dermatol 1968;80:17–23.
245. Melli MC, Giorgini S, Sertoli A. Occupational dermatitis in a bee-keeper. Contact Dermatitis 1983;9:427–428.
246. Rothenborg HW. Occupational dermatitis in bee-keepers due to poplar resins in beeswax. Arch Dermatol 1967;95:381–384.
247. Balachandran C, Srinivas CR, Shenoy SD, Edison KP. Occupational dermatosis in coconut palm climbers. Contact Dermatitis 1992;26:143.
248. Cardullo AC, Ruszkowski AM, DeLeo VA. Allergic contact dermatitis resulting from sensitivity to citrus peel, geraniol, and citral. J Am Acad Dermatol 1989;21(part 2):395–397.
249. Salvaggio JE, O'Neil CE. Occupational asthma caused by organic dusts and chemicals. In: Proceedings of the XII International Congress on Allergology and Clinical Immunology. St. Louis: CV Mosby, 1986, 486–490.
250. Bruun E. Allergy to coffee. Acta Allergol 1957;11:150–154.
251. Layton LL, Greene FC, Panzani R, Corse JW. Allergy to green coffee. J Allergy 1965;36:84–91.
252. Zuskin E, Valic F, Skuric Z. Respiratory function in coffee workers. Br J Ind Med 1979;36:117–122.
253. Uragoda CG. Symptoms among chili grinders. Br J Ind Med 1967;24:162–164.
254. Weiner A. Bronchial asthma due to organic phosphate insecticide. Ann Allergy 1961;19:397–401.
255. Figley KD, Rawling FFA. Castor bean: an industrial hazard as a contaminant of green coffee dust and used burlap bags. J Allergy 1950;21:545–553.
256. Bernton HS. An occupational sensitization—a hazard to the coffee industry. JAMA 1973;223:1146–1147.
257. Zuskin E, Valic F, Kanceljak B. Immunological and respiratory changes in coffee workers. Thorax 1981;36:9–13.
258. Lehrer SB, Karr RM, Salvaggio JE. Extraction and analysis of coffee bean allergens. Clin Allergy 1978;8:217–226.
259. Lehrer SB, Karr RM, Salvaggio JE. Analysis of coffee bean and castor bean allergens using RAST inhibition. Clin Allergy 1981;11:357–366.
260. Osterman K, Johansson SGO, Zetterstrom O. Diagnostic tests in allergy to green coffee. Allergy 1985;40:336–343.
261. Dosman JA. Chronic obstructive pulmonary disease and smoking among grain workers. Ann Intern Med 1977;87:784–786.
262. Ramazzini B. De morbis artificum diatriba. Chicago: University of Chicago Press, 1940.
263. Herbert FA, Woytowich V, Schram E, Baldwin D. Respiratory profiles of grain handlers and sedentary workers. Can Med Assoc J 1981;125:46–50.
264. Broder I, Mintz S, Hutcheon M, et al. Comparison of respiratory variables in grain elevator workers and civic outside workers of Thunder Bay, Canada. Am Rev Respir Dis 1979;119:193–203.
265. Chan-Yeung M, Ashley MJ, Grzybowski S. Grain dust and the lungs. Can Med Assoc J 1978;118:1271–1274.
266. doPico GA, Flaherty D, Bhansali P, Chavaje N. Grain fever syndrome induced by airborne grain dust. J Allergy Clin Immunol 1982;69:435–443.
267. Warren P, Cherniack RM, Tse KS. Hypersensitivity reactions in grain dust. J Allergy Clin Immunol 1974;53:139–149.
268. Chan-Yeung M, Wong R, MacLean L. Respiratory abnormalities among grain elevator workers. Chest 1979;75:461–467.
269. doPico GA, Jacobs S, Flaherty D, Rankin J. Pulmonary reaction to durum wheat; a constituent of grain dust. Chest 1982;81:55–61.
270. Olenchock SA, Mull JC, Major P. Extracts of airborne grain dust activate alternative and classical complement pathways. Ann Allergy 1980;44:23–28.
271. Chan-Yeung M, Chan H, Salari H, Wall R, Tse KS. Grain-dust extract induced direct release of mediators from human lung tissue. J Allergy Clin Immunol 1987;80:279–284.
272. Chan-Yeung M, Enarson D, Grzybowski S. Grain dust and respiratory health. Can Med Assoc J 1985;133:969–973.
273. Blands J, Diamant B, Kailos P, Kallos-Deffner L, Lowenstein

H. Flour allergy in bakers. Int Arch Allergy Appl Immunol 1976;52:392–409.

274. Baldo BA, Krilis S, Wrigley CW. Hypersensitivity to inhaled flour allergens. Comparison between cereals. Allergy 1980;35:45–56.

275. Bjorksten F, Backman A, Jarvinen KAJ, et al. Immunoglobulin E specific to wheat and rye flour proteins. Clin Allergy 1977;7:473–483.

276. Wilbur RD, Ward GW. Immunologic studies in a case of baker's asthma. J Allergy Clin Immunol 1976;58:366–372.

277. Sutton R, Skerritt JH, Balbo BA, Wrigley CW. The diversity of allergens involved in baker's asthma. Clin Allergy 1984;14:93–107.

278. Block G, Tse KS, Kijek K, Chan H, Chan-Yeung M. Baker's asthma: studies of cross-antigenicity between different cereal grains. Clin Allergy 1984;14:177–185.

279. Prichard MG, Ryan G, Walsh BJ, Musk AW. Skin test and RAST responses to wheat and common allergens and respiratory diseases in bakers. Clin Allergy 1985;15:203–210.

280. Thiel H, Ulmer WNT. Baker's asthma: development and possibility of treatment. Chest 1980;78(suppl):400–405.

281. Bousquet J, Campos J, Michel F-B. Food intolerance to honey. Allergy 1984;39:73–75.

282. Burrell R, Rylander R. A critical review of the role of precipitins in hypersensitivity pneumonitis. Eur J Respir Dis 1981;62:332–343.

283. Jackson E, Welch KMA. Mushroom worker's lung. Thorax 1970;25:25–30.

284. Craig DB, Donevan RE. Mushroom worker's lung. Can Med Assoc J 1970;102:1289–1293.

285. Chan-Yeung M, Grzybowski S, Schonell ME. Mushroom worker's lung. Am Rev Respir Dis 1972;105:819–822.

286. Stewart CJ. Mushroom worker's lung—two out-breaks. Thorax 1974;29:252–257.

287. Schulz KH, Felten G, Hausen BM. Allergy to the spores of Pleurotus florida. Lancet 1974;5:29.

288. Lockey SD. Mushroom worker's pneumonitis. Ann Allergy 1974;33:282–288.

289. Stewart CJ, Pickering CAC. Mushroom worker's lung. Lancet 1974;23:317.

290. Oury M, Hocquet P, Simard C, et al. Fibrose pulmonaire chez un champignonniste. Rev Fr Mal Respir 1974;2:594–608.

291. Noster U, Hausen BM, Felten G, Schulz KH. Pilzzuchter-lunge durch Speisepilzsporen. Dtsch Med Wochenschr 1976;101:1241–1245.

292. Stolz JL, Arger PH, Benson JM. Mushroom worker's lung disease. Radiology 1976;119:61–63.

293. Gilliland JL. Mushroom-worker's lung: report of case. J Am Osteopath Assoc 1980;79:411–414.

294. Johnson WM, Kleyn JG. Respiratory disease in a mushroom worker. J Occup Med 1981;23:49–51.

295. Marland P, Tabait J, Bersay CL, et al. Le poumon du champignonniste. Pumon-Coeur 1982;38:371–376.

296. Phillips MS, Robinson AA, Higgenbottam TW, Calder IN. Mushroom compost worker's lung. J R Soc Med 1987;80:674–677.

297. Cox A, Folgering HTM, van Griensven LJLD. Extrinsic allergic alveolitis caused by spores of the oyster mushroom Pleurotus ostreatus. Eur Respir J 1988;1:466–468.

298. Lacey J. Allergy in mushroom workers. Lancet 1974;1:366.

299. Sastre J, Ibanez MD, Lopez M, Lehrer SB. Respiratory and immunological reactions of Shiitake mushroom workers. Clin Allergy 1990;20:13–19.

300. Nakumura S, Yamaguchi M, Oishi M, Hayama T. Studies on the buckwheat allergose report. 1. On the cases with the buckwheat allergose. Allerg Immunol 1974–1975;20–21:449–456.

301. Butcher BT, O'Neil CE, Reed MA, Salvaggio JE, Weill H. Development and loss of toluene diisocyanate (TDI) reactivity: immunologic, pharmacologic, and provocative inhalation challenge studies. J Allergy Clin Immunol 1982;70:231–235.

302. Dickie HA, Rankin J. Farmer's lung: an acute granulomatous interstitial pneumonitis occurring in agricultural workers. JAMA 1958;167:1069–1076.

303. Reed CE, Sosman A, Barbie RA. Pigeon breeder's lung. JAMA 1965;193:261–265.

304. Pepys J. Hypersensitivity diseases of the lung due to fungi and other organic dusts. Monogr Allergy 1969;4:1–147.

305. Chmelik F, doPico G, Reed C, Dickie H. Farmer's lung. J Allergy Clin Immunol 1974;54:180–188.

306. Thorpe SC, Kemeny DM, Panzani R, Lassof MH. Allergy to castor bean. Its relationship to sensitization to common inhalant allergens (atopy). J Allergy Clin Immunol 1988;82:62–66.

307. Pepys J, Jenkins PA. Precipitins (F.L.H.) tests in farmer's lung. Thorax 1965;20:21–35.

308. Lopez M, Salvaggio JE. Diagnostic methods in occupational lung disease. Clin Rev Allergy 1986;4:289–302.

309. Maibach HI, Epstein E. Contact dermatitis. In: Middleton E Jr, Reed CE, Ellis FF, eds. Allergy, principles and practice, 2nd ed. St. Louis: CV Mosby, 1983, 1313–1339.

310. Davies RJ, Green M, McShofield NM. Recurrent nocturnal asthma after exposure to grain dust. Am Rev Respir Dis 1976;114:1011–1019.

311. Townley RJ, Hopp RJ. Inhalation methods for the study of airway responsiveness. J Allergy Clin Immunol 1987;80:111–124.

312. Chai H, Farr RS, Froelich LA. Standardization of inhalation challenge. J Allergy Clin Immunol 1975;56:323–327.

313. Lam S, Wong R, Chan-Yeung M. Non-specific bronchial reactivity in occupational asthma. J Allergy Clin Immunol 1979;63:28–34.

314. Mapp CE, Polato R, Maestrelli P, Hendrick DJ, Fabbri LM. Time course of the increase in airway responsiveness associated with late asthmatic reactions to toluene diisocyanate in sensitized subjects. J Allergy Clin Immunol 1985;75:568–572.

315. Hargreave FE, Dolovich J, O'Byrne PM, Ramsdale EH, Daniel EE. The origin of airway hyperresponsiveness. J Allergy Clin Immunol 1986;78:825–832.

316. Chan-Yeung M. Evaluation of impairment/disability in patients with occupational asthma. Am Rev Respir Dis 1987;135:950–951.

317. Chan-Yeung M, Schulzer M, MacLean L, Dorken E, Grzybowski S. Epidemiologic health survey of grain elevator workers in British Columbia. Am Rev Respir Dis 1980;121:329–337.

318. doPico GA, Reddan W, Anderson S, Flaherty D, Smalley E. Acute effects of grain dust exposure during a work shift. Am Rev Respir Dis 1983;128:399–404.

319. Butcher BT, Hammad YY, Hendrick DJ. Occupational asthma: identification of the agent. In: Gee JBL, ed. Occupational lung disease. New York: Churchill Livingstone, 1984, 111–140.

320. Schumacher MJ, Tait BD, Holmes MC. Allergy to murine

antigens in a biological research institute. J Allergy Clin Immunol 1981;68:310.

321. Paggiaro PL, Loi AM, Rossi O, *et al*. Follow-up study of patients with respiratory disease due to toluene diisocyanate (TDI). Clin Allergy 1984;14:463–469.

322. Hudson P, Cartier A, Pineau L, *et al*. Follow-up of occupational asthma caused by crab and various agents. J Allergy Clin Immunol 1985;76:682–688.

323. Turjanmaa K. Allergy to natural rubber latex: a growing problem (review). Ann Med 1994;26:297–300.

324. Hamann CP. Latex hypersensitivity: an update (review). Allergy Proc 1994;15:17–20.

325. Slater JE. Allergic reactions to natural rubber (review). Ann Allergy 1992;68:203–209.

326. Warpinski JR, Folgert J, Cohen M, Bush RK. Allergic reactions to latex: a risk factor for unsuspected anaphylaxis. Allergy Proc 1991;12:95–102.

327. Chan-Yeung M. Immunologic and non-immunologic mechanisms in asthma due to Western red cedar *(Thuja plicata)*. J Allergy Clin Immunol 1982;70:32–37.

328. Banks DE, Rando RJ. Recurrent asthma induced by toluene diisocyanate. Thorax 1988;43:660–662.

Part Three

ADVERSE REACTIONS
TO FOOD ADDITIVES

22

SULFITES

Steve L. Taylor
Robert K. Bush
Julie A. Nordlee

Sulfites or sulfiting agents include sulfur dioxide (SO_2), sulfurous acid (H_2SO_3), and any of several inorganic sulfite salts that may liberate SO_2 under their conditions of use. The inorganic sulfite salts include sodium and potassium metabisulfite ($Na_2S_2O_5$, $K_2S_2O_5$), sodium and potassium bisulfite ($NaHSO_3$, $KHSO_3$), and sodium and potassium sulfite (Na_2SO_3, K_2SO_3). Sulfites have a long history of use as food ingredients, although potassium sulfite and sulfurous acid are not permitted to be used in food (1). Sulfites may occur naturally in many foods, especially fermented foods such as wines (1, 2). In addition, they have long been used as ingredients in pharmaceuticals (3, 4).

In recent years, questions have arisen about the safety of the continued use of sulfites in foods and drugs. These concerns were voiced following the independent observations in 1981 by David Allen in Australia and Donald Stevenson and Ronald Simon in the United States of the role of sulfites in triggering asthmatic reactions in some sensitive individuals (5–7). While it is now apparent that sulfite sensitivity affects only a small subgroup of the asthmatic population (7–9), concerns remain because sulfite-induced asthma can be severe—even life-threatening—in sensitive individuals.

As a consequence of the concerns related to sulfite-induced asthma, the use of sulfites in foods and drugs has changed considerably over the past 10 years. Sulfites have been replaced in some products, and the search for effective alternatives continues; in addition, the levels of sulfites used have been reduced in other products. Federal regulations have further restricted some uses of sulfites. Nevertheless, the sulfite-sensitive individual must stay alert to avoid inadvertent exposure to sulfites.

Clinical Manifestations of Sulfite Sensitivity

A host of adverse reactions have been attributed to sulfiting agents, as reported to the U.S. Food and Drug Administration (10). These effects include diarrhea, abdominal pain and cramping, nausea and vomiting, urticaria, pruritus, localized angioedema, difficulty in swallowing, faintness, headache, chest pain, loss of consciousness, "change in body temperature," "change in heart rate," and nonspecific rashes. In most instances, diagnostic challenges were not undertaken to confirm the reported adverse reaction. For normal individuals, exposure to sulfiting agents appears to pose little risk. Toxicity studies in normal volunteers showed that ingestion of 400 mg of sulfite daily for 25 days had no adverse effect (11).

NONASTHMATIC RESPONSES TO SULFITES

Various authors have suggested adverse reactions involving several organ systems, but for the most part these effects have not been substantiated by double-blind, placebo-controlled provocation studies. Schmidt *et al.* (12) posited that sulfiting agents may have caused the appearance of a cardiac arrhythmia in a patient given intravenous dexamethasone. This relationship was never confirmed by appropriate challenge, however. Hallaby and Maddocks (13) attributed central nervous system toxicity to the absorption of sodium bisulfite from peritoneal dialysis solutions. Wang *et al.* (14) described eight patients who developed chronic neurological defects after receiving an epidural anesthetic agent that contained sodium bisulfite as a preservative. Using an animal model, they demonstrated that the sulfiting agent produced a similar defect. Whether the clinical manifestation in humans was directly attributable to the bisulfite ingredient is unknown. In a preliminary report, Flaherty and coworkers (15) presented a patient who appeared to have hepatotoxicity as manifested by changes in liver function tests following challenge with potassium metabisulfite.

Other adverse reactions suggestive of a hypersensitivity response have been observed in nonatopic individuals. Epstein (16) described a patient who developed contact sensitivity through exposure to sulfiting agents used in a restaurant; the patient's condition was later confirmed by appropriate patch testing. Belchi-Hernandez *et al.* (17) reported a single case of sulfite-induced urticaria induced by ingestion of sulfited foods and beverages. The role of sulfites was confirmed by double-blind, placebo-controlled challenge, although the pathogenic mechanism involved was not identified. Two patients have been reported (18) who presumably experienced urticaria and angioedema after ingesting sulfiting agents. On open challenge with potassium metabisulfite, one of the individuals experienced generalized urticaria. The study was not repeated using a double-blind procedure. Another individual described in the literature reportedly developed urticaria after administration of sulfited medications (19), although the reaction was not confirmed by challenge. Huang and Frazier (20) presented an individual who developed palmar and plantar pruritus, general urticaria, laryngeal edema, and severe abdominal pain with fulminant diarrhea after ingesting sulfiting agents. In an uncontrolled challenge with a local anesthetic containing 0.9 mg of sodium metabisulfite, the patient experienced palmar pruritus but no generalized urticaria.

ROLE OF SULFITES IN ANAPHYLAXIS

Anaphylactic-like events have been characterized in several individuals, although appropriate confirmatory testing generally was not performed. Prenner and Stevens (21) described a nonasthmatic individual who developed urticaria, pruritus, and angioedema after eating sulfited foods in a restaurant. A single-blind, non–placebo-controlled challenge with sodium metabisulfite produced nausea, coughing, and erythema of the patient's skin. Clayton and Busse (22) reported a patient who developed anaphylaxis after ingesting wine. An open challenge with wine reproduced the patient's symptoms of urticaria, angioedema, and hypotension. While this instance represents a possible case of sulfite sensitivity, specific testing with sulfites was not conducted, nor was any association with sulfiting agents in wine recognized.

Sokol and Hydick (23) identified a single case of sulfite-induced anaphylaxis presenting with urticaria, angioedema, nasal congestion, and nasal polyp swelling that was later confirmed by multiple single-blind, placebo-controlled oral challenge trials. The patient, who had a history of similar food-related reactions, also produced a positive skin test to sulfite, and histamine could be released from her basophils following incubation with sulfites. Yang *et al.* (24) described three patients with systemic anaphylactic symptoms (rhinorrhea with asthma in one; urticaria with asthma in the second; asthma only in the third) confirmed by sulfite challenge. These three patients had positive skin tests to sulfites, and two of the three had positive Prausnitz-Kustner tests. One individual subsequently died, allegedly after ingestion of sulfited food.

In addition, systemic adverse reactions have been attributed to intravenous and inhalation administration of sulfiting agents contained in pharmaceutical agents (25). While receiving bronchodilator therapy with isoetharine, an asthmatic subject developed acute respiratory failure that required mechanical ventilation. The patient subsequently experienced erythematous flushing with urticaria upon intravenous administration of metaclopramide, which contained a sulfiting agent. In placebo-controlled oral provocation with sodium metabisulfite, this patient developed flushing without urticaria, as well as a significant decrease in pulmonary function. Jamieson *et al.* (26) performed inhalation challenge in a patient with presumed sulfite sensitivity. They observed intense pruritus, tingling of the mouth, nausea, chest tightness, and a feeling of impending doom, which would suggest that nonasthmatic responses can be reproduced by sulfite challenge. No placebo challenge was undertaken, however.

Schwartz (27) described two nonasthmatic subjects who developed abdominal distress and hypotension associated with oral challenge with potassium metabisulfite. Placebo-controlled challenges proved negative, however. Wuthrich (28) conducted single-blind, placebo-controlled challenges with sodium bisulfite in 245 patients with suspected sulfite sensitivity. Fifty-seven (15%) of the challenges were positive, including 17 patients with urticaria/angioedema, 7 patients with rhinitis, and 5 patients with local anesthetic reactions. Thus, nonasthmatic manifestations resembling anaphylaxis with multiple-system involvement may occur as an adverse reaction to sulfite.

Studies have been undertaken to determine whether sulfiting agent sensitivity frequently causes idiopathic anaphylaxis (29, 30). Sonin and Patterson (29) conducted sodium metabisulfite challenges on 12 individuals with idiopathic anaphylaxis, nine of whom reported episodes associated with restaurant meals. None of the patients responded to the challenge. One additional patient with chronic idiopathic urticaria and restaurant-associated symptoms was also challenged; this individual also failed to react to the challenge. Meggs *et al.* (30) studied 25 patients with idiopathic anaphylaxis. Two of the individuals reacted on single-blind challenge; after repeating the sulfite and placebo challenge, one of these patients was subsequently found not to be sulfite-sensitive. Another individual appeared to react on repeated challenge and not to placebo. Institution of a sulfite-free diet had no effect on this patient's subsequent episodes. Furthermore, studies by Meggs' group in eight individuals with systemic mastocytosis failed to demonstrate any reactions to sulfite challenge.

Thus, while many adverse reactions have been ascribed to sulfiting agents, the risk appears to be rather low for the nonatopic, nonasthmatic subject. Properly performed double-blind placebo-controlled challenges will be necessary to confirm whether sulfite sensitivity was responsible in suspected adverse reactions.

THE ROLE OF SULFITING AGENTS IN ASTHMA

Although sulfiting agents play a very limited and somewhat controversial role in the production of nonasthmatic adverse reactions, their role in the production of bronchospasm and severe asthma is better established. Kochen (31) was among the first to suggest that ingestion of sulfited food can cause bronchospasm. He described a child with mild asthma who repeatedly experienced coughing, shortness of breath, and wheezing when exposed to dehydrated fruits treated with sulfur dioxide that were packaged in hermetically sealed plastic bags. No direct challenge studies were conducted to confirm this observation, however. Single-dose, open challenges without placebo control performed in a group of asthmatics by Freedman (32, 33) suggested that sulfiting agents could trigger asthma. Eight of 14 subjects with a history of wheezing following consumption of sulfited orange drinks were shown to experience changes in pulmonary function upon administration of an acidic solution containing 100 ppm of sodium metabisulfite.

The role of sulfite sensitivity in asthma became more widely recognized after reports of Stevenson and Simon (6) and Baker *et al.* (5). The initial studies of Stevenson and Simon (6) demonstrated that placebo-controlled oral challenges with potassium metabisulfite could produce significant changes in pulmonary function in certain asthmatics. Their first subjects had steroid-dependent asthma. In addition to their asthmatic response, these individuals experienced systemic symptoms of flushing, tingling, and faintness following sulfite challenges. Work by Baker *et al.* (5) in two steroid-dependent asthmatics showed that oral ingestion and intravenous administration of sulfites could cause significant bronchoconstriction, to the point of becoming a respiratory arrest. In a preliminary study, Baker and Allen (34) reported a spectrum of asthmatic responses to sulfite, including an immediate decline in pulmonary function occurring 1 to 5 minutes after ingestion of an acidic metabisulfite solution and a delayed response occurring 20 to 30 minutes after ingestion of solid foods treated with sulfiting agents. Other patients responded to parenteral medications containing sulfiting agents administered through an intravenous route. In addition, some patients were believed to have chronic asthma caused by continuous ingestion of sulfited foods. Although anecdotal and clinical oral challenge studies as well as parenteral administration challenges support the observation that sulfites can provoke acute bronchoconstriction (both the immediate and delayed responses), data to support the continuous response have not been forthcoming.

Exposure to sulfiting agents may occur through ingestion and other routes. Sulfur dioxide generated from sulfited foods or drugs may be inhaled. Werth (35) described an asthmatic individual who developed wheezing, flushing, and diaphoresis upon inhaling the vapors from a bag of dried apricots. The patient did not respond to ingested metabisulfite in capsule form, but reacted to inhalation of nebulized metabisulfite in distilled water. Reports have described several patients who suffered paradoxical responses to the inhalation of bronchodilator solutions. Koepke *et al.* (36, 37) demonstrated that sodium bisulfite used as a preservative in bronchodilator solutions was capable of producing bronchoconstriction. Other studies from this group (38) confirmed that the concentration of metabisulfite contained in bronchodilator solutions could potentially generate 0.8 to 1.2 ppm of sulfur dioxide. Four of 10 subjects who tested negative to a capsule challenge with metabisulfite reacted upon inhalation, whereas 10 nonasthmatic controls did not respond.

In addition to sulfiting agents administered intravenously, orally, or via inhalation, patients may react to the topical application of sulfiting agents. Schwartz and Sher (39) reported an individual who experienced a 25% decrease in FEV_1 after application of one drop of a 0.75 mg/mL potassium metabisulfite solution to the eye. This patient had previously experienced episodes of bronchoconstriction from the use of eye drops containing sulfite preservatives for the treatment of glaucoma.

Asthmatic subjects may develop bronchoconstriction in response to a wide variety of stimuli. Interestingly, a patient has been described (40) who failed to respond to typical triggers of bronchoconstriction, including inhalation of methacholine and cold air hyperventilation, but who nevertheless experienced increased airway resistance and decreased

specific airway conductance following oral challenge with potassium metabisulfite. The significance of this response remains unknown, as no changes in other parameters of pulmonary function, including FEV_1, were observed.

The potential for fatal reactions from sulfite exposure has been confirmed (10, 24, 41). In many instances, individuals who supposedly died from an adverse reaction to sulfite had not undergone appropriate diagnostic challenges. Nonetheless, competent investigators observed that severe bronchoconstriction, hypotension, and loss of consciousness can occur, demonstrating the potential for fatal reactions in some subjects—particularly those with steroid-dependent asthma.

Prevalence

ADULT POPULATION

The prevalence of adverse reactions to sulfiting agents is not precisely known. Although attempts have been made to establish the prevalence of sulfite sensitivity in asthmatic subjects, the nature of the population studied and the challenge methods employed means that only estimates of prevalence are possible. Simon *et al.* (9) examined the prevalence of sensitivity to ingested metabisulfite in a group of 61 adult asthmatics. None indicated a history of sulfite sensitivity. After challenges were conducted with potassium metabisulfite capsules and solutions, a placebo-controlled challenge was used to confirm positive responses. Five of 61 patients (8.2%) experienced a 25% or greater decline in FEV_1 upon challenge.

Koepke and Selner (42) conducted open challenges with sodium metabisulfite in 15 adults with a history of asthma after ingestion of sulfited foods and beverages. One of 15 patients (7%) showed a 28% decline in FEV_1; no confirmatory challenge was conducted. In a larger study by Buckley *et al.* (43), 134 patients underwent single-blind challenges with potassium metabisulfite capsules. Of these subjects, 4.6% were suspected of having sulfite sensitivity. In these three studies, the population consisted of a large portion of steroid-dependent asthma patients being treated at major referral centers, although sulfite sensitivity was diagnosed in several mild asthmatics as well (7). Thus, the prevalence estimated from these observations may not be applicable to the asthma population as a whole. In addition, Wuthrich (28) challenged 87 suspected, sulfite-sensitive asthmatics with capsules containing sodium bisulfite (5–200 mg doses). Fifteen of the 87 asthmatics (17.2%) reacted to these sulfite challenges, but the steroid dependency of this study population was not determined. Because subjects were selected for suspected sulfite sensitivity, the results of this study cannot be used to assess the prevalence of sulfite sensitivity in the overall population of asthmatics.

In the largest study reported to date, Bush et al. (8) conducted capsule and neutral solution sulfite challenges in 203 adult asthmatics. None was selected based on a history of sulfite sensitivity. Of these patients, 120 were not receiving corticosteroids, while 83 were steroid-dependent. Of the non–steroid-dependent group, only one experienced a 20% or greater decline in FEV_1 after single-blind and confirmatory double-blind challenge. The steroid-dependent asthma group had a higher response rate, estimated at approximately 8.4%. The prevalence in the asthmatic population as a whole was less than 3.9%, with steroid-dependent asthmatic patients appearing to face the greatest risk.

PEDIATRIC POPULATION

Limited studies have been conducted in children. Towns and Mellis (44) evaluated 29 children, aged 5.5 to 14 years, with moderate to severe asthma. Seven subjects had a history suggestive of sulfite sensitivity. Challenges were conducted with placebo on one day and with sequential administration of sodium metabisulfite in capsule and solution form on a second day. Nineteen of the 29 subjects showed a decrease in the peak expiratory flow rate varying from 23% to 72%, while peak expiratory flow rates with placebo were either unaffected or dropped 19%. When the 20% decline in peak expiratory flow rate was viewed as a positive response, 66% of these children were considered to be sulfite-sensitive. Subsequently, the patients were instructed to avoid sulfited foods for three months. No overall significant improvement appeared in the patients' asthma as a

result of this avoidance diet. Friedman and Easton (45) studied 51 children, aged 5 to 17 years. Eighteen of 51 (36%) showed a 20% or greater decrease in FEV_1 when provoked with potassium metabisulfite in an acidic solution, although placebo challenges in these individuals showed only one responder. No differences in steroid use were noted between responders and nonresponders. Steinman et al. (46) evaluated 37 asthmatic children and determined that 8 (22%) responded to double-blind challenges of sulfited apple juice with a 20% or greater decline in FEV_1. An additional 8 children were considered to experience a reaction to sulfite when the criterion for a positive response was changed to a 10% or greater decrease in FEV_1. In contrast, a study by Boner et al. (47) determined that only 4 of 56 asthmatic children (7%) responded to single-blind challenges with sulfite in capsules and/or solutions. Furthermore, the sulfite-sensitive individuals displayed no additional change in bronchial reactivity as assessed by methacholine challenges conducted after sulfite reactions. In this study, a positive response was defined as a 20% decline in FEV_1.

Whether sulfite sensitivity really occurs more frequently in children has yet to be definitively established. Differences in challenge procedures (capsule versus acidic beverage solutions) may account for the observed differences. Nonetheless, the overall prevalence of sulfiting agent sensitivity—particularly in adult asthmatics—is small but significant. Steroid dependency appears to pose a risk, particularly for the adult asthmatic.

Mechanisms

The mechanisms of sulfiting agent sensitivity remain unknown. Depending upon the route of exposure, a number of possible mechanisms have been hypothesized. Asthmatics are known to respond with significant bronchoconstriction upon inhalation of less than 1.0 ppm of sulfur dioxide (48). Fine and coworkers (49) demonstrated that bronchoconstriction developed in asthmatics who inhaled sulfur dioxide and bisulfite (HSO_3^-), but not sulfite ($SO_3^=$). Alteration of airway pH itself did not cause bronchoconstriction. Thus, depending on pH and the ionic species, asthmatics may respond to various forms of sulfite. Some asthmatics also respond to either oral or inhalation challenge with sulfite, although inhalation appears more apt to produce a bronchoconstrictive response (50). Considerable variability in the response to capsule and acidic challenges with sulfiting agents has been observed as well (51). When challenged on repeated occasions, the same group of individuals may not consistently show a bronchoconstrictatory response. Therefore, attempts have been made to understand the nature of this variable response more fully.

INHALATION DURING SWALLOWING

Delohery *et al.* (52) studied 10 sulfite-sensitive asthmatic subjects. All of the subjects reacted to an acidic metabisulfite solution when it was administered as a mouthwash or swallowed, but not when it was instilled through a nasogastric tube. These same individuals, however, did not respond with changes in pulmonary function when they held their breath while swallowing the solution. Ten non–sulfite-sensitive asthmatics showed no response to the mouthwash or swallowing challenge. Researchers hypothesized that some individuals respond to these forms of challenge because they inhale sulfur dioxide during the swallowing process.

LINKAGE WITH AIRWAY HYPERREACTIVITY

Because asthmatics respond to various stimuli (airway irritants) at concentrations lower than normal individuals (i.e., they exhibit airway hyperresponsiveness), attempts have been made to link sulfite sensitivity with airway responsiveness to histamine and methacholine. Australian investigators (52), for example, were unable to demonstrate a relationship between the degree of airway responsiveness to inhaled histamine and the presence of sulfite sensitivity.

Our group attempted to induce sulfite sensitivity in a group of 16 asthmatic subjects (unpublished). After the provocative dose of methacholine producing a 20% decrease in FEV_1 was established, a sulfite challenge using an acidic sulfite solution was then instigated to identify any sulfite sensitivity. Prior to challenge, 3 of the 16 subjects reacted to the sulfiting agent with a 20% decrease in FEV_1. One week after this challenge, the patients underwent bronchial challenge with an antigen to which they exhibited sensitivity. Twenty-four hours later, the patients returned for a repeat methacholine challenge, followed by a second sulfite challenge 24 hours later. After the antigen challenge, only one additional subject showed a response to sulfiting agent that had not been present before the antigen challenge. No significant increase was observed in airway response to methacholine. Thus, this study did not link airway hyperreactivity and sulfite sensitivity. Similar negative results were obtained in a study of asthmatic children (47).

CHOLINERGIC REFLEX

Because sulfur dioxide may produce bronchoconstriction through cholinergic reflex mechanisms, preliminary studies have examined the effect of atropine and other anticholinergic agents (53). Inhalation of atropine blocked the airway response to sulfiting agents in three of five subjects and partially inhibited the response in two of these individuals. Doxepin, which possesses both anticholinergic and antihistaminic properties, had protective effects in three of five individuals. In a study on sheep, inhaled metabisulfite induced bronchoconstriction that could be prevented by pretreatment with either ipratropium bromide or nedocromil sodium, but not by chlorpheniramine (54). Sulfite-induced bronchoconstriction in these sheep was also associated with a ninefold increase in immunoreactive kinins. Consequently, Mansour *et al.* (54) concluded that sulfite-induced bronchoconstriction in sheep involves stimulation of bradykinin B_2-receptors with subsequent activation of cholinergic mechanisms. Studies in guinea pigs suggest that capsaicin-sensitive sensory nerves may play a role in sulfite-induced bronchoconstriction (55).

POSSIBLE IgE-MEDIATED REACTIONS

Adverse reactions to sulfites appear most commonly in atopic individuals, and studies have attempted to identify an immunologic basis for these reactions. Patch tests in patients with contact dermatitis (17) suggest a delayed hypersensitivity mechanism in those individuals. Precipitating antibodies to sulfites (21) or alterations in complement activity (25) have not been detected.

A more likely explanation centers on the presence of an IgE-mediated response. Prenner and Stevens (21) observed a positive scratch skin test to an aqueous solution of sodium bisulfite at 10 mg/mL in a patient. This patient also exhibited a dramatic response with intradermal testing at the same concentration. Three nonsensitive control subjects had negative skin tests. In the five subjects studied by Stevenson and Simon (6), none showed positive skin tests. A patient of Twarog and Leung (25), however, showed a positive intradermal skin test response to an aqueous solution of bisulfite at 0.1 mg/mL; controls tested negative with 1.0 mg/mL of the same solution. Meggs et al. (30) reported that a patient developed wheezing when skin tests were carried out with sodium bisulfite at 100 μg/mL. As noted earlier, Yang et al. (24) identified several asthmatic subjects who had either positive prick or intradermal skin tests to sulfites. In addition, Boxer et al. (56) described two cases with positive skin tests with positive oral challenges to sulfiting agents. Selner et al. (57) reported positive intradermal and skin puncture tests with 0.1 mg/mL and 10 mg/mL potassium metabisulfite solutions, respectively, in a sulfite-sensitive asthmatic subject. The subject also exhibited a positive intradermal skin test with a 0.1 mg/mL solution of acetaldehyde hydroxysulfonate, while two nonsensitive control subjects had negative skin tests. These observations suggest the possibility of an IgE-mediated mechanism.

Further evidence for an IgE-mediated mechanism is based on the results of passive transfer tests (Prausnitz-Kustner transfer). Several investigators have successfully transferred skin test reactivity to nonsensitive subjects with sera taken from sulfite-sensitive individuals (21, 24, 58). The effect was eliminated by heating the sera to 56 °C for 30 minutes (58). Other such studies have not demonstrated similar results (25).

These data suggest the presence of a serum factor (IgE). To date, specific IgE antibodies to sulfiting agents or sulfiting agents conjugated to human serum albumin have not been demonstrated (56, 58). The ability of sulfiting agents to produce mediator release from mast cells or basophils in the absence of IgE

has been investigated. Histamine release from mixed peripheral blood leukocytes could not be shown in the five subjects studied by Stevenson and Simon (6). Simon and Wasserman (58) also found inconsistencies in leukocyte histamine release from peripheral blood leukocytes of an individual who had a positive skin test. In contrast, Twarog and Leung (25) found that 20% of the total histamine was released from peripheral blood leukocytes in one patient at concentrations of 10^{-3} to 10^{-7} M sodium bisulfite. Cells from control subjects did not release histamine. Moreover, the histamine release was enhanced by preincubating the patient's serum with sodium bisulfite. Sokol and Hydick (23) observed that incubation with sulfites elicited 37% histamine release from basophils in the case of their single patient.

Similarly, reports of inconsistencies in the measurement of mast cell or basophil mediators in the peripheral blood have surfaced. Schwartz (27) did not observe any rise in plasma histamine levels in patients experiencing hypotension and gastrointestinal response on sulfite challenge. Likewise, Altman et al. (59) failed to find changes in serum neutrophil chemotactic activity in sulfite-sensitive individuals. In contrast, Meggs et al. (30) noted a significant rise in plasma histamine levels in two of seven subjects with systemic mastocytosis undergoing a sulfite challenge. No clinical response was observed in these patients, however. In a skin test-positive asthmatic, a tripling of plasma histamine level was observed during an asthmatic response to sulfite challenge. When challenged intranasally with 5 mg of potassium metabisulfite in distilled water, four subjects with asthma or rhinitis attributed to sulfite exposure demonstrated increased histamine levels in nasal lavage fluid 7.5 minutes after challenge (60). Similar results were obtained in chronic rhinitis control subjects, although the histamine levels generally fell below those found in the patients with sulfite sensitivity (60).

Indirect evidence for a role of mast cell mediators in the production of bronchoconstriction due to sulfiting agents has also been found. Friedman (33) mentions that inhaled sodium cromolyn prevented the asthmatic response to acidic solutions of sulfite. In preliminary studies, Simon et al. (53) found that inhaled cromolyn inhibited sulfite-induced asthma in four of six subjects and partially inhibited the response in the other two subjects. Schwartz (61) reported that oral cromolyn at a dose of 200 mg blocked an asthmatic response to an oral sulfite challenge in a single individual.

SULFITE OXIDASE DEFICIENCY

Other possible mechanisms for sulfite sensitivity have been suggested as well. Simon (62) has proposed that a deficiency in sulfite oxidase, an enzyme that metabolizes sulfite to sulfate, may promote the adverse reactions. Six subjects found to be sulfite-sensitive by provocative challenge exhibited less sulfite oxidase activity in skin fibroblasts compared with normal controls. It should be noted, however, that the major source of sulfite oxidase activity in humans resides in the liver. Further investigations have not been reported.

Diagnosis

The diagnosis of sulfite sensitivity cannot be established by the patient's history alone. Our group (8) was unable to correlate the presence of a positive sulfite challenge with the patient's history, and vice versa. The diagnosis of sulfite sensitivity should, therefore, be made only in individuals who demonstrate an objective response upon appropriate challenge.

Skin testing—by both prick and scratch methods—has identified some individuals with positive responses (24, 56). In contrast, some individuals who have equally severe bronchospastic or other reactions had negative skin tests.

DIAGNOSTIC CHALLENGES

Because diagnostic challenges represent the only effective confirmatory technique and because such challenges may pose significant risk to sensitive subjects, patients must be informed of the risks involved. Physicians instituting such provocation procedures should have available all equipment necessary for the treatment of a severe bronchospastic or anaphylactic reaction, including airway intubation and mechanical

ventilation. The end point for objective assessment of reactivity should be ascertained before the challenge begins. Such measures might include changes in airway function in asthmatics or the appearance of urticaria in patients with this type of response. Patients may be challenged with capsules, neutral solutions, or acidic solutions of metabisulfite. Some protocols previously reported in the literature are shown in Tables 22.1 (63) and 22.2 (63). Currently, a capsule challenge is the preferred option as most sulfite exposure is likely to involve bound forms of sulfites in foods rather than solutions.

When conducting challenges in a single-blind fashion, positive results should be confirmed via a double-blind procedure. Moreover, if a placebo day and an active challenge day are conducted on two

Table 22.1
Capsule and Neutral-Solution Metabisulfite Challenge

Preparing the patient and collecting preliminary data
- Withhold aerosol sympathomimetics and cromolyn sodium for 8 hours and antihistamines for 24 to 48 hours before pulmonary function testing.
- Measure pulmonary function: Forced expiratory volume in 1 second (FEV_1) must be greater than or equal to 70% of predicted normal value and greater than or equal to 1.5 L in adults. (Test contraindicated in patients with an FEV_1 below those levels. Standards for children have not been defined.)

Performing the single-blind challenge
- Administer placebo (powdered sucrose) in capsule form. Measure FEV_1.
- Administer capsules containing 1, 5, 25, 50, 100, and 200 mg of potassium metabisulfite at 30-minute intervals. Measure FEV_1 30 minutes after administering each dose and if the patient becomes symptomatic.
- If no response, administer 1, 10, and 25 mg of potassium metabisulfite in water–sucrose solution at 30-minute intervals. Measure FEV_1 30 minutes after each dose and if symptoms occur. Positive response is indicated by a decrease in FEV_1 of 20% or more.

Performing the double-blind challenge
- Perform challenge and placebo procedures on separate days, in random order.
- Placebo day: Administer only sucrose in capsules and solution. Measure FEV_1 30 minutes after each dose and if patient becomes symptomatic.
- Challenge day: Same protocol as single-blind challenge day.

Protocol used in the University of Wisconsin prevalence study. Perform this test only where the capability for managing severe asthmatic reactions exists. Stop challenge sequence after a positive response is obtained. (63)

Table 22.2
Acid-Solution Metabisulfite Challenge

Preparing the patient and collecting preliminary data
- Withhold aerosol sympathomimetics and cromolyn sodium for 8 hours and antihistamines for 24 to 48 hours before pulmonary function testing.
- Measure pulmonary function: Forced expiratory volume in 1 second (FEV_1) must be greater than or equal to 70% of predicted normal value and greater than or equal to 1.5 L in adults. (Test contraindicated in patients with an FEV_1 below those levels. Standards for children have not been defined.)

Performing the bisulfite challenge
- Dissolve 0.1 mg of potassium metabisulfite in 20 mL of a sulfite-free lemonade crystal solution. Have the patient swish the solution around for 10 to 15 seconds, then swallow.
- Measure FEV_1 10 minutes after the first dose. Administer 0.5, 1, 5, 10, 15, 25, 50, 75, 100, 150,* and 200* mg per 20 mL of the solution at 10-minute intervals. Measure FEV_1 10 minutes after each incremental increase in dose. Positive response is signified by a decrease in FEV_1 of 20% or more.

*Doses in excess of 100 mg are likely to produce nonspecific bronchial reactions in asthmatics due to the high levels of free SO_2 generated.
Protocol investigated by the Bronchoprovocation Committee–American Academy of Allergy, Asthma and Immunology. Perform this test only where the capability for managing severe asthmatic reactions exists. Stop challenge sequence after a positive response. (63)

separate occasions, the possibility of order effects on the results must be considered. For example, if a patient receives placebo on the first day and experiences no response, he or she may experience a reaction on the subsequent challenge day regardless of whether placebo or active challenge with sulfite is administered. To overcome this possibility, the order of administration of active and placebo challenges should be randomized and a third challenge day, either active or placebo, potentially instituted.

Treatment

AVOIDANCE OF SULFITED FOODS AND DRUGS

Sulfite-sensitive individuals should avoid sulfite-treated foods (64, 65) and drugs (63, 66) that have been shown to trigger the response. Because individuals may vary in their sensitivity to sulfited foods, it may be necessary to perform challenges with foods containing sulfites to determine which ones the patient can tolerate.

Some bronchodilator solutions, subcutaneous lidocaine, intravenous corticosteroids, and intravenous metaclopramide may pose a risk for sensitive subjects. Many pharmaceutical companies are aware of this possibility, however, and are taking steps to eliminate sulfiting agents in their products. A partial list of sulfited medications appears in Table 22.3. Package inserts for suspect medications should be consulted for the latest information.

USE OF INJECTABLE EPINEPHRINE

Although some forms of epinephrine contain sulfite used as a preservative, administration of this drug has not been shown to cause a reaction in sulfite-sensitive individuals. Apparently epinephrine's action overcomes any adverse effects attributable to the preservative. Thus, patients who are inadvertently exposed to sulfites typically find self-administration of epinephrine useful. Self-injection with an automatic dispenser of epinephrine, delivering 0.3 mL of a 1:1000 solution (0.3 mg) for adults, is available (Epi-Pen, Center Laboratories, Port Washington, New

Table 22.3
Some Antiasthmatic Preparations Containing Sulfites

Epinephrine	Adrenaline, Parke-Davis
	Ana-Kit, Hollister-Stier
	Epi-Pen, Center
	Micronefrin, Bird (aerosol)
	AsthmaNefrin, Menley & James (aerosol)
Isoetharine HCl	Bronkosol, Sanofi Winthrop
	Isoetharine HCl, Roxane
Isoproterenol	Isuprel solution, Sanofi Winthrop (aerosol)
	Isoproterenol parenteral solution, Abbott (injectable)
Hydrocortisone	Hydrocortone phosphate-inj., MSD
Dexamethasone	Decadron LA-inj., MSD
	Decadron phosphate-inj., MSD
	Dalalone LA-inj., Forest
	Decajet-inj., Mayrand
	Dexone-inj., Keene
Prednisolone	Hydeltrasol-inj., MSD
	Kay-Pred-SP-inj., Hyrex

Consult package insert for latest information.

York). A similar device available for children delivers 0.15 mL of a 1 : 1000 solution of epinephrine.

USE OF BLOCKING AGENTS

Limited studies have been conducted with a variety of agents that may block the responses to sulfite, including cromolyn sodium, atropine, doxepin, and vitamin B_{12} (53, 67). Although these treatments have demonstrated beneficial effects in limited numbers of patients, they remain investigational and cannot be recommended for standard use.

SULFITE TEST STRIPS

Chemically treated strips to test foods for sulfite content are available. Both false-positive and false-negative reactions have been encountered using these devices, so they have not proved to be always reliable (68).

A better understanding of the mechanisms involved in sulfiting agent sensitivity would allow for more specific interventions to treat and perhaps prevent these reactions.

Food and Drug Uses

FOODS

Sulfites are added to many different types of foods for several distinct technical purposes (Table 22.4). The key technical attributes of sulfites in foods include the inhibition of enzymatic browning, the inhibition of nonenzymatic browning, antimicrobial actions, dough conditioning effects, antioxidant purposes, bleaching applications, and a host of other uses characterized as processing aids (1). Some uses of sulfites have now been restricted by federal regulatory actions, as will be described later in this chapter. In many food products, sulfites serve multiple purposes. In white wines, for example, their primary function is to prevent bacterial growth and acetic acid formation; an important secondary effect is to prevent browning (1). Because of their important technical attributes, sulfites are utilized in an enormous number of specific applications in a wide variety of foods. Several reviews have appeared that provide more details on these applications (1, 69).

Given the wide variety of applications for sulfites in foods, a broad range of use levels and residual sulfite concentrations can also be found in foods (Table 22.5). Residual sulfite concentrations in foods can range from undetectable (less than 10 ppm) to more than 2000 ppm (mg SO_2 equivalents per kg of food). Although sulfite-sensitive asthmatics vary in their degree of sensitivity to ingested sulfites, all such individuals can tolerate some sulfite. Certainly, the more highly sulfited foods pose the greatest hazard to sulfite-sensitive asthmatics.

Inhibition of Enzymatic Browning and Other Enzymatic Reactions

Sulfites can inhibit numerous enzymatic reactions, including those involving polyphenoloxidase, ascorbate oxidase, lipoxygenase, peroxidase, and thiamine-dependent enzymes (1, 70). The inhibition of polyphenoloxidase helps to control enzymatic browning, which occurs to varying degrees and at variable rates on the surfaces of cut fruits (especially apples and pears) and vegetables (especially potatoes), at the edges of shredded lettuce, and in guacamole. In the

Table 22.4
Technical Attributes of Sulfites in Foods

Technical Attribute	Examples of Specific Food Applications
Inhibition of enzymatic browning	Fresh fruits and vegetables*
	Salads*
	Guacamole*
	Shrimp (black spot formation)
	Prepeeled raw potatoes
Inhibition of nonenzymatic browning	Dehydrated potatoes
	Other dehydrated vegetables
	Dried fruits
Antimicrobial actions	Wines
	Corn wet-milling to make cornstarch, corn syrup
Dough conditioning	Frozen pie crust
	Frozen pizza crust
Antioxidant action	No major U.S. applications
Bleaching effect	Maraschino cherries
	Hominy

* No longer allowed by U.S. Food and Drug Administration.

Table 22.5
Estimated Total SO$_2$ Level as Consumed for Some Sulfited Foods

≥ 100 ppm
Dried fruit (excluding dark raisins and prunes)
Lemon juice (nonfrozen)
Lime juice (nonfrozen)
Wine
Molasses
Sauerkraut juice
Grape juice (white, white sparkling, pink sparkling, red sparkling)

50–99.9 ppm
Dried potatoes
Wine vinegar
Gravies, sauces
Fruit topping
Maraschino cherries

10.1–49.9 ppm
Pectin
Shrimp (fresh)
Corn syrup
Sauerkraut
Pickled peppers
Pickled cocktail onions
Pickles/relishes
Corn starch
Hominy
Frozen potatoes
Maple syrup
Imported jams and jellies
Fresh mushrooms

≤ 10 ppm

Malt vinegar	Sugar (especially beet sugar)
Dried cod	Gelatin
Canned potatoes	Coconut
Beer	Fresh fruit salad
Dry soup mix	Domestic jams and jellies
Soft drinks	Crackers
Instant tea	Cookies
Pizza dough (frozen)	Grapes
Pie dough	High-fructose corn syrup

Adapted from The re-examination of the GRAS status of sulfiting agents. Life Science Research Office, Federation of American Societies for Experimental Biology. January 1985.

presence of oxygen, polyphenoloxidase catalyzes the oxidation of mono- and ortho-diphenols in these fruits and vegetables to quinones. The quinones can cyclize, undergo further oxidation, and condense to form brown pigments. Black spot formation in shrimp comprises a similar type of reaction, in which tyrosinase (a type of polyphenoloxidase) catalyzes the oxidation of the amino acid, tyrosine, in the shrimp tissue.

The mechanism of action of sulfites in inhibition of enzymatic browning appears to be complex (1). Sulfites may directly inhibit the polyphenoloxidase (1). They may also react with intermediate products, especially the quinones, formed during the browning reaction, thereby preventing the ultimate formation of the brown pigments (70). Sulfites also act as reducing agents that promote the conversion of the quinones back to the original phenols.

The amount of sulfites necessary to prevent enzymatic browning varies according to the level of activity exhibited by the polyphenoloxidase, the nature and concentration of the substrate, the desired period of control, and the presence of other inhibitors or controlling factors. When only monophenols such as tyrosine are present, fairly low levels of sulfite can produce an effect (as in potatoes and shrimp). When diphenols are present (as in guacamole and cut fruit), much higher concentrations of sulfites may be necessary. The concentrations of these phenolic substrates in fruits and vegetables vary widely, with high levels found in guacamole and rather low levels present in lettuce. Sulfites do not irreversibly inhibit enzymatic browning, so the required concentrations of sulfites remain dependent on the length of time that the reaction must be inhibited.

The FDA has prohibited many of the uses of sulfites for the control of enzymatic browning. Several alternatives exist for the control of enzymatic browning (1). Because polyphenoloxidase is dependent on oxygen, exclusion of oxygen through modified atmosphere packaging is a viable alternative. The use of acidulents (e.g., citric, acetic, or erythorbic acids) to slow the activity of the enzyme and the addition of reducing agents (e.g., ascorbic acid) to convert the quinones back to phenols are the most common alternatives; these techniques are often used in combination. Blanching of the fruits or vegetables can also inactivate the enzyme—but then the products are no longer fresh. Freezing slows the activity of polyphenoloxidase markedly. For this reason, frozen potatoes do not require the addition of appreciable levels of sulfite, unlike fresh or refrigerated potatoes. This freezing effect also avoids the necessity of adding sulfites to other fruits and vegetables. Alternatives to sulfites for prepeeled raw potatoes and shrimp have proved more difficult to develop due to the level of activity of the enzymes, the long period of inhibition desired, and especially the ability of sulfite to penetrate into subsurface tissue. Recently, 4-hexylresorcinol has been identified as an effective alternative in shrimp and other foods (71, 72).

Inhibition of Nonenzymatic Browning

Nonenzymatic browning is a term used to describe a family of diverse reactions that commonly involve the formation of carbonyl intermediates and, ultimately, brown polymeric pigments. The final pigments formed closely resemble those produced by enzymatic browning; the key difference is the lack of any enzyme to catalyze these reactions. Examples of nonenzymatic browning include the reaction between amino acids and reducing sugars and the carmelization of sugar. Specific food applications in which sulfites are used to control nonenzymatic browning include dehydrated potatoes, other dehydrated vegetables, dried fruits, white wines, white grape juice, nonfrozen lemon and lime juices, coconut, pectin, and some varieties of vinegar.

Sulfites control nonenzymatic browning by reacting with any of the carbonyl intermediates or substrates for this reaction (1, 73). Once bound to sulfites, the carbonyls can no longer condense to form the brown pigments. The stability of the carbonyl–sulfite reaction products varies widely, ranging from virtually irreversible to readily reversible. The sulfite level necessary to control nonenzymatic browning likewise varies with the nature of the carbonyls formed and the stability of the carbonyl–sulfite reaction products. Where unstable products result, more sulfite is needed.

No effective alternatives to sulfite for the inhibition of nonenzymatic browning have been identified despite intensive efforts (1). The removal of sugars by fermentation, application of glucose oxidase, changes in formulation, or leaching can produce the desired effect, but have obvious limitations because the resulting products would be dramatically altered. Acids can slow, but not stop, nonenzymatic browning.

Acidification has limitations as well because of the long shelf life of some of the affected products.

Antimicrobial Actions

Sulfites are not widely used in foods for their antimicrobial actions. In a few food processes, however, sulfites play a crucial role in the inhibition of undesirable bacteria (1, 74). In winemaking, sulfites allow the yeast to ferment sugar to ethanol while preventing the growth of undesirable bacteria that would lead to the formation of acetic acid. In corn wet-milling, the corn kernels are soaked in a sulfited steep liquor. The sulfite dissociates interactions between corn germ proteins and the starchy endosperm, thereby facilitating the removal of the starch. Another extraordinarily important function of the sulfites in corn wet-milling is the prevention of bacterial growth in the steep liquor. In addition, SO_2 is widely used during the transport and storage of table grapes to prevent mold growth (75). In general, sulfites work much more effectively against bacteria and molds than they do against yeasts.

The mechanism of antimicrobial action of sulfites is not well understood (1). Acidic pHs enhance the antimicrobial activity of sulfites, suggesting that H_2SO_3 may be the active sulfite form in producing the antimicrobial effects. The amount of sulfites necessary to prevent undesirable microbial growth depends on the nature of the substrate, the length of time that growth inhibition is required, and the degree of binding between sulfites and other food components. Certain wine components (such as acetaldehyde and pyruvate) bind strongly to sulfites, and these bound forms of sulfite do not provide effective antimicrobial properties. Thus, sufficient sulfite must be added to wines to preserve enough free sulfite to prevent bacterial growth. In corn wet-milling, the sulfite concentrations in the steep liquor are relatively high, but nearly all of the sulfite is removed following further purification of the corn starch and corn syrup. With table grapes, distribution of the fruit is not allowed unless residual sulfites have dissipated to nondetectable levels.

While sulfites have few applications in foods for antimicrobial purposes, suitable alternatives have proved difficult to find. The wide spectrum of antimicrobial activity of sulfites is appealing in both corn wet-milling and winemaking. Other antimicrobial agents approved for use in foods have a narrower spectrum of activity and represent ineffective replacements for sulfites. In table grapes, the gaseous nature of SO_2 is indispensable and replacement is, therefore, unlikely.

Dough Conditioning

Sulfites were widely used as dough conditioners in the baking industry, especially in frozen pizza doughs and pie crusts (1). Most of these sulfite uses have now been discontinued. Occasionally, these substances are used in crackers, cookies, biscuits, and tortilla shells. Sulfites act by breaking the cystine disulfide bonds that are prevalent in the gluten fraction of the dough (76). The levels of sulfite required for dough conditioning are relatively low. Some dough formulations do not require sulfites, and such options are growing in favor.

Antioxidant Uses

Sulfites are not used in the United States to prevent oxidative rancidity of fats because other additives are favored for this application. Sulfites are used for this purpose in other countries, especially in meat products. In contrast, it is illegal to add sulfites to meats in the United States. (The ability of sulfites to inhibit enzymatic and nonenzymatic browning might also be described as an antioxidative effect.) At one time, sulfites were routinely added to beer to prevent undesirable, oxidative flavor changes (74), but they are no longer used in U.S. beers.

Bleaching Actions

Sulfites have major applications in the bleaching of cherries for the production of maraschino cherries and glace fruit and the bleaching of hominy (1). Other minor bleaching uses include the bleaching of pectins and the development of translucency in orange, lemon, grapefruit, and citron peel (1). In other products, their bleaching effects are considered detrimental to quality. Relatively high concentrations of sulfites are necessary to produce the bleaching effect, although further processing removes much of the sulfite from these products. Consequently, exposure to sulfites from these foods is minimal. No alternative bleaching agents have been identified.

DRUGS

Sulfites are added to many pharmaceutical products (4, 77). Table 22.3 contains a list of drugs intended for asthmatics that may contain sulfites. With the increased concern over sulfite-induced asthma, these substances have been removed from some drugs in recent years—especially from drugs intended for asthmatics. Sulfites are used in drugs intended for oral, topical, respiratory, and internal use.

Sulfites have two primary functions as drug ingredients. First, they act as antioxidants, typically preventing the oxidation of one or more of the active drug ingredients. Second, they prevent nonenzymatic browning, which involves the reactions of reducing sugars with amino acids or amines. The addition of sulfites prevents these reactions, which can occur in enteral feeding solutions and dextrose solutions. The latter stages of the nonenzymatic browning reaction involve the condensation of quinones. Epinephrine can undergo a similiar reaction that diminishes its potency. Consequently, sulfites are routinely added to epinephrine to prevent such condensation reactions.

The usage levels of sulfites in pharmaceutical products vary from 0.1% to 1.0%, although a few products may contain higher concentrations. Exposure to sulfites via drugs can be high but would be sporadic in most cases. The active ingredients of the drug may, in a few cases, counteract the effects of sulfite in sulfite-sensitive individuals. Until recently, sulfites were common additives in certain bronchodilators but, except in a few rare cases (36, 78), the bronchodilating effect of the active ingredient overwhelms the bronchoconstricting effect of sulfite. As noted earlier, epinephrine easily overwhelms the bronchoconstricting effects of sulfites. Thus, sulfite-containing epinephrine should never be denied to or avoided by a sulfite-sensitive asthmatic because it can act as a life-saving antidote (77, 79).

Many existing alternatives could replace sulfites as antioxidants in pharmaceutical products. These alternative formulations have been widely adopted in drugs commonly used by asthmatics. On the other hand, alternatives do not exist for sulfites for the prevention of nonenzymatic browning. The development of effective alternatives for this purpose will be extremely difficult. Sulfite-sensitive individuals should stay alert to the possible presence of sulfites in medications and seek out alternative formulations. The exception comprises epinephrine, which can be administered if necessary to sulfite-sensitive individuals.

Fate of Sulfites in Foods

SO_2 and its sulfite salts are extremely reactive in food systems. The wide range of technical attributes of sulfites in foods is a direct result of this reactivity. Thus, these substances often react with a variety of food components. A dynamic equilibrium exists between free sulfites and the many bound forms of sulfite (1). Thus, the fate of these food additives will vary widely, depending on the nature of each individual food.

SO_2 and the sulfite salts readily dissolve in water and, depending upon the pH of the medium, can exist as sulfurous acid (H_2SO_3), bisulfite ion (HSO_3^-), or sulfite ion ($SO_3^=$) (66). All of these forms react with a variety of food components, with the extent and reversibility of these reactions relating to pH. At acidic pHs (pH of less than 4.0), SO_2 can be released as a gas from a sulfite-containing food or solution. Thus, sulfites can actually be lost from foods, albeit only under acidic conditions.

Sulfites readily react with food constituents including aldehydes, ketones, reducing sugars, proteins, amino acids, vitamins, nucleic acids, fatty acids, and pigments, to name but a few (1). The extent of any reaction between sulfite and some food component is dependent on the pH, temperature, sulfite concentration, and reactive components present in the food matrix. An equilibrium always exists between free and bound sulfites, although the reversibility of the reactions varies over a wide range (1, 69). Some reactions, such as between acetaldehyde and sulfite to form acetaldehyde hydroxysulfonate, are virtually irreversible. Other reactions, such as between the anthocyanin pigments of fruits and sulfite, reverse

themselves readily. The binding of sulfite by various food constituents diminishes the concentration of free sulfite in the food. While the dissociable, bound forms of sulfite can serve as reservoirs of free sulfite in the food, irreversible reactions tend to remove sulfite permanently from the pool of free sulfite. The desirable actions of sulfites in foods frequently depend on free sulfite, so the concentration of the pool of free sulfite represents a critically important factor in technical effectiveness. Therefore, treatment levels for specific food applications aim to provide an active, residual level of free sulfite throughout the shelf life of the product.

A comprehensive discussion of the possible reactions between sulfites and food constituents lies beyond the scope of this chapter. An entire book has been written on the subject of the chemistry of sulfites in foods (69). Suffice it to say that the fate of sulfite in individual food products is dynamic, extraordinary complex, and difficult to predict with any degree of precision.

In lettuce, high concentrations of sulfite (500 to 1000 ppm) have been recommended to prevent enzymatic browning. Because lettuce consists mostly of cellulose and water, the sulfite has few components with which to react. Consequently, most of the sulfite added to lettuce lingers in the form of free inorganic sulfite (80). Lettuce is unique in this regard, as most foods contain substances that readily react with sulfites. In most foods, therefore, the bound forms of sulfite would predominate.

Likelihood of Reactions to Sulfited Foods

Few trials have attempted to evaluate the sensitivity of sulfite-sensitive asthmatics to sulfited foods. Based on the suspected mechanisms of sulfite-induced asthma, one might predict that acidic foods and beverages capable of generating SO_2 gas would be more hazardous than other forms of sulfited foods. Clinical challenges with acidic solutions of sulfite in lemon juice or some other vehicle appear to support this conclusion (52, 79). In all foods, the fate of sulfite may be an important determinant of the degree of hazard faced by the sulfite-sensitive consumer. Little evidence currently exists, however, regarding the hazard levels posed by the various forms of foodborne sulfite. The overall concentration of residual sulfite in the food also represents an important determinant of the likelihood of a reaction.

Clinical challenges have documented several features of sulfite-induced asthma. First, all sulfite-sensitive asthmatics exhibit some tolerance for ingested sulfite. The threshold levels vary from one patient to another, ranging from approximately 0.6 mg of SO_2 equivalents (1 mg of $K_2S_2O_5$) to levels greater than 100 mg of SO_2 equivalents (200 mg of $K_2S_2O_5$). Second, clinical challenges have confirmed that free, inorganic sulfite presents a hazard to sulfite-sensitive asthmatics. Third, more asthmatics will respond to inhalation of SO_2 or ingestion of acidic sulfite solutions than to ingestion of sulfite in capsules.

From these facts, several predictions can be made about the likelihood of reactions to sulfited foods among sulfite-sensitive asthmatics. First, reactions will be more likely and probably more severe to highly sulfited foods such as lettuce, dried fruit, and wines. Certainly, no evidence exists to implicate foods with low levels of residual sulfite (less than 10 to 50 ppm) in adverse reactions in sensitive individuals (81). Second, foods containing a high proportion of free inorganic sulfite may offer greater risks than foods in which the bound forms of sulfite predominate. Sulfited lettuce is certainly the best example of a food with a high proportion of free inorganic sulfite (80). This prediction assumes, however, that the bound forms of sulfite are less hazardous than free inorganic sulfite—an assumption that has not been clinically established. Finally, one might predict that acidic foods or beverages containing sulfites would pose greater danger than other sulfited foods. Examples of these hazardous foods would include wines, white grape juice, nonfrozen lemon and lime juices, and possibly lettuce treated with an acidic salad freshener solution. These predictions appear to match the practical experiences of sulfite-sensitive asthmatics.

Few experiments have been conducted to test these predictions. Halpern et al. (82) tested 25 nonselected asthmatics with 4 oz of white wine containing 160 mg of SO_2 equivalents per liter. Because patients were not prescreened for sulfite sensitivity, the results of this clinical trial are difficult to evaluate. Only 1 of the 25 patients exhibited reproducible symptoms with the wine challenge, however.

Howland and Simon (83) conclusively demonstrated that sulfited lettuce can trigger asthmatic reactions in confirmed sulfite-sensitive asthmatics. The five patients in this trial were exposed to 3 oz of lettuce containing about 500 ppm of SO_2 equivalents. All of these patients had documented reactions to sulfite ingested in capsule form. Taylor et al. (64) confirmed the reactivity of sulfite-sensitive asthmatics to ingestion of sulfited lettuce, including one subject who responded to only acidic solution challenges of sulfite.

In their study, Taylor et al. (64) assessed the sensitivity of eight sulfite-sensitive asthmatics to a variety of sulfited foods, including lettuce, shrimp, dried apricots, white grape juice, dehydrated potatoes, and mushrooms. Results were confirmed by double-blind, capsule–beverage challenges. Despite the positive double-blind challenges, four of these patients failed to respond to any of the sulfited foods or beverages. The other four patients experienced bronchoconstriction after ingesting sulfited lettuce, although this test was the only positive food challenge for the acidic beverage reactor. Curiously, this patient did not react adversely to a challenge with white grape juice, which is an acidic, sulfited beverage. Two of the remaining three patients also reacted to dried apricots and white grape juice; the third patient did not complete these challenges. Only one of the three patients reacted to challenges with dehydrated potatoes and mushrooms; in the case of the dehydrated potatoes, however, her response to multiple double-blind challenges was not consistent. None of these patients responded to sulfited shrimp.

While these results were somewhat confusing, they illustrated that sulfite-sensitive asthmatics will not react equivalently to the ingestion of all sulfited foods. The likelihood of a response could not be predicted on the basis of the dose of residual SO_2 equivalents in the sulfited foods. The nature of the sulfite present in these foods varied widely. In lettuce, sulfite levels are high and free inorganic sulfite predominates (80). In white grape juice and especially dried apricots, sulfite levels are high, the foods are acidic, and sulfite may be bound to reducing sugars (1, 64). In dehydrated potatoes, sulfite levels are intermediate, the food is not acidic, and sulfite is typically bound to starch (1, 64). In mushrooms, sulfite levels are low and variable, but the form of sulfite remains unknown. In shrimp, sulfite levels are intermediate, the food is not acidic, and sulfite is probably bound to protein (1, 64). The likelihood of a reaction to a sulfited food depends on several factors: the nature of the food, the level of residual sulfite, the sensitivity of the patient, and (perhaps) the form of residual sulfite and the mechanism of sulfite-induced asthma (64).

Detection of Sulfited Foods

A comprehensive discussion of the methods for the detection of sulfite residues in foods lies beyond the scope of this chapter, although the subject has been extensively reviewed elsewhere (1, 69). The numerous procedures available include distillation–titration, ion chromatography, polarography, enzymatic oxidation with sulfite oxidase, and gas chromatography (1, 69). These procedures are highly specialized and should be undertaken only by skilled analytical chemists. One of these procedures, the Monier-Williams distillation–titration procedure, probably represents the method of choice because it has been officially sanctioned by the Association of Official Analytical Chemists (84). None of the available methods has the ability to measure all forms of sulfite in foods, including free inorganic sulfite plus the many bound forms of sulfite (1). Most of these methods aim to detect free sulfite plus some of the reversibly bound forms of sulfite. While they are termed methods for measuring total SO_2, they actually measure "subtotal SO_2." A few procedures intended to measure only free inorganic sulfite in foods are used on rare occasions (1, 80). Because clinicians do not know which forms of sulfites in foods pose hazards to sulfite-sensitive asthmatics, it would be impossible to develop a procedure that would detect only clinically relevant forms of sulfite. Instead, in the absence of information on the hazardous forms of sulfite, the focus has been on

measuring as much of the residual sulfite—both free and bound—as possible.

Avoidance Diets

As noted earlier, the most common treatment for individuals with sulfite-induced asthma is the avoidance of sulfite in the diet. Of course, asthmatics with a low threshold for sulfites must take greater care to avoid these substances than individuals with higher thresholds. Certainly, all sulfite-sensitive asthmatics should be instructed to avoid the more highly sulfited foods, which are defined as having in excess of 100 ppm of SO_2 equivalents (Table 22.5). Individuals with lower thresholds for sulfite might best be advised to remove all sulfited foods from their diets, although adherence to such diets can prove difficult. Packaged foods containing more than 10 ppm residual SO_2 equivalents must declare the presence of sulfites or one of the specific sulfiting agents on their labels. Thus, sulfite-sensitive consumers should be able to avoid significantly sulfited foods by careful perusal of the labels. They must also be instructed that the terms sulfur dioxide, sodium or potassium bisulfite, sodium or potassium metabisulfite, and sodium sulfite indicate the presence of sulfites or sulfiting agents. Some sulfite-sensitive individuals may know that they can safely consume certain foods declaring sulfite on the labels because the amount of available sulfite in that particular food falls below their threshold doses. Such patients should be warned that the concentration of residual sulfite in any specific food is variable and that continued consumption might occasionally elicit an adverse response. No absolute evidence exists to suggest that sulfite-sensitive individuals need to avoid foods having less than 10 ppm residual SO_2 equivalents.

While the avoidance of sulfited packaged foods is relatively straightforward, restaurant foods pose a more difficult challenge. The FDA has banned sulfite from fresh fruits and vegetables in restaurants, but other sulfited foods in restaurants remain unlabeled. With the banning of sulfites from salad bar items, many of the problems with sulfite-induced asthma in restaurants disappeared. The major continuing problem centers on sulfited potatoes. Sulfite-sensitive individuals should be instructed to avoid all potato products in restaurants except baked potatoes with the skins intact.

Regulatory Restrictions

The FDA, Bureau of Alcohol, Tobacco and Firearms (BATF), and Environmental Protection Agency (EPA) have moved to regulate certain uses of sulfite following the discovery of sulfite-sensitive asthma. FDA initially moved to require the declaration of sulfites on the label of foods when sulfite residues exceeded 10 ppm; BATF followed suit with wines. FDA then banned the use of sulfites from fresh fruits and vegetables other than potatoes. This ban affected lettuce, cut fruits, guacamole, mushrooms, and many other applications, especially the once-common practice of sulfiting fresh fruits and vegetables placed in salad bars. Potatoes remain the sole exception to the ban of sulfite use on fresh fruits and vegetables. In these actions, FDA has not distinguished between uses that result in low levels of residual sulfite and uses that create much higher levels. Under EPA restrictions, imported table grapes must be detained at their port of entry until sulfite residues can no longer be detected. FDA has also enacted a regulation specifying the allowable sulfite residue levels in shrimp.

The actions should help to protect sulfite-sensitive individuals from hazards associated with sulfited foods. Unfortunately, at this time, the FDA has taken no action to limit the use of sulfites in drugs. Certainly, any regulation is only as effective as its enforcement, so sulfite-sensitive individuals and their physicians should remain alert to avoid inadvertent exposures.

Conclusion

Sulfite sensitivity primarily affects a relatively small subgroup of the asthmatic population. The symptoms of sulfite-induced asthma can, on occasion, prove quite severe and even life-threatening. Sulfite sensitivity should ideally be diagnosed with a double-blind bronchoprovocation protocol. Many unknowns remain regarding sulfite-induced asthma, including the mechanism of the illness and the likelihood of reactions to specific sulfited foods. Reactions to sulfited foods certainly derive in part from the concentration of residual sulfite in the food and the degree of sensitivity exhibited by the individual patient. In addition, the form of sulfite in the food and the mechanism of the sulfite-induced reaction may affect the likelihood of a response to a specific sulfited food.

Sulfite-sensitive asthmatics should be instructed to avoid highly sulfited foods. The FDA and other U.S. federal regulatory agencies have moved to protect sulfite-sensitive asthmatics from unlabeled uses of sulfites in foods. Nevertheless, sulfites continue to be used in many foods and drugs, and sensitive individuals must be cautious to avoid inadvertent exposures.

REFERENCES

1. Taylor SL, Higley NA, Bush RK. Sulfites in foods: uses, analytical methods, residues, fate, exposure assessment, metabolism, toxicity, and hypersensitivity. Adv Food Res 1986;30:1–76.
2. Eschenbruch R. Sulfite and sulfide formation during wine-making—a review. Am J Enol Vitic 1974;25:157–161.
3. Simon RA. Adverse reactions to drug additives. J Allergy Clin Immunol 1984;74:623–630.
4. Settipane GA. Sulfites in drugs: a new comprehensive list. N Engl Reg Allergy Proc 1986;7:543–545.
5. Baker GJ, Collett P, Allen DH. Bronchospasm induced by metabisulfite-containing foods and drugs. Med J Aust 1981;2:614–616.
6. Stevenson DD, Simon RA. Sensitivity to ingested metabisulfites in asthmatic subjects. J Allergy Clin Immunol 1981;68:26–32.
7. Simon RA. Pulmonary reactions to sulfites in foods. Pediatr Allergy Immunol 1992;3:218–221.
8. Bush RK, Taylor SL, Holden K, Nordlee JA, Busse WW. The prevalence of sensitivity to sulfiting agents in asthmatics. Am J Med 1986;81:816–820.
9. Simon RA, Green L, Stevenson DD. The incidence of ingested metabisulfite sensitivity in an asthmatic population. J Allergy Clin Immunol 1982;69:118 (abstract).
10. Tollefson L. Quarterly report on consumer complaints on sulfiting agents. U.S. Department of Health and Human Services Memorandum, April 2, 1986, 1–7.
11. Hotzel D, Muskat E, Bitsch I, Aign W, Althoff JD, Cremer HD. Thiamin-mangel und unbedenklichkeit von sulfit fur den menschen. Int Z Vitaminforsch 1969;39:372–383.
12. Schmidt GB, Meier MA, Sadove MS. Sudden appearance of cardiac arrhythmias after dexamethasone. JAMA 1972; 221:1402–1404.
13. Hallaby SF, Mattocks AM. Absorption of sodium bisulfite from peritoneal dialysis solutions. J Pharm Sci 1965;54:52–55.
14. Wang BC, Hillman DE, Spielholz NI, Turndorf H. Chronic neurological deficits and Nescaine-CE—an effect of the anesthetic, 2-chloroprocaine, or the antioxidant, sodium bisulfite? Anesth Analg 1984;63:445–447.
15. Flaherty M, Stormont JM, Condemi JJ. Metabisulfite (MBS)-

associated hepatotoxicity and protection by cobalamins (B12). J Allergy Clin Immunol 1985;75:198 (abstract).

16. Epstein E. Sodium bisulfite. Contact Dermatitis Newsletter 1970;7:115.

17. Belchi-Hernandez J, Florido-Lopez JF, Estrada-Rodriquez JL, Martinez-Alzamora F, Lopez-Serrano C, Ojeca-Casas JA. Sulfite-induced urticaria. Ann Allergy 1993;71:230–232.

18. Habernicht HA, Preuss L, Lovell RG. Sensitivity to ingested metabisulfites: cause of bronchospasm and urticaria. Immunol Allergy Prac 1983;5:25–27.

19. Riggs BS, Harchelroad FP Jr, Poole C. Allergic reaction to sulfiting agents. Ann Emerg Med 1986;77:129–131.

20. Huang AS, Fraser WM. Are sulfite additives really safe? (letter). N Engl J Med 1984;311:542.

21. Prenner BM, Stevens JJ. Anaphylaxis after ingestion of sodium bisulfite. Ann Allergy 1976;37:180–182.

22. Clayton DE, Busse W. Anaphylaxis to wine. Clin Allergy 1980;10:341–343.

23. Sokol WN, Hydick IB. Nasal congestion, urticaria, and angioedema caused by an IgE-mediated reaction to sodium metabisulfite. Ann Allergy 1990;65:233–237.

24. Yang WH, Purchase ECR, Rivington RN. Positive skin tests and Prausnitz-Kustner reactions in metabisulfite-sensitive subjects. J Allergy Clin Immunol 1986;78:443–449.

25. Twarog FJ, Leung DYM. Anaphylaxis to a component of isoetharine (sodium bisulfite). JAMA 1982;248:2030–2031.

26. Jamieson DM, Guill MF, Wray BB, May JR. Metabisulfite sensitivity: case report and literature review. Ann Allergy 1985;54:115–121.

27. Schwartz HJ. Sensitivity to ingested metabisulfite: variations in clinical presentation. J Allergy Clin Immunol 1983;71:487–489.

28. Wuthrich B. Sulfite additives causing allergic or pseudo-allergic reactions. In: Miyamoto T, Okuda M, eds. Progress in allergy and clinical immunology. Vol. 2. Seattle: Hogrefe & Huber, 1992, 339–344.

29. Sonin L, Patterson R. Metabisulfite challenge in patients with idiopathic anaphylaxis. J Allergy Clin Immunol 1985;75:67–69.

30. Meggs WJ, Atkins FM, Wright R, Fishman M, Kaliner MA, Metcalfe DD. Failure of sulfites to produce clinical responses in patients with systemic mastocytosis or recurrent anaphylaxis: results of a single-blind study. J Allergy Clin Immunol 1985;76:840–846.

31. Kochen J. Sulfur dioxide, a respiratory tract irritant, even if ingested (letter). Pediatrics 1973;52:145–146.

32. Freedman BJ. Asthma induced by sulphur dioxide, benzoate and tartrazine contained in orange drinks. Clin Allergy 1977;7:407–415.

33. Freedman BJ. Sulphur dioxide in foods and beverages: its use as a preservative and its effect on asthma. Br J Dis Chest 1980;74:128–134.

34. Baker GJ, Allen DH. The spectrum of metabisulfite induced asthmatic reactions, their diagnosis and management. Aust NZ Med J 1982;12:213 (abstract).

35. Werth GR. Inhaled metabisulfite sensitivity (letter). J Allergy Clin Immunol 1982;70:143.

36. Koepke JW, Christopher KL, Chai H, Selner JC. Dose-dependent bronchospasm from sulfites in isoetharine. JAMA 1984;251:2982–2983.

37. Koepke JW, Staudenmayer H, Selner JC. Inhaled metabisulfite sensitivity. Ann Allergy 1985;54:213–215.

38. Koepke JW, Selner JC, Dunhill AL. Presence of sulfur dioxide in commonly used bronchodilator solutions. J Allergy Clin Immunol 1983;72:504–508.

39. Schwartz H, Sher TH. Bisulfite intolerance manifest as bronchospasm following topical dipirefrin hydrochloride therapy for glaucoma (letter). Arch Ophthalmol 1985;103:14–15.

40. Schwartz HJ, Sher TH. Metabisulfite sensitivity in a patient without hyperactive airways disease. Immunol Allergy Prac 1986;8:17–20.

41. Tsevat J, Gross GN, Dowling GP. Fatal asthma after ingestion of sulfite-containing wine (letter). Ann Intern Med 1987;107:263.

42. Koepke JW, Selner JC. Sulfur dioxide sensitivity. Ann Allergy 1982;48:258 (abstract).

43. Buckley CE III, Saltzman HA, Sieker HO. The prevalence and degree of sensitivity to ingested sulfites. J Allergy Clin Immunol 1985;75:144 (abstract).

44. Towns SJ, Mellis CM. Role of acetyl salicylic acid and sodium metabisulfite in chronic childhood asthma. Pediatrics 1984; 73:631–637.

45. Friedman ME, Easton JG. Prevalence of positive metabisulfite challenges in children with asthma. Pediatr Asthma Allergy Immunol 1987;1:53–59.

46. Steinman HA, Le Roux M, Potter PC. Sulphur dioxide sensitivity in South African asthmatic children. S Afr Med J 1993;83:387–390.

47. Boner AL, Guerise A, Vallone G, Fornari A, Piacentinin F, Sette L. Metabisulfite oral challenge: incidence of adverse responses in chronic childhood asthma and its relationship with bronchial hyperreactivity. J Allergy Clin Immunol 1990;85:479–483.

48. Boushey HA. Bronchial hyperreactivity to sulfur dioxide: physiologic and political implications. J Allergy Clin Immunol 1982;69:335–338.

49. Fine JM, Gordon T, Sheppard D. The roles of pH and ionic species in sulfur dioxide- and sulfite-induced bronchoconstriction. Am Rev Respir Dis 1987;136:1122–1126.

50. Schwartz HJ, Chester E. Bronchospastic responses to aerosolized metabisulfite in asthmatic subjects: potential mechanisms and clinical implications. J Allergy Clin Immunol 1984;74:511–513.

51. Lee RJ, Braman SS, Settipane GA. Reproducibility of metabisulfite challenge. J Allergy Clin Immunol 1986;77:157 (abstract).

52. Delohery J, Simmul R, Castle WD, Allen DH. The relationship of inhaled sulfur dioxide reactivity to ingested metabisulfite sensitivity in patients with asthma. Am Rev Respir Dis 1984;130:1027–1032.

53. Simon R, Goldfarb G, Jacobsen D. Blocking studies in sulfite-sensitive asthmatics (SSA). J Allergy Clin Immunol 1984;73:136 (abstract).

54. Mansour E, Ahmed A, Cortes A, Caplan J, Burch RM, Abraham WM. Mechanisms of metabisulfite-induced bronchoconstriction: evidence for bradykinin B_2-receptor stimulation. J Appl Physiol 1992;72:1831–1837.

55. Bannenberg G, Alzori L, Xue J, Auberson S, Kimlund M, Ryrfeldt A, Lundberg JM, Moldeus P. Sulfur dioxide and sodium metabisulfite induce bronchoconstriction in isolated perfused and ventilated guinea pig lung via stimulation of capsaicin-sensitive sensory nerves. Respiration 1994;61:130–137.

56. Boxer MB, Bush RK, Harris KE, Patterson R, Pruzansky JJ, Yang WH. The laboratory evaluation of IgE antibody to meta-

bisulfites in patients skin test positive to metabisulfite. J Allergy Clin Immunol 1988;82:622–626.

57. Selner J, Bush R, Nordlee J, Wiener M, Buckley J, Koepke J, Taylor S. Skin reactivity to sulfite and sensitivity to sulfited foods in a sulfite sensitive asthmatic. J Allergy Clin Immunol 1987;79:241 (abstract).

58. Simon RA, Wasserman SI. IgE-mediated sulfite-sensitive asthma. J Allergy Clin Immunol 1986;77:157 (abstract).

59. Altman LC, Sprenger JD, Ayars GH, Marshall S, Johnson LE, Koenig J, Pierson WE. Neutrophil chemotactic activity (NCA) in sulfite sensitive patients. Ann Allergy 1985;55:234 (abstract).

60. Ortolani C, Mirone C, Fontana A, Folco GC, Miadonna A, Montalbetti N, Rinaldi M, Sala A, Tedeschi A, Valente D. Study of mediators of anaphylaxis in nasal wash fluids after aspirin and sodium metabisulfite nasal provocation in intolerant rhinitis patients. Ann Allergy 1987;59:106–112.

61. Schwartz HJ. Observations on the use of oral sodium cromoglycate in a sulfite sensitive asthmatic subject. Ann Allergy 1986;57:36–37.

62. Simon RA. Sulfite sensitivity. Ann Allergy 1986;56:281–288.

63. Bush RK. Sulfite and aspirin sensitivity: who is most susceptible? J Respir Dis 1987;8:23–32.

64. Taylor SL, Bush RK, Selner JC, Nordlee JA, Weiner MB, Holden K, Koepke J, Busse WW. Sensitivity to sulfited foods among sulfite-sensitive subjects with asthma. J Allergy Clin Immunol 1988;81:1159–1167.

65. Nagy SM, Teuber SS, Loscutoff SM, Muruphy PJ. Clustered outbreak of adverse reactions to a salsa containing high levels of sulfites. J Food Protect 1995;58:95–97.

66. Bush RK, Taylor SL, Busse W. A critical evaluation of clinical trials in reactions to sulfites. J Allergy Clin Immunol 1986;78:191–202.

67. Anibarro B, Caballero MT, Garcia-Ara MC, Diaz-Pena JM, Ojeda JA. Asthma with sulfite intolerance in children: a blocking study with cyanocobalamin. J Allergy Clin Immunol 1992;90:103–109.

68. Nordlee JA, Naidu SG, Taylor SL. False positive and false negative reactions encountered in the use of sulfite test strips for the detection of sulfite-treated foods. J Allergy Clin Immunol 1988;81:537–541.

69. Wedzicha B. Chemistry of sulphur dioxide in foods. Barking, England: Elsevier Applied Science Publishers, 1984.

70. Haisman DR. The effect of sulphur dioxide on oxidizing enzyme systems in plant tissues. J Sci Food Agric 1974;25:803–810.

71. Otwell WS, Iyengar R, McEvily AJ. Inhibition of shrimp melanosis by 4-hexylresorcinol. J Aquatic Food Prod Technol 1992;1:53–65.

72. Monsalve-Gonzalez A, Barbosa-Conovas GV, Cavalieri RP, McEvily AJ, Iyengar R. Control of browning during storage of apple slices preserved by combined methods: 4-hexylresorcinol as anti-browning agent. J Food Sci 1993;797–800.

73. McWeeny DJ, Knowles ME, Hearne JF. The chemistry of non-enzymatic browning in foods and its control by sulphites. J Sci Food Agric 1974;25;735–746.

74. Roberts AC, McWeeny DJ. The uses of sulphur dioxide in the food industry—a review. J Food Technol 1972;7:221–238.

75. Nelson KE. Effects of in-package sulfur dioxide generators, package liners, and temperature on decay and desiccation of table grapes. Am J Enol Vitic 1983;34:10–16.

76. Wade P. Action of sodium metabisulphite on the properties of hard sweet biscuit dough. J Sci Food Agric 1972;23:333–336.

77. Smolinske SC. Review of parenteral sulfite reactions. Clin Toxicol 1992;30:597–606.

78. Simon RA. Reactivity to inhaled Bronkosol in sulfite sensitive asthmatics (SSA). J Allergy Clin Immunol 1985;75:145 (abstract).

79. Simon RA. Sulfite sensitivity. Ann Allergy 1987;59:100–105.

80. Martin LB, Nordlee JA, Taylor SL. Sulfite residues in restaurant salads. J Food Prot 1986;49:126–129.

81. Taylor SL, Bush RK, Busse WW. The sulfite story. Assoc Food Drug Off Quart Bull 1985;49:185–193.

82. Halpern GM, Gershwin E, Ough C, Fletcher MP, Nagy SM. The effect of white wine upon pulmonary function of asthmatic subjects. Ann Allergy 1985;55:686–690.

83. Howland WA, Simon RA. Restaurant-provoked asthma: sulfite sensitivity? J Allergy Clin Immunol 1985;75:145 (abstract).

84. Helrich K, ed. Official methods of analysis of the Association of Official Analytical Chemists, 15th ed. Arlington, VA: Association of Official Analytical Chemists, 1990, 1157–1158.

23

MONOSODIUM GLUTAMATE

Katharine M. Woessner
Ronald A. Simon

Glutamic acid is a nonessential amino acid that constitutes approximately 20% of dietary protein. When added to foods in the form of a sodium, potassium, or calcium salt, glutamate enhances the palatability of foods. Ikeda first documented the unique taste- and flavor-enhancing qualities of monosodium glutamate (MSG) in 1909 (1) after isolating it from the seaweed *Laminaria japonica,* which has been used for centuries in Japanese cooking as a flavor enhancer. Its characteristic taste, umami, is imparted through its stereochemical structure, monosodium L-glutamate; the D-isomer has no characteristic taste. Glutamate is produced commercially by hydrolysis of plant and vegetable protein. After the hydrolysis is complete, sodium, potassium, or calcium is added to form amino acid salts. MSG is also produced by fermentation of beetroot pulp or sugarcane. It is then purified to 98% purity. MSG is known as hydrolyzed vegetable protein (HVP) when other amino acid salts are present. Table 23.1 lists FDA-approved names for MSG.

Normal dietary intake of MSG is approximately 1 g/day in its free form. An additional 0.55 g/day comes from added MSG (2). Some foods, such as tomatoes (0.34% MSG), Parmesan cheese (1.5% MSG), and soy sauce (1.3% MSG), contain naturally high levels of MSG (3). In the body, the turnover rate for MSG is 5 to 10 g per hour (3). Glutamate is metabolized in a number of ways, including oxidative deamination, transamination, decarboxylation, and amidation (4). MSG is readily transaminated to alpha-ketoglutarate, which is converted to energy via the Krebs cycle (4). Studies on humans indicate that MSG ingested with meals results in only a very small increase in plasma glutamate concentration when compared with the levels achieved when it is consumed while dissolved in water or consommé (5). The presence of metabolizable carbohydrates appears to greatly reduce the levels of free glutamate in plasma after meals, even those containing very high levels of MSG. Stegink *et al.* have shown that when plasma levels are increased by huge doses of MSG (more than 5 g) in the absence of food, they return to basal levels in less than two hours (6).

In the late 1960s, concerns were raised regarding possible toxicity associated with MSG. Olney reported MSG toxicity in the nervous systems of rodents when glutamate was given in large amounts by nondietary routes to neonatal mice (7). Olney was able to demonstrate glutamate-induced hypothalamic neuronal necrosis. This lesion resulted in functional alteration of the reproductive capability and body weight regulation in the mice. Around the time of these studies, large amounts of MSG were routinely being added to infant formulas in the United States. After these data became available, however, manufacturers of infant formula voluntarily removed MSG from their products. In 1970, Adamo and Ratner were unable to produce this lesion in the mature rat (8). Furthermore, the glutamate-induced neuronal necrosis cannot be induced in the neonatal rodent when the glutamate is incorporated in the diet even at very high concentrations (9). Additional studies in other animal species, including the dog, rabbit, and monkey, conducted by Heywood and Worden have consistently shown no neurological lesions, even though the daily intakes of glutamate were as high as 42 g/kg body weight (10).

Neuroendocrine effects of high-dose glutamate administration have been demonstrated in rodents,

Table 23.1
FDA-Approved Labeling for MSG (as of 1995)

MSG
Hydrolyzed vegetable protein (HVP)
Hydrolyzed plant protein (HPP)
Kombu extract
Natural flavoring
Flavor

---

including a reduction in hypothalamic GHRH release and pituitary GH secretion as well as an increase in serum LH levels (11–13). Such effects have not been shown in humans, and the implications of these findings remain unknown. Acute toxicity of glutamate has been determined with a LD_{50} value of 16–20 g/kg body weight (14). No evidence to date suggests MSG-associated carcinogenicity or teratogenicity (15–19). In fact, the FDA at the time this chapter was prepared classified MSG generally as safe (GRAS). The Joint FAO/WHO Expert Committee on Food Additives has evaluated MSG and has determined that no numerical limitation is necessary for its use in food (20). The amount of MSG that can be added to foods is limited only by its palatability.

The controversy surrounding MSG as a food additive first came to the fore in 1968, when Dr. Kwok wrote a letter to the *New England Journal of Medicine* detailing a set of symptoms he experienced when eating at Chinese restaurants (21). He described the experience of numbness of the back of the neck, general weakness, and palpitations. This set of symptoms, named the Chinese restaurant syndrome (CRS), has been most closely associated with MSG over the years. Since 1968, MSG has been suggested as a cause of bronchospasm, angioedema, headache, shudder attacks in children, hyperactivity in children, and even convulsions.

Chinese Restaurant Syndrome

As defined by Settipane, a restaurant syndrome is an adverse reaction to foods occurring within 20 minutes of ingestion, frequently while patients are still dining in restaurants (22). After Dr. Kwok's letter in 1968, a series of anecdotes implicated MSG as the agent responsible for the Chinese restaurant syndrome. The triad of symptoms that now defines CRS includes paresthesia and burning sensations of the neck, chest, and limbs, palpitations, and a sensation of weakness. In 1968, Schaumburg reported that his own experiences included tightening of facial muscles, lacrimation, periorbital fasciculation, numbness of the neck and hands, palpitations, and syncope occurring within 20 minutes of eating Chinese food on separate occasions, with symptoms resolving spontaneously in 45 minutes. He reported having as many as eight experiences per day without sequelae (23). Anecdotes of Chinese meal-induced symptoms prompted studies to determine the etiology of this condition. Over the past 20 years, numerous human challenge studies have been conducted in an attempt to determine the association of MSG with the clinical entity of the CRS.

In one of the first challenge studies with MSG (24), Schaumburg *et al.* found an oral dose–response curve to MSG and concluded that all of the subjects they tested would eventually experience the sensory phenomena if they ingested enough MSG. Double-blind studies by Kenney (1979) and Kenney and Tidball (1972) identified individuals who experienced symptoms specific to MSG on a relatively regular basis but only when the MSG was given in amounts or concentrations far greater than that normally encountered in a regular diet (25, 26). Double-blind studies from Italy and the United Kingdom found no difference between the sensation experienced after MSG or placebo (27–29).

In general, challenge studies with MSG pose a difficult challenge because of the distinct taste properties of MSG, which makes adequate blinding hard to achieve. Interpretation of some reported challenge studies has been hampered by the lack of a food vehicle. As outlined previously, the metabolism of MSG is greatly enhanced by the presence of metabolizable carbohydrates, which characterizes most dietary encounters with MSG. Extrapolation of food-free challenges to "in-use" situations may not be valid (30).

Despite the difficulties in studying the effects of MSG, it does appear that large, single doses of MSG in fasting subjects can sometimes elicit certain sensations including light-headedness, muscle tightness, weakness of the upper extremities, tingling and warmth of the skin, and mild burning sensations (21, 22). These symptoms appear within 15 to 20 minutes of ingestion and last 15 to 60 minutes. The entire triad of defining symptoms has been found only very rarely despite numerous clinical studies. This finding has been reflected in studies investigating the actual prevalence of CRS in the general population. Reif-Lehrer conducted a questionnaire study of the prevalence of CRS in 1977 and found that 25% of respondents reported adverse symptoms when eating Chinese food (31). This study has been criticized for containing too much subjective bias, however. Kerr et al. tried to eliminate such bias by conducting a much more objective questionnaire among medical students and employees of the Harvard University Medical Center (32). The questionnaire listed 18 food-associated symptoms, of which only 3 were associated with the CRS. None of the respondents reported experiencing a typical CRS response to Chinese restaurant meals. Kerr's group identified only 6.6% of responses as probable CRS. As the clinical studies have shown, the actual incidence of CRS appears to be quite low.

The pathophysiology of the CRS has not been elucidated. It is clearly *not* the result of an IgE-mediated process. Many theories have been put forth to explain the condition. Ghadimi et al. proposed that the symptoms of CRS are linked to an increase in acetylcholine (33); this group was able to show an attenuation of symptoms in subjects pretreated with atropine. Gajalakshmi et al. lent further support to this theory when they demonstrated MSG's ability to produce spasmogenic effects on the isolated guinea pig ileum (34); these effects were also blocked by atropine. Glutamic acid is a precursor to acetylcholine, which may account for these findings. Folkers et al. suggested that vitamin B_6 deficiency may play a role in the development of CRS (35, 36). Kenney has suggested that the clinical symptoms result from esophageal dysfunction or reflux esophagitis (37). More recently, Scher and Scher have proposed that nitric oxide production may play an active role in the pathogenesis of MSG-induced CRS (38).

Asthma

Several reports have suggested that MSG can provoke bronchospasm. In 1981, Allen and Baker reported their experience with two young women who had developed life-threatening asthma after ingestion of MSG in meals from a Chinese restaurant (39). The asthma developed 12 to 14 hours after ingestion of the MSG-containing meals. Allen and Baker performed single-blind, oral challenge studies on both patients and found that 2.5 g MSG capsules resulted in asthma 11 to 12 hours after ingestion. In a subsequent paper, Allen et al. detailed their experiences with 12 other patients who had MSG-induced asthma (40). Once again, these patients were studied in a single-blind, placebo-controlled protocol. Many details of the challenge were omitted from the paper. Seven of the 12 patients had symptoms within 1 to 2 hours of MSG ingestion. Asthma was substantially delayed in the remaining patients, for as long as 12 hours. These patients were moderate to severe, steroid-dependent asthmatics. For the challenge protocol, theophylline was discontinued 12 hours before the first challenge (placebo) and was held back throughout the MSG challenge (days 1–3). It is not clear from the data presented which patients also received inhaled beta agonists before the challenges. The delayed nature of the asthmatic response after challenge brings into question whether the response resulted from MSG ingestion or reflected other factors, such as a falling serum theophylline level. Furthermore, the study relied on an effort-dependent peak flow meter to measure flow rates in a single-blind study in which the patients might attempt to validate their bias toward Chinese restaurant-associated bronchospasm as being due to MSG.

Other investigators have failed to demonstrate MSG-induced asthma in double-blind challenges. Schwartzstein et al. found no exacerbation of asthma from MSG in 12 asthmatics challenged with 25 mg MSG/kg body weight (41). This study involved mild asthmatics who had no history of MSG or Chinese restaurant meal-induced symptoms. In addition, the doses of MSG were lower than those used in Allen and Baker's study. Moneret-Vautrin published a report of delayed bronchospasm occurring in 2 of 30 asthmatics challenged with MSG (42). Evidence of broncho-constriction was defined by a 15% decline in peak flow rate determinations. If the same criteria for bronchospasticity found in the Allen and Baker paper (20% decline from baseline or "the lowest value recorded during placebo single blind challenge") were applied to Moneret-Vautrin's subjects, the two patients would not fit the definition of a positive response, as the decline in peak expiratory flow rate was less than 20% (40). The two patients of Moneret-Vautrin would, therefore, not be considered MSG-reactors.

At this point, it cannot be decided with certainty whether ingestion of MSG can induce bronchospasm in a subset of patients. Studies with greater numbers of patients, including those with a history of Chinese restaurant-induced symptoms, and adequate double-blind, placebo-controlled protocols are needed to ascertain the impact of MSG on asthma with more assurance.

Urticaria and Angioedema

Very few case reports of MSG-induced angioedema or urticaria have appeared in the literature. A report by Squire in the *Lancet* described a 50-year-old man with recurrent angioedema of the face and extremities that was temporally related to ingestion of a soup mix high in MSG (43). A single-blind, placebo-controlled challenge with the soup base resulted in angioedema 24 hours after the challenge. In a graded challenge using only MSG, angioedema was provoked 16 hours after challenge. Details of the challenge and concurrent medication use were not reported, which makes interpretation of the results difficult.

Botey *et al.* published a report detailing five children with urticaria or angioedema that they concluded was due in part to MSG (44). The authors did not provide pertinent clinical details about the children's concomitant medication use and the nature of the reactions they attributed to MSG ingestion. Four of the five children originally presented with urticaria that was believed to be secondary to medication. One child presented with atopic dermatitis. The children underwent 50 mg and 100 mg MSG challenges in single-blinded fashion. One out of the five developed urticaria 1 hour after oral MSG challenge. A second child developed urticaria 2 hours after challenge with 100 mg MSG. A third patient developed urticaria 12 hours after MSG challenge. The remaining children did not develop urticaria after the challenge.

Reports in the literature of possible MSG-induced urticaria or angioedema do not clarify whether MSG was necessarily the inciting agent. Evaluation of possible MSG-induced urticaria or angioedema must be approached in a double-blind, placebo-controlled protocol to obtain more information regarding the role of MSG in these processes.

REFERENCES

1. Ikeda K. On the taste of the salt of glutamic acid (new seasonings). J Tokyo Chem Soc 1909;820–836.
2. Filer LJ, Stegink LD, eds. A report of the proceedings of a MSG workshop held August 1991. Critical Reviews Food Science and Nutrition 1994;34:159–174.
3. Giacometti T. Free and bound glutamate in natural products. In: Filer LJ, Garattini S, Kare MR, Reynolds WA, Wurtman RJ, eds. Glutamic acid: advances in biochemistry and physiology. New York: Raven Press, 1979, 25–34.
4. Meisler A. Biochemistry of glutamate, glutamine and glutathione. In: Filer LJ, Garattini S, Kare MR, Reynolds WA, Wurtman RJ, eds. Glutamic acid: advances in biochemistry and physiology. New York: Raven Press, 1979, 69–84.
5. Stegink LD, Bell E, Daabees TT, Anderson DW, Wilbur LZ, Filer LJ. Factors influencing utilization of glycine, glutamate and aspartate in clinical products. In: Blackburn JL, Grant JP, Young VP, eds. Amino acids: metabolism and medical applications. Massachusetts: John Wrist, 1983, 123–141.
6. Stegink LD, Filer LJ, Baker GL, Mueller SM, Wu-Rideout M. Factors affecting plasma glutamate levels in normal adult subjects. In: Filer LJ, Garattini S, Kare MR, Reynolds WA, Wurtman RJ, eds. Glutamic acid: advances in biochemistry and physiology. New York: Raven Press, 1979, 333–351.
7. Olney JW. Brain lesions, obesity and other disturbances in mice treated with monosodium glutamate. Science 1969;164:719–723.
8. Adamo NG, Ratner A. Monosodium glutamate: lack of effects on brain and reproductive function in rats. Science 1970;169:673–674.
9. Takasaki Y. Studies on brain lesions after administration of monosodium L-glutamate to mice. II. Absence of brain damage following administration of monosodium L-glutamate in the diet. Toxicology 1979;9:307–318.
10. Heywood R, Worden AN. Glutamate toxicity in laboratory animals. In: Filer LJ, Garattini S, Kare MR, Reynolds WA, Wurtman RJ, eds. Glutamic acid: advances in biochemistry and physiology. New York: Raven Press, 1979, 203–215.
11. Wakabayashi I, Hatano H, Minami S, Tonegawa Y, Akira S,

Sugihara H, Ling NC. Effects of neonatal administration of monosodium glutamate on plasma growth hormone (GH) response to GH-releasing factor in adult male and female rats. Brain Res 1986;372:361–366.

12. Olney JW, Cicero TJ, Meyer ER, DeGubaneff T. Acute glutamate-induced elevations in serum testosterone and luteinizing hormone. Brain Res 1976;112:420–424.

13. Filer LJ, Stegink LD, eds. A report of the proceedings of an MSG workshop held August 1991. Crit Rev Food Sci Nutr 1994;34:159–174.

14. Morikyi H, Ichimura M. Acute toxicity of monosodium L-glutamate in mice and rats. Pharmacometrics 1979;5:433–436.

15. Shibata MA, Tanaka H, Kawabe M, Sano M, Hagiwara A, Shira T. Lack of carcinogenicity of monosodium L-glutamate in Fischer 344 rats. Food Chem Toxicol 1995;33:383–389.

16. Ebert AG. The dietary administration of L-monosodium glutamate, DL-monosodium glutamate and L-glutamic acid to rats. Toxicol Let 1979a;3:71–78.

17. Ebert AG. The dietary administration of monosodium glutamate or glutamic acid to c-57 black mice for two years. Toxicol Let 1979;3:65–70.

18. Owen G, Cherry CP, Prentice DE, Worden AN. The feeding of diets containing up to 10% MSG to beagle dogs for two years. Toxicol Let 1978;1:217–219.

19. Ishidate M Jr, Sofuni T, Yoshikawa K, Hayashi M, Nohmi T, Sawada M, Matsuoka A. Primary mutagenicity screening of food additives currently used in Japan. Food Chem Toxicol 1984;22:623–636.

20. WHO. L-glutamate acid and its ammonium, calcium, monosodium and potassium salts. In: Toxicological evaluation of certain food additives. 31st meeting of the Joint FAR/WHO expert committee on food additives. WHO Food Additive Series Number 22. 1988:97.

21. Kwok RHM. Chinese restaurant syndrome. N Engl J Med 1968;178:796.

22. Settipane GA. The restaurant syndromes. New Eng Allerg Proc 1987;8:39–46.

23. Schaumburg HH, Byck R. Sin cib-syn: accent on glutamate. N Engl J Med 1968;279:105.

24. Schaumburg HH, Byck R, Gersrl R, Mashman JH. Monosodium L-glutamate: its pharmacology and role in the Chinese restaurant syndrome. Science 1969;163:826–828.

25. Kenney RA. Placebo controlled studies of human reaction to oral monosodium L-glutamate. In: Filer LJ, Garattini S, Kare MR, Reynolds WA, Wurtman RJ, eds. Glutamic acid: advances in biochemistry and physiology. New York: Raven Press, 1979, 363–373.

26. Kenney RA, Tidball CS. Human susceptibility to oral monosodium L-glutamate. Am J Clin Nutr 1972;25:140–146.

27. Morselli PL, Garattini S. Monosodium glutamate and the Chinese restaurant syndrome. Science 1970;227:611–612.

28. Zanda G, Franciosi P, Tognoni G, Rizzo M, Stander SM, Morselli PL, Garattini S. A double blind study on the effects of monosodium glutamate in man. Biomed 1973;19:202–204.

29. Gore ME, Salmon PR. Chinese restaurant syndrome, fact or fiction. Lancet 1980;1:251–252.

30. Tarasoff L, Kelly MF. Monosodium L-glutamate: a double blind study and review. Food Chem Toxic 1993;31:1019–1035.

31. Reif-Lehrer L. A questionnaire study of the prevalence of Chinese restaurant syndrome. Fed Am Soc Exp Biol 1977;36:1617–1623.

32. Kerr GR, Wu-Lee M, El-Lozy M, McGandy R, Stare FJ. Prevalence of the Chinese restaurant syndrome. J Am Diet Assoc 1979b;75:29–33.

33. Ghadimi H, Kumar S, Abaci F. Studies on monosodium glutamate ingestion. I. Biochemical explanation of the Chinese restaurant syndrome. Biochem Med 1971;5:447–456.

34. Gajalakshmi BS, Thiagarajah C, Yahya GM. Parasympathomimetic effects of monosodium glutamate. Ind J Physiol Pharm 1977;21:55–61.

35. Folkers K, Shizukuishi S, Scudder SL. Biochemical evidence for a deficiency of vitamin B_6 in subjects reacting to monosodium L-glutamate by the Chinese restaurant syndrome. Biochem Biophys Res Comm 1981;100:972–977.

36. Folkers K, Shizukuishi S, Willis R. The biochemistry of vitamin B_6 is basic to the cause of the Chinese restaurant syndrome. Hoppe-Seyler's Z Physiol Chem 1984;365:405–414.

37. Kenney RA. The Chinese restaurant syndrome: an anecdote revisited. Food Chem Toxicol 1986;24:351–354.

38. Scher W, Scher BM. A possible role for nitric oxide in glutamate (MSG)-induced Chinese restaurant syndrome, glutamate-induced asthma, 'hot-dog headache,' pugilistic Alzheimer's disease and other disorders. Med Hypoth 1992;38:185–188.

39. Allen DH, Baker GJ. Chinese restaurant asthma. N Engl J Med 1981;278:796.

40. Allen DH, Delohery J, Baker GJ. Monosodium L-glutamate induced asthma. J Aller Clin Immun 1987;80:530–537.

41. Schwartzstein RM, Kelleher M, Weinberger SE, Weiss JW, Drazen JM. Airway effects of monosodium glutamate in subjects with chronic stable asthma. J Asthma 1987;24:167–172.

42. Moneret-Vautrin DA. Monosodium glutamate induced asthma: a study of the potential risk in 30 asthmatics and review of the literature. Alergie Immun 1987;19:29–35.

43. Squire EN. Angioedema and MSG. Lancet 1987;1:988.

44. Botey J, Cozzo M, Marin A, Eseverri JL. Monosodium glutamate and skin pathology in pediatric allergology. Allerogol Immunopath 1988;16:425–428.

24

TARTRAZINE, AZO, AND NONAZO DYES

Donald D. Stevenson

*T*en coal tar derivatives are currently under the Food Dye and Coloring Act (FD&C) for use as dyes in food, drink, and color coding of pills and tablets (1, 2). All of these dyes contain aromatic rings and some contain azo linkages ($-N:N-$). Examples of azo dyes include tartrazine (FD&C yellow no. 5) (Fig. 24.1), sunset yellow (FD&C yellow no. 6), ponceau (FD&C red no. 4), and carmoisine (FD&C red no. 2). Amaranth (FD&C red no. 5) was banned in the United States in 1975 during a controversy about its alleged carcinogenesis. By contrast, the nonazo dyes do not contain the $-N:N-$ linkage. Members of this group include brilliant blue (FD&C blue no. 1) (Fig. 24.2), erythrosine (FD&C red no. 3), and indigotin (FD&C blue no. 2). Although all azo and nonazo dyes are present in the diets of most developed nations, controversy exists as to whether such exposure constitutes a threat to the user (2). Are these dyes safe, or are certain subpopulations peculiarly vulnerable to these dyes? Alternatively, as some claim, should all "unnatural" coal tar derivatives be banned from human diet because "chemicals" are bad?

In 1984, Simon (2) thoroughly reviewed this subject and concluded that the evidence that azo and nonazo dyes caused immediate hypersensitivity reactions was largely speculative. For the purposes of clarity and brevity, this chapter particularly focuses upon the azo-dye tartrazine (FD&C yellow no. 5) because of the availability of a large body of literature on this substance and its alleged adverse effects. Effects of other azo and nonazo dyes are also mentioned when relevant. In 1958, Speer (1) stated that "agents used in artificial coloring were the cause of asthma in sick children." The data supporting this claim were not presented. In 1959, Lockey (3) reported three patients with a history of rash that occurred after ingestion of yellow-color-coded drugs.

The author conducted unblinded oral challenges with dilute solutions of tartrazine and concluded that the various types of events observed over the ensuing hours must have been induced by the tartrazine solutions.

Since the 1950s, physicians have published a series of articles that attempted to link ingestion of tartrazine or other artificial coal tar dyes with a variety of adverse reactions. In some papers, details are limited or obscure, particularly with respect to selection of patient populations for study; administering or withholding antiurticarial or antiasthmatic medications during the dye challenges; the dosages of dyes used in challenges; and the criteria by which the authors judged the appearance of an adverse effect. Most studies described adverse events occurring in either the respiratory or the cutaneous systems. A few studies, however, mixed the responses together.

This chapter is organized into a section dealing with urticaria associated with tartrazine and other dyes; a section dealing with asthma associated with tartrazine and other dyes; a section on hyperkinesis associated with tartrazine; and a section on miscellaneous adverse reactions.

Urticarial Reactions Associated with Tartrazine and Other Dyes

After Lockey's original description of cutaneous reactions to tartrazine (3), the idea began to emerge that tartrazine might be responsible for hives in various populations of patients, particularly those with chronic urticaria. Juhlin and his coworkers (4) reported a prevalence of tartrazine-associated urticaria that ranged between 49% and 100% after ingestion

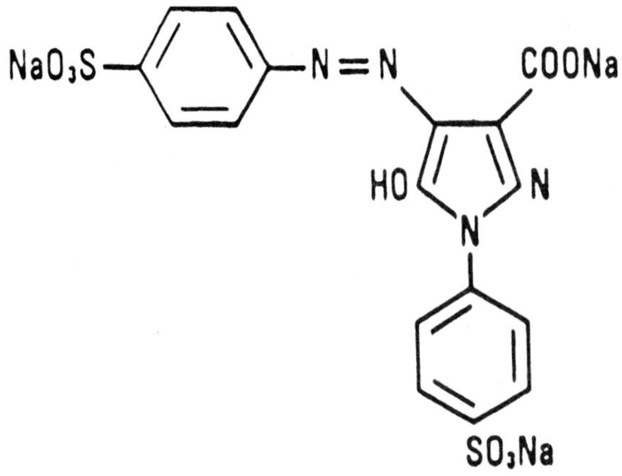

Figure 24.1

An example of an azo dye (tartrazine or FD&C yellow no. 5). Note azo linkages.

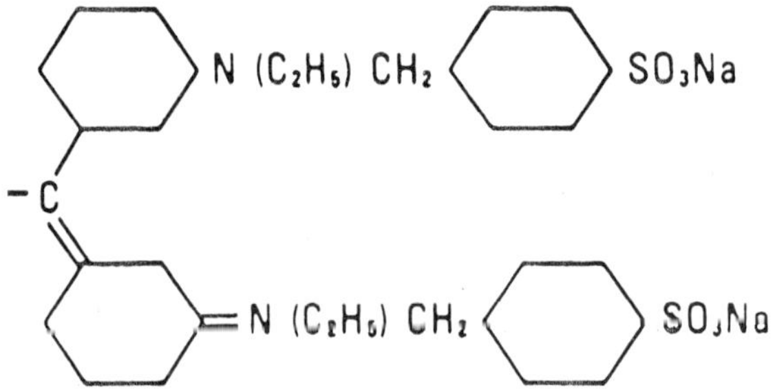

Figure 24.2

An example of a nonazo dye (brilliant blue or FD&C blue no. 1).

of 1 to 18 mg of tartrazine; others subsequently reported smaller reaction rates (5, 6). In the largest series, reported in 1981, Juhlin (7) claimed that 18 of 179 (10%) chronic urticaria patients experienced a flare of urticaria after single-blind challenges with 0.1 to 10 mg tartrazine. In these papers, problems in the design and interpretation of positive reactions immediately become apparent. Antihistamines were probably withheld on the morning of the challenge. The single-blind challenge sequence always guaranteed ingestion of placebo, followed by aspirin and then tartrazine. A spontaneous flare of urticaria following withdrawal of antihistamine was more likely to be ascribed to aspirin, tartrazine, or both, as these materials were always ingested last. In the first article (4), Juhlin and his group reported an incidence ranging from 49% to 100% provocation of urticaria by tartrazine in their study populations; ten years later, however, they reported that the prevalence had decreased to 10% (7). It is difficult to understand how the urticaria population in the same country could change so dramatically in its response to tartrazine, even assuming that tartrazine ingestion declined somewhat.

Doeglas (8), Thune and Granholt (9), and Gibson and Clancy (10) reported tartrazine-induced cutaneous reactions in 21%, 30%, and 34%, respectively, of patient populations afflicted with chronic urticaria

who also had "cross-reactivity with aspirin." Neither of the first two challenge studies was a double-blind, placebo-controlled procedure. In the last study, the authors rechallenged 3 of the 26 reactors one year later and none "reacted." Were these patients initially sensitive to tartrazine but later lost their sensitivity, or did the challenges one year earlier produce spontaneous urticaria falsely ascribed to provocation by tartrazine?

In 1975, Settipane and Pudupakkam (11) conducted a double-blind challenge study of 2 chronic urticaria patients and 18 others who reported urticaria after ingesting aspirin. In 1 of the 2 patients with chronic urticaria, tartrazine challenge was associated with a flare of urticaria. In the aspirin-sensitive group, 2 of 18 (11%) subjects developed urticaria after ingesting between 0.22 and 0.44 mg of tartrazine (the amount of dye found in a color-coded capsule or pill). Further extension of these investigations produced a 1976 report of tartrazine challenges in 38 patients with chronic urticaria (12), 10 of whom had a history of aspirin-sensitive urticaria. Antihistamines were withheld and tartrazine challenge dosage was 0.22 mg. During double-blind, placebo-controlled challenges, 3 of 38 (8%) subjects experienced a tartrazine-associated flare of urticaria. Interestingly, 2 of 3 tartrazine reactors also gave a history of aspirin sensitivity.

Of the nine studies described above, only three were double-blinded. Seven studies identified chronic urticaria, and patients were incompletely described in two other studies. Antihistamine therapy was withheld in five studies, although the timing of the withdrawal relative to the beginning of tartrazine challenges was not clearly stated. The other four studies did not provide information with respect to pretreatment with antihistamines during the challenges. Likewise, the presence or absence of aspirin-induced urticaria is difficult to extract from these manuscripts. Nevertheless, in at least three studies, tartrazine was reported to induce urticaria in patients who were shown to be insensitive to aspirin during oral challenge studies.

In 1986, Stevenson and associates (13) reported tartrazine challenge studies in patients with urticaria. Screening single-blind, placebo-controlled tartrazine challenges were conducted using tartrazine doses of 25 or 50 mg in opaque capsules. If urticarial lesions increased during an initial single-blind challenge, the protocol called for double-blind, placebo-controlled rechallenge. Nineteen patients, selected because of a suspicion that tartrazine in food, drink, or medications produced or worsened their urticaria, underwent tartrazine ingestive challenges in the outpatient clinic. Nine patients gave a history of daily urticaria of six weeks or more duration and were taking antihistamines daily; these medications were continued before and during the challenges. For the 10 patients with acute intermittent urticaria, antihistamines were not administered in the 72 hours before or during the challenges. At the time challenges started, all patients were free of any urticaria or angioedema. Patients who had urticarial lesions on the morning of challenge were challenged at a later time. A positive cutaneous response was defined by the appearance of urticarial lesions or angioedema during the 24 hours after the ingestive challenge.

One of the 19 patients developed urticarial lesions during her single-blind challenge after ingestion of 25 mg of tartrazine. Five days later, a double-blind, placebo-controlled challenge with tartrazine was conducted and again was associated with generalized urticaria, which appeared 30 minutes after ingestion of 25 mg of tartrazine. Interestingly, during a subsequent challenge with 650 mg of aspirin, this patient did not develop any adverse effects (including urticaria). Furthermore, of the remaining 18 patients who did not react to tartrazine, 5 subsequently developed urticaria during oral aspirin challenges. In another group of 5 aspirin-sensitive urticaria patients, inpa-

tient challenges with tartrazine failed to provoke cutaneous reactions. These same 5 patients then underwent aspirin challenges and developed urticaria and angioedema within hours. Thus, in this study (13), the only patient reacting to tartrazine was insensitive to aspirin.

Murdoch and associates (14) challenged 24 patients whose urticaria appeared to remit on a diet free of dyes and additives. During double-blind, placebo-controlled challenges, 15 patients failed to react to any challenge substance. Four reacted to aspirin, two reacted to sodium benzoate, and three reacted to a panel of azo dyes (tartrazine, sunset yellow, amaranth, and carmoisine). These latter three subjects were then investigated via double-blind, placebo-controlled challenges during hospital admissions. Two of the three reacted to each of the azo dyes on four separate days, after receiving doses of 0.5, 5, 50, and 150 mg at four-hour intervals. The third patient did not react while in the hospital. For all four azo dyes, plasma and urinary histamine increased during the dye-associated urticaria in the two patients who reacted; similar increases appeared in the third patient, who reported only sweating during the in-house challenges. In addition, prostaglandins were recovered in the urine from all three patients. This study carefully documents that azo-dye–associated urticaria developed and that histamine release and prostaglandin synthesis occurred simultaneously. Furthermore, shock organ responsiveness was variable (the third patient failed to react to ingestion of any dyes when admitted to the hospital for challenge studies).

In conclusion, yellow dye no. 5 (tartrazine) and several other azo dyes can provoke urticaria in a few patients. Documentation of urticarial reactions to nonazo dyes is not available. It seems unlikely that tartrazine or other azo dyes are responsible for continued provocation of chronic urticaria in the vast majority of patients who suffer from this disease. In the studies by Stevenson *et al.* (13) and Murdoch *et al.* (14), urticaria patients with known aspirin-sensitive urticarial reactions did not experience cross-reactivity with tartrazine. This finding suggests that cross-sensitivity between aspirin and tartrazine does not exist. Based upon the disparate chemical structures of azo and nonazo dyes and aspirin, immune cross-recognition appears unlikely to occur.

Asthma Associated with Tartrazine and Other Dyes

In 1958, Speer (1) stated that tartrazine and other chemical dyes caused asthma in some children. This theory was first tested and reported by Chafee and Settipane in 1967 (15), In one patient, using a double-blind, placebo-controlled challenge protocol, six FD&C approved dyes or a placebo were introduced at the beginning of six consecutive days. Unfortunately, objective parameters for an asthmatic reaction were not used, and the physical location of the patient during the 24 hours of the challenge was not described. Nevertheless, when the code was later broken, "coughing" appeared on the day that the patient took yellow dye no. 5 (tartrazine).

Samter and Beers attempted to link aspirin intolerance to tartrazine-induced asthmatic reactions (16, 17). In their first report (16), 80 patients with asthma underwent unknown types of oral challenges with unknown dosages of tartrazine and three "reacted." Of the 80 patients, 40 were identified as being aspirin-intolerant. In their second report, 14 of 182 (8%) asthmatic patients were reported to have reacted to tartrazine (17). The report does not indicate how many subjects were aspirin-sensitive, by what criteria this fact was established, and how many of the 14 experienced urticaria or asthma during the tartrazine challenges.

In 1975, Settipane and Pudupakkam carried out double-blind, placebo-controlled challenges involving 20 asthmatic patients (11). Three of these 20 patients (15%) experienced a 20% or greater decline in forced expiratory volume in 1 second (FEV_1). The challenge dosages of tartrazine were less than 0.44 mg, an amount found in capsules and tablets but considerably less than that encountered in foods and drinks. Whether asthma medications were withheld during the challenges was not stated in the report.

Stenius and Lemola (18) conducted oral challenges with small dosages of tartrazine (0.1 to 10 mg). Following ingestion of tartrazine, 25 of 114 (22%) unselected asthmatics experienced a simultaneous 20% or more decline in peak flow rates. In the same study, a separate population of 25 aspirin-sensitive asthmatics underwent tartrazine challenges, and 12 (50%) reacted with bronchospasm, based on the same criteria of a decline in peak flow rates. It is now generally agreed that measurement of airway obstruction by peak flow devices is less reproducible than timed volume measurements (19, 20). Most investigators who conduct challenge studies requiring repetitive measurements of lung function use FEV_1 values obtained with a wedge spirometer.

Even for investigators who used FEV_1 determinations, however, controversy exists as to what changes in FEV_1 values represent evidence of an asthmatic response. One investigator conducted tartrazine challenges and used a decline of FEV_1 of only 14% as evidence for an asthmatic reaction (21), whereas other investigators have used either a 20% or 25% decline in FEV_1 values. FEV_1 values vary between 0% and 15% in some asthmatic patients because of airway hyperirritability. Rarely, FEV_1 values change by as much as 43% in patients with unstable airways during placebo challenges (22). To interpret any changes in lung function values that occur after ingestion of a test substance, the investigator must first establish, during an 8-hour day of placebo challenges, that FEV_1 values remain stable.

Spector and coworkers conducted one of the largest studies investigating the prevalence of tartrazine sensitivity in asthmatic patients (23). In their study, bronchodilators were withheld for 6 to 12 hours before beginning double-blind, oral challenges with one provoking substance administered per day. A 20% or greater decline of FEV_1 values was considered to indicate a bronchospastic reaction. Tartrazine provoking dosages ranged from 1 to 50 mg. Of the 44 asthmatic patients proven to have aspirin idiosyncrasy during oral aspirin challenges, 11 (25%) also experienced a greater than 20% decline in FEV_1 values on the days when tartrazine was ingested. By contrast, none of 233 aspirin-tolerant patients experienced similar declines in FEV_1 values after ingesting tartrazine. The report stated that, of the 11 patients who met their criteria for a positive reaction to tartrazine, "five did not undergo placebo challenges" (i.e., did not have a proven baseline day of bronchial stability before testing other substances including tartrazine). These authors concluded that cross-idiosyncrasy between aspirin and tartrazine exists, occurring in one-fourth of their aspirin-sensitive patients but none of their aspirin-tolerant asthmatic subjects.

Vedantham and associates offered the first study of tartrazine sensitivity in children (24). In spite of Speer's (1) 1958 statement, Vedantham's group was unable to document tartrazine sensitivity in 5 aspirin-sensitive or 49 aspirin-tolerant asthmatic children. During challenges, the authors continued to treat their patients with theophylline, cromolyn, and corticosteroids. This challenge protocol was sensitive enough to detect 5 aspirin-sensitive asthmatic patients during standard oral challenges with aspirin, where FEV_1 values declined by 20% or more.

The most revealing study on this subject was conducted by Weber and colleagues (25). Using oral aspirin challenges, they identified 13 of 44 asthmatic patients as having aspirin sensitivity. After challenge with tartrazine (in doses ranging from 2.5 to 25 mg) and withholding morning bronchodilators, 7 of 44 patients experienced a 20% or greater decline in FEV_1 values during the four hours after tartrazine ingestion. Challenges were repeated in the same 7 patients at least one week later. This time, the patients' usual bronchodilators were administered along with their tartrazine challenges. During these repeat studies, FEV_1 values did not decline, supporting the conclusion that these patients were never sensitive to tartrazine. These patients were also challenged with six other azo and nonazo dyes. None experienced an asthmatic reaction.

Weber *et al.* conducted the first study that clearly documented the ability of bronchodilators to affect the rate of "reactions" (25). The expected controversy resulting from this study has generated two schools of thought. The first states that withholding bronchodilators allows tartrazine to provoke asthma and that administering bronchodilators blocks the target organ response to tartrazine. The second school maintains that "tartrazine provocation" is, in reality, a false-positive, spontaneous asthmatic event, generated by withholding bronchodilators in asthmatics with unstable airways. Adherents to the second position contend that tartrazine-induced asthma is so minimal that it cannot overcome standard broncho-

dilators, and thus bears no resemblance to ASA-induced reactions. If the condition exists at all, these observers say, it has little if any consequence.

In a study by Tarlo and Broder where bronchodilators were continued, 1 of 26 aspirin-tolerant asthmatics had a wheezing reaction and a greater than 20% decline in FEV_1 values after tartrazine challenge (26). The authors stated that this patient's asthma did not improve when he was placed on a rigid tartrazine-free diet. In 1986, Stevenson and associates challenged 150 known aspirin sensitive asthmatics with tartrazine in dosages of 25 and 50 mg (13). During single-blind screening challenges, 6 of 150 (4%) patients experienced a 20% or greater decline in FEV_1 values. When these patients returned for repeat double-blind, placebo-controlled challenges, however, none experienced any changes in FEV_1 values. Bronchodilators were continued during the challenge studies and all patients experienced asthmatic responses during standard oral aspirin challenges, proving that they were aspirin-sensitive and that bronchodilators did not block asthmatic reactions to aspirin. Stevenson and colleagues extended this work, challenging an additional 44 ASA-sensitive asthmatics with tartrazine. Again, none reacted to tartrazine (27). In a single-blind challenge study in children, 0 of 10 reacted to tartrazine even though bronchodilators were withheld (28). In a study by Morales (29), 1 of 47 patients experienced changes in FEV_1 values after tartrazine challenge. Repeat challenges were not conducted. In a large multinational study of known aspirin-sensitive adult asthmatics, 4 of 156 patients experienced a 25% or greater decline in FEV_1 values after ingesting 25 mg of tartrazine (30). When rechallenged under double-blind protocol, all four patients were confirmed to have a decline in FEV_1 of 25% or more. A full day of placebo challenges were not reported as part of the double-blind protocol. The authors did pretreat patients with bronchodilators "as needed." The authors of this study are well-known investigators in the clinical study of aspirin and cross-reacting drugs and chemicals, and have extensive experience in oral challenge procedures.

Whether tartrazine-induced reactions have actually occurred in asthmatic patients, as suggested above (30), or whether investigators have, in fact, reported spontaneous asthma activity coinciding with ingestion of tartrazine, continues to inspire controversy. A review of the available literature shows that the strongest relationship between reported tartrazine sensitivity and aspirin-sensitive asthma exists between the high prevalence of unstable airways and antiasthmatic drug dependence in ASA-sensitive asthmatic patients. Much, if not all, of the available literature that reported tartrazine-induced asthmatic reactions probably reported unstable airways, often in patients deprived of their morning bronchodilators. Such interpretations are supported by the reports of six research groups (13, 24–29) and the fact that tartrazine does not inhibit cyclooxygenase (31), a pharmacologic characteristic shared by all cross-reacting nonsteroidal anti-inflammatory drugs and aspirin (32).

A final possibility—particularly in view of the multicenter report from Europe (30)—is that immediate hypersensitivity reactions to tartrazine, which have been associated with urticaria (13, 14), could occasionally induce respiratory reactions through IgE-mediated mechanisms. Under such circumstances, any relationship to aspirin sensitivity would be purely coincidental. This problem might be even more vexing if the offending chemical (or antigen) was not tartrazine itself but either a contaminant or a metabolite. Aminopyrazolone, which is a weak inhibitor of cyclooxygenase and a potential hapten, or p-azobenzenesulfonate, could function in this role (33, 34). Thus, rather than reacting to tartrazine, the patient may be responding to a contaminating chemical. Alternatively, a rare patient, with an unusual metabolic pathway that transformed tartrazine into a different metabolite, may react to that metabolite.

None of these ideas has been supported by clear biochemical investigations and all remain speculations to be proved or disproved. The final answer on this subject must wait until all of these facts are available. In view of the extensive reports of negative challenges to tartrazine (13, 24–29), however, it is difficult to recommend that aspirin-sensitive asthmatic patients should always avoid tartrazine or any of the azo or nonazo coal tar dyes. If a physician is suspicious of such reactions, he or she should specifically demonstrate that a dye induces asthmatic reactions during properly controlled oral challenges.

Anaphylaxis and Dye Ingestion

A case report of a patient who developed angioedema, wheezing, urticaria, and dizziness one hour after taking a Premarin tablet from a new refill generates interesting questions about dye ingestion (35). The new tablets were a slightly different shade of maroon. Investigation revealed that the manufacturer had changed the dye formulation from FD&C red no. 3 and FD&C yellow no. 6 to FD&C red no. 40 and FD&C yellow no. 27. A puncture prick test from a suspension of the new Premarin (including the dyes) induced a wheal-and-flare cutaneous response. Prick tests to Premarin without dyes proved negative.

Hyperkinesis and Tartrazine

Hyperkinesis and learning impairment have been attributed to the ingestion of tartrazine in children (36, 37). Great controversy has emerged over whether such reactions even exist (38). The literature has been characterized by inconclusive results, largely because findings have been confounded by logistic and methodologic difficulties, the use of imprecise definitions of hyperactivity, and poor reliability of behavioral outcome measures. Furthermore, it has proved difficult to segregate responding children from a heterogeneous population and to study such children with any degree of comparability. Placebo effects, as detected by vigilant parents, have consistently reflected parental attitudes and bias.

Nevertheless, studies suggest that some children may experience adverse psychologic or psychomotor effects from these dyes. Swanson and Kinsbourne challenged 40 children with as much as 150 mg of tartrazine and then tested them with paired associate learning tests (39). The performances of the hyperactive children were impaired on the day of dye ingestion when compared with placebo days. Control children did not experience any differences in behavior regardless of whether they ingested dyes or placebos.

One study examined 220 children referred because of suspected dye-induced behavioral problems. Based upon clinical interviews by the author, 55 were entered into a study (40). After six weeks of a Feingold diet (38), 40 (73%) patients were reported by the parents to have exhibited improved behavior. In 14 of these 40 children, the parents claimed strong clusters of abnormal behaviors associated with ingestion of foods containing azo colorings. Eight of these 14 highly selected and suspected children agreed to participate in a double-blind, crossover study, employing a single-subject, repeated-measures design. Subjects were maintained on a diet free of synthetic dyes and additives. They were challenged daily for 18 weeks with either placebo (particularly during lead in and washouts) or 50 mg of either tartrazine or carmoisine, each for 2 separate weeks. When the codes were broken, 2 of 8 subjects showed excellent correlation between dye ingestion and behavioral changes, including increased activity, irritability, low frustration tolerance, short attention span, aggressiveness, and sleep disturbance. Both subjects were boys who had mild atopic disease that did not flare with dye ingestion. The remaining 6 subjects showed some behavioral changes that did not correlate with dye ingestion. This study is instructive because it demonstrates the size of the denominator (220 suspected children) required to identify a correlation between dye and behavior in even a few study subjects (2 children). Additionally, a significant study effort was initiated in a highly selected population. Even in the 2 "reactors," however, one cannot predict with any certainty that such correlations would always occur at other times and under other circumstances. Therefore, although tartrazine and carmoisine dye ingestion were associated with behavioral changes in 2 highly selected children, this observation does not definitively prove that dyes caused the described psychologic activity.

The authors extended their studies and reported a group of 24 out of 800 suspected dye-reacting children (41). A dose–response effect in the 24 patients, evidenced by restlessness, irritability, and sleep disturbance, was observed; when daily doses exceeded 10 mg, the duration of the effect was prolonged. Even though all 800 referred children were suspected to be dye-sensitive by parents and or physicians, tests showed that only 24 (3%) were dye-sensitive. Thus, although dye-induced hyperkinesis appears to exist in some cases, the claim that dyes are responsible for adverse behavior in large numbers of children is not supported by carefully conducted studies (40, 41, 42).

Other Reactions to Tartrazine and Azo Dyes

Three reports have detailed tartrazine ingestion associated with purpura (43–45). In these reports involving seven patients, the mechanisms appeared to be allergic vasculitis (hypersensitivity vasculitic or angiitis). Leukocytoclastic vasculitis has been reported as a consequence of cutaneous vasculitic reactions to dyes (46). Contact dermatitis to tartrazine has also been documented (47–49). It is clear that other coal tar derivatives can function as skin sensitizers as well, as in the textile dye manufacturing process (50).

In a small study of 12 children with atopic dermatitis, tartrazine-induced dermatitis was suspected. During double-blind, placebo-controlled oral challenges with tartrazine (50 mg) on three separate occasions, no dermatitis reactions were observed (51). The notion that dietary dyes induce headaches is a popular theory that has not been proved true during placebo-controlled, oral challenge studies (52).

Conclusions

Although a few well-designed and -implemented studies have been conducted, others that attempted to link coal tar dyes with short-term adverse effects have not been of high quality. After sifting through the maze of claims, the paucity of documented adverse effects caused by azo and nonazo dyes becomes apparent. Except for a rare patient who experiences urticaria, mild asthma, anaphylaxis, cutaneous vasculitis, and contact dermatitis, and considering the massive exposure, these dyes appear extraordinarily safe. No cross-reactivity occurs between aspirin and tartrazine or other coal tar dyes. Hyperactivity may occasionally occur after ingestion of dyes, but the massive media exposure for these rare events again appears inappropriate. In point of fact, the majority of claims against these dyes are mistaken identity, association, or misdirected blame.

REFERENCES

1. Speer K. The management of childhood asthma. Springfield, IL: Charles C. Thomas, 1958, 23.

2. Simon RA. Adverse reactions to drug additives. J Allergy Clin Immunol 1984:74;623–630.

3. Lockey SD. Allergic reactions due to F.D. and C. yellow #5 tartrazine, an aniline dye used as a coloring agent in various steroids. Ann Allergy 1959:17;719–725.

4. Juhlin L, Michaelsson G, Zetterstrom O. Urticaria and asthma induced by food and drug additives in patients with aspirin sensitivity. J Allergy Clin Immunol 1972:50;92–102.

5. Michaelsson G, Juhlin L. Urticaria induced by preservatives and dye additives in food and drugs. Brit J Derm 1973:88;525–532.

6. Ros A, Juhlin L, Michaelsson G. A follow up study of patients with recurrent urticaria and hypersensitivity to aspirin, benzoates and azo dyes. Brit J Derm 1976:95;19–27.

7. Juhlin L. Recurrent urticaria: clinical investigation of 330 patients. Brit J Derm 1981:104;369–381.

8. Doeglas HMG. Reactions to aspirin and food additives in patients with chronic urticaria, including physical urticarias. Brit J Derm 1975:93;135–143.

9. Thune P, Granholt A. Provocation tests with antiphlogistica and food additives in recurrent urticaria. Dermatogica 1975:151;360–364.

10. Gibson A, Clancy R. Management of chronic idiopathic urticaria by the identification and exclusion of dietary factors. Clin Allergy 1980:10;699–705.

11. Settipane GA, Pudupakkam RK. Aspirin intolerance III: subtypes, familial occurrence and cross-reactivity with tartrazine. J Allergy Clin Immunol 1975:56;215–221.

12. Settipane GA, Chafee H, Postman M, Levine MI. Significance of tartrazine sensitivity in chronic urticaria of unknown etiology. J Allergy Clin Immunol 1976:57;541–546.

13. Stevenson DD, Simon RA, Lumry WR, Mathison DA. Adverse reactions to tartrazine. J Allergy Clin Immunol 1986:78;182–191.

14. Murdoch D, Pollock I, Young E, Lessof MH. Food additive induced urticaria: studies of mediator release during provocation tests. J Royal College Phys 1987:4;262–266.

15. Chafee FH, Settipane GA. Asthma caused by F.D. and C. approved dyes. J Allergy 1967:40;65–72.

16. Samter M, Beers RF. Concerning the nature of the intolerance to aspirin. J Allergy 1967:40;281–293.

17. Samter M, Beers RF. Intolerance to aspirin. Ann Int Med 1968:68;975–983.

18. Stenius BSM, Lemola M. Hypersensitivity to acetylsalicylic acid (ASA) and tartrazine in patients with asthma. Clin Allergy 1976:6;119–127.

19. Kory RC, Hamilton LH. Evaluation of spirometers used in pulmonary function studies. Am Rev Respir Dis 1963:87;228–236.

20. Fitzgerald MX, Smith AA, Gaensler EA. Evaluation of electronic spirometers. N Engl J Med 1973:289;1283–1286.

21. Freedman BJ. Asthma induced by sulfur dioxide, benzoate and tartrazine contained in orange drinks. Clin Allergy 1977:7;407–415.

22. Stevenson DD. Oral challenges to detect aspirin and sulfite sensitivity in asthma. NER Allergy Proc 1988:9;135–142.

23. Spector SL, Wangaard CH, Farr RS. Aspirin and concomitant idiosyncrasies in adult asthmatic patients. J Allergy Clin Immunol 1979:64;500–506.

24. Vedantham P, Menon MM, Bell TD, Bergin D. Aspirin and tartrazine oral challenge: incidence of adverse response in chronic childhood asthma. J Allergy Clin Immunol 1977:60;8–13.

25. Weber RW, Hoffman M, Raine DA, Nelson IIS. Incidence of bronchoconstriction due to aspirin, azo dyes, non-azo dyes and preservatives in a population of perennial asthmatics. J Allergy Clin Immunol 1979:64;32–37.

26. Tarlo SM, Broder I. Tartrazine and benzoate challenge and dietary avoidance in chronic asthma. Clin Allergy 1982:12;303–312.

27. Stevenson DD, Simon RA, Lumry WR, Mathison DA. Pulmonary reactions to tartrazine. Pediatr Allergy Immunol 1992:3;222–227.

28. Hariparsad D, Wilson N, Dixon C, Silverman M. Oral tartrazine challenge in childhood asthma: effect on bronchial reactivity. Clin Allergy 1984:14;81–87.

29. Morales MC, Basomba A, Palaez A, Villalmanzo IG, Campos A. Challenge tests with tartrazine in patients associated with intolerance to analgesics. Clin Allergy 1985:15;55–59.

30. Virchow CH, Szczeklik A, Bianco S, Schmitz-Schumann M, Juhl E, Robuschi M, Damonte C, Menz G, Serwonska M. Intolerance to tartrazine in aspirin-induced asthma: results of a multicenter study. Resp 1988:53;20–23.

31. Gerber JG, Payne NA, Oelz O, Nies S, Oates JA. Tartrazine and the prostaglandin system. J Allergy Clin Immunol 1979:63;289–294.

32. Mathison DA, Stevenson DD. Hypersensitivity to nonsteroidal anti-inflammatory drugs; indications and methods for oral challenge. J Allergy Clin Immunol 1979:64;669–676.

33. Johnson HM, Smith BG. Haptenic relationships of p-azobenzensulfonate and some structurally related food dyes. Immunochem 1972:9;253–260.

34. Miller K. Sensitivity to tartrazine. Br Med J 1982:285;1597–1601.

35. Caucino JA, Armenaka M, Rosensteich DL. Anaphylaxis associated with a change in Premarin dye formulation. Ann Allergy 1994:72;33–35.

36. Feingold BF. Hyperkinesis and learning disabilities linked to artificial food flavors and colors. Am J Nurs 1975:75;797–803.

37. Collins-Williams C. Clinical spectrum of adverse reactions to tartrazine. J Asthma 1985:22;139–143.

38. David TJ. Reactions to dietary tartrazine. Arch Dis Child 1987:62;119–122.

39. Swanson JM, Kinsbourne M. Food dyes affect performance of hyperactive children on a laboratory learning test. Science 1980:207;1485–1491.

40. Rowe KS. Synthetic food colourings and hyperactivity: a double-blind crossover study. Aust Pediatr J 1988:24;143–147.

41. Rowe KS, Rowe KJ. Synthetic food coloring and behavior: a dose response effect in a double-blind, placebo-controlled, repeated measures study. J Pediatr 1994:125;691–698.

42. Podell RN. Food, mind and mood. Hyperactivity revisited. Postgrad Med 1985:78;119–122.

43. Criep LH. Allergic vascular purpura. J Allergy Clin Immunol 1971:48;7–12.

44. Michaelsson G, Pettersson L, Juhlin L. Purpura caused by food and drug additives. Arch Dermatol 1974:109;49–53.

45. Kubba R, Champion RH. Anaphylactoid purpura caused by tartrazine and bensoates. Br J Dermatol 1975:93(suppl);61–68.

46. Lowry MD, Hudson CF, Callen JP. Leukoctoclastic vasculitis caused by drug additives. J Am Acad Dermatol 1994:30;854–855.

47. Roeleveld CG, Van Ketel WG. Positive patch test to the azo-dye tartrazine. Contact Derm 1976:2;180–183.

48. Theirbach MA, Geursen-Reitsma AM, van Joost T. Sensitization to azo dyes. Contact Derm 1992:27;22–26.

49. Wuthrich B. Adverse reactions to food additives. Ann Allergy 1993:71;379–384.

50. Hatch KL, Maibach HI. Textile dermatitis. J Am Acad Dermatol 1995:32;631–639.

51. Devlin J, David TJ. Tartrazine in atopic dermatitis. Arch Dis Child 1992:67;709–711.

52. Diamond S, Pager J, Freitag FG. Diet and headache. Is there a link? Postgrad Med 1986:79;279–286.

25

ADVERSE REACTIONS TO BENZOATES AND PARABENS

Donald W. Jacobsen

*B*enzoic acid and sodium benzoate (benzoates) are widely used as antimycotic and antibacterial preservatives in foods and beverages. To a much lesser extent, the methyl, *n*-propyl, *n*-butyl, and *n*-heptyl esters of *para*-hydroxybenzoic acid (hereafter referred to as parabens) are employed as preservatives in a limited number of foods and beverages. Parabens, however, are used extensively as preservatives in pharmaceuticals and cosmetics. Benzoic acid, sodium benzoate, methylparaben, propylparaben, and heptylparaben are approved as direct food additives by the U.S. Food and Drug Administration and have GRAS (generally recognized as safe) status. In 1982 (Table 25.1), nearly 3000 tons of sodium benzoate and 3 tons of benzoic acid were used as direct food additives by food and beverage producers in the United States. Less than 7 tons of parabens were used in that same year. Adverse reactions to benzoates, parabens, and other food additives have been reviewed by Simon and Stevenson (1).

Benzoates as Food and Beverage Additives

Benzoates have been used as preservatives in foods and beverages since the early 1900s. With current annual consumption by worldwide food industries exceeding 10 million pounds, they continue to be one of the most commonly used additives. The benzoates have a broad range of antimicrobial and antimycotic activities, exhibit little or no toxicity in the concentrations used in food applications, and are relatively inexpensive to produce.

The effectiveness of benzoates as preservatives was demonstrated by an outbreak of diarrhea and hemolytic uremic syndrome due to *Escherichia coli* O157:H7 in Massachusetts (2). This organism was also responsible for a serious outbreak involving 400 cases and at least one death in the Pacific Northwest when undercooked hamburger was served at a fast-food restaurant chain (3). In the Massachusetts outbreak, 23 cases of *E. coli* O157:H7 infection were identified, 4 of whom had hemolytic uremic syndrome. The infections were probably caused by drinking nonpasteurized and unpreserved apple cider. Survival studies of *E. coli* O157:H7 in apple cider suggest that the outbreak might not have occurred if 0.1% sodium benzoate had been used as a preservative (2, 4).

PHYSICAL, CHEMICAL, AND ANTIMICROBIAL PROPERTIES OF THE BENZOATES

The structures of benzoic acid, sodium benzoate, and closely related congeners are shown in Figure 25.1. Benzoic acid is a white crystalline solid with a melting point of 122 °C and limited water solubility (0.34 g/100 mL at 23 °C) (6). The pKa of benzoic acid is 4.19, and saturated solutions have a pH of about 2.8. Sodium benzoate is a white crystalline powder that readily dissolves in water (approximately 56 g/100 mL), resulting in a slightly alkaline solution (approximately pH 8) (7). When sodium benzoate is dissolved in acidic solutions, it is partially converted to the free acid. Benzoates appear most effective as antimicrobial and antimycotic agents at acidic pH. For this reason, benzoic acid is believed to be the active agent in the prevention of spoilage.

Table 25.1
Use of Benzoates and Parabens as Food Additives in the United States

Additive	CFR Entry[a]	Status	Max. Level[b]	Usage (lb)[c]
Benzoic acid	21CFR184.1021	GRAS	0.1%	6690
Sodium benzoate	21CFR184.1733	GRAS	0.1%	5,660,000
Methylparaben	21CFR184.1490	GRAS	0.1%	7840
Propylparaben	21CFR184.1670	GRAS	0.1%	5660
Heptylparaben	21CFR172.145	GRAS	12–20 ppm	

[a] Code of Federal Regulation, April 1, 1988.
[b] Maximum level permitted in food.
[c] 1982 Poundage update of food chemicals (Food and Nutrition Board Commission on Life Sciences, National Research Council. Washington, DC: National Academy Press, 1984) (5); data for heptylparaben unavailable.

NATURAL OCCURRENCE AND METABOLISM

Benzoates are widely distributed in nature in the form of the free acid or as simple salts, esters, and amides. They occur naturally in prunes, cinnamon, cloves, tea, anise, and many berries. Raspberries and cranberries contain up to 0.05% by weight (6, 8). The closely related salicylates (2-hydroxybenzoic acid) are widely distributed in the plant kingdom (9) and have been suspected as the cause of chronic urticaria, angioedema, and asthma. Aspirin (acetylsalicylic acid) intolerance in patients with these conditions has inspired many investigations.

Orally administered benzoic acid and its sodium salt are rapidly absorbed through the intestine and transported to the liver. In mitochondria, as well as other sites, benzoate is converted to a thioester with coenzyme A to form benzoyl-CoA (reaction 1). The latter product then reacts with glycine to form hippuric acid (reaction 2)

$$\text{Benzoic acid} + \text{coenzyme A} \rightarrow \text{benzoyl-CoA} + \text{water} \quad (1)$$

$$\text{Benzoyl-CoA} + \text{glycine} \rightarrow \text{hippuric acid} + \text{CoA} \quad (2)$$

which is excreted in the urine. The daily excretion of hippuric acid in the urine averages about 0.7 g. Early studies by Kingsbury (10) and Quick (11) and more recent studies by Schachter (12) demonstrated the efficiency and near-quantitative behavior of this pathway. Benzoyl glucuronide, which is formed by the reaction between benzoate and uridine diphosphate glucuronate (UDP-GlcUA; reaction 3), is also excreted

$$\text{Benzoate} + \text{UDP-GlcUA} \rightarrow \text{benzoyl glucuronide} \quad (3)$$

when large oral doses (more than 5 g) are administered (11, 13).

Sodium benzoate is used to treat infants with inborn errors of the urea cycle enzymes by reducing or preventing hyperammonemia (14). The doses required may prove cytotoxic to the liver (15), however, which could explain the higher survival rates for patients treated with sodium phenylacetate or sodium

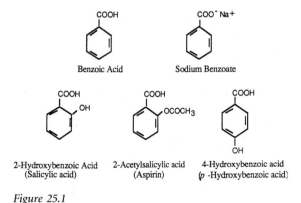

Figure 25.1

Benzoates and closely related congeners.

phenylbutyrate (16). Sodium benzoate is also used to manage seizures in infants with nonketotic hyperglycinemia (17).

Adverse Reactions to Benzoates

The acute and chronic effects of orally administered benzoates in humans have been observed for more than 100 years. Because large oral doses were found to be well tolerated in the general population, sodium benzoate was widely used as a diagnostic and therapeutic agent. In the treatment of rheumatic disease, sodium benzoate was administered in doses that ranged from 25 to 60 g without apparent major side effects. Bryan utilized as much as 25 g of sodium benzoate to assess renal function and liver damage (18). A liver function test using 6 g of oral sodium benzoate (or 1.5 to 2.0 g intravenously) was established by Quick in 1933 (19). This test was used extensively to evaluate liver function in thyroid disease (20), pregnancy (21), mental illness (22, 23), and many other conditions (24–27). Although severe systemic reactions to orally administered benzoate were extremely rare, short-term and usually mild gastrointestinal complaints appeared occasionally.

In 1944, Kinsey and Wright reported an "anaphylactoid type" reaction in a 24-year-old male who had received a 6 g oral dose of sodium benzoate to evaluate liver function (28). Onset of symptoms occurred four hours after the patient received the dose and included severe chest pains, extreme dyspnea, orthopnea, and elevated blood pressure. The patient went into shock and became semicomatose. Two days later, after the patient had stabilized, a second hippuric acid excretion study was conducted with 6 g of orally administered sodium benzoate. Within four hours, the patient experienced identical symptoms. He also developed a granulocytopenia within three days after receiving this second dose of sodium benzoate. Although the patient appeared to exhibit an intolerance to the benzoate, the effect may have related to a seriously impaired liver.

During the last 20 years, numerous reports of adverse reactions to benzoates and other additives in foods and beverages have appeared. The majority of these reports have come from Northern European countries and usually concern small groups of patients suffering from chronic urticaria or asthma. Oral provocation tests using open, single-blind, and limited, double-blind protocols were typically used to establish hypersensitivity. The offending additives reportedly induced urticaria with or without angioedema, asthma, rhinitis, and purpura (allergic vasculitis).

Studies in the United Kingdom and Denmark have attempted to determine the prevalence of food additive intolerance in large populations. The U.K. study, which surveyed an estimated 30,000 individuals by questionnaire, followed by clinical assessment, found that 0.01% to 0.23% of the general population had intolerance to food additives (29, 30). The Danish study involved 4274 children between the ages of 5 to 16 years, who responded to a questionnaire (86%) (31). Based on clinical assessment of a study group of 271 students and results from a parallel study involving 335 children referred to hospital allergy clinics (32), it was estimated that 1% to 2% of Danish children were intolerant to food additives. These large studies in the United Kingdom and Denmark have been compared and contrasted by Madsen (33).

The mechanism of benzoate-induced hypersensitivity reactions remains unknown. Early studies suggested that sodium benzoate and other food additives directly stimulated tritiated thymidine incorporation in peripheral blood lymphocytes in vitro (34) and stimulated the production of leukocyte inhibitory factor by peripheral blood mononuclear cells (35). In more recent studies, sodium benzoate appeared to stimulate release of histamine and 6-keto-prostaglandin $F_{1\alpha}$ from the gastric mucosa after an oral provocation test in patients suffering from asthma, atopic dermatitis, and chronic urticaria (36); it also stimulated release of angiotensin I and II into the urine after oral provocation in patients with a history of food additive or drug hypersensitivity (37). The classification of chronic idiopathic urticaria as an autoimmune disease is supported by evidence identifying IgG anti-IgE antibodies in patients (38). The mechanism by which benzoates might serve as sensitizers in this situation is not understood, however.

HYPERSENSITIVITY REACTIONS IN CHRONIC URTICARIA–ANGIOEDEMA

The prevalence of adverse reactions to benzoates in patients who suffer from chronic urticaria has inspired numerous investigations during the past 20 years [earlier studies are reviewed in (39)]. Shortly after the pioneering work of Samter and Beers (40, 41) on intolerance to aspirin, Juhlin and associates investigated the sensitivity of aspirin-intolerant patients to p-hydroxybenzoate (50–100 mg) and sodium benzoate (250–500 mg) via oral provocation testing (42). The benzoates—particularly p-hydroxybenzoate—induced urticaria in five of seven patients, suggesting that individuals with chronic urticaria might have a greater sensitivity to these additives found in foods and beverages. In Michaëlsson and Juhlin's study of 52 patients with recurrent urticaria or angioedema, they found that 27 (52%) subjects reacted to sodium benzoate and/or p-hydroxybenzoic acid after oral provocation (43). Sixteen patients reacted to both compounds. Subjective (urticaria) versus objective (itchy skin) symptoms were distinguished. In these single-blind studies, only asymptomatic patients were challenged and testing was usually initiated with a placebo (lactose) challenge.

A low prevalence of intolerance to p-hydroxybenzoic acid (2 of 32 subjects) and sodium benzoate (3 doses of 150 mg delivered every 60 minutes, with positive reactions in 4 of 41 patients) was reported by Thune and Granholt after oral challenge in a series of 100 patients with chronic urticaria (44). Doeglas (45) screened 131 patients for aspirin intolerance (31 positive), then further tested them by oral challenge for hypersensitivity to p-hydroxybenzoic acid (50 and 100 mg) and sodium benzoate (250 and 500 mg). Positive reactions (urticaria or angioedema) occurred in 4 of 23 and 5 of 22 patients tested, respectively. No clear-cut distribution of positive reactions consisting of pressure, cholinergic, and chronic idiopathic urticaria appeared within subgroups.

In a study involving 111 patients with chronic urticaria, Warin and Smith (29) reported that 5% reacted to p-hydroxybenzoic acid (50 and 200 mg) and 11% to sodium benzoate (50 and 500 mg). Their challenge protocol involved serial testing of tartrazine, benzoates, yeast extract, penicillin G, and aspirin with kaolin or lactose placebo administered between test compounds. Antihistamine use was continued during the study, which could explain the lower prevalence (5%–11%) in comparison with an earlier study in which antihistamines were discontinued three days prior to challenge (26).

Kaaber found a low prevalence of hypersensitivity (3%) to sodium benzoate (250 and 500 mg) after oral provocation testing in 65 patients with chronic urticaria (46), while the prevalence was reported to be 25% in a similar group of 24 patients (47). August reported that 33 of 86 patients with chronic urticaria gave positive reactions to tartrazine and sodium benzoate administered either separately or individually (48). Based on the data provided for 22 patients, 12 (55%) responded to sodium benzoate (50 and 500 mg) when the doses were administered separately. Wüthrich and Hächi-Hermann (49) tested 33 aspirin-intolerant patients with chronic urticaria and found that 18% (6 of 33 subjects) experienced positive reactions to sodium benzoate (250 mg) or p-hydroxybenzoic acid (250 mg), which closely agrees with the results of an earlier study by Doeglas (45). Follow-up studies on patients with chronic urticaria conducted by Ros and coworkers (50) indicated that the prevalence of benzoate hypersensitivity was nearly 60% (44 of 75 patients). The same group had previously reported a prevalence of 44% (43). Only two out of 75 patients reacted to benzoate only; the vast majority were hypersensitive to at least one other compound (azo dye or aspirin), and many exhibited sensitivity to all three compounds.

Studies performed by Juhlin during 1974–1978 showed that the prevalence of benzoate hypersensitivity was 11% in 172 patients subjected to oral provocation tests (51). In 18% of those challenged, the diagnosis was uncertain; in addition, 71% were reported to be negative responders. Previous studies by Juhlin's group indicated that the prevalence of benzoate hypersensitivity ranged from 44% to nearly 60% (43, 50). The investigators suggested that the more recent lower prevalence data reflected a change in the type of patient (i.e., more refractory to treatment) referred to their clinic and greater public awareness of the problem as a result of federal regulations requiring additive labeling, which led to fewer referrals of patients with true benzoate hypersensitivity. The more recent protocol appears to differ from the previous protocol in that the evaluation of the oral provocation tests was carried out by "several doctors," which resulted in a higher percentage of uncertain diagnoses.

Using a selected group of patients with chronic idiopathic urticaria, Gibson and Clancy performed oral provocation tests only after stabilization had been achieved with an exclusionary diet (52). Most patients became stable within several days to two weeks after beginning the diet. The patients were then challenged with a battery of agents, beginning with a lactose placebo. New compounds were tested every 48 hours. The prevalence of benzoate hypersensitivity in this group was 52% (34 of 65 subjects). Four of the benzoate-positive patients were placed on an exclusionary diet for another 12 months and then rechallenged; three of four remained positive to benzoate.

A group of 25 pediatric patients (18 to 153 months of age) presenting with clinical symptoms of food allergy were subjected to oral provocation tests after two days on an additive-free diet (53). A battery protocol was employed, with a new compound being tested every 24 hours. The prevalence of benzoate sensitivity in these patients was 40% (10 of 25 subjects). Although the group contained 8 patients originally presenting with urticaria, the report did not identify these patients, as well as the others presenting with different symptoms. Benzoic acid and sorbic acid, which are used as preservatives in salad dressing, apparently caused the induction of a mild perioral contact urticaria in 18 of 20 normal children after smearing the food around their faces (54). The reactions were transient and disappeared within 30 to 60 minutes. Benzoates (especially benzoic acid) are capable of inducing nonimmunological contact urticaria in adults as well (55). Because antihistamines do not block the reactions, vasoactive mediators other than histamine appear to be responsible for the induction of contact urticaria (56).

Studies by Ortolani and associates found that 21% (14 of 67) of a patient group with chronic urticaria–angioedema were intolerant to benzoic acid (57). The patients followed an additive-free elimination diet for three weeks prior to testing. Although

not explicitly detailed in their protocol, open challenge studies were initially conducted with benzoic acid (50 and 500 mg) dissolved in water. Positive responders were then rechallenged in a double-blind fashion with capsules containing benzoic acid or lactose. The relatively high prevalence of benzoic acid hypersensitivity reported in this group correlated with a high incidence of cross-reactivity to aspirin. No benzoic acid-induced hypersensitivity reactions were observed in 30 aspirin-intolerant asthmatics.

Studies by Genton and colleagues also support the notion that the urticarial patient population is intolerant to the benzoates (58). In a study involving 17 patients with chronic urticaria, 20% (5 of 17) proved intolerant to successive doses of sodium benzoate (10, 50, 250, and 500 mg) in oral provocation tests. Supramanian and Warner obtained a similar result in a pediatric population presenting with recurrent or persistent urticaria and angioedema (59). Using double-blind, oral provocation tests with a battery of additives presented at 4-hour intervals, 15% (4 of 27) of the patients tested positive to sodium benzoate (100 mg). Of the 43 children who participated in the study, 24 responded positively to one or more of the additives used in the study. These substances included tartrazine (11 positive responses in 43 patients), sunset yellow (10 of 36), amaranth (4 of 37), indigo carmine (3 of 19), carmoisine (0 of 12), monosodium glutamate (3 of 36), sodium metabisulfite (1 of 12), and, interestingly, aspirin (1 of 42).

While many studies suggest that the prevalence of intolerance to benzoates ranges from 10% to 20% in patients with chronic urticaria, other studies have produced different numbers. Garcia and coworkers found a very low prevalence of sodium benzoate (50 and 500 mg) intolerance (1 of 80 subjects) in a group of 80 patients with chronic urticaria (60).

The role that foods and food additives play in atopic dermatitis in children was investigated by van Bever and colleagues (61). In this study, 25 children classified by Hanifin and Lobitz (62) as having severe atopic dermatitis were studied by double-blind, placebo-controlled oral challenges with foods, food additives, and acetylsalicylic acid and tyramine. The children were hospitalized and stabilized after receiving an elemental diet via a nasogastric tube for one to two weeks. Of the 24 children challenged with food, all but one exhibited positive reactions to one or more of the foods (milk, soya, egg, and wheat). Six of the children were challenged with food additives: sodium benzoate (100 mg), tartrazine (0.1 mg), monosodium glutamate (100 mg), and sodium metabisulfite (10 mg). Acetylsalicylic acid (100 mg) and tyramine (20 mg) were also studied. All of the subjects reacted positively to at least one additive and either acetylsalicylic acid or tyramine. Three children had positive reactions to sodium benzoate that consisted of exacerbations of existing skin symptoms, and one of these children had associated abdominal pain. No respiratory symptoms were observed after challenge with food or food additives, and no child reacted to placebo (elemental diet).

HYPERSENSITIVITY REACTIONS IN ASTHMA

The prevalence of hypersensitivity to benzoates in the asthmatic population is unknown because most of the few studies that have been conducted were not adequately placebo-controlled nor were double-blind techniques utilized. In 1967, Chafee and Settipane suggested that sodium benzoate might have been responsible for the provocation of asthma in a patient who consumed a dye-free multiple-vitamin preparation preserved with benzoate (63). Using placebo controls and double-blind oral provocation methodology, this patient was shown to be hypersensitive to tartrazine (FD&C yellow no. 5). The authors speculated that compounds with an aromatic ring structure and carboxylate group (e.g., tartrazine and benzoate) might be capable of provoking attacks in asthmatic patients.

Juhlin and associates were able to provoke asthma in three aspirin-sensitive patients with either sodium benzoate or p-hydroxybenzoic acid using a single-blind battery challenge approach in which a new compound was introduced daily (42). A single placebo test was conducted on variable days. In a study involving 53 chronic asthmatics, Rosenhall and Zelterström (64) reported that 21 patients (40%) were intolerant to sodium benzoate (50 and 200 mg) and, to a lesser extent, p-hydroxybenzoic acid (50 and 200 mg). These single-blind, single-placebo (lactose)

studies utilized peak expiratory flow to assess airway responses (a 20% or greater decrease was considered positive) after oral administration of the test compounds.

In a series of 30 adult subjects with perennial severe asthma reported by Hoffman (65), only one reacted to sodium benzoate (and p-hydroxybenzoic acid). Seven out of 19 reacted to aspirin, and no positive reactions to tartrazine or other colorants were observed. The studies were "rigorously controlled" and conducted by double-blind challenges. Freedman undertook oral provocation tests in 14 asthmatic patients who had histories of exacerbations after the ingestion of carbonated orange drinks containing sulfite, sodium benzoate, and tartrazine (66). In the initial survey of 272 asthma patients, 30 (11%) reported an intolerance to orange drinks. Eight of the 14 patients reacted to sulfite, 4 reacted to sodium benzoate, 1 reacted to tartrazine, and 4 had no response to any of the compounds. Three of the benzoate responders also reacted to sulfite. The criterion for a positive reaction was a decrease in forced expiratory volume (1 second) (FEV_1) of 12% below basal level. These single-blind studies apparently were not placebo-controlled. In a study reported by Rosenhall (67, 68), the prevalence of intolerance to aspirin, sodium benzoate, and tartrazine in 504 patients with asthma or rhinitis was 21%. Twelve positive (2%) and 39 suspected positive (6%) oral challenge tests were reported out of 589 tests conducted with sodium benzoate (50, 200, and 400 mg) and p-hydroxybenzoic acid (50, 200, and 400 mg). The actual number of patients with benzoate intolerance was not reported, but probably did not exceed 5% of the total patient population studied. The tests were initiated with a placebo control, and test doses were administered every 20 minutes until signs and symptoms appeared. The study was performed in a single-blind fashion.

Weber and coworkers found that intolerance to benzoates rarely caused clinically significant bronchoconstriction in moderately severe perennial asthmatics (69). In a study of 43 patients, two were found to be hypersensitive to sodium benzoate/p-hydroxybenzoic acid (maximum dose, 250 mg each) in single-blind challenge studies. Only 1 of 43 patients (2%) gave a positive response to benzoates when retested by a double-blind, placebo-controlled method. Positive responses were defined as a decrease in FEV_1 of 25% or greater from baseline. Bronchodilator medication was not withheld in the majority of patients studied, as a number of false-positive reactions were obtained early in the study with patients whose medications were withheld prior to the challenge. The prevalence of aspirin intolerance in this study was 44% based on history in 7 patients and open challenge studies in 13 patients. The prevalence of tartrazine sensitivity was 16% (7 of 44 subjects) in open challenges but fell to 0% in double-blind studies.

Østerballe and colleagues conducted open oral provocation tests on 46 children with perennial asthma using capsules containing eight different dyes, benzoates (sodium benzoate, 50 and 100 mg; *p*-hydroxybenzoic acid, 50 and 100 mg), and aspirin (70). Eleven of 46 patients gave positive reactions (greater than 20% decrease in peak pulmonary flow) during the open challenges. Subsequent retesting of the 11 patients using a double-blind, placebo-controlled protocol produced only three positive responders. Tarlo and Broder found only one subject with sodium benzoate intolerance in a double-blind study involving 28 patients (3%–4%) with chronic asthma (71). Medications were not withheld, and a decline in FEV_1 of 20% from baseline was considered a positive response.

Moneret-Vautrin and associates described an asthmatic patient who suffered an anaphylactoid reaction while being prepared for polypectomy (72). Sodium benzoate present in diazepam administered to the patient was suspected as the cause of the reaction. Unspecified oral challenges gave positive results with both sodium benzoate (100 mg) and methylparaben (10 mg).

Genton *et al.* (58) performed oral provocation tests with sodium benzoate (10–500 mg) on 17 asthmatic patients using a single-blind, random-placebo protocol and found only one responder (6%). A 20% drop in peak flow rate was considered a positive reaction in patients who were maintained on an additive-free diet for 14 days prior to testing. Drugs were continued in some patients to maintain their stability. Garcia *et al.* tested 62 patients with steroid-dependent intrinsic asthma with sodium benzoate (500 mg) and found no intolerance after defining a

fall in FEV_1 of 20% or greater as significant (60). Finally, Steinman and Weinberg evaluated the effects of soft-drink preservatives on South African asthmatic children by questionnaire and found that approximately 8% were intolerant to drinks containing sodium benzoate as the sole preservative and 20% were intolerant to drinks containing a mixture of benzoate and sulfite (73).

HYPERSENSITIVITY REACTIONS IN PURPURA

The incidence of allergic vascular purpura (also known as allergic vasculitis or Chonlein-Henoch purpura) caused by intolerance to benzoates and other food additives remains unknown. It is probably exceedingly infrequent in the general population and is rare even in susceptible groups (e.g., chronic asthmatics). Intolerance to tartrazine in butter that manifested as vascular purpura was suspected by Criep in a 22-year-old patient with a family history of bronchial asthma (74). Double-blind, placebo-controlled oral challenges confirmed a hypersensitivity to tartrazine. Michaëlsson and coworkers reported that three out of seven patients with allergic vascular purpura were intolerant to oral sodium benzoate or *p*-hydroxybenzoic acid that was administered in a single-blind test along with an initial lactose placebo (75). All medications were withheld three days prior to testing. One of the three benzoate responders also exhibited sensitivity to aspirin and tartrazine. One of the other two patients was sensitive to new coccine and tartrazine. Kubba and Champion (76) described an asthmatic patient who developed purpura on the legs after oral challenge (methods unspecified) with tartrazine (1 mg), sodium benzoate (50 mg), and methylparaben (methyl-4-hydroxybenzoate; 50 mg). Her asthma did not change during the provocation tests.

THE MELKERSSON-ROSENTHAL SYNDROME

Food allergy and sensitization or intolerance to sodium benzoate and other food additives have been implicated in the etiology of the Melkersson-Rosenthal syndrome as, in some cases, dietary restriction has alleviated or prompted remission of the symptoms (77–81). This rare disorder is characterized by chronic orofacial granulomatosis (particularly of the lips), peripheral facial paralysis, and fissuring of the tongue. It is reportedly more common in atopic patients (78, 80).

In a 34-year-old male patient, symptoms were triggered by sodium benzoate (50 mg) and tartrazine (5 mg) after double-blind, oral challenge tests (79). Elimination of sodium benzoate and tartrazine from the patient's diet led to progressive improvement and complete remission lasting at least one year. Another patient with the Melkersson-Rosenthal syndrome had positive 20 minute, closed-patch testing reactions to cinnamaldehyde and benzoic acid (81). On the other hand, 45% of the control subjects (9 of 20) showed positive reactions to these compounds in similar tests. Nevertheless, the patient's condition improved by avoiding foods containing these additives.

Morales and coworkers investigated six subjects with Melkersson-Rosenthal syndrome as diagnosed both clinically and histologically (82). The patients included five females and one male, ranging in age from 38 to 50 years (mean age = 42 years). Comprehensive prick skin tests gave negative results in these patients. In addition, double-blind, placebo-controlled oral challenge tests, spaced at least 72 hours apart, were conducted with the following compounds: sodium benzoate (250 mg); monosodium glutamate (300 mg); tartrazine (30 mg); sulfites (90 mg); erythrosine (15 mg); paraoxibenzoate (250 mg); lactose (100 mg); acetylsalicylic acid (360 mg); and annate (15 mg). The oral challenges were also negative in these patients. Thus, this study found no evidence of atopy and no evidence of hypersensitivity to sodium benzoate or other food additives.

Parabens as Food Additives

The parabens, which are straight-chain alkyl esters of *p*-hydroxybenzoic acid (4-hydroxybenzoic acid), include methylparaben, ethylparaben, propylparaben, butylparaben and heptylparaben (Fig. 25.2). The widespread use of parabens as antimicrobial agents in pharmaceuticals, cosmetics, and food began in

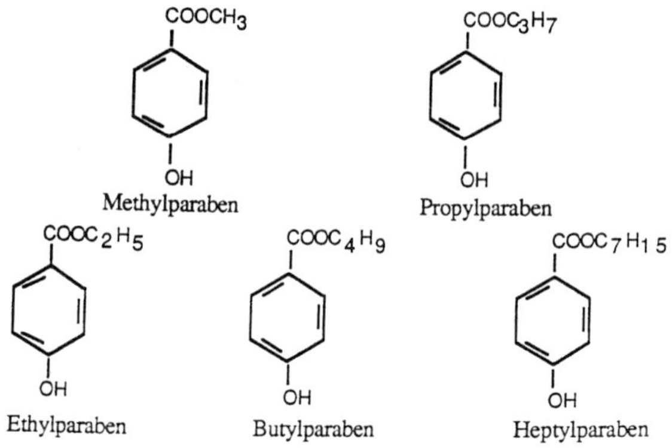

Figure 25.2

The paraben family of food additives.

Europe in the 1920s and later spread to the United States in the 1930s, where they were used as preservatives (primarily in pharmaceuticals and cosmetics). Methylparaben and propylparaben are also approved for use as antimicrobial agents in foods such as processed vegetables, baked goods, fats and oils, and seasonings, to name just a few. They are present in amounts ranging from 0.0001% to 0.10%.

PHYSICAL, CHEMICAL, AND ANTIMICROBIAL PROPERTIES OF PARABENS

The parabens are white crystalline or powder solids that have practically no odor or taste (Fig. 25.2). Their melting points decrease with increasing length of the alkyl chain (e.g., methylparaben, 131 °C; propylparaben, 97 °C). They have limited water solubility that also decreases with increasing alkyl chain length (e.g., methylparaben, 0.25 g/100 mL at 25 °C; propylparaben, 0.04 g/100 mL at 25 °C) (83). Bacteriocidal activity increases with increasing paraben alkyl chain length. The parabens provide effective antimicrobial properties over a much broader pH range than benzoic acid, which is active primarily at acidic pH (84). Because methylparaben is an effective antimicrobial agent against psychotropic (cold-tolerant) bacteria (85), it is frequently used to preserve chilled convenience foods.

NATURAL OCCURRENCE
AND METABOLISM

Parabens are not described as occurring naturally in plants or animals even though the parent compound, p-hydroxybenzoic acid, is produced by certain fungi. The acute and chronic toxicity, carcinogenicity, teratogenicity, mutagenicity, and metabolism was extensively reviewed by the Life Sciences Research Office of the Federation of American Society for Experimental Biology for the Food and Drug Administration in 1972. It concluded that "there was no short-term toxicological consequences in the rat, rabbit, cat, dog or man, and no long-term toxicological consequences in rats, of consuming the parabens in amounts greatly exceeding those currently consumed in the normal diet of the U.S. population" (86). Recent studies have shown, however, that parabens can inhibit the release of lysosomal enzymes by mitogen-stimulated peripheral blood lymphocytes in vitro at concentrations ranging from 0.06 mmol/L for butylparaben to 0.25 to 0.50 mmol/L for the other parabens (87).

The parabens are rapidly absorbed and hydrolyzed to the free acid p-hydroxybenzoic acid. Glycine, glucuronic acid, and sulfuric acid conjugates are then formed and eliminated in the urine, along with the free acid. Thus, the later stages of paraben metabolism mimic the metabolism of the benzoates as described earlier. The pathways for paraben metabolism in animals and humans were elucidated in the 1920s and 1930s. These studies, as well as studies on contact sensitivity and sensitization, have been reviewed (88).

Adverse Reactions to Parabens

An extensive body of literature dating back to 1940 describes paraben-induced contact dermatitis in patients using topical pharmaceuticals and cosmetics containing parabens as preservatives (88). In contrast, only a few reports have appeared that describe adverse reactions to parabens used as food additives. In a study involving 37 patients with chronic urticaria, Thune and Granholt reported that five individuals (14%) reacted to an oral paraben mixture of methyl-, ethyl-, and propylparaben (50 mg each) that was combined in a single capsule (44). The validity of this study can be questioned because the clinical protocol was not described. Kaminer and coworkers described a delayed hypersensitivity reaction consisting of an urticarial maculopapular rash over the entire body (except face) to orally administered haloperidol containing methylparaben in a 17-year-old male psychiatric patient (89). In the presence of methylparaben, the patient's lymphocytes inhibited guinea pig macrophage migration (90). In a group of 25 pediatric patients presenting with recurrent urticaria, angioedema, asthma, and other conditions suspected of being caused by food allergy, Ibero et al. (53) observed positive reactions to orally administered methylparaben (5 and 50 mg) in only three individuals (12%) using the single-blind battery protocol developed by Michaëlsson and Juhlin (43). As described earlier, 10 patients in the Ibero study had positive provocation tests with sodium benzoate.

Diagnosing Hypersensitivity to Benzoates and Parabens

Although the prevalence of intolerance to benzoates and parabens in the general population is unknown, it is probably very low given the extensive worldwide use of benzoates and parabens for many decades. That certain groups of individuals—namely, those with asthma, chronic urticaria–angioedema, rhinitis, and purpura—might be predisposed toward hypersensitivity reactions with benzoates and parabens has not been firmly established, even though many investigators have reported a high prevalence of additive intolerance in selected study groups. Most studies assessing food additive intolerance have used either open or single-blind protocols. Stevenson and colleagues, for example, have shown that patients who tested positive to tartrazine in a single-blind study failed to demonstrate positive reactions when tested by a double-blind protocol (91).

The study by Lahti and Hannuksela on intolerance to benzoic acid clearly illustrates the necessity of conducting double-blind, placebo-controlled challenges (92). A group of 150 dermatological patients presenting with urticaria ($n = 29$), atopy (atopic eczema, allergic rhinitis, or asthma, $n = 32$), and other skin diseases ($n = 118$) were challenged with oral benzoic acid (500 mg) or lactose (500 mg) in gelatin capsules given on two consecutive days using a double-blind, placebo-controlled protocol. Both objective and subjective symptoms were recorded for 24 hours after the patients received their test capsules. The range of objective and subjective symptoms observed in all patients receiving benzoic acid was 3% to 7% and 25% to 28%, respectively. The corresponding figures for patients receiving the placebo were 6% to 14% and 17% to 28%. Thus, no significant difference was observed between benzoic acid and lactose. Although not reported, any correlation between benzoic acid responders and placebo responders (if present) would have been an interesting result to report. This study clearly indicates the need to conduct double-blind protocols when attempting to determine the prevalence of food additive intolerance in a specific patient population.

Patient selection for oral provocation studies also plays an important role as pointed out by Podell's critique (93) of the Genton *et al.* (58) study of food additive intolerance in chronic urticaria and asthma. Patients were selected on the basis of a history of (1) suspected reactions to aspirin or food additives, (2) resistance to treatment, and (3) unexplained exacerbations. They were then placed on a two-week, additive-free diet and told to stop taking nonsteroidal anti-inflammatory drugs. All of the patients showed significant declines in symptoms prior to their oral provocation tests, which suggests that this improvement may have comprised another criterion for selection. As suggested by Podell, the authors may have selected out a rare group of "diet-responsive individuals" who were unrepresentative of the general urticaria/asthma population. Of the 33 single-blind, single-placebo challenges conducted with sodium benzoate, 6 (18%) were positive. One wonders what outcome might have resulted if the studies had been conducted using a double-blind, multiple-placebo protocol. Simon has reviewed techniques used in food additive oral provocation tests (94), while Yunginger has compared the diagnostic value of skin tests, im-

munoassays, and provocative challenge tests for food and food additive hypersensitivity (95).

Other factors likely to affect the outcome of oral provocation tests with benzoates and parabens include: (1) withholding of antihistamines, bronchodilators, and other medications prior to testing; (2) disguising test compounds in appropriate vehicles; (3) using solid (capsule) versus dissolved test compounds (the oral mucosa may be hyperreactive); (4) the frequency of multiple-dose administration and the possible development of tolerance; and (5) establishing a post-challenge observation period that is long enough to include delayed reactions.

REFERENCES

1. Simon RA, Stevenson DD. Adverse reactions to food and drug additives. In: Middleton E, Reed CE, Ellis EF, Adkinson NF, Yunginger JW, Busse WW, eds. Allergy: principles and practice. 4th ed. Mosby, 1993, 1687–1704.
2. Besser RE, Lett SM, Weber JT, et al. An outbreak of diarrhea and hemolytic uremic syndrome from Escherichia coli O157:H7 in fresh-pressed apple cider. J Am Med Assoc 1993;269:2217–2220.
3. Deresinski S. From hamburgers to hemolysis: Escherichia coli O157:H7. Infect Dis Alert 1993;12:81–84.
4. Zhao T, Doyle MP, Besser RE. Fate of enterohemorrhagic Escherichia coli O157:H7 in apple cider with and without preservatives. Appl Environ Microbiol 1993;59:2526–2530.
5. Food and Nutrition Board Commission of Life Sciences, National Research Council. 1982 Poundage update of Food Chemicals, Committee on Food Additive Survey Data. Washington, DC: National Academy Press, 1984.
6. Williams AE. Benzoic acid. In: Kirk-Othermer Encyclopedia of Chemical Technology. 3rd ed. New York: Wiley-Interscience, 1978, 778–792.
7. Lueck E. Antimicrobial food additives. New York: Springer-Verlag, 1980.
8. Juhlin E. Intolerance to food additives. In: Marzulli FM, Maibach HI, eds. Advances in modern toxicology, vol. 4. Dermatotoxicology and pharmacology. New York: J. Wiley, 1977, 455–463.
9. Swain AR, Dutten SP, Truswell AS. Salicylates in foods. J Am Diet Assoc 1985;85:950–959.
10. Kingsbury FB. The synthesis and excretion of hippuric acid. The glycine factor. Proc Soc Exp Biol Med 1923;20:405–408.
11. Quick AJ. The conjugation of benzoic acid in man. J Biol Chem 1931;92:65–85.
12. Schachter D. The chemical estimation of acyl glucuronides and its application to studies on the metabolism of benzoate and salicylate. J Clin Invest 1957;36:297–302.
13. Williams RT. The metabolism of aromatic acids. In: Williams RT, ed. Detoxication mechanisms. 2nd ed. London: Chapman & Hall, 1959, 348–389.
14. Batshaw ME, Monahan PS. Treatment of urea cycle disorders. Enzyme 1987;38:242–250.

15. Oyanagi K, Kuniya Y, Nagao M, Tsuchiyama A, Nakao T. Cytotoxicities of sodium benzoate in primary culture of hepatocytes from adult rat liver. Tohoku J Exp Med 1987;152:47–51.

16. Brusilow SW, Horwich AL. Urea cycle enzymes. In: Scriver CR, Beaudet AL, Sly WS, Valle D, eds. The metabolic and molecular bases of inherited disease. 7th ed. New York: McGraw-Hill, 1995, 1187–1232.

17. Wolff JA, Kulovich S, Yu AL, Qiao C-N, Nyhan WL. The effectiveness of benzoate in the management of seizures in nonketotic hyperglycinemia. Amer J Dis Child 1986;140:596–602.

18. Bryan AW. Clinical and experimental studies on sodium benzoate. The value of the sodium benzoate test of renal function and the effect of injury of the liver on hippuric acid synthesis. J Clin Invest 1925;2:1–33.

19. Quick AJ. The synthesis of hippuric acid: a new test of liver function. J Med Sci 1933;185:630–635.

20. Bartels EC. Liver function in hyperthyroidism as determined by the hippuric acid test. Ann Intern Med 1938;12:652–674.

21. Hirsheimer A. The hippuric acid excretion test in pregnancy. Am J Obst Gynec 1939;37:363–376.

22. Quastel JH, Wales WT. Faulty detoxication in schizophrenia: abnormal excretion of hippuric acid after administration of sodium benzoate. Lancet 1940;1:402–403.

23. Davies DR, Wales AIC, Hughes TPE. Faulty detoxication in mental disorder. Lancet 1940;1:403–405.

24. Lipschutz EW. A modification of the hippuric acid liver function test. Am J Digest Dis 1939;6:197–199.

25. Londe S, Probstein JG. The hippuric acid liver function test in children. J Pediatrics 1941;18:371–384.

26. Campbell DA. Some observations on the Quick hippuric acid test on hepatic function. Surgery 1942;11:195–197.

27. Quick AJ. The clinical application of the hippuric acid and prothrombin tests. Am J Clin Path 1940;10:222–233.

28. Kinsey RE, Wright DO. Reaction following ingestion of sodium benzoate in a patient with severe liver damage. J Lab Clin Med 1944;29:188–196.

29. Young E, Patel S, Stoneham M, Rona R, Wilkinson JD. The prevalence of reaction to food additives in a survey population. J R Coll Physicians Lond 1987;21:241–247.

30. Pollock I, Warner JO. A follow-up study of childhood food additive intolerance. J R Coll Physicians Lond 1987;21:248–250.

31. Fuglsang G, Madsen C, Saval P, Østerballe O. Prevalence of intolerance to food additives among Danish school children. Pediatr Allergy Immunol 1993;4:123–129.

32. Fuglsang G, Madsen C, Halken S, Jørgensen M, Østergaard PA, Østerballe O. Adverse reactions to food additives in children with atopic symptoms. Allergy 1994;49:31–37.

33. Madsen C. Prevalence of food additive intolerance. Hum Exp Toxicol 1995;13:393–399.

34. Valverde E, Vich JM, Garcia-Calderon JV, Garcia-Calderon PA. In vitro simulation of lymphocytes in patients with chronic urticaria induced by additives and food. Clin Allergy 1980;10:691–698.

35. Warrington RJ, Sauder PJ, McPhillips S. Cell-mediated immune responses to artificial food additives in chronic urticaria. Clin Allergy 1986;16:527–533.

36. Schaubschlager WW, Becker W-M, Schade U, Zabel P, Schlaak M. Release of mediators from human gastric mucosa and blood in adverse reactions to benzoate. Int Arch Allergy Appl Immunol 1991;96:97–101.

37. Hermann K, Rittweger R, Ring J. Urinary excretion of angiotensin I, II, arginine vasopressin and oxytocin in patients with anaphylactoid reactions. Clin Exp Allergy 1992;22:845–853.

38. Greaves MW. Urticaria: new molecular insights and treatments. J R Coll Physicians Lond 1992;26:199–203.

39. Juhlin L. Incidence of intolerance to food additives. Int J Dermatol 1980;19:548–551.

40. Sampter M, Beers RF. Concerning the routine intolerance to aspirin. J Allergy 1967;40:281–293.

41. Sampter M, Beers RF. Concerning the routine intolerance to aspirin. Ann Intern Med 1968;68:975–983.

42. Juhlin L, Michaëlsson G, Zetterström O. Urticaria and asthma induced by food-and-drug additives in patients with aspirin hypersensitivity. J Allergy Clin Immunol 1972;50:92–98.

43. Michaëlsson G, Juhlin L. Urticaria induced by preservatives are dye additives in food and drugs. Br J Dermatol 1973;88:525–532.

44. Thune P, Granholt A. Provocation tests with antiphlogistic and food additives in recurrent urticaria. Dermatologica 1975;151:360–367.

45. Doeglas HMG. Reactions to aspirin and food additives in patients with chronic urticaria, including the physical urticarias. Br J Dermatol 1975;93:135–144.

46. Kaaber K. Farvestoffer og konserveringsmidler ved kronisk urticaria. Vaerdien af provokationsforsog og eliminationsdiaet. Ugeskr Laeger 1978;140:1473–1476.

47. Meynadier J, Guillhou JJ, Levanture N. Chronic urticaria. Etiologic and therapeutic evaluation of 150 cases. Ann Dermatol Venereol 1979;106:153–158.

48. August PJ. Successful treatment of urticaria due to food additives with sodium cromoglycate and exclusion diet. In: Pepys J, Edward AM, eds. The mast cell: its role in health and disease. Kent, England: Pitman Medical, 1979, 584–590.

49. Wüthrich B, Hächi-Hermann D. Zur ätiologie der urticaria: sine retrospecktive studie amband von 316 consekutiven fallen. Z Hautkr 1980;55:102–111.

50. Ros A-M, Juhlin L, Michaëlsson G. A following study of patients with recurrent urticaria and hypersensitivity to aspirin, benzoates and azo dyes. Br J Dermatol 1976;95:19–24.

51. Juhlin L. Recurrent urticaria: clinical investigation of 330 patients. Br J Dermatol 1981;104:369–381.

52. Gibson A, Clancy R. Management of chronic idiopathic urticaria by the identification and exclusion of dietary factors. Clin Allergy 1980;10:699–704.

53. Ibero M, Esverri JL, Barroso C, Botey J. Dyes, preservatives and salicylates in the induction of food tolerance and/or hypersensitivity in children. Allergol Immunopathol (Madr) 1982;10:263–268.

54. Clemmensen O, Hjorth N. Perioral contact urticaria from sorbic acid and benzoic acid in a salad dressing. Contact Dermatitis 1982;8:1–6.

55. Nethercott JR, Lawrence MJ, Roy A-M, Gibson BL. Airborn contact urticaria due to sodium benzoate in a pharmaceutical manufacturing plant. J Occupational Med 1984;26:734–736.

56. Lahti A. Non-immunologic contact urticaria. Acta Derm Venereol 1980;50(suppl 91):1–49.

57. Ortolani C, Pastorello E, Luraghi MT, Della Torre F, Bellani M, Zanussi C. Diagnosis of intolerance to food additives. Ann Allergy 1984;53:587–591.

58. Genton D, Frei PC, Pecored A. Value of oral provocation tests to aspirin and food additives in the routine investigation of asthma and chronic urticaria. J Allergy Clin Immunol 1985;76:40–45.

59. Supramaniam G, Warner OJ. Artificial food additive intolerance in patients with angio-oedema and urticaria. Lancet 1986;907–909.

60. Garcia HJ, Alvarez JMN, Selles FJS, Aleman JAP. Reacciones adversas a conservatines alimentarios. Allergol Immunopathol (Madr) 1986;14:55–63.

61. van Bever HP, Docx M, Stevens WJ. Food and food additives in severe atopic dermatitis. Allergy 1989;44:588–594.

62. Hanifin JM, Lobitz WC. Newer concepts of atopic dermatitis. Arch Dermatol 1977;113:663–670.

63. Chafee RH, Settipane GA. Asthma caused by FD & C approved dyes. J Allergy 1967;40:65–72.

64. Rosenhall L, Zetterström O. Asthma provoked by analgesics, food colorants and food preservatives. Lakartidningen 1973;70:1417–1419.

65. Hoffman M. Challenges with aspirin, FD and C dyes, and preservatives in asthma. J Allergy Clin Immunol 1976;57:206–207 (abstract).

66. Freedman BJ. Asthma induced by sulphur dioxide, benzoate and tartrazine contained on orange drinks. Clin Allergy 1977;7:407–415.

67. Rosenhall L. Hypersensitivity to analgesics, preservatives and food colorants in patients with asthma or rhinitis. Acta Universitatis Upsaliensis 1977;269.

68. Rosenhall L. Evaluation of intolerance to analgesics, preservatives and food colorants with challenge test. Eur J Respir Dis 1982;634:410–419.

69. Weber RW, Hoffman M, Rane DA, Nelson HS. Incidence of bronchoconstrictions due to aspirin, azo dyes, non-azo dyes, and preservatives in a population of perennial asthmatics. J Allergy Clin Immunol 1979;64:32–37.

70. Østerballe O, Taudoroff E, Haahr J. Intolerance to aspirin, food-colouring agents and food preservatives in childhood asthma. Ugeskr Laeger 1979;141:1908–1910.

71. Tarlo SM, Broder I. Tartrazine and benzoate challenge and dietary avoidance in chronic asthma. Clin Allergy 1982;12:303–312.

72. Moneret-Vautrin DA, Moeller R, Malingrey L, Laxenaire MC. Anaphylactoid reaction to general anaesthesia: a case of intolerance to sodium benzoate. Anaesth Intens Care 1982;156–157.

73. Steinman HA, Weinberg EG. The effects of soft-drink preservatives on asthmatic children. South African Med J 1986;70:404–406.

74. Criep LH. Allergic vascular purpura. J Allergy Clin Immunol 1971;48:7–12.

75. Michaëlsson G, Pettersson L, Juhlin L. Purpura caused by food and drug additives. Arch Dermatol 1974;109:49–52.

76. Kubba R, Champion RH. Anaphylactoid purpura caused by tartrazine and benzoates. Br J Dermatol 1975;93(suppl):61–62.

77. Patton DW, Ferguson MM, Forsyth A, James J. Oro-facial granulomatosis: a possible allergic basis. Br J Oral Maxillofac Surg 1985;23:235–242.

78. Sweatman MC, Tasker R, Warner JO, Ferguson MM, Mitchell DN. Oro-facial granulomatosis. Response to elemental diet and provocation by food additives. Clin Allergy 1986;16:331–338.

79. Pachor ML, Ubani G, Cortina P, et al. Is the Melkersson-Rosenthal syndrome related to the exposure to food additives? Oral Surg Oral Med Oral Pathol 1996;67:393–395.

80. Lamey PJ, Lewis MA. Oral medicine in practice: orofacial allergic reactions. Br Dent J 1990;168:59–63.

81. McKenna KE, Walsh MY, Burrows D. The Melkersson-Rosenthal syndrome and food additive hypersensitivity. Br J Dermatol 1994;131:921–922.

82. Morales C, Penarrocha M, Bagan JV, Burches E, Pelaez A. Immunological study of Melkersson-Rosenthal syndrome. Lack of response to food additive challenge. Clin Exp Allergy 1995;25:260–264.

83. Chichester DF, Tanner FW. Antimicrobial food additives. In: Handbook of food additives. 2nd ed. Cleveland: CRC Press, 1972, 115–184.

84. Aalto TR, Firman MC, Rigler NE. p-Hydroxybenzoic acid esters as preservatives. I. Uses, antibacterial and antifungal studies, properties and determination. J Am Pharm Assoc 1953;42:449–457.

85. Moir CJ, Eyles MJ. Inhibition, injury, and inactivation of four psychotrophic foodborne bacteria by the preservatives methyl p-hydroxybenzoate and potassium sorbate. J Food Protect 1992;55:360–366.

86. Schmidt AM. Methylparaben and propylparaben. Affirmation of GRAS status of direct human food ingredients. Fed Register 1973;38:20048–20050.

87. Bairati C, Goi G, Lombardo A, Tettamanti G. The esters of p-hydroxybenzoate (parabens) inhibit the release of lysosomal enzymes by mitogen-stimulated peripheral human lymphocytes in culture. Clin Chim Acta 1994;224:147–157.

88. Final report on the safety assessment of methylparaben, ethylparaben, propylparaben and butylparaben. J Am College Toxicol 1984;3:147–209.

89. Kaminer Y, Apter A, Tyano S, Livni E, Wijsenbeek H. Delayed hypersensitivity reaction to orally administered methylparaben. Clin Pharm 1982;1:169–470.

90. Rajapakse DA, Glynn LE. Macrophage migration inhibition test using guinea pig macrophages and human lymphocytes. Nature 1970;226:857–858.

91. Stevenson DD, Simon RA, Lumry WR, Mathison DA. Adverse reactions to tartrazine. J Allergy Clin Immunol 1986;78(suppl 1, part 2):182–191.

92. Lahti A, Hannuksela M. Is benzoic acid really harmful in cases of atopy and urticaria? Lancet 1986;1055.

93. Podell RN. Unwrapping urticaria. The role of food additives. Postgrad Med 1985;78:83–97.

94. Simon RA. Adverse reactions to food additives. New Engl Regional Allergy Proc 1986;7:533–542.

95. Yunginger JW. Proper application of available laboratory tests for adverse reactions to foods and food additives. J Allergy Clin Immunol 1986;78:220–223.

26

ADVERSE REACTIONS TO THE ANTIOXIDANTS BUTYLATED HYDROXYANISOLE (BHA) AND BUTYLATED HYDROXYTOLUENE (BHT)

Richard W. Weber

Foods containing vegetable or animal fat turn rancid through chemical changes induced by exposure to oxygen, heat, moisture, or the action of enzymes. The rapidity with which rancidity develops depends on the source and storage conditions of the fats or oils. The structure of unsaturated fats includes carbon–carbon double bonds, and these sites are susceptible to the chemical changes causing rancidity. Saturated fats are more resistant. Vegetable oils include more unsaturated fats, but also contain naturally occurring protective antioxidants such as tocopherols. Animal fats are more saturated, but have lower amounts of natural antioxidants, and therefore face a greater risk for spoilage (1, 2). These same factors may cause fruits and vegetables to lose their freshness and change colors—a condition known as the "browning effect." Antioxidants block these events, and may even restore "freshness" in some cases.

The phenolic antioxidants butylated hydroxyanisole (BHA) and butylated hydroxytoluene (BHT) are used in a large number of foods that contain oil and fat. Other chemicals having antioxidant activity are frequently combined with BHA or BHT to enhance their activity: such agents include propyl gallate, citric acid, phosphoric acid, and ascorbic acid. Additionally, tocopherols are antioxidants that are used commonly in baked goods, cereals, soups, and milk products. The members of this group of closely related compounds have varying amounts of vitamin E action, and about eight forms occur naturally in foods such as vegetable oils, cereals, nuts, and leafy vegetables.

BHA and BHT are synthetic compounds and do not occur in nature. BHT (also termed 2,6-di-*tert*-butyl-4-methylphenol or 2,6-di-*tert*-butyl-*p*-cresol) is manufactured from *p*-cresol and isobutylene (3). BHA represents a mixture of two isomers: 85% 2-*tert*-butyl-4-methoxyphenol and 15% 3-*tert*-butyl-4-methoxyphenol (Fig. 26.1) (4). BHT was initially patented in 1947. Both of these substances were originally developed as antioxidants for petroleum and rubber products, but were quickly discovered to have effective antioxidant properties in animal fats.

In 1949, BHA appeared on the new Class IV perservative positive (allowed) list of the Health Protection Branch of Health and Welfare Canada. Usage was restricted to levels less than 0.02% (5). Animal studies from BHA manufacturers were submitted to the U.S. Food and Drug Administration in 1954 and 1955, and marketing permission was granted prior to the 1958 Food Additives Amendment. As a result, BHA and BHT were granted "generally recognized as safe" (GRAS) status and no additional studies were required. A number of items on the GRAS list have come under further scrutiny, however, and BHA and BHT remain on the list with provisional status. The FDA limits their use in food, either alone or in combination with other antioxidants, to 0.02% or less of the total fat and oil content (1).

These compounds are commonly added to various foods, cosmetics, and pharmaceuticals to prevent oxidation of unsaturated fatty acids, and are considered more potent than other antioxidants. Also, they

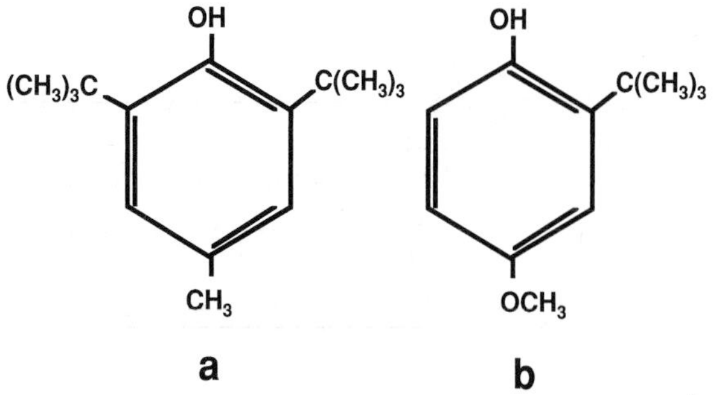

Figure 26.1

(a) Butylated hydroxytoluene (BHT, 2,6-di-*tert*-butyl-4-methylphenol). (b) Butylated hydroxyanisole (BHA, 2-*tert*-butyl-4-methoxyphenol). Commercial BHA also contains 15% 3-*tert*-butyl-4-methoxyphenol.

are less expensive than some other antioxidants, costing $1–$5/lb, as opposed to, for example, nordihydroguaiaretic acid (NDGA) at $25–$30/lb (5). BHA is used more often than BHT because it offers greater stability at higher temperatures. Both substances are employed in breakfast cereals, chewing gum, snack foods, vegetable oils, shortening, potato flakes, granules and chips, enriched rice, and candy (1). By 1970, the total amount of BHT used in foods was near 600,000 pounds, or twice the amount used in 1960. By 1976, the annual U.S. production of BHT totaled 19.81 million pounds, of which 10.95 million pounds went for nonfood uses and 8.86 million pounds for food use. In addition to human food, BHT is added to animal feeds, such as fish meal included in poultry feed (3). Passive food exposure to these antioxidants also occurs through their use in food-packaging materials such as pressure-sensitive adhesives, paper and cardboard, lubricants, and sealing gaskets for food containers (1, 3).

The U.S. average daily intake per person of BHT alone was estimated as 2 mg in 1970, while intake in the United Kingdom was estimated at half that amount (3). Given today's greater reliance of the North American diet on processed, packaged foods, substantially larger daily intakes of BHA and BHT have been measured recently. In 1986, the mean intakes for BHA ranged from 0.13 to 0.39 mg/kg body weight/day. The intake for teenage males was 12.12 mg/person/day, with the average for both sexes of all ages at 7.40 mg/person/day (5). Presumably, current intakes are even higher. In 1974, the Joint Food and Agriculture Organization of the United Nation/World Health Organization Expert Committee on Food Additives recommended 0.5 mg/kg body weight as the acceptable daily intake of BHA, BHT, or the combination of the two (4).

Toxicology

Despite the ease with which these antioxidants passed muster at the FDA, animal toxicology studies have revealed a variety of adverse events associated with BHA and BHT. These reactions may well be related to their actions as antioxidants. BHA and BHT act as lipid-soluble chain-breaking agents, delaying lipid peroxidation by scavenging intermediate radicals such as lipid peroxyls (6). In the process, however, the antioxidant loses a hydrogen atom, thus becoming a radical. The antioxidant radical generally appears less reactive than the peroxyl free radical, but under some circumstances can show pro-oxidant properties, frequently due to interactions with iron ions.

Single doses of BHT have been reported to induce interstitial pneumonitis and pulmonary fibrosis in mice, although BHA and other antioxidants did not appear to produce the same effect (7). This BHT effect can be potentiated by oxygen given early (but not late) (8, 9). Additionally, high-dose corticosteroids may significantly worsen lung damage if given early, while late administration may alleviate the injury (10, 11). Whether the lung injury is mediated through some unique property of BHT, rather than through an antioxidant pathway remains unclear: It does appear that the extent of damage depends on several factors, interweaving both dose and timing. Recent research demonstrates that distinct mouse strain differences appear in the chronic response to BHT, part of which may be due to cytochrome P_{450} conversion of BHT to the more pneumotoxic metabolite *tert*-butyl hydroxylated BHT (BHT-BuOH) (12). CXB H mice became tolerant to the chronic administration of BHT, while Balb/cBy mice showed a chronic inflammatory process with activated alveolar macrophages and increased lung tumor multiplicity. Acute effects demonstrated two- to fivefold decreases in protein kinase Cα and calpain II (calcium-dependent protease isozyme II).

In recent years, the impact of dietary antioxidants on cancer prevention has received much scientific and media attention. BHA and BHT have been shown to both prevent and enhance tumor development in different systems. BHA, BHT, and NDGA have been shown to decrease skin tumor promotion by 12-O-tetradecanoylphorbol-13-acetate (TPA), benzoyl peroxide, and ultraviolet light. BHA achieves this result through decreased gene expression of ornithine decarboxylase, an indicator of skin tumor promotion and hyperproliferation (13). BHT, however, increased the incidence of liver tumors in male C3H mice (14). The same study showed increased colon cancer in Balb/c mice following one chemical carcinogen (dimethylhydrazine), but not another (methylnitrosourea). BHA, on the other hand, appeared to protect against the acute liver toxicity of a colon-specific carcinogen, methylazoxymethanol acetate (15). In contrast, high-dose BHA has been shown to produce cancers of the forestomach in rats (5). Because humans do not have a forestomach, and doses about 10,000 times higher than likely human consumption were used in this study, the FAO/WHO Joint Expert Committee, after a review of the data, concluded that the benefits of BHA outweighed the potential risks (5).

Using human lymphocytes, Klein and Bruser demonstrated BHT cytotoxicity with concentrations greater than 100 μg/mL (16). At 50 μg/mL, BHT inhibited the mixed lymphocyte reaction, but not PHA stimulation. A synergistic effect of PHA suppression was seen with coincubation with either cortisol or prednisolone.

In mouse studies, BHA inhibited several microsomal enzymes, but long-term administration also induced specific P$_{450}$ cytochrome enzymes (17). In humans, BHA administered at 0.5 mg/kg body weight for 10 days had no appreciable effects on biotransformation capacity (18). Antipyrine and paracetamol (acetaminophen) metabolism were unaffected. Urinary excretion of BHA metabolites was significantly increased on days 3 and 7 as compared with day 1, suggesting either an inhibition of BHA metabolizing enzymes or bioaccumulation of BHA and/or its metabolites in the body.

Asthma/Rhinitis

Despite a wealth of animal toxicology literature on these antioxidants, only scattered reports exist indicating adverse reactions to BHA and BHT in humans. In 1973, Fisherman and Cohen reported on seven patients with either asthma, vasomotor rhinitis with or without nasal polyps, or a combination of the two, who were suspected of intolerance to BHA and BHT (19). No clinical details were given, nor were the reasons that BHA and BHT were suspected to cause difficulty detailed. These patients were identified following open challenge with capsule ingestion of 125 to 250 mg of BHA/BHT and reproduction of symptoms of worsening vasomotor rhinitis, headache, flushing, asthma, conjunctival suffusion, dull retrosternal pain radiating to the back, diaphoresis, or somnolence. No objective measures were noted. BHA/BHT intolerance was also associated with a doubling of a Duke earlobe bleeding time (termed the "sequential vascular response" by the authors) in all cases. No rationale for the reported effect on the bleeding time was given, other than a supposed similarity to aspirin intolerance. In a follow-up paper published in the same year dealing with aspirin cross-reactivity, these authors reported finding 21 patients with intolerance to BHA/BHT as identified via the bleeding time, of whom 17 had clinical symptoms on challenge. No clinical details were given in this later paper (20).

The following year, in an unsuccessful attempt to duplicate Fisherman and Cohen's initial findings, Cloninger and Novey performed a similar study using oral ingestion of 300 to 850 mg BHA in five asthmatics and two rhinitics (21). They reported that the baseline earlobe bleeding time was not reproducible to the degree suggested by the previous authors. None of the patients had clinical exacerbations, changes in peak flows, or more than a 50% change in the bleeding times; a non–dose-related effect of drowsiness was noted in four of seven patients. Cloninger and Novey, therefore, questioned the validity of clincal BHA intolerance as well as the validity and reproducibility of the sequential vascular response. Parenthetically, Goodman and colleagues, in a case of well-documented BHA/BHT-induced chronic urticaria (discussed below), could not demonstrate a positive effect of BHA 250 mg or placebo on the earlobe bleeding time in either the patient or two controls (22).

Weber and colleagues found no asthmatic responses (greater than 25% drop in FEV$_1$) in 43 moderately severe perennial asthmatics undergoing single-blind capsule challenges with sequential doses of 125 mg and 250 mg of BHA and BHT (23). This group represented a subset of a larger study where single-blind challenges were validated by subsequent double-blind challenges. Aspirin sensitivity was documented in 44% of the patients, and reactivity to *p*-hydroxybenzoic acid, sodium benzoate, or azo or nonazo dyes in 2% to 5%. In one unpublished case, a drop of pulmonary function followed double-blind challenge with 250 mg of BHT in a patient having food anaphylaxis and oral allergy syndrome, but this finding was not validated with additional blinded challenges. Thus, at the present time, no reports of challenges with either BHA or BHT have resulted in well-documented, reproducible asthmatic responses.

Urticaria

In 1975, Thune and Granholt reported on 100 patients with recurrent urticaria evaluated with provocative food additive challenges (24). Sixty-two patients had positive challenges, with two-thirds reacting to multiple substances. Positivity rates for individual dyes, preservatives, or anti-inflammatory drugs ranged from 10% to 30%. Most reactions occurred within 1 to 2 hours, with a number occurring between 12 and 20-plus hours. Six of 47 (12.7%) reacted to BHA, and 6 of 43 (13.9%) reacted to BHT; it is unclear whether these were the same six patients. Test doses were given in 2 or 3 increments, with the total dose of BHA and BHT reaching 17 mg. The provocative challenges were not blinded, nor did the authors state criteria used to determine a positive response.

In 1977, Fisherman and Cohen reported the results of provocative oral or intradermal challenges of a large number of suspected agents on the bleeding time (their "sequential vascular response") in the assessment of 215 patients with chronic urticaria (25). Medications were withdrawn 12 hours prior to challenge, with the exception of hydroxyzine, which was withheld for 72 hours. Intolerance was found in 19 patients with challenges of 250 to 500 mg of BHA and BHT. Some details on four reactors challenged with 250 mg each of BHA and BHT were provided in a table in the published report. In addition to doubling of the earlobe bleeding time, two developed nasal congestion and three had urticaria, although it is not clear whether this effect represented an increase over baseline. These authors believed that they had determined "single or partial etiologies" in 203 of the 215 patients (94.4%), an astounding success rate in a clinical entity known for its resistance to defining a cause. Obviously, the same criticism based on the lack of a conceivable mechanism and the nonreproducibility of the test by other investigators holds for these authors' urticaria evaluations as well as the asthma challenges.

In a review on urticaria in 1977, Juhlin mentioned the results of provocative challenges with a mix of BHA and BHT in 130 urticaria patients (26). Incremental doses of 1, 10, and 50 mg each of BHA and BHT resulted in nine positive and five suspected positive challenges (6.9% to 10.8%). Details on the nature of the patients' symptoms, criteria for positive responses, or the blinding of the challenges were not given. Four years later, Juhlin published the results of an evaluation of 330 patients with recurrent urticaria (27). He used a 15-day, single-blind challenge battery of dyes, preservatives, and placebo. Antihistamines were withheld for 4 to 5 days before the challenge sequence commenced. Testing was carried out when patients had "no or slight symptoms." Tests were judged to be positive if "clear signs of urticaria or angio-oedema" occurred within 24 hours. Slightly less than half of the 330 patients (156) received a BHA/BHT challenge with cumulative doses of 1, 10, 50, and 50 mg given (total dose 111 mg). Fifteen percent had positive reactions, and 12% had equivocal reactions. Lactose placebo was given in two doses on days 1, 3, 9, and 12, although the order was modified. Active substances were given in single to six divided doses at hourly intervals. Most patients did not undergo the entire challenge schedule; in particular, one-third did not receive a placebo challenge.

Hannuksela and Lahti published the results of an extensive double-blind challenge study in 1986 (28). They evaluated 44 patients with chronic urticaria of greater than 2 months' duration, 91 atopic dermatitis patients, and 123 patients with resolved contact dermatitis. They used wheat starch as their placebo rather than lactose because of Juhlin's reports of positive responses to lactose placebo. Patients were challenged to sodium metabisulfite (9 mg), benzoic acid (200 mg), BHA and BHA mixture (50 mg each), and beta carotene and beta-apo-carotenal mixture (200 mg each). In cases of positive reactions, challenges were repeated 4 days later to validate the response; challenges were rated as positive if the patient responded both times, and as equivocal if the repeat proved negative. Of the 44 urticaria patients, none had reproducible positive reactions to BHA/BHT, and two responded to the first challenge but not the second. The same response occurred with the atopic dermatitis patients in that two experienced equivocal reactions to BHA/BHT. None of the contact dermatitis patients reacted to the antioxidants. One urticaria patient had reproducible responses to the wheat placebo, and another to benzoic acid; a third urticaria subject experienced an equivocal response to metabisulfite. One atopic dermatitis patient had positive reactions to carotenal/carotene, and another had an equivocal reaction to metabisulfite. One contact dermatitis patient had an equivocal reaction to the wheat placebo (a second challenge was not performed). The authors contrasted their results to those obtained by Juhlin, and cited challenge differences to explain their lack of responses. They also wondered whether a prolonged refractory period following the initial positive challenges could account for the negative follow-up trials, as they had waited only 4 days. In summary, however, the authors suggested that ordinary amounts of food additives generally do not provoke urticaria or influence atopic dermatitis (28).

In 1990, Goodman and colleagues reported the first double-blind, placebo-controlled, multiple-challenge protocol documenting the link of BHA and BHT with chronic urticaria. The demonstration of symptom aggravation did not rest on single challenges; instead, two patients with chronic urticaria and angioedema of 3 to 4 years' duration underwent oral challenges with several agents performed 2 to 3 times for verification. The patients had demonstrated improvement on restricted diets, but had lost 20 to 30 pounds in the process. Both patients were admitted, placed on an elemental diet formula, and observed for 5 to 7 days to establish baseline activity. The patients' pruritus severity was then evaluated, and skin lesions were ranked from 0 to 4+ based on degree of body distribution. Only challenges inducing lesions within 12 hours of ingestion and involving generalized lesions or an entire extremity or body area were considered positive responses. Lesions appeared 12 to 24 hours after the challenges were considered equivocal. A mixture of 125 mg each of BHA and BHT was given, with 250 mg of each antioxidant given 2 to 4 hours later if no major reaction had occurred. One patient was also challenged to BHA 250 mg alone. Placebo capsules consisted of either dextrose or lactose. The patients were also challenged to sodium benzoate, p-hydroxybenzoic acid, tartrazine, and other azo dyes. Both patients reacted within 1 to 6 hours to BHA and BHT, at all times, and did not react to the other additives or placebo on numerous trials. No delayed reactions occurred past 6 hours.

One patient had been routinely ingesting oatmeal for breakfast that contained BHA and BHT. Both patients were placed on diets specifically avoiding BHA and BHT, resulting in sustained diminution of frequency and severity of urticaria. At seven years follow-up, the first patient continued to adhere to his diet rigidly, and noted exacerbations of his urticaria when unexpected exposures occurred. At one year follow-up, the other patient also continued to follow his diet, noting only two minor exacerbations, again after ingesting foods containing BHA and BHT. These two episodes lasted less than 12 hours and required no medication. Each patient returned to his pre-illness weight and was able to resume his normal occupation.

The first patient assessed had serial plasma determinations throughout the challenge period for CH_{50}, activated C_3 and factor B, and PGE2, $PGF_{2\alpha}$, and dihydroxyketoPGF$_{2\alpha}$. Blood was drawn at baseline, at half-hour intervals after the first dose to 2 hours, and at hourly intervals until 6 hours after the second dose. After the initial challenges were completed with the first patient and the code broken, both the patient and two normal controls underwent an additional double-blind session, using BHA (250 mg) and placebo. This step was taken to evaluate the predictive value of the sequential vascular response test (SVR) of Fisherman and Cohen. As noted earlier, this test is basically an earlobe bleeding time, but has been advanced as a diagnostic for adverse reactions to BHA/BHT, as well as aspirin and other chemicals. Prick skin tests with serial dilutions of BHA, BHT, sodium salicylate, and OHBA were also performed, and proved uniformly negative.

Serial complement and prostaglandin determinations during the challenges were unrewarding. CH$_{50}$ was seen to decrease 30% to 35% randomly on both placebo and active compound days. Activated C_3 and factor B were sporadically elevated on four occasions—twice with placebo and once during the pre-challenge baseline period. The prostaglandin levels decreased as the day progressed, regardless of whether the patient received placebo or active compound. The authors, therefore, could not demonstrate any changes with positive challenges in the prostaglandins measured. Despite the extensive evaluation, the mechanism of action remains uncertain. An immunological process was not supported by the inconsistent changes in complement components, negative immediate skin tests, and lack of vasculitis on biopsy. The strict elimination diets did not totally ablate lesions in either patient. The antioxidants may have acted as potentiators of an underlying unrelated process, similar to the action of aspirin in chronic urticaria (29). Serial earlobe bleeding times were all unchanged with both placebo and BHA in the patient and control subjects, despite the patient's brisk urticarial response to the BHA.

Osmundsen reported a case of contact urticaria related to BHT contained in plastic folders (30). Contact with the folders on unbroken skin resulted in a strong urticarial reaction within 20 minutes. The patient had positive wheal and flare responses to 1% BHA and BHT in ethanol.

The importance of these antioxidants in causing or aggravating chronic urticaria is not clear, and the true incidence of urticarial adverse reactions to BHA/BHT remains unknown. Identification of provokers in a disease of waxing and waning nature may be difficult: Are reactions truly causally related, or do they represent only spontaneous exacerbations of the process? This issue becomes especially critical when a background of urticarial activity persists during challenges. A clear definition of what constitutes a positive reaction becomes essential in such cases. Additionally, the observer rating the severity of the reaction must be blinded as well as the subject, as he or she is equally susceptible to expectation bias. The studies of Thune and Granholt, and Juhlin fail to meet both of these standards (24, 26, 27). The 13% to 15% incidence of BHA/BHT reactions reported in these studies most likely represents an overestimate. Preliminary results of single-blind, placebo-controlled food additive panel challenges at Scripps Clinic have been unrewarding (31). In evaluating more than 20 chronic urticaria patients, challenge with a panel including tartrazine, potassium metabisulfite, monosodium glutamate, aspartame, sodium benzoate, methylparaben, BHA, BHT, and sunset yellow (FD&C yellow no. 6) has revealed no responders. It is hoped that larger numbers will ultimately be reported. Additionally, the importance of double-blinding in such studies has been pointed out by Weber and colleagues, and reenforced by Stevenson and associates (23, 32). In the former study, of 15 patients who reacted to dyes or preservatives on open challenge, only 3 responded under repeat double-blind conditions.

Dermatitis

A variety of nonurticarial skin eruptions have been attributed to food additives. Contact dermatitis may appear in response to a large number of food additives—especially antioxidants, spices, gums, and waxes. Evidence for such responses can be objectively obtained through patch testing for delayed hypersensitivity.

Tosti and colleagues reported two cases of contact dermatitis due to BHA in topical agents for psoriasis and eczema (33). Patch testing was positive for BHA but negative for BHT in both cases. The concentration of BHA in the preparations was 0.1% and 0.2%, respectively. In their 1987 report, the authors cited 14 cases of BHA contact dermatitis in the literature. Contact sensitivity to latex gloves constitutes an ever-increasing problem; one recent report, however, revealed sensitivity not to the usual rubber allergens, but to antioxidants, one of which was BHA (34). Acciai and coworkers found one case of contact dermatitis from BHA in a pastry cook during their investigation of 72 caterers with eczema (35). An evaluation of contact sensitivity in 69 women with pruritus vulvae revealed patch positivity of clinical significance in 40 (58%); one of these women also demonstrated sensitivity to BHA (2% in petrolatum) (36). Thus, in some cases, once the hypersensitivity has been initiated through cutaneous exposure, dermatitis symptoms could be flared by ingestion of the causative agent. Roed-Petersen and Hjorth found four patients with eczematous dermatitis who had positive patch tests to both BHA and BHT (37). Dietary avoidance of the antioxidants resulted in remissions in two patients. When challenged with ingestion of 10 to 40 mg BHA or BHT, both patients experienced exacerbations of the dermatitis.

Cutaneous vasculitis from food additives in chewing gum has been induced by ponceau (FD&C red no. 4), and also by BHT (38, 39). The case of acute urticarial vasculitis due to BHT was reported in 1986 by Moneret-Vautrin and associates. Biopsy revealed a heavy perivascular lymphoid infiltrate of the upper dermis, with immunofluorescence revealing IgM, C1q, C_3, C_9, and fibrinogen. Lesions resolved after use of the chewing gum was discontinued. A series of single-blind challenges showed that the lesions returned with ingestion of BHT but not other ingredients.

Mechanisms

The reports of Roed-Petersen and Hjorth, Osmundsen, and Moneret-Vautrin suggest that certain adverse reactions to BHA and BHT may be mediated through immunological mechanisms in addition to the mechanism seen in typical delayed hypersensitivity contact disorders. Histamine release from leukocytes has been

described following contact with ASA, benzoate, BHA/BHT, and azo dyes (40). The authors studied 12 urticaria patients as well as 18 healthy subjects. BHA and BHT each caused histamine release one time in an urticaria patient, but four healthy subjects reacted to BHT only and one to BHA only, raising questions about the clinical relevance of these in vitro tests. These studies suggest that immune effector cells are probably involved in at least some adverse effects and that different mechanisms are operant. The majority of data to date, however, does not support the hypothesis that these responses are immunologically specific reactions.

Several authors have suggested that adverse cutaneous reactions in humans to BHA or BHT are akin to skin lesions induced by aspirin and nonsteroidal anti-inflammatory drugs, and represent alterations in the arachidonic acid–prostaglandin cascade. At present, no data support such an action of the phenolic antioxidants. The evaluation of the single patient by Goodman and associates did not reveal obvious perturbations of prostaglandin metabolites despite clinical exacerbation (22). It appears reasonable that BHA and BHT are acting in these circumstances in a pharmacological manner, but the mode of action remains elusive.

Unsubstantiated Effects

In addition to the purported adverse effects of BHA and BHT advanced by Fisherman and Cohen based on the nonreproducible earlobe bleeding time prolongation, these two antioxidants have gained notoriety in the health food lay press as agents capable of prolonging life. Claims for their benefit in increasing lifespan are apparently based on mouse studies performed 25 years ago (3). Unfortunately, these studies produced somewhat contradictory results, and it appears unclear whether the improved lifespan in the mice might not also be achieved by consumption of an optimum normal diet. Recommendations have been made for the ingestion of 2 g of BHT daily as a counteragent for disordered nutrition, age-related problems, and genital herpes (4). As pointed out by Llaurado, however, the dosing recommended by these health food advocates is only an order of magnitude (i.e., tenfold) lower than the lethal concentration noted in certain rat toxicology studies (4). Obviously, such careless dosing is to be strongly discouraged.

Summary

BHA and BHT are food additives found in a variety of foods, but to greatest degree in foods that contain larger amounts of fats or oils that may become rancid. These phenolic antioxidants are also added to plastic or paper products that may come in contact with food items, as well as to cosmetics and medicinals to which the skin or mucosa may be exposed. They continue to be widely used despite concerns over animal toxicity studies. Their continued provisional status on the GRAS list reflects the fact that such toxicology studies in animals have employed greatly larger doses than those utilized in the food industry. Nevertheless, consumption has appeared to be creeping up during the past two decades.

Adverse reactions in humans to date are best substantiated in the skin. Delayed hypersensitivity contact dermatitis through a variety of occupational or medicinal exposures is well documented, but not common. The true incidence of antioxidant sensitivity in chronic urticaria is presently unknown. High reaction rates of adverse reactions to food additives have not been substantiated by carefully conducted double-blind studies. Despite earlier reports suggesting a 10% to 15% incidence of BHA/BHT intolerance in chronic urticaria patients, this finding appears to reflect deficiencies in study design. A number of positives most likely were due to random fluctuations of disease activity, and not true reactions to the antioxidants or other food additives. To date, no convincing reports of human respiratory adverse responses have surfaced. Therefore, the true prevalence of adverse reactions to BHA and BHT remains unclear.

Oral challenges—preferably double-blind—remain the ideal approach to verifying suspected adverse reactions to these antioxidants. The recommended schedule involves a truncated incremental challenge. The doses used may be considered high, greatly exceeding an average daily intake. Such doses are more likely to provide a definitive reaction, however. Clinical relevance can then be ascertained by elimination of the incriminated agent from the diet. Such doses, while appropriate for urticaria evaluations, could prove dangerous if the challenge is intended to provoke possible asthmatic responses.

Considering the lack of success in identifying causes in chronic urticaria, a search for additive sensitivity is probably warranted, even given the anticipated low yield. Strict elimination diets or the use of elemental formulas are difficult to maintain and poorly tolerated by patients. Open or single-blind challenges could identify possible aggravants, which should then be further authenticated with double-blind testing. The diet restrictions could then be rationally addressed.

REFERENCES

1. Lecos C. Food preservatives: a fresh report. FDA Consumer 1984;4:23–25.
2. Jukes TH. Food additives. N Engl J Med 1977;297:427–430.
3. Babich H. Butylated hydroxytoluene (BHT): a review. Environ Res 1982;29:1–29.
4. Llaurado JP. The saga of BHT and BHA in life extension myths. J Amer Coll Nutrition 1985;4:481–484.
5. Lauer BH, Kirkpatrick DC. Antioxidants: the Canadian perspective. Toxicol Ind Health 1993;9:373–382.
6. Halliwell B, Gutteridge JMC, Cross CE. Free radicals, antioxidants, and human disease: where are we now? J Lab Clin Med 1992;119:598–620.
7. Omaye ST, Reddy KA, Cross CE. Effect of butylated hydroxytoluene and other antioxidants on mouse lung metabolism. J Toxicol Environ Health 1977;3:829–836.
8. Williamson D, Esterez P, Witschi H. Studies on the pathogenesis of butylated hydroxytoluene-induced lung damage in mice. Toxicol Appl Pharmacol 1978;43:577–587.
9. Haschek WM, Reiser KM, Klein-Szanto AJP, et al. Potentiation of butylated hydroxytoluene-induced acute lung damage by oxygen: cell kinetics and collagen metabolism. Am Rev Respir Dis 1983;127:28–34.
10. Hakkinen PJ, Schmoyer RL, Witschi HP. Potential of butylated-hydroxytoluene-induced acute lung damage by oxygen; effects of prednisolone and indomethacin. Am Rev Respir Dis 1983;128:648–651.
11. Kehrer JP, Klein-Szanto AJP, Sorensen EMB, Pearlman R, Rosner MH. Enhanced acute lung damage following corticosteroid treatment. Am Rev Respir Dis 1984;130:256–261.
12. Miller ACK, Dwyer LD, Auerbach CE, Miley FB, Dinsdale D, Malkinson AM. Strain-related differences in the pneumotoxic effects of chronically administered butylated hydroxytoluene on protein kinase C and calpain. Toxicol 1994;90:141–159.
13. Taniguchi S, Kono T, Mizuno N, et al. Effects of butylated hydroxyanisole on ornithine decarboxylase activity and its gene

expression induced by phorbol ester tumor promoter. J Invest Dermatol 1991;96:289–291.

14. Lindenschmidt RC, Tryka AF, Goad ME, Witschi HP. The effects of dietary butylated hydroxytoluene on liver and colon cancer development in mice. Toxicol 1986;38:151–160.

15. Reddy BS, Furuya K, Hanson D, Dibello J, Berke B. Effect of dietary butylated hydroxyanisole on methylazoxymethanol acetate-induced toxicity in mice. Fd Chem Toxicol 1982; 20:853–859.

16. Klein A, Bruser B. The effect of butylated hydroxytoluene, with and without cortisol, on stimulated lymphocytes. Life Sci 1992;50:883–889.

17. Peng R-X, Lewis KF, Yang CS. Effects of butylated hydroxyanisole on microsomal monooxygenase and drug metabolism. Acta Pharmacol Sinica 1986;7:157–161.

18. Verhagen H, Maas LM, Beckers RHG, et al. Effect of subacute oral intake of the food antioxidant butylated hydroxyanisole on clinical parameters and phase-I and phase-II biotransformation capacity in man. Human Toxicol 1989;8:451–459.

19. Fisherman EW, Cohen G. Chemical intolerance to butylated-hydroxyanisole (BHA) and butylated-hydroxytoluene (BHT) and vascular response as an indicator and monitor of drug intolerance. Ann Allergy 1973;31:126–133.

20. Fisherman EW, Cohen GN. Aspirin and other cross-reacting small chemicals in known aspirin intolerant patients. Ann Allergy 1973;31:476–484.

21. Cloninger P, Novey HS. The acute effects of butylated hydroxyanisole ingestion in asthma and rhinitis of unknown etiology. Ann Allergy 1974;32:131–133.

22. Goodman DL, McDonnell JT, Nelson HS, Vaughan TR, Weber RW. Chronic urticaria exacerbated by the antioxidant food additives, butylated hydroxyanisole (BHA) and butylated hydroxytoluene (BHT). J Allergy Clin Immunol 1990;86:570–575.

23. Weber RW, Hoffman M, Raine DA Jr, Nelson HS. Incidence of bronchoconstriction due to aspirin, azo dyes, non-azo dyes, and preservatives in a population of perennial asthmatics. J Allergy Clin Immunol 1979;64:32–37.

24. Thune P, Granholt A. Provocation tests with antiphlogistic and food additives in recurrent urticaria. Dermatologica 1975;151:360–367.

25. Fisherman EW, Cohen GN. Chronic and recurrent urticaria: new concepts of drug-group sensitivity. Ann Allergy 1977; 39:404–414.

26. Juhlin L. Clinical studies on the diagnosis and treatment of urticaria. Ann Allergy 1977;39:356–361.

27. Juhlin L. Recurrent urticaria: clinical investigation of 330 patients. Br J Dermatol 1981;104:369–381.

28. Hannuksela M, Lahti A. Peroral challenge tests with food additives in urticaria and atopic dermatitis. Int J Dermatol 1986;25:178–180.

29. Moore-Robinson M, Warin RP. Effect of salicylates in urticaria. Br Med J 1967;4:262–264.

30. Osmundsen PE. Contact urticaria from nickel and plastic additives (butylhydroxytoluene, oleylamide). Contact Dermatitis 1980;6:245–254.

31. Manning ME, Stevenson DD, Mathison DA. Reactions to aspirin and other nonsteroidal anti-inflammatory drugs. Immunol Allergy Clin N Am 1992;12:611–631.

32. Stevenson DD, Simon RA, Lumry WR, Mathison DA. Adverse reactions to tartrazine. J Allergy Clin Immunol 1986;78:182–191.

33. Tosti A, Bardazzi F, Valeri F, Russo R. Contact dermatitis from butylated hydroxyanisole. Contact Dermatitis 1987;17:257–258.

34. Rich P, Belozer ML, Norris P, Storrs FJ. Allergic contact dermatitis to two antioxidants in latex gloves: 4,4'-thiobis (6-tert-butyl-meta-cresol) (Lowinox 44S36) and butylhydroxyanisole. Allergen alternatives for glove-allergic patients. J Am Acad Dermatol 1991;24:37–43.

35. Acciai MC, Brusi C, Francalanci S, Giorgini S, Sertoli A. Allergic contact dermatitis in caterers. Contact Dermatitis 1993;28:48.

36. Lewis FM, Harrington CI, Gawkrodger DJ. Contact sensitivity in pruritus vulvae: a common and manageable problem. Contact Dermatitis 1994;31:264–265.

37. Roed-Petersen J, Hjorth N. Contact dermatitis from antioxidants: hidden sensitizers in topical medications and foods. Br J Dermatol 1976;94:233–241.

38. Veien NK, Krogdahl A. Cutaneous vasculitis induced by food additives. Acta Dermatol Venereol 1991;71:73–74.

39. Moneret-Vautrin DA, Faure G, Bene MC. Chewing-gum preservative induced toxidermic vasculitis. Allergy 1986;41:546–548.

40. Murdoch RD, Lessof MH, Pollock I, Young E. Effects of food additives on leukocyte histamine release in normal and urticaria subjects. J Royal Coll Phys Lond 1987;21:251–256.

27

URTICARIA, ANGIOEDEMA, AND ANAPHYLAXIS PROVOKED BY FOOD ADDITIVES

John V. Bosso
Ronald A. Simon

*M*any different agents are added to the food that we consume (1); estimates are that the number of additives ranges from 2000 to 20,000. These substances include preservatives, stabilizers, conditioners, thickeners, colorings, flavorings, sweeteners, and antioxidants. Despite the multitude of additives known, only a surprisingly small number have been associated with hypersensitivity reactions.

A number of investigators have suggested that a significant population of patients with chronic urticaria and angioedema have symptoms related to the ingestion of food additives. The incidence of reactions to additives in patients with chronic urticaria and angioedema remains unknown, due primarily to the lack of properly and rigorously controlled studies.

Table 27.1 lists the food additives that have been suspected in association with adverse reactions. In this chapter, these additives are discussed in detail as they relate to urticaria and angioedema, as well as to anaphylaxis or anaphylactoid reactions.

General Considerations and Descriptions of Certain Food Additives

A brief overview of selected food additives follows. For additional information, the reader is referred to Chapters 22 through 28 in this text.

DYES

Dyes approved under the Food Dye and Coloring Act (FD&C) are coal tar derivatives, the best known of which is tartrazine (FD&C yellow no. 5). In addition to tartrazine, the group of azo dyes includes ponceau (FD&C red no. 4) and sunset yellow (FD&C yellow no. 6). Amaranth (FD&C red no. 5) was banned from use in the United States in 1975 because of claims related to carcinogenicity. Nonazo dyes include brilliant blue (FD&C blue no. 1), erythrosine (FD&C red no. 3), and indigotin (FD&C blue no. 2).

SULFITES

Sulfites and the burning of sulfur-containing coal have been used for centuries to preserve food. In addition, sulfiting agents (including sulfur dioxide and sodium or potassium sulfite, bisulfite, or metabisulfite) are used by the fermentation industry to sanitize containers and to inhibit the growth of undesirable microorganisms. Sulfites act as potent antioxidants, which explains their widespread use in foods as preventives against oxidative discolorations (browning) and as fresheners. Many packaged foods, including fresh and frozen cellophane-wrapped fruits and vegetables, processed grain foods (crackers and cookies), and citrus-flavored beverages, may contain sulfites; the highest levels, however, occur in potatoes (any peeled variety), dried fruits (apricots and white raisins), and possibly shrimp and other seafoods,

Table 27.1
Additives Suspected in Association with Adverse Reactions

FD&C dyes
Azo dyes
  Tartrazine (FD&C yellow no. 5)
  Sunset yellow (FD&C yellow no. 6)
  Ponceau (FD&C red no. 4)
  Amaranth (FD&C red no. 5)
Nonazo dyes
  Brilliant blue (FD&C blue no. 1)
  Erythrosine (FD&C red no. 3)
  Indigotin (FD&C blue no. 2)

Parabens
Parahydroxybenzoic acid
  Methylparaben
  Ethylparaben
  Butylparaben
Sodium benzoate

Butylated hydroxyanisole (BHA)

Butylated hydroxytoluene (BHT)

Nitrates

Nitrites

Monosodium glutamate (MSG)

Sulfites
Sulfur dioxide
  Sodium sulfite
  Sodium bisulfite
  Sodium metabisulfite
  Potassium bisulfite
  Potassium metabisulfite

Aspartame (NutraSweet)

which may be sprayed after unloading on the dock. Sulfites are listed as ingredients in prepared and packaged foods or drinks that contain at least 10 parts per million (ppm) SO_2 equivalents. In 1986, the FDA banned the use of sulfites on foods marketed as fresh.

PARABENS

Parabens are aliphatic esters of parahydroxybenzoic acid; they include methyl-, ethyl-, propyl-, and butylparabens. Sodium benzoate is a closely related substance usually reported to cross-react with these compounds. These agents, which are widely used as preservatives in both foods and drugs, are well recognized as causes of severe contact dermatitis.

MONOSODIUM GLUTAMATE

Glutamic acid is a nonessential, dicarboxylic amino acid that constitutes 20% of dietary protein. Glutamate occurs naturally in some foods in significant amounts: 100 g of Camembert cheese, for example, contains as much as 1 g of monosodium glutamate (MSG). The greatest exposure to MSG, however, occurs through its role as a flavor enhancer. MSG is added to a wide variety of foods by both manufacturers and restaurateurs. Approximately 75 years ago, a Japanese chemist established that MSG produces the flavor-enhancing properties of seaweed, a traditional component of Japanese cooking. Large amounts of MSG are frequently added to Chinese, Japanese, and other Southeast Asian cooking. As much as 6 g of MSG may be ingested in a highly seasoned oriental meal, and a single bowl of wonton soup may contain 2.5 g of MSG. MSG may be found in manufactured meat and chicken products. It has been reported to provoke a syndrome that occurs within hours of eating. The syndrome characterized by headache, a burning sensation along the back of the neck, chest tightness, nausea, and sweating. Recently, a trend toward reducing MSG use in oriental cooking has emerged, likely in response to consumer dissatisfaction related to the occurrence of the syndrome in relation to some oriental meals.

ASPARTAME

Aspartame (NutraSweet) is a dipeptide composed of aspartic acid and the methyl ester of phenylalanine. This low-calorie artificial sweetener is 180 times sweeter than sucrose.

BUTYLATED HYDROXYANISOLE AND BUTYLATED HYDROXYTOLUENE

Butylated hydroxyanisole (BHA) and butylated hydroxytoluene (BHT) are antioxidants used in cereal and other grain products.

NITRATES

Nitrates and nitrites are widely used preservatives. Their popularity stems from both flavoring and color-

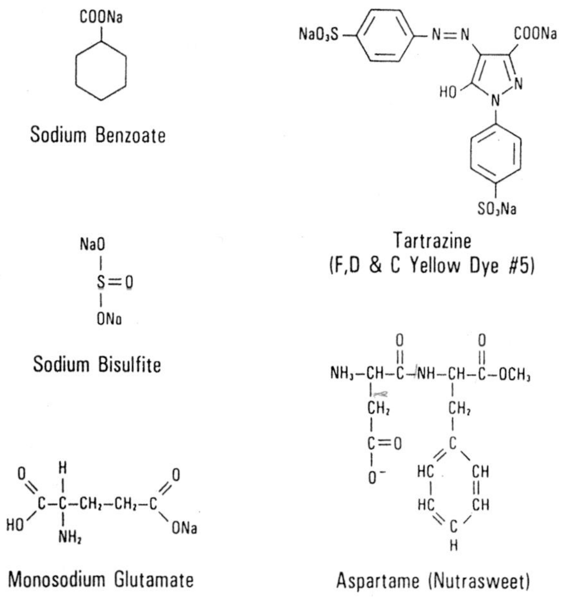

Figure 27.1

Chemical structures of some food additives.

ing attributes. These agents are found mostly in processed meats such as frankfurters and salami (2).

Mechanism of Food Additive-Induced Urticaria, Angioedema, and Anaphylaxis

To date, the mechanisms underlying additive-induced urticaria and angioedema have not yet been elucidated. It seems reasonable to postulate, however, that multiple mechanisms are responsible for these adverse reactions given the heterogeneity of chemical structures found among these additives (Fig. 27.1).

IMMEDIATE (IgE-MEDIATED) HYPERSENSITIVITY

Additives would have to act as haptens to create a response mediated by immunoglobulin E (IgE). Only a few reports have suggested IgE-mediated reactions, notably to sulfites and parabens. Instead, the over-

whelming majority of these reactions are not of the immediate hypersensitivity type. In fact, many cases of additive-provoked urticaria occur as late as 24 hours after challenge, arguing against an IgE-mediated mechanism.

In 1976, Prenner and Stevens reported an anaphylactic reaction occurring after the ingestion of food sprayed with sodium bisulfite (3). Minutes after eating lunch at a restaurant, a 50-year-old male experienced generalized urticaria and pruritus, swelling of the tongue, difficulty with swallowing, and tightness in his chest. He responded promptly to treatment with subcutaneous epinephrine. Subsequently, the patient's prick skin test and an intradermal test gave positive results (with negative controls). The authors were able to demonstrate passive transfer, via Prausnitz-Küstner testing, to a nonatopic subject. Yang and associates also described one patient with a history of sulfite-provoked anaphylaxis (4). A borderline result was obtained via intradermal skin test, followed by a positive response to single-blind, oral provocation challenge with 5 mg of potassium metabisulfite. This patient's cutaneous reactivity was also passively transferred via the Prausnitz-Küstner reaction. Yang's group was, however, unable to elicit positive responses to challenges in nine patients with histories of hives related to eating restaurant food. In addition, Sokol and Hydick reported a case of sulfite-induced anaphylaxis that provided evidence for a specific IgE-mediated mechanism (5). Despite these isolated reports, IgE-mediated immediate hypersensitivity reactions to sulfites (possibly via a hapten mechanism) appear to occur only rarely.

Studies of neutrophil chemotactic factor of anaphylaxis have failed to demonstrate an increase in this mast cell mediator post-challenge in subjects with negative metabisulfite skin tests, suggesting that mast cell degranulation is not associated with non–IgE-mediated sulfite reactions (6). Cromolyn pretreatment did not ablate an urticarial reaction in an individual sensitive to potassium metabisulfite (7). In the overwhelming majority of cases, the mechanisms behind sulfite-provoked urticaria, angioedema, and anaphylaxis (or anaphylactoid reactions) remain unknown.

At least three cases of apparent IgE-mediated, paraben-induced urticaria and angioedema have been reported (8, 9). All of these cases concerned reactions to benzoates used as pharmaceutical preservatives. The three patients had positive skin test responses to parabens, but negative results when exposed to the drugs themselves minus the paraben preservatives. These subjects, however, could tolerate oral benzoates in their diets without reactions.

DELAYED (TYPE IV) HYPERSENSITIVITY

Another suggested mechanism focuses on delayed hypersensitivity. Studies in this area have been few in number and often poorly designed. Warrington and coworkers measured the release of a T-lymphocyte-derived leukocyte-migration inhibition factor in response to incubation with tartrazine, sodium benzoate, and aspirin (acetylsalicylic acid) in vitro using peripheral blood mononuclear cells from patients with chronic urticaria, with or without associated additive or aspirin sensitivity (10). Significant production of the inhibitory factor occurred in response to tartrazine and sodium benzoate in individuals with chronic additive-induced urticaria. The groups of patients studied (four patients per group) exhibited sensitivity to tartrazine, sodium benzoate, and aspirin as determined either by response to elimination diet alone or by challenge-proved sensitivity. In this study, the potential for false-positive reactions on the basis of response to diet alone created a problem. Essentially no details of the challenge procedure were given.

Valverde and associates studied in vitro lymphocyte stimulation in 258 patients with chronic urticaria, angioedema, or both, using a series of food extracts and additives that included tartrazine, benzoic acid, and aspirin (11). They found positive stimulation (using the lymphocyte transformation test) to additives in 18.4% of subjects. After the patients were placed on a diet that excluded the offending additives, 62% had total remission of symptoms and 22% had partial remission. The investigators concluded that this response to diet lent credence to the lymphocyte transformation test as an in vitro diagnostic test for chronic urticaria and angioedema related to food additives. No provocation challenges were performed in this study, however.

No conclusions regarding the presence or absence of a delayed-type hypersensitivity mechanism in additive-provoked urticaria can be made from the studies described above. It seems reasonable to conclude that a reaction occurring between 30 minutes and 6 hours (most reactions began within the first 6 hours) is not typical of a type IV mechanism.

CYCLOOXYGENASE, ASPIRIN, AND TARTRAZINE

The subject of tartrazine sensitivity remains controversial. Many claims of cross-reactivity between aspirin and tartrazine have been made; estimates of its incidence based on earlier studies range from 21% to 100% (12–16). In a double-blind, placebo-controlled study of tartrazine sensitivity in urticaria patients that utilized objective reaction criteria (and withheld antihistamines for 72 hours prior to challenge), only 1 of 24 patients experienced urticaria after challenge with 50 mg of tartrazine (17). When challenged with 975 mg of aspirin, this patient did not react, suggesting that cross-reactivity between aspirin and tartrazine may not occur. An earlier double-blind, placebo-controlled crossover challenge with 0.22 mg of tartrazine found sensitivity in 8% of patients (3 of 38) with chronic urticaria and 20% of patients (2 of 10) with aspirin intolerance (15). This dose of tartrazine is similar to that used to color medication tablets, but remains far less than that typically encountered in the diet. The report did not mention, however, whether antihistamines were withheld during the challenges.

No convincing evidence has been found to prove that tartrazine inhibits the enzyme cyclooxygenase (in the arachidonic acid cascade), an often-suggested mechanism for aspirin sensitivity. In addition, tartrazine (Fig. 27.1) and acetylsalicylic acid have dissimilar chemical structures. The mechanism of tartrazine sensitivity has not been well studied and remains unknown.

NEUROLOGICALLY MEDIATED HYPERSENSITIVITY

Considerable evidence exists that MSG has both neuroexcitatory and neurotoxic effects in animals (18) and humans (19). Neurologically mediated urticarias have been previously described (20). Several factors—including heat, exercise, and stress—may induce cholinergically mediated urticaria. This mechanism represents a theoretical basis for MSG-induced urticaria, possibly via release of cutaneous neuropeptides.

ANTICOAGULATION

Zimmerman and Czarnetzki in 1986 sought to disprove claims by earlier investigators that changes in the bleeding time play an important role in diagnosing anaphylactoid reactions to aspirin, other nonsteroidal anti-inflammatory drugs (NSAIDs), and food additives (21). They measured bleeding time, prothrombin time, and partial thromboplastin times in 10 patients with histories of anaphylactoid reactions to these drugs and various food additives. Challenges were not placebo-controlled, nor did the report include any mention of whether the challenges were blinded. Nevertheless, the investigators found no correlation between patients' reactions and the aforementioned coagulation parameters.

Thus, aside from a small number of case reports describing IgE-mediated reactions to sulfites and parabens, the overwhelming majority of additive-induced urticaria, angioedema, and anaphylactic reactions involve mechanisms that have not been elucidated. Further properly controlled studies in this area are clearly needed.

Food Additive Challenge Studies in Patients with Urticaria

PATIENT SELECTION

Selection of patients for study may include three types of subjects: (1) all available patients with chronic urticaria (or only those with chronic idiopathic urticaria); (2) patients with histories suggestive of food additive-provoked urticaria; or (3) patients who have responded to a diet free of commonly implicated additives. The percentage of positive reactors will depend on the group selected. This variability adds more confusion to the already difficult task of comparing results from differing studies.

ACTIVITY OF URTICARIA AT THE TIME OF STUDY

The relative degree of activity or inactivity of urticaria or angioedema at the time of challenge appears to affect the ability to obtain cutaneous responses to food additives. Challenges performed on patients with active urticaria are more likely to yield false-positive results. Challenges performed on patients whose urticaria is in remission, on the other hand, are more likely to yield false-negative results. In a study by Mathison and colleagues, only 1 of 15 patients whose urticaria was in remission experienced a reaction to aspirin, whereas 7 of 10 patients with active urticaria reacted to aspirin (22). These challenges were performed using objective reaction criteria, and the reactions observed were then compared with a baseline observation.

MEDICATIONS

Several studies made no reference to whether medications—particularly antihistamines—were continued or withheld during challenges. Several caveats must be considered when interpreting challenge studies that do mention these important details: (1) discontinuation of antihistamines immediately before or within 24 hours of challenge often generates more false-positive results; (2) continuation of antihistamines during challenges may block milder additive-induced cutaneous responses and, therefore, give more false-negative results; and (3) subjects become increasingly likely to experience breakthrough urticaria as the interval from the last antihistamine dose to the "positive challenge" increases. Such results would be even more confusing if placebo-controlled challenges preceded additive challenges.

REACTION CRITERIA

There often is no period of baseline observation made by the investigators for comparison with reaction data. Most challenge studies performed to date have employed a loosely defined and rather subjective means to define urticarial responses. The reaction criteria could simply consist of "clear signs of urticaria developing within 24 hours." The studies by Stevenson *et al.* (17) and Mathison *et al.* (22), in contrast, utilized an objective system of scoring urticarial responses.

PLACEBO CONTROLS

We cannot overemphasize the use of placebo-controlled studies in additive challenges. Studies without placebo controls are essentially useless in assessing positive urticarial challenge responses. Nevertheless, a surprising number of reported additive challenge studies do not employ placebo controls. Even in many placebo-controlled studies, the placebo was always the first challenge, followed by aspirin, and finally by an additive. Thus, a spontaneous flare of urticaria was least likely to coincide with the first placebo challenge. We also question the validity of having only a single placebo in challenge studies that test large numbers of additives. Clearly, a need exists for multiple placebos and randomization of placebo usage in the order of challenges.

BLINDING

Among the most important features of any protocol for food additive challenge is a double-blind challenge, as urticaria may be exacerbated by stress. In addition, it is necessary to eliminate observer bias given the subjective nature of positive responses. Open challenges represent useful tools for "ruling out" additive-associated reactions. Positive challenge responses, on the other hand, need double-blinded confirmation before they can be accepted as "true positives."

Multiple Additive Challenges in Patients with Chronic Urticaria

EXAMPLES OF STUDIES WITH LESS STRINGENT DESIGN CRITERIA

One of the earliest additive challenge studies in patients with chronic urticaria was reported by Doeglas (23). In the study, seven (30.4%) subjects reacted to tartrazine and "four or five" (17.4% or 22.7%) reacted to sodium benzoate. Placebo-controlled challenges were not performed. In another study, Thune and

Granholt reported that 20 of 96 patients reacted to tartrazine, 13 of 86 reacted to sunset yellow, 5 of 7 reacted to parabens, and 6 of 47 reacted to BHA and BHT (24). Furthermore, in the group of patients with chronic idiopathic urticaria, 62 of the 100 patients challenged reacted to at least 1 of the 22 different agents used. The challenges were not placebo-controlled, however, so any conclusions about the incidence of reactions to a particular agent derived from this study would be difficult to support.

In a study of 330 patients with recurrent urticaria, Juhlin performed single-blind challenges using multiple additives and a single placebo, which always preceded the additive challenges (25). He found that one or more positive reactions occurred in 31% of patients tested. Reaction criteria were relatively subjective in this study. In fact, 33% of patients had reactions judged to be "uncertain" because, as the author stated, "Judging whether a reaction is positive or negative is not always easy." Furthermore, if patients reacted to the lactose placebo, retesting employed a wheat starch placebo. Questionable reactors were retested. If the repeat test gave a positive result, the first test was assumed to be positive as well; the same logic applied for negative retesting.

Supramaniam and Warner described 24 of 43 children as reacting to one or more additives used in their double-blind challenge study (26). No baseline observation period was established, however, and only one placebo was interspersed among the nine additives used for challenge. Furthermore, no mention was made about whether antihistamines were withheld prior to or during challenges.

In 1985, Genton and coworkers performed single-blind additive challenges on 17 patients with chronic urticaria or angioedema (27). The patients were placed on a 14-day elimination diet (free of food additives) before challenges, and medications were discontinued at the beginning of the diet. Of the 17 patients in the study, 15 reacted to at least one of the six additives used for challenge.

EXAMPLES OF STUDIES WITH MORE STRINGENT DESIGN CRITERIA

In 1988, Ortolani and associates reported 396 patients with recurrent chronic urticaria and angioedema

(28); this report represented a follow-up to a study performed in 1984 (29). Double-blind, placebo-controlled, oral food provocations were performed on patients that had experienced significant remissions while following an elimination diet. The diet was maintained, but medications were discontinued during challenges. The report did not describe the timing of discontinuation of medications. On the basis of history alone, 179 patients were considered for an elimination diet for suspected food or food additive intolerance; only 135 patients ultimately participated in the study. Only 8 of 87 patients that significantly improved on the diet after 2 weeks gave positive responses to food challenges. Of the 79 patients with negative responses to food challenge, 72 underwent double-blind, placebo-controlled, oral food additive provocations. Twelve of these patients experienced positive responses to challenges with one or more additives. Many of these patients naturally reacted to two or three additives. Five of the 16 patients with positive responses to aspirin challenges gave positive responses to additive challenges; four of these subjects tested positive to sodium salicylate.

The similarity in chemical structure observed between aspirin and sodium salicylate supports the finding of cross-reactivity between them. The doses used (greater than 400 mg) in the sodium salicylate challenge, however, far exceed the levels encountered in most conventional diets. Considering that the proposed mechanisms for reactions to additives such as tartrazine, sodium benzoate, and sulfites differ so dramatically, skepticism about the validity of the positive challenge results in this study is warranted. Furthermore, although a patient's history provides an important consideration in assessing food sensitivity, it usually represents a poor indicator of a possible additive hypersensitivity, as patients usually remain unaware of all additives that they consume daily. Elimination of more than 50% of the original study population may have been proper for food-sensitivity determinations, but was not justified for selection of patients for additive challenges.

Hannuksela and Lahti challenged 44 chronic urticaria patients with several food additives, including sodium metabisulfite, BHA or BHT, beta-carotene, and benzoic acid in a prospective, double-blind, placebo-controlled study (30). Only 1 of the 44 patients had a positive response to challenge, reacting positively to benzoic acid. Another patient also reacted to the placebo challenge. All medications were discontinued 72 hours before the first challenge and during the study. Patients were not placed on an additive-free diet prior to the challenge. The challenge dose of metabisulfite was quite low—only 9 mg. Similarly, Kellett and associates noted that approximately 10% of 44 chronic idiopathic urticaria patients reacted to benzoates, tartrazine, or both, but 10% of the subjects reacted to placebo challenges (31).

ELIMINATION DIET STUDIES

An alternative strategy for investigating food additive-induced urticaria involves the elimination of all additives from the diet and the observation of its effects on hives. Unfortunately, there are no reported blinded or placebo-controlled studies of this nature. In uncontrolled studies, Ros and coworkers reported an additive-free diet to be "completely helpful" in 24% of patients with chronic urticaria; 57% of patients were deemed "much improved," and 19% were "slightly better" or experienced no change in their urticaria (32). Rudzki and associates reported that 50 of 158 patients responded to a diet that eliminated salicylates, benzoates, and azo dyes (33). These studies did not address the question of which, if any, additives constituted the cause of the problem.

In another study, Gibson and Clancy found that 54 of 76 patients who underwent a 2-week, additive-free diet "responded" (34). They then challenged the responders with individual additives. Although the challenges were controlled, the patients always received the placebo first. No mention was made of whether the challenges were blinded. A diet that eliminated the offending additive was then continued for 6 to 18 months, followed by repeat challenge. All three patients who initially responded positively to tartrazine challenge had negative results upon rechallenge, as did one of the four patients with initially positive responses to benzoate challenges. Thus, despite this approach, the incidence of additive sensitivity in urticaria remains unknown.

Reports of Single Food Additive Challenge Studies

SULFITES

The reports by Prenner and Stevens (3) and Yang *et al.* (4), discussed earlier, both presented single cases of sulfite-provoked anaphylaxis and gave skin test and Prausnitz-Küstner transfer evidence to suggest that an IgE-mediated mechanism played a role in these reactions. In addition, Yang *et al.* performed a single-blind oral challenge. Their patient responded positively to a challenge with 5 mg of potassium metabisulfite.

In 1980, Clayton and Busse (35) described a nonatopic female who developed generalized urticaria that progressed to life-threatening anaphylaxis within 15 minutes of drinking wine. Her symptoms were not reproduced by ingestion of other alcoholic beverages. This case may have involved sulfite-provoked urticaria and anaphylaxis.

Habenicht and coworkers described two patients who experienced several episodes of urticaria and angioedema after consuming restaurant meals (36). Only one of these individuals underwent a single-blind oral challenge with potassium metabisulfite. Generalized urticarial lesions developed in this patient within 15 minutes of receiving the 25 mg challenge dose. No placebo challenge was performed. Avoidance of potential sulfite sources apparently resolved this patient's recurrent symptoms.

Schwartz reported two patients with restaurant-related symptoms who underwent oral challenges with metabisulfite (37). Both subjects had symptoms temporally related to ingestion of salads: weakness, a feeling of dissociation from the body, dizziness, borderline hypotension, and bradycardia. These signs and symptoms are more consistent with vasovagal reactions than with anaphylaxis. One report has described a patient who received less than 2 mL of procaine (Novocaine) with epinephrine administered subcutaneously by her dentist (38). Within several minutes, she developed flushing, a sense of warmth, and pruritus, followed by scattered urticaria, dyspnea, and anxiety. Skin tests of various local anesthetics and sulfite proved negative. Thirty minutes after receiving a single-blind, oral dose of 10 mg of sodium bisulfite, she developed "a sense of fullness in her head, nasal congestion, and a pruritic erythematous blotchy eruption." No respiratory symptoms developed, and the investigators did not observe any pulmonary function test abnormalities. This patient was able to tolerate local anesthetics without epinephrine. Importantly, this patient did not describe a history of food related symptoms. Furthermore, the usual dose of aqueous epinephrine (Adrenalin) contains only 0.3 mg of sulfite and local anesthetics contain only as much as 2 mg/mL of sulfite. Thus, the usual doses—even in the most sensitive persons—would not provoke reactions. The mechanism of this patient's reaction cannot be definitively linked to sulfite and likely comprised a vasomotor response to the effects of epinephrine.

A double-blind, placebo-controlled challenge that reproduced urticaria after challenge with 25 mg of potassium metabisulfite was reported by Belchi-Hernandez *et al.* (7). Skin tests were negative in this subject.

Two reports have demonstrated the inability to provoke reactions to sulfites in patients with idiopathic anaphylaxis, some of whom had histories of restaurant-associated symptoms (39, 40). In a study describing food-related skin testing in 102 patients with idiopathic anaphylaxis, only one patient was found to have metabisulfite sensitivity (41). In addition, the authors have performed sulfite-ingestion challenges in 25 patients with chronic idiopathic urticaria and angioedema without a reaction (unpublished observations). At present, sulfite-induced urticaria, angioedema, or anaphylaxis appears to be a rare phenomenon.

TARTRAZINE/AZO DYES

Murdoch *et al.* found at least 2 of 24 patients who developed hives after ingesting a panel of four azo dyes, including tartrazine (42). As previously indicated, Stevenson found that only 1 of 24 aspirin-sensitive subjects undergoing double-blind challenge with 50 mg tartrazine developed urticaria (17). It appears, therefore, that tartrazine and other azo dyes rarely induce urticaria. The tartrazine-sensitive individual identified in Stevenson's study did not react to a blinded challenge with doses of aspirin of as much as 975 mg, suggesting a lack of cross-reactivity between tartrazine and aspirin.

ASPARTAME

Two cases of aspartame-provoked urticaria and angioedema have been reported. In these individuals, their hives emerged only after aspartame's 1983 approval as a sweetener in carbonated beverages. Both patients reported the onset of urticaria within 1 hour of ingesting aspartame-sweetened soft drinks. Double-blind, placebo-controlled challenges reproduced urticaria with doses of aspartame (25–75 mg) that fall below the amount contained in typical 12-ounce cans (100–150 mg) (43).

In a well-publicized multicenter, randomized, placebo-controlled crossover study, Geha *et al.* (44) challenged 21 subjects with histories of a temporal (minutes to hours) association between aspartame ingestion and urticaria/angioedema. These subjects were identified after an extensive recruiting process spanning four years. Only four urticarial reactions were observed—two following aspartame consumption and two following placebo ingestion. Doses used ranged as high as 600 mg of aspartame.

BHA AND BHT

In a double-blind, placebo-controlled study, Goodman *et al.* (45) challenged two patients with chronic idiopathic urticaria who experienced remissions after following dye- and preservative-elimination diets. Both patients noted significant exacerbations of their urticaria after challenge with BHA and BHT. Subsequent avoidance of foods containing these antioxidants resulted in marked abatement of the frequency, severity, and duration of urticaria episodes. Long-term follow-up revealed urticarial flares after dietary indiscretion, but an otherwise quiescent disease.

MONOSODIUM GLUTAMATE

Squire described a 50-year-old man with recurrent angioedema of the face and extremities that was related to a history involving ingestion of a soup containing MSG (46). A single-blind, placebo-controlled challenge with the soup base resulted in "a sensation of imminent swelling" within a few hours, with visible angioedema emerging 24 hours after the challenge. In a graded challenge with only MSG, angioedema occurred 16 hours after challenge with a dose of 250 mg. Avoidance of MSG led to extended remission. Details of the challenge were not reported, nor did the author mention whether medications were withheld during challenges.

Food Additive Sensitivity in Chronic and Recurrent Urticaria/Angioedema (CRUA)

Malamin and Kalimo performed prick and scratch skin tests on 91 individuals with CRUA, utilizing a panel of 18 food additives and preservatives. A positive response was defined as a wheal greater than or equal to the size of the histamine control. Twenty-six percent of subjects had at least one positive skin test as compared with 10% of 247 non-urticaria control subjects. Ten of the 24 CRUA patients with positive skin tests underwent oral provocation with the additives that gave the positive skin test results. Details of the challenge procedure were not provided. Only one patient reacted, experiencing an urticarial reaction to benzoic acid (47). The activity level of the patient's prechallenge urticaria was not noted.

In a study now under way at Scripps Clinic and Research Foundation, patients with chronic urticaria are undergoing challenges with a panel of food additives. The additive panel consists of tartrazine, potassium metabisulfite, MSG, aspartame, sodium benzoate, methylparaben, BHA, BHT, and FD&C yellow no. 6. To date, no positive reactors have been identified among more than 40 patients (unpublished observations).

Volonakis and colleagues performed an extensive analysis of etiologic factors in 226 children with chronic urticaria. Elimination of food additives and double-blind, placebo-controlled challenges performed with a panel of four additives (tartrazine, sodium benzoate, nitrates, and sorbic acid) plus aspirin resulted in an overall incidence of 2.6% of cases attributable to these additives (6 of 226 subjects). Half of these patients (3 of 226, or 1.3%) reacted to aspirin (a known exacerbator of chronic urticaria) and the remaining 3 subjects (1.3%) reacted to tartrazine. No benzoate, nitrate, or sorbic acid reactions occurred among their subjects (48).

Miscellaneous Case Reports

Anecdotal single case reports exist for anaphylactic reactions to sodium benzoate (49), annotto dye (50) (orange–yellow coloring extracted from the seeds of the tree *Bixa orellana*), and carmine (51, 52) (an insect-derived red dye that gives Campari Liqueur its characteristic color; often designated E120).

Acute urticaria associated with leukocytoclastic vasculitis and eosinophilia was induced by a single placebo-controlled challenge with 50 mg sodium bisulfite in a subject suffering from recurrent urticaria and angioedema of unclear etiology. Blinded challenges were performed during a symptom-free period, followed by biopsy confirmation of the leukocytoclasis. Conscious avoidance of sulfites reduced the frequency of subsequent reactions dramatically (53).

Recommendations for Food Additive Challenge Protocols in Patients with Chronic Urticaria

A review of the literature on food additive challenges in patients with chronic urticaria leads to the overwhelming conclusion that more rigorously conducted studies are needed. With the use of more objective criteria and stringent design, more meaningful conclusions may be drawn regarding the true incidence of food additive-induced urticaria, angioedema, and anaphylaxis. Our recommendations for future additive challenge protocols in patients with chronic urticaria or angioedema are presented in the following sections.

PATIENT SELECTION

In view of the ubiquitous and frequent dietary exposure to food additives, the study population should be selected from patients with chronic "idiopathic" urticarias or angioedema, unless the study is intended to examine another defined subgroup of patients with chronic urticaria or angioedema (e.g., patients with a positive history or patients responsive to an elimination diet). The diagnosis of chronic idiopathic urticaria or angioedema should be made in subjects with recurrent urticaria of at least 6 weeks' duration without indentifiable cause. The condition should be documented by a thorough history and physical examination as well as a chest radiograph, complete blood cell count and differential chemistry panel, urine analysis, thyroid function testing, thyroid autoantibodies, erythrocyte sedimentation rate, hepatitis B serology, antinuclear antibody level, rheumatoid factor, serum protein electrophoresis, stool specimen for ova and parasites, and skin biopsy (54). In addition, appropriate challenges should be conducted to ascertain any physical urticarias. After a negative workup, a patient's urticaria may then be considered idiopathic.

ACTIVITY OF URTICARIA

Urticaria should be in an active phase (e.g., some lesions should have appeared within 1 month prior to challenge), as food additives may not only provoke urticaria de novo, but also exacerbate ongoing urticaria, as is true with aspirin (22).

MEDICATIONS

Antihistamines should be withheld for 3 to 5 days prior to the challenges, if possible. For patients with intractable symptoms, antihistamines should be tapered to the minimal effective dose. Although corticosteroids are not generally recommended for the treatment of chronic urticaria or angioedema, when necessary their use should also be tapered to the minimal effective dose.

DIET

Patients should be placed on a diet free of all additives included in the challenge protocol at least 1 week prior to challenge. The patient should continue on this diet during the challenge protocol period.

REACTION CRITERIA

Reaction criteria should be as objective as possible. The "rule of nines" used for assessing thermal burns provides a useful method for estimating skin surface area. On each of the 11 divided areas of the body, the investigator assigns a score of 0 to 4 and then derives a total score (0 to 44 points). A positive urticarial response may be defined as either an absolute increase in the total score of 9 points or an increase of more than 300% from the baseline score determined immediately before challenge. A positive angioedema response may be defined as a relative increase in size of more than 50% in the body part affected.

BASELINE OBSERVATION

Prior to any challenges, skin scores should be recorded at the same intervals during a baseline period of observation as during challenges. The appropriate length of the baseline observation period depends on factors such as the activity of the patient's urticaria, the interval of time between discontinuation of antihistamines and the challenges, and the length of the challenge protocol.

In general, one day of pure observation with skin scoring should be followed by one day of single-blind placebo challenge with skin scoring, except perhaps in patients who are completely free of hives at challenge (in this instance, one day of placebo challenge should prove sufficient). Skin scores on those two days should not vary by more than 3 points or 30% (whichever is greater) before proceeding to additive and further placebo challenges.

PLACEBO CONTROLS

Placebo challenge should be conducted in a randomized fashion. In addition, at least an equal number of placebo and active challenges should be undertaken. Screening challenges may be performed without placebo. Positive reactors must undergo a placebo-controlled protocol, however.

Table 27.2
Suggested Maximum Doses for Additives
Used in Challenge Protocols

Tartrazine	50 mg
Sulfites	200 mg
MSG	5 g
Aspartame	150 mg
Parabens/benzoates	100 mg

BLINDING

Challenges should be conducted in a double-blind manner. Coded opaque capsules will serve for this purpose. The code should not be broken until the completion of all challenges. Screening challenges may be performed open or single-blinded. Any "positive challenges" should be confirmed with a double-blind protocol.

ADDITIVE DOSES

The additive doses used in challenge protocols should reflect natural exposure to each agent. Suggested limits for some common additives are listed in Table 27.2. Starting doses should be individualized depending on the patient's history, but usually consist of 1/100 of the maximum dose. Challenges must be performed with informed consent and in a setting where unexpected severe reactions may be appropriately treated.

Conclusion

Unfortunately, only a small number of well-designed clinical studies have been conducted in the area of food additive-provoked urticaria, angioedema, and anaphylaxis. The incidence of such reactions remains unknown. It appears to be a rare phenomenon, however, despite many investigators' claims. Except for a small number of case reports describing IgE-mediated reactions to sulfites and parabens, the mechanisms responsible for such reactions are unclear at present.

More well-designed trials must be carried out before any definitive conclusions can be reached regarding the incidence or pathogenesis of food additive-induced urticaria, angioedema, and anaphylaxis.

REFERENCES

1. Collins-Williams C. Intolerance to additives. Ann Allergy 1983;51:315–316.
2. Simon RA. Adverse reactions to food additives. N Engl Regional Allergy Proc 1986;7:533–542.
3. Prenner BM, Stevens JJ. Anaphylaxis after ingestion of sodium bisulfite. Ann Allergy 1976;37:180–182.
4. Yang W, Purchase E, Rivington RN. Positive skin tests and Prausnitz-Küstner reactions in metabisulfite-sensitive subjects. J Allergy Clin Immunol 1986;78:443–449.
5. Sokol WN, Hydick IB. Nasal congestion, urticaria and angioedema caused by an IgE mediated reaction to sodium metabisulfite. Ann Allergy 1990;65:233–238.
6. Sprenger JD, Altman LC, Marshall SG, Pierson WE, Koenig JQ. Studies of neutrophil chemotactic factor of anaphylaxis in metabisulfite sensitivity. Ann Allergy 1989;62:117–121.
7. Belchi-Hernandez J, Florido-Lopez JF, et al. Sulfite induced urticaria. Ann Allergy 1993;71:230–232.
8. Nagel JE, Fuscaldo JT, Fireman P. Paraben allergy. JAMA 1977;237:1594–1595.
9. Aldrete JA, Johnson DA. Allergy to local anesthetics. JAMA 1969;207:356–357.
10. Warrington RJ, Sauder PJ, McPhillips S. Cell-mediated immune responses to artificial food additives in chronic urticaria. Clin Allergy 1986;16:527–533.
11. Valverde E, Vich JM, Garcia-Calderone JV, Garcia-Calderone PA. In vitro stimulation of lymphocytes in patients with chronic urticaria induced by additives and food. Clin Allergy 1980;10:691–698.
12. Juhlin L, Michaelsson G, Zetterstrom O. Urticaria and asthma induced by food and drug additives in patients with aspirin sensitivity. J Allergy Clin Immunol 1972;50:92–98.
13. Michaelsson G, Juhlin L. Urticaria induced by preservatives and dye additives in food and drugs. Br J Dermatol 1973;88:525–532.
14. Ros A, Juhlin L, Michaelsson G. A follow-up study of patients with recurrent urticaria and hypersensitivity to aspirin, benzoates and azo dyes. Br J Dermatol 1976;95:19–24.
15. Settipane GA, Pudupakkam RK. Aspirin tolerance. III. Subtypes, familial occurrence and cross-reactivity with tartrazine. J Allergy Clin Immunol 1975;56:215–221.
16. Settipane GA, Chafee FH, Postman M, Levine MI. Significance of tartrazine sensitivity in chronic urticaria of unknown etiology. J Allergy Clin Immunol 1976;57:541–546.
17. Stevenson DD, Simon RA, Lumry WR, Mathison DA. Adverse reactions to tartrazine. J Allergy Clin Immunol 1986;78:182–191.
18. Blake JL, Lawrence N, Bennet J, Robinson S, Bowers CY. Late endocrine effects of administering monosodium glutamate to neonatal rats. Neuroendocrinology 1978;26:220–223.
19. Allen DH, Van Nunen S, Loblay R, Clark L, Swain A. Adverse reactions to foods. Med J Aust (Suppl) September 1984.
20. Casale TB, Sampson HA, Hanifin J. Guide to physical urticarias. J Allergy Clin Immunol 1988;82:758–763.
21. Zimmerman RE, Czarnetzki BM. Changes in the coagulation system during pseudoallergic anaphylactoid reactions to drugs and food additives. Int Arch Allergy Appl Immunol 1986;81:375–377.
22. Mathinson DA, Lumry WR, Stevenson DD, Curd JG. Aspirin in chronic urticaria and/or angioedema: studies of sensitivity and desensitization. J Allergy Clin Immunol 1982;69:135 (abstract).
23. Doeglas HM. Reactions to aspirin and food additives in patients with chronic urticaria, including the physical urticarias. Br J Dermatol 1975;93:135–144.
24. Thune P, Granholt A. Provocation tests with anti-phlogistica and food additives in recurrent urticaria. Dermatologica 1975;151:136–167.
25. Juhlin L. Recurrent urticaria: clinical investigation of 330 patients. Br J Dermatol 1981;104:369–381.
26. Supramaniam G, Warner JO. Artificial food additive intolerance in patients with angio-oedema and urticaria. Lancet 1986;2:907–910.
27. Genton C, Frei PC, Pecoud A. Value of oral provocation tests to aspirin and food additives in the routine investigation of asthma and chronic urticaria. J Allergy Clin Immunol 1985;76:40–45.
28. Ortolani C, Pastorello E, Fontana A, et al. Chemicals and drugs as triggers of food-associated disorder. Ann Allergy 1988;60:358–366.
29. Ortolani C, Pastorello E, Luraghi MT, Della-Torre F, Bellani M, Anzussi C. Diagnosis of intolerance to food additives. Ann Allergy 1984;53:587–591.
30. Hannuksela M, Lahti A. Peroral challenge tests with food additives in urticaria and atopic dermatitis. Int J Dermatol 1986;25:178–180.
31. Kellett JK, August PJ, Beck MH. Double-blinded challenge tests with food additives in chronic urticaria. Br J Dermatol 1984;111(suppl):32.
32. Ros AM, Juhlin L, Michaelsson G. A follow-up study of patients with recurrent urticaria and hypersensitivity to aspirin, benzoates and azo dyes. Br J Dermatol 1976;95:19–24.
33. Rudzki E, Czubalski K, Grzywa Z. Detection of urticaria with food additive intolerance by means of diet. Dermatologica 1980;161:57–62.
34. Gibson A, Clancy R. Management of chronic idiopathic urticaria by the identification and exclusion of dietary factors. Clin Allergy 1980;10:699–704.
35. Clayton DE, Busse W. Anaphylaxis to wine. Clin Allergy 1980;10:341–343.
36. Habenicht HA, Preuss L, Lovell RG. Sensitivity to ingested metabisulfites: cause of bronchospasm and urticaria. Immunol Allergy Pract 1983;5:243–245.
37. Schwartz HJ. Sensitivity to ingested metabisulfite: variations in clinical presentation. J Allergy Clin Immunol 1983;71:487–489.
38. Schwartz HJ, Sher TH. Bisulfite sensitivity manifesting as allergy to local dental anesthesia. J Allergy Clin Immunol 1985;75:525–527.
39. Sonin L, Patterson R. Metabisulfite challenge in patients with idiopathic anaphylaxis. J Allergy Clin Immunol 1985;75:67–69.

40. Meggs WJ, Atkins FM, Wright RH. Sulfite challenges in patients with systemic mastocytosis or unexplained anaphylaxis. J Allergy Clin Immunol 1985;75:144.

41. Stricker WE, Anorve-Lopez E, Reed CE. Food skin testing in patients with idiopathic anaphylaxis. J Allergy Clin Immunol 1986;77:516–519.

42. Murdoch RD, Pollock I, Young E, et al. Food additive induced urticaria: studies of mediator release during provocation tests. J R Coll Phys London 1987;21:262.

43. Kulczycki A. Aspartame-induced urticaria. Ann Intern Med 1986;104:207–208.

44. Geha R, Buckley CE, Greenberger P, et al. Aspartame is no more likely than placebo to cause urticaria/angioedema: results of a multicenter, randomized, double-blind, placebo-controlled, crossover study. J Allergy Clin Immunol 1993;92:513–520.

45. Goodman DL, McDonnell JT, Nelson HS, Vaughn TR, Weber RW. Chronic urticaria exacerbated by the antioxidant food preservative, butylated hydroxyanisole (BHA) and butylated hydroxytoluene (BHT). J Allergy Clin Immunol 1990;86:570–575.

46. Squire EN. Angio-oedema. In: Allergy, principles and practice. Lancet 1987;1:988.

47. Malamin G, Kalimo K. The results of skin testing with food additives and the effect of an elimination diet in chronic and recurrent urticaria and recurrent angioedema. Clin Exp Allergy 1989;19:539–543.

48. Volonakis M, Katsarou-Katsari A, Stratigos J. Etiologic factors on childhood chronic urticaria. Ann Allergy 1992;69:61–65.

49. Michils A, et al. Anaphylaxis with sodium benzoate. Lancet 1991;337:1424–1425.

50. Nish WA, et al. Anaphylaxis to annatto dye: a case report. Ann Allergy 1991;66:129–131.

51. Kagi MK, Wüthrich B, Johansson SGO. Campari–orange anaphylaxis due to carmine allergy. Lancet 1994;344:60–61.

52. Beaudouin E, et al. Food anaphylaxis following ingestion of carmine. Ann Allergy 1995;74:427–430.

53. Wüthrich B, Kägi MK, Hafner J. Disulfite-induced acute intermittent urticaria with vasculitis. Dermatology 1993.

54. Kaplan A. Urticaria angioedema. In: Middleton E, Reed CE, Ellis EF, eds. Allergy, principles and practice, 3rd ed. St. Louis: CV Mosby, 1988, 1377–1401.

28

ASTHMA AND FOOD ADDITIVES

Howard J. Schwartz

*F*ood additives are essentially non-nutritive substances intentionally added to foods. They have been a continuing source of concern to the public as potential causes of behavioral or allergic reactions, especially given the increased use of synthetic additives (1). Food additives, which are present in food supplies in small amounts, improve appearance, texture, and storage capabilities of foods. They include coloring agents, anticaking agents, preservatives, emulsifiers, stabilizers, synthetic flavors, and antioxidants. Although such substances are generally regarded as safe by the Food and Drug Administration (FDA), public concern has been stimulated by a few case reports that may or may not be scientifically sound and by many scientifically unfounded claims alleging a causal role for various food additives in a variety of physical and psychosocial diseases. While well-designed studies are difficult to conduct in any area, they can be carried out in this field. This chapter will review principles with which this subject should be studied and will review and summarize published data.

The proper establishment of a cause–effect relationship between an agent and a disease state is an issue that has concerned all subspecialties in medicine. One set of guiding principles originated in the work of Robert Koch; utilizing a modified version of Koch's postulates can work very well in allergic disease states. First, one must identify and try to isolate the alleged cause of the illness. Second, attempts should be made to remove that factor from the patient's environment and properly evaluate whether any subsequent improvement occurs in the patient's symptoms. Third, one can reintroduce the presumed cause to the patient and observe whether symptoms recur. A parallel strategy is employed in studies using allergen provocation testing in appropriately selected subjects.

With these steps, one can study the possible role of food additives in a patient's illness.

We all consume both a wide variety and at times a large amount of these agents without any effect. Because only a very small number of hypersensitivity reactions from these agents have been reported, the clinician is obligated to approach a patient concerned about the role of food additives in causing or aggravating asthma with caution.

Asthma is an illness of great complexity. Each patient's asthma can result from multiple possible causes. The disease also displays spontaneous clinical variability. It is currently reasonable to define asthma as a disease of reversible eosinophilic bronchitis. Clinical triggers include immunologic and non-immunologic stimuli that impact a hyperresponsive airway. Thus, the precise assignment of a direct cause–effect relationship of any one patient's asthma to any one trigger is fraught with difficulty, and needs to be done with scientific rigor—otherwise the patient will suffer from poorly founded observations that could lead to poorly based therapeutic maneuvers.

From the point of view of an allergist–immunologist, food additives should be viewed as simple chemicals/drugs. To evaluate whether they have a causal role in an illness, their possible pharmacologic effects should be considered and the claimed clinical effect scientifically classified, using a system such as that developed by the Committee on Adverse Reactions to Foods of the American Academy of Allergy and Immunology (2). This system includes the following definitions:

Adverse reaction: A clinically abnormal response attributed to an ingested food substance or food additive.
Food hypersensitivity: An immunologic hypersensi-

tivity or truly "allergic" reaction resulting from the ingestion of a food substance or additive, which occurs only in some patients and which is usually unrelated to the amount of food ingested.

Food allergy: A term that should be used in its strictest sense—as a synonym for food hypersensitivity; it is frequently overused and often applied to any adverse reaction to an ingestion of a food or food additive in both the medical and the lay literature.

Food idiosyncrasy: A quantitatively abnormal response to a food substance or additive differing in its physiologic or pharmacologic effects. This response resembles a hypersensitivity reaction but does not involve an immune mechanism.

Food intolerance: A physiologic response in the recipient of ingested food substances or additives that is not proven to be immunologic in nature. This response could include idiosyncratic, pharmacologic, metabolic, or toxic food reactions.

Food poisoning: An adverse reaction to a food resulting from a natural noxious constituent of the food or a microorganism, parasitic or toxic contaminant of a food. May include a toxic reaction to a food substance or additive.

Food sensitivity: A general term implying an adverse reaction as a result of an ingested food substance or additive.

Food toxicity: Direct action of a food substance or additive upon the recipient. Non-immune release of chemical mediators may lead to symptoms that mimic a food hypersensitivity reaction.

Pharmacologic food reaction: A drug reaction in the recipient as a result of chemicals in ingested food substances or additives.

Metabolic food reaction: A metabolic response in the recipient to ingested food substances or additives.

Types of Food Additives

The twentieth century has brought major changes for the food industry, as the vast majority of the public no longer lives within easy reach of food sources.

Food is now produced in massive quantities and transported to all parts of the world before use. It would be virtually impossible to safely process, package, ship, store, and display preservative-free foods on supermarket shelves for long periods of time. Thus, aside from enhancing flavor and appearance, antimicrobials and antioxidants are added to keep food from spoiling, to prevent rancidity, and to inhibit development of off-colors and flavors.

Since the late 1930s, the FDA has been reviewing the additives used in foods in an effort to ensure the safety of the ongoing use of such agents in foods and drugs. Among the many agents used, the FDA continues to allow the widespread use of benzoates, parabens, gallates, butylated hydroxyanisole (BHA), butylated hydroxytoluene (BHT), citric acid, phosphoric acid, and ascorbic acid.

Ascorbates and related chemicals are used as antioxidants. They generally have not been suggested as possible causes of asthma or other adverse reactions.

BHA and BHT are antioxidants used in many foods to retard rancidity. Like ascorbates, they have not been reported as causing asthma in either the general or allergic populations.

Benzoic acid and benzoates are antimicrobial food additives that continue to be regarded as generally safe for use in a wide variety of foods and beverages at a maximum level of 0.1%. These agents have, however, been implicated as causes of human disease. Most often these reports involve patients with chronic urticaria (3), but in rare instances they appear to be involved in asthmatic reactions (4, 5).

Parabens have been used for more than 50 years as antimicrobial agents. They have occasionally been implicated as causes of eczematous or contact dermatitis reactions, but have not been regarded as causes of asthma in any case reports on the subject of additive-induced asthma.

Propionic acid and its salts have been used for many years, blending with emulsifying agents and proving useful in many cheese products and baked goods as antimicrobials. They continue to be regarded as safe and have not been implicated as causes of asthma.

Gallates, which are useful antioxidants and sorbates, and which function as antimicrobial preservatives, are widely used, especially in packaged foods. They have not been implicated as causes of human asthma.

Tocopherols are antioxidant preservatives that incidentally contribute varying amounts of vitamin E to the human diet. They have not been reported as causing asthma in humans.

Colors

Among the coloring agents used in the food industry, the agent tartrazine (FD&C yellow no. 5) has most often been implicated as a cause of allergies, especially urticaria and asthma (3, 6). Chaffee and Settipane incriminated it as a cause of recurrent severe asthma in a patient receiving a drug containing tartrazine (4). Fishman (7) and Lockey (8) have also described individual patients with clinically severe attacks of asthma following tartrazine ingestion. Clinical occurrence of these reactions appears, however, to be rare (9).

Flavoring agents, especially the glutamates (e.g., monosodium glutamate), have been most often associated with headaches and other symptoms, including flushing (10). Allen has described occasional cases of asthma caused by ingestion of glutamate. This relationship has been tested by oral provocation challenge (11–13).

Sweeteners, especially saccharin (14) and aspartame (15), have rarely been recognized as causing acute urticaria in individual cases. No reports of asthmatic reactions with either of these agents are known.

Sulfiting agents (including sulfites, bisulfite, metabisulfite, and sulfur dioxide) have been used for centuries as antioxidants and sanitizing agents in beverages, foods, and even drugs (16). During the past 10 years, it has been widely recognized that severe potentially fatal attacks of asthma and anaphylaxis can occur in a significant number of persons (17–21). The use of these agents remains widespread, but somewhat restricted since this problem has been recognized.

Prevalence

The prevalence of asthmatic reactions to food additives in either the general population or the allergy-prone population (i.e., atopics) is unknown. Estimates of the frequency of all types of adverse reactions to food additives in the general population derive from challenge tests in highly selected groups, with calculations leading to a presumed prevalence; this method is fraught with inaccuracy, however. A prevalence study in the United Kingdom utilized questionnaires in more than 11,000 households regarding possible intolerance to food or food additives (22). Positive respondents were later interviewed in detail, and those with a possible additive intolerance were asked to enter a double-blind, placebo-controlled challenge. Based on the tests, the occurrence of food additive intolerance in the general population was estimated to range between 0.01% and 0.26%. None of the subjects had asthmatic reactions.

Two Danish studies have been carried out to estimate the prevalence of intolerance to food additives in school children, aged 5 to 16. In these two studies, a total of 606 children were challenged openly with food additives. Only 2 had asthma (23, 24).

It can also be inferred from several other studies (25, 26) that such reactions are rare. Stenius et al. (27) reported that 25 of 140 asthmatic patients had a positive bronchoconstrictor response to challenge with tartrazine, although only 9 of these patients gave a clinical history suggesting a cause–effect relationship between ingestion of foods or drugs known to contain tartrazine and aggravation of their asthma. Genton et al. (28) tested 17 asthmatic patients (by oral provocation methods) with tartrazine, benzoate, sorbate, glutamate, and sulfur dioxide in various doses. Only 1 positive response was found in 34 tests done with tartrazine, 1 positive of 33 tests performed with benzoate, and 4 positives of 25 subjects tested with sulfur dioxide. No positive tests using sorbate or glutamate were obtained in 21 and 19 challenges, respectively. Freedman (5) found that 11% of 272 patients with asthma gave a history suggestive of food additive reactions. Four of 30 such patients underwent oral provocation tests with sulfur dioxide, benzoate, and tartrazine. Eight patients reacted to sulfur dioxide, 4 reacted positively to benzoate, and 1 reacted to tartrazine. Tarlo *et al.* (29) found only 1 positive tartrazine challenge and 1 positive benzoate challenge in double-blind studies involving 28 patients with chronic asthma. On the basis of such studies, it can be inferred that significant reactions to additives are rare. Even in the well-studied area of sulfite reactivity, only 5% of all asthmatics are estimated to be sulfite-intolerant (17, 18).

Subsets of asthmatics may possibly be especially subject to adverse additive reactions. Spector and colleagues (30) performed oral challenges in more than 200 asthmatic patients with tartrazine and aspirin. Eleven of 277 experienced a significant response, with a fall in first-second forced expiratory volume (FEV_1) of greater than 20%. This result indicates a prevalence of approximately 4% in the entire asthmatic population studied. Although other investigators have suggested that certain subsets of asthmatics are more likely to have sensitivity to one or another food additive (31), little further data exist to prove this point. Weber and colleagues (32) and Vendanthan *et al.* (33) failed to find positive provocation tests to tartrazine despite testing a population of patients including those with aspirin intolerance. The issue of whether subset populations of asthmatics may have unusual susceptibility to aggravation of their asthma by ingestion of additives is, at this time, a moot point (34).

Mechanisms

The mechanisms underlying asthmatic reactions caused by food additives are not understood. Immunologic reactions involving either IgE or IgG antibodies have been proposed. Sensitization and reexposure are not merely potential consequences of oral ingestion (eating/drinking) but can involve inhalation as well. Cooking, pouring, and serving foods and beverages give ample opportunities for the inhalation of both the primary foods and the additives contained in the foods being served. Some sulfite reactions have been explained as the result of eructation of sulfur dioxide vapor from the stomach (20).

Non-immunologic reactions leading to asthmatic attacks may also occur. Tartrazine-induced asthma at one time was thought to be limited to patients who are aspirin-sensitive. In a classic review of aspirin intolerance, Samter and Beers pointed out that benzoates and tartrazine appear in foods that have been implicated as having asthmagenic effects in aspirin-sensitive patients (31). Juhlin *et al.* (35) and Stenius *et al.* (27) have reported asthmatic reactions to tartrazine challenges in aspirin-sensitive patients, but their criteria for positive reactions and the manner with which the challenges were conducted leave some doubts as to the validity of their results.

Settipane *et al.* carried out double-blind, placebo-controlled challenges with tartrazine in 38 patients with a history of aspirin-induced asthma; although the highest challenge dose was only 0.44 mg, 3 of these patients experienced a significant fall in pulmonary function (36). Spector and colleagues (30) found that 11 patients who had positive provocation tests to tartrazine also had positive provocation tests to aspirin; they did not find tartrazine sensitivity in an asthmatic patient without aspirin sensitivity. Tarlo and Broder (29) found that 1 of 28 asthmatic subjects had a positive challenge on double-blind, oral challenge with tartrazine and benzoate. Stevenson *et al.* (9) and Vandanthan *et al.* (33) have been unable to document tartrazine-induced asthma in a series of oral provocation challenges in 150 adults (9) and 54 children (33). Thus, although it originally seemed that tartrazine-sensitive asthmatic responses might be explained by non-immunologic mechanisms charged with producing aspirin-induced asthma, the coexistence of these two sensitivities appears questionable and the shared mechanism is doubtful.

Samter and Beers also pointed out that sodium benzoate was used as a preservative, which was implicated as the trigger causing attacks of asthma in the aspirin-sensitive asthmatics they studied. Rosenhall (25) found only 1 of 504 patients who reacted to oral benzoate challenge, and Weber *et al.* (32) found only 1 of 43 patients who reacted to benzoate challenge. Again, given such limited data, shared mechanisms of causality cannot be claimed or supported.

Although the use of sulfites in foods and beverages dates back for centuries, recognition of sulfiting agents as causes of acute asthma and anaphylaxis date only from the 1970s (37). Studies utilizing open challenge, as well as single- and double-blind challenge methods have been reported that leave no doubt as to the significance of sulfites in causing asthma—albeit only in a minority of cases.

The pathogenesis of these sulfite-induced reactions remains unknown. Several case reports have suggested that IgE-mediated hypersensitivity is involved (37, 38). On the other hand, many cases appear to be non–IgE-mediated and may involve other pathways, including sulfite oxidase deficiency (39) and reflex bronchoconstriction via parasympathetic nervous system pathways (40).

Diagnosis

The diagnosis of additive-induced asthma rests upon the ability to take an exquisitely detailed history of the clinical attacks of asthma, with special attention paid to the events and ingestants preceding the attack. Food additives should be considered a possible triggering factor in a patient with asthma if the patient indicates in his or her history that symptoms were precipitated after ingesting any foods or beverages. If symptoms appear to be provoked by several different foods or drinks, the possibility of a common food additive should be considered and further investigated. This history must then be followed by a great deal of "homework" on the part of both the patient and the physician, during which time the potential triggers are itemized and ranked as to likelihood of causality. Diagnostic methods involve a trial of additive avoidance or blinded additive challenge. Dietary manipulation and specific additive avoidance may lead to clinical improvement, which may be sufficient to prove causality for the patient. This finding does not constitute scientifically sufficient proof and, if appropriate, specific, double-blind and controlled oral challenges can be carried out. These tests must be conducted with great care to avoid (or control) a potential serious adverse effect of the challenge on the patient, so they must be performed under considerable control and only if warranted. Allergy skin testing or in vitro searches for evidence of additive specific IgE are unlikely to be helpful clinically, as appropriate test reagents are not available. At best, these research procedures have limited value.

Treatment

Simply stated, the cornerstone of treating additive induced asthma is avoidance. Immunotherapy has no place in the treatment of such patients. It may also be necessary to place patients at risk on drug therapy on either a chronic basis or to be used prior to meals which the patient has not prepared.

Summary

Chemical additives of all sorts are used in the modern food supply, and, in most cases, are also found in pharmaceutical preparations. They may affect one or more food characteristics, including color, taste, and texture, or act to preserve freshness and inhibit contamination. It is not surprising that a few patients may exhibit allergic or idiosyncratic intolerance responses to one or more of these agents. The mechanisms by which additives cause asthma is essentially unknown. Fortunately, additive-induced asthma is rare, and most susceptible patients can be managed with diet control and drug therapy. The concerned physician must take great care not to magnify the frequency or severity of this problem.

REFERENCES

1. Smith JM. Adverse reactions to food and drug additives. European J of Clin Nutr 1991;45(suppl 1):17–21.
2. Anderson JA, Sogn DD, eds. Adverse reactions to foods. AAAI and NIAID Report, NIH Publication No. 84-2442, U.S. Department of Health and Human Services, Public Health Service, National Institutes of Health 1994.
3. Michaelson G, Juhlin L. Urticaria induced by preservative and dye additives in foods and drugs. Brit J Dermat 1973;88:525–532.
4. Chaffee FH, Settipane GA. Asthma caused by FD&C approved dyes. J Allergy 1967;40:65–72.
5. Freedman BJ. Asthma induced by sulfur dioxide, benzoate and tartrazine contained in orange drinks. Clin Allergy 1977;7:407–415.
6. Lockey SD. Allergic reactions due to FD&C yellow no. 5 tartrazine, an aniline dye used as a coloring and identifying agent in various steroids. Ann Allergy 1959;17:719–721.
7. Fishman AE. Suspected aminophylline causes of asthma: three case reports. Ann Allergy 1974;33:161–163.
8. Lockey SD. Reactions to hidden agents in foods and drugs can be serious. Ann Allergy 1975;35:239–242.
9. Stevenson DD, Simon BA, Lumry WR, Matheson DA. Adverse

reactions to tartrazine. J Allergy Clin Immunol 1986;78:182–191.

10. Kerr GR, Wu-Lee M, El-Lozy M, McGandy R, Stare FJ. Prevalence of the "Chinese restaurant syndrome." J Am Diet Assoc 1979;75:29–33.

11. Allen DH, Baker GJ. Chinese restaurant asthma. N Engl J Med 1981;305:1154–1155.

12. Allen DH, Delohery J, Baker GJ, Wood R. Monosodium glutamate induced asthma. J Allergy Clin Immunol 1983;71:98 (abstract).

13. Koepke JW, Selner JC. Combined monosodium glutamate/metabisulfite induced asthma. J Allergy Clin Immunol 1986;77:158 (abstract).

14. Miller R, White LW, Schwartz HJ. A case of episodic urticaria due to saccharin ingestion. J Allergy Clin Immunol 1974;53:240–242.

15. Kulczycki A Jr. Aspartame induced urticaria. Ann Int Med 1986;104:207–208.

16. Schwartz HJ. Observations on the uses and effects of sulfiting agents in foods and drugs. Immunol Allergy Practice 1984;6:302–307.

17. Simon RA, Green L, Stevenson DD. The incidence of metabisulfite sensitivity in an asthmatic population. J Allergy Clin Immunol 1982;69:118 (abstract).

18. Bush RK, Taylor SL, Holden K, Nordlee JA, Busse WW. Prevalence of sensitivity to sulfiting agents in asthmatic patients. Am J Med 1986;81:816–820.

19. Gunnison AF, Jacobsen DW. Sulfite hypersensitivity. A critical review. CRC Crit Rev Toxicol 1987;17:185–214.

20. Simon RA. Sulfite sensitivity. Ann Allergy 1986;56:281–288.

21. Bush RK, Taylor SL, Busse W. A critical evaluation of clinical trials in reactions to sulfites. J Allergy Clin Immunol 1986;78:191–202.

22. Young E, Patel S, Stoneham M, Rona R, Wilkinson JD. The prevalence of reaction to food additives in a survey population. JR Call Physicians 1987;21:241–247.

23. Fuglsang G, Madsen C, Saval P, Oterballe O. Prevalence of intolerance to food additives among Danish school children. Pediatr Allergy Immunol 1993;4:123–129.

24. Fuglsang G, Madsen C, Hallsen S, Jorgensen M, Ostergaard PA, Osterballe O. Adverse reactions to food additives in children with atopic symptoms. Allergy 1994;49:31–37.

25. Rosenhall L. Evaluation of intolerance to analgesics, preservatives and food colorants with challenge tests. Eur J Resp Dis 1982;63:410–419.

26. Taylor SL, Bush RK, Selner JC, Nordlee JA, Wiener MB, Holden K, Koepke JW, Busse WW. Sensitivity to sulfited foods among sulfite-sensitive subjects with asthma. J Allergy Clin Immunol 1988;81:1159–1167.

27. Stenius BS, Lemola M. Hypersensitivity to aspirin and tartrazine in patients with asthma. Clin Allergy 1976;6:119–129.

28. Genton C, Frei PC, Pe'Coud A. J Allergy Clin Immunol, 1985;76:40–45.

29. Tarlo SM, Broder I. Tartrazine and benzoate challenge and dietary avoidance in chronic asthma. Clin Allergy 1982;12:303–312.

30. Spector SL, Wangaar CH, Farr RJ. Aspirin and concomitant idiosyncrasies in adult asthmatic patients. J Allergy Clin Immunol 1979;64:500–506.

31. Samter M, Beers RF. Intolerance to aspirin: clinical studies and considerations of its pathogenesis. Ann Intern Med 1968;68:975–983.

32. Weber RW, Hoffman M, Raine DA Jr, Nelson HS. Incidence of bronchoconstriction due to aspirin, azo dyes and non-azo dyes and preservatives in a population of perennial asthmatics. J Allergy Clin Immunol 1979;64:32–37.

33. Vedanthan PK, Menon MM, Bell TD, Bergin D. Aspirin and tartrazine oral challenge: incidence of adverse response in chronic childhood asthma. J Allergy Clin Immunol 1977;62:608–613.

34. Moneret-Vautrin DA. Monosodium glutamate-induced asthma; study of the potential risk of 30 asthmatics and review of the literature. Allerg-Immunol (Paris) 1987;19:29–35.

35. Juhlin L, Michaelson G, Zetterstrom O. Urticaria and asthma induced by foods and drug additives in patients with aspirin hypersensitivity. J Allergy Clin Immunol 1972;50:92–98.

36. Settipane GA, Pudupakkam RK. Aspirin intolerance. III. Subtypes familial occurrence and cross reactivity with tartrazine. J Allergy Clin Immunol 1975;56:215–221.

37. Prenner BM, Stevens JJ. Anaphylaxis after ingestion of sodium bisulfite. Ann Allergy 1976;37:180–182.

38. Twarog FJ, Leung DY. Anaphylaxis to a component of isoetharine (sodium bisulfite). JAMA 1982;248:2030–2032.

39. Jacobsen DW, Simon RA, Singh M. Sulfite oxidase deficiency and cobalamin protection in sulfite sensitive asthmatics. J Allergy Clin Immunol 1984;73:135 (abstract).

40. Sheppard D, Wong WS, Vehara CF, Nadel JA, Boushey HA. Lower threshold and greater bronchomotor responsiveness of asthmatic subjects to sulfur dioxide. Am Rev Resp Dis 1980;122:873–878.

Part Four

CONTEMPORARY TOPICS IN ADVERSE REACTIONS TO FOODS

29

PHARMACOLOGIC FOOD REACTIONS

James L. Baldwin

Many foods contain a variety of either naturally occurring or added components that provide pharmacologic or drug-like activity (1). When consumed in moderation, however, only a small number of substances have been identified that account for the majority of clinically apparent adverse pharmacologic reactions attributed to foods. This chapter focuses on the most common endogenous substances implicated in pharmacologic reactions to foods and discusses, where possible, the mechanisms involved, prevention, and treatment strategies.

Definitions and Characteristics

Pharmacologic food reactions have been defined as adverse reactions to foods or food additives that result from naturally derived or added chemicals that produce drug-like or pharmacologic effects in the host (2). Unlike type I allergic food reactions, which affect only a selected group of atopic patients, pharmacologic food reactions can potentially be elicited in a wider, more diverse group of individuals. The dose or quantity ingested necessary to elicit a clinically apparent reaction typically varies among individuals and even in the same individual over time. It may depend on metabolic differences, concurrent medication usage, food freshness, and food preparation.

Pharmacologic substances in foods can mediate their effects via either direct or indirect routes. In the direct route, the food substance interacts directly with host tissue to exert an effect. In the indirect route, the food substance activates one or more of the host's endogenous mediator systems, which in turn exerts the effect on the host tissue. Differences in host tissue and/or host mediator system susceptibility at the time of ingestion are two factors that can contribute to the variability of these reactions.

Endogenous Substances Responsible for Pharmacologic Food Reactions

The different classes of endogenous substances responsible for pharmacologic reactions to foods are shown in Figure 29.1. Vasoactive amines constitute the largest class of substances responsible for pharmacologic reactions to foods. Methylxanthines make up a second class of food components having pharmacologic activity. Finally, several unrelated food components with pharmacologic activity, such as capsaicin, ethanol, and myristicin, have been identified.

Vasoactive Amines

The vasoactive amines include dopamine, histamine, norepinephrine, phenylethylamine, serotonin, tryptamine, and tyramine. Of these substances, dopamine, histamine, phenylethylamine, serotonin, and tyramine may be present in appreciable amounts in foods, thereby producing clinically apparent pharmacologic effects.

HISTAMINE

The diamine histamine is perhaps the best known of the vasoactive amines present in, and responsible for, pharmacologic reactions to foods. Because of histamine's significant contribution to the pathophysiology of atopic disease, histamine-induced pharmacologic food reactions are frequently confused with food allergic reactions.

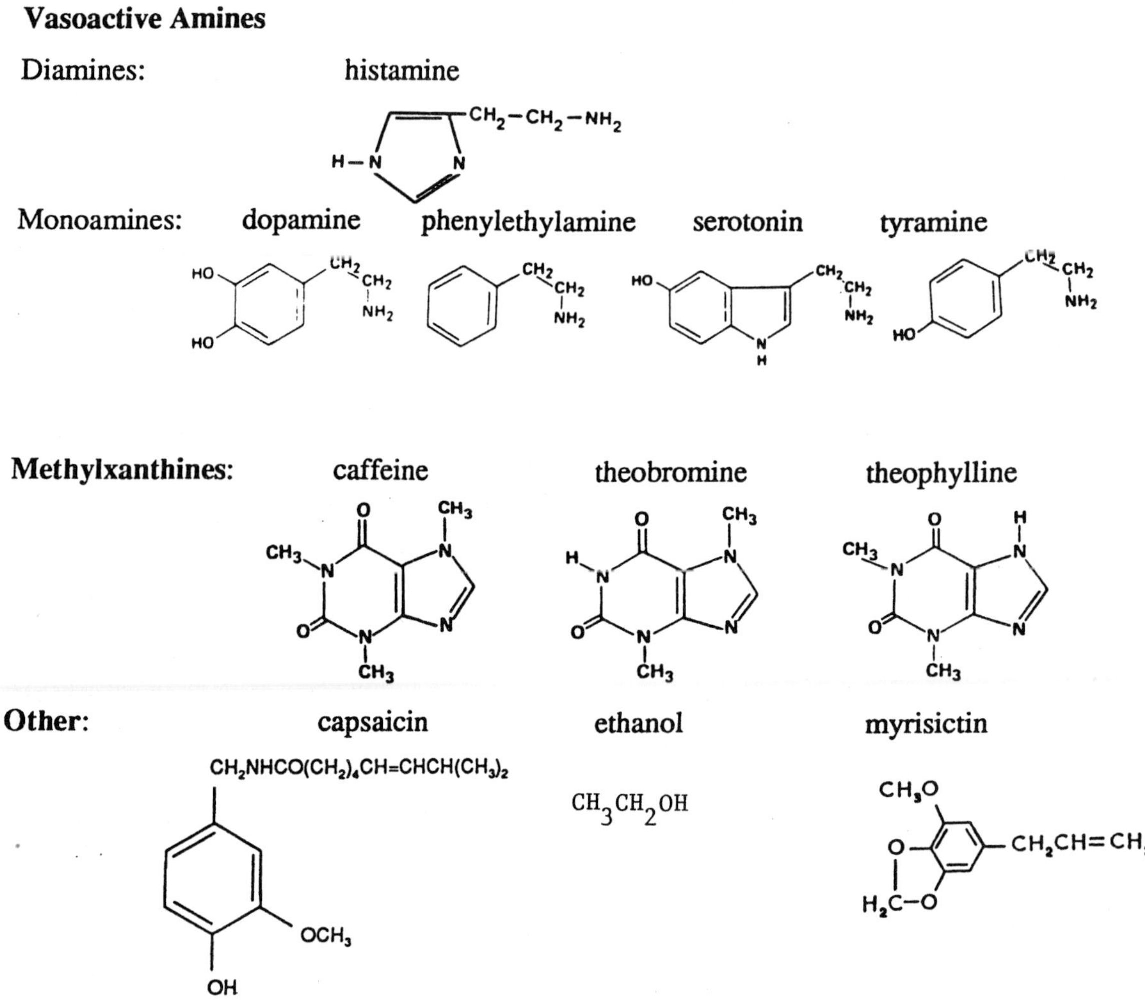

Vasoactive Amines

Figure 29.1

Endogenous substances responsible for pharmacologic food reactions.

Synthesis

Histamine is synthesized in nature by the decarboxylation of its amino acid precursor histidine. This synthesis is catalyzed by the enzyme histidine decarboxylase and other enzymes that are widely distributed in nature. Canine intestinal bacteria may be capable of decarboxylation of dietary histidine to form histamine (3). Likewise, marine bacteria contaminating inappropriately refrigerated scombroid fish may convert the histidine present to histamine

(4, 5). The wide distribution of enzymes capable of decarboxylating histidine to histamine partially accounts for the presence of histamine in many foods.

Physiologic Effects

Histamine mediates its effects on tissues through H_1 receptors, H_2 receptors, or both. The subsequent tissue responses to histamine, summarized in Table 29.1, can present following any type I hypersensitivity reaction in which histamine is released from mast

Table 29.1
Physiologic Responses Elicited by Histamine

Response Mediated by H$_1$ Receptors
Smooth muscle contraction
Increased vascular permeability
Mucous gland secretion

Responses Mediated by H$_2$ Receptors
Gastric acid secretion
Inhibition of basophil histamine release
Inhibition of lymphokine release

Responses Mediated by H$_1$ and H$_2$ Receptors
Vasodilatation
   Hypotension
   Flush
   Headache
Tachycardia

cells and/or basophils through an IgE-dependent mechanism. A clinically similar physiologic response can be noted in non–IgE-dependent pharmacologic food reactions in which histamine is either present in the food ingested or released from tissue stores due to some intrinsic histamine-releasing ability of the food ingested. The IgE- and non–IgE-dependent histamine-mediated events both occur within minutes of ingestion of the culpable food, and can prove clinically indistinguishable.

The physiologic effects of an oral ingestion of histamine depend upon a number of factors, including individual susceptibility (6), metabolism, and dose ingested.

Certain subjects are known to exhibit particular sensitivity to elevation of plasma histamine. For example, in response to elevated plasma histamine, acute bronchospasm can occur in asthmatics and coronary artery spasm can develop in patients with variant angina pectoris (7, 8). Histamine-induced migraine can also be inhibited by H$_2$ receptor blockade (9). Elevations in plasma and urinary histamine have been described following ingestion of a high-histamine-content food. Consequently, susceptible patients might be at particularly high risk for developing adverse events following ingestion of a high-histamine-content food.

Adverse responses to histamine, including abdominal cramping, flushing, headache, palpitations, and hypotension, appear to be a roughly dose-dependent phenomena. It has been suggested that ingestion of 25 to 50 mg of histamine may precipitate headache, whereas 100 to 150 mg may induce flushing (10). These values are only rough estimates, however, and scombroid toxicity has been described with ingestion of as little as 2.5 mg of histamine (11). Although sensitivity and specificity of different histamine assays may account for some of the discrepancies, it is clear that individual susceptibility and factors affecting metabolism play prominent roles in clinical responses as well.

Metabolism

The duration of histamine's effect depends upon its metabolism. In normal physiology, conversion of histamine to its major inactive metabolites by either histamine methyltransferase or diamine oxidase (DAO) generally occurs rapidly (12, 13). Figure 29.2 shows the two routes of histamine metabolism. Prolonged binding of histamine from normal dietary sources to H$_1$ and H$_2$ receptors is uncommon, and symptoms rarely occur with such incidental ingestions. When large ingestions of histamine such as in cases of scombroid poisoning occur, however, the metabolic capacity is exceeded and a multitude of histamine mediated effects are observed. Experimental administration of large oral quantities of histamine yields similar clinical responses (14).

Although methylation appears to comprise the primary route for metabolism of histamine administered by both the oral and intravenous routes, DAO is important as well. DAO is present in the intestinal mucosa in almost all mammalian species examined (15). Ingestion of a histamine-containing meal along with ingestion of drugs that inhibit DAO can produce histamine-induced symptoms. Pigs pretreated with the potent DAO inhibitor aminoguanidine and fed a high-histamine-content meal experienced severe clinical histamine-induced signs including, in some cases, shock and death. Conversely, pigs fed the same meal without pretreatment were generally asymptomatic (16). Isoniazid is a potent DAO inhibitor and, when combined with a histamine-containing meal, has resulted in severe histamine-induced symptoms (17, 18). In vitro experiments have shown a number of drugs (e.g., chloroquine, pentamidine, clavulanic acid, dobutamine, pancuronium, imipenam, and oth-

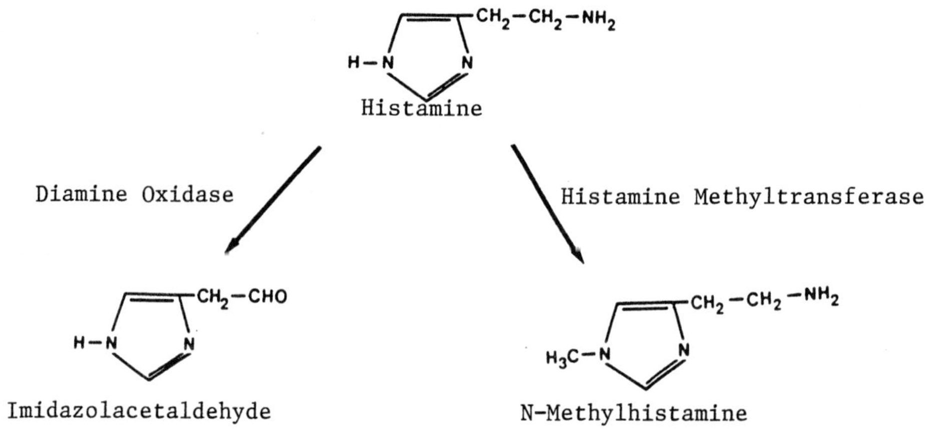

Figure 29.2

Histamine metabolism.

Histamine-Containing Foods

ers) to be potent human intestinal mucosal DAO inhibitors. The in vivo clinical relevance of these findings remains uncertain (16).

Histamine-Containing Foods

Accurate measurement of the histamine content of foods has proved difficult to obtain because of the lack of both specificity and sensitivity of the bioassays and chemical assays used. Certain foods are generally accepted as having a higher histamine content than others (19, 20). Three cheeses (Parmesan, blue, and Roquefort), two vegetables (spinach and eggplant), two red wines (Chianti and Burgundy), yeast extract, and scombroid fish have histamine content adequate to raise post-prandial 24-hour urinary histamine levels (19). For this reason, dietary histamine restrictions are recommended for patients undergoing 24-hour urinary histamine determinations.

Several symptoms generally attributed to monosodium glutamate resemble those associated with histamine toxicity. Using a radioenzymatic assay technique, the histamine content of several common oriental dishes, condiments, and basic ingredients was measured. Although the amount of histamine in individual food portions was determined to fall below the level generally thought necessary to induce symptoms, consumption of multiple portions could result in ingestion of enough histamine to produce symptoms (21).

Scombroid Poisoning

It has been well documented that histamine poisoning can result from ingestion of foods with a high histamine content. The prototype for this type of histamine toxicity is *scombroid poisoning*. Marine bacteria decarboxylate histidine present in improperly refrigerated scombroid fish such as tuna, mackerel, skipjack, and bonito and nonscombroid fish such as mahi mahi, bluefish, amberjack, herring, sardines, marlin, and anchovies, thereby increasing the histamine content of these fish. Ingestion of such fish can result in symptoms of scombroid poisoning, including flushing, sweating, nausea, vomiting, abdominal cramps, diarrhea, headache, palpitations, urticaria, dizziness, a metallic, sharp, or peppery taste, and, in severe cases, hypotension and bronchospasm (11, 22). These symptoms, which usually begin within an hour of ingestion of such fish and last for several hours, have been definitively linked to histamine in spoiled fish (11). The FDA has established a hazard concentration for histamine poisoning of greater than 450 $\mu g/100$ g tuna (23). Levels from 2.5 to 250 mg histamine/100 g fish have been reported in most cases of scombroid poisoning. Treatment is supportive and includes H_1

and H_2 receptor blockade. Improper warming between the time that the fish is caught and when it is prepared can lead to histamine production sufficient to cause poisoning. Scombroid poisoning can be prevented only by proper handling and refrigeration of fish (22, 24).

Histamine-Releasing Foods

Some foods without significant histamine content have been said to contain substances capable of triggering degranulation of tissue mast cells with resultant histamine release. Substances thought to be responsible for this histamine-releasing activity include enzymes in foods, such as trypsin, and other agents from both animal and vegetable sources, such as peptone. Foods with this unproven intrinsic histamine-releasing capacity include egg white, crustaceans, chocolate, strawberries, ethanol, tomatoes, and citrus fruits (25).

MONOAMINES

Monoamines of dietary significance include dopamine, phenylethylamine, serotonin, and tyramine. Of these substances, phenylethylamine and tyramine account for the majority of pharmacologic reactions, although adverse effects of both dopamine- and serotonin-containing foods have been reported as well. These vasoactive monoamines are found in the greatest amounts in fermented foods.

Synthesis

Naturally occurring amino acids are converted into the vasoactive monoamines by a number of microorganisms that possess the amino acid decarboxylases necessary for this conversion. For example, tyrosine is the precursor for both dopamine and tyramine, while phenylalanine is the precursor for phenylethylamine and tryptophan is the precursor for serotonin. Amine production by these microorganisms varies depending upon a variety of different conditions, including pH, temperature, and NaCl content (26).

Metabolism

The vasoactive monoamines are metabolized by the enzyme monoamine oxidase (MAO), which includes two subtypes: MAO-A and MAO-B. The genes for both MAO-A and MAO-B have been mapped to the short arm of the X chromosome (Xp11.23) (27), and appear to be derived from a duplication of a common ancestral gene (28). MAO is found in a variety of tissues, where it is localized to the outer membrane of mitochondria. It catalyzes the oxidative deamination of a variety of neurotransmitters as well as the monoamines having dietary significance. Dopamine and tyramine can be metabolized by both MAO-A and MAO-B. The polar amines (serotonin, epinephrine, and norepinephrine) are metabolized primarily by MAO-A, whereas the nonpolar amine phenylethylamine is metabolized primarily by MAO-B (29).

SPECIFIC MONOAMINES

Tyramine

Many fermented foods contain tyramine derived from the bacterial decarboxylation of tyrosine. Foods with particularly high levels of tyramine include Camembert and cheddar cheeses, yeast extract, wine (especially Chianti), pickled herring, fermented bean curd, fermented soya bean, soy sauces and miso soup, and chicken liver. Smaller, but still detectable amounts are present in avocados, bananas, figs, red plums, eggplant, and tomato (30–32).

Although tyramine exerts an indirect sympathomimetic effect by releasing endogenous norepinephrine (33), dietary tyramine usually does not cause detectable clinical effects. Two instances where dietary tyramine is thought to be responsible for adverse clinical effects involve migraine headache and the hypertensive crisis experienced by patients receiving concurrent treatment with MAO inhibitors.

Foods and beverages containing tyramine have been linked to vascular headache in some patients with food-induced migraine. In one study employing double-blind, placebo-controlled challenges in 45 patients with food-induced migraine, 75 of 94 tyramine (125 mg) challenges (80%) evoked a migraine, whereas only 5 of 60 placebo challenges (8%) were followed by migraine (34). Several other studies, however, have failed to demonstrate a relationship between migraine and tyramine (35, 36).

As noted earlier, ingestion of foods and beverages

containing large quantities of tyramine can lead to headache and hypertensive crisis in patients being treated with MAO inhibitors (31). Monoamine oxidase found in the gastrointestinal tract normally metabolizes dietary monoamines readily. When MAO inhibitors block MAO function, however, exogenous dietary monoamines are absorbed and release endogenous norepinephrine. The resulting pressor effect is linked to palpitations, severe headache, and hypertensive crisis. Prevention of such an episode can be averted by avoiding foods rich in tyramine and other monoamines. Treatment involves slow intravenous administration of the alpha-adrenergic antagonist phentolamine, which is given until blood pressure stabilizes.

Dopamine

Dopamine exerts both an indirect sympathomimetic effect, by releasing endogenous norepinephrine, and a direct sympathomimetic effect, by interacting with alpha and beta-1 adrenoreceptors. Although tyramine in foods and beverages accounts for the majority of MAO inhibitor-associated hypertensive crises, dopamine present in fava beans or broad beans can also precipitate such a crisis. Avoidance of those foods is recommended for patients taking MAO inhibitors (31).

Phenylethylamine

Like the other monoamines, phenylethylamine may be found in several fermented foods and beverages, especially gouda and Stilton cheeses and red wine. Unlike the other monoamines, however, phenylethylamine is also found in chocolate (30, 37).

Several mechanisms have been implicated in producing phenylethylamine's action (38, 39). It appears likely that phenylethylamine, like tyramine, primarily exerts an indirect sympathomimetic effect by releasing endogenous norepinephrine. Consequently, phenylethylamine has been implicated in both food-induced migraine (40) as well as MAO inhibitor-associated hypertensive crisis (31).

Serotonin (5-Hydroxytryptamine)

Serotonin is found in highest concentrations (greater than 3.0 μg/g) in certain fruits, vegetables, and nuts, including banana, kiwi, pineapple, plantain, plum, tomato, walnuts, and hickory nuts (30, 41). Serotonin is present in moderate amounts (0.1 to 3.0 μg/g) in avocados, dates, grapefruit, cantaloupe, honeydew, black olives, broccoli, eggplant, figs, spinach, and cauliflower (41). The only non-plant foods with significant amounts of serotonin are certain mollusks, especially octopus (30).

Serotonin acts on at least two distinct receptors and a variety of cell types. Its actions are complex and exhibit wide species and receptor variability. Two major effects attributed to serotonin are skeletal muscle vasodilation with flushing and both intracranial and extracranial vasoconstriction. Although these effects are often seen with endogenous serotonin production from carcinoid tumors, dietary serotonin does not appear to produce any immediate clinical symptoms, even in patients concurrently taking MAO inhibitors. In fact, oral feeding of serotonin equivalent to as many as 30 bananas failed to elicit clinical symptoms (42). The urinary excretion of the major metabolite of serotonin, 5-hydroxyindoleacetic acid (5-HIAA), increases following ingestion of large amounts of serotonin. In this circumstance, a false diagnosis of carcinoid tumor may be entertained. Consequently, patients collecting 24-hour urine for 5-HIAA measurement should avoid serotonin-containing foods.

Although not proven, dietary serotonin has been implicated in a form of endomyocardial fibrosis seen in Uganda, similar to the endomyocardial fibrosis noted in patients with the carcinoid syndrome (43). It appears that this entity is no longer a major health problem (41).

Methylxanthines

The three dietary methylxanthines are caffeine, theophylline, and theobromine. All are methylated derivatives of xanthine, which is a dioxypurine. Theobromine is extremely weak physiologically, as compared with theophylline and caffeine. While all methylxanthine-containing beverages and foods contain caffeine, theophylline is present in only very small amounts in these foods and beverages, and theobro-

Table 29.2
Some Physiologic Effects of the Methylxanthines

Central Nervous System:	Psychostimulation (anxiety, insomnia)
Cardiovascular:	Increased contractility, blood pressure, pulse; increased cerebrovascular resistance
Respiratory:	Relaxation of respiratory smooth muscle; increased diaphragm contractility
Renal:	Diuretic effect
Gastrointestinal:	Decreased lower esophageal sphincter pressure; increased gastric secretion, nausea
Skeletal Muscle:	Increased contractility

mine is present in significant amounts in only cocoa and chocolate products. Consequently, caffeine accounts for most of the adverse responses from dietary methylxanthine consumption. This section will, therefore, focus on dietary caffeine and its effects.

PHYSIOLOGIC EFFECTS

By far the most common physiologic effect of the methylxanthines involves stimulation of the central nervous system (CNS). The methylxanthines also exert effects on the cardiovascular, respiratory, gastrointestinal, renal, and musculoskeletal systems (44). These effects are outlined in Table 29.2.

MECHANISM OF ACTION

The mechanism of action of the methylxanthines has been studied in various systems (44). At least three mechanisms of action have been suggested. Initial investigations focused on the ability of these agents to inhibit the enzyme phosphodiesterase. In many systems studied, however, it appears that under physiologic conditions this mechanism plays a minor role at best. In the CNS, the methylxanthines appear to act as adenosine antagonists, producing excitation by blocking adenosine's inhibitory effects. In addition, caffeine has been shown to compete for binding at the benzodiazepine site of central chloride channels, causing excitation by limiting activation of these channels (45).

ABSORPTION, DISTRIBUTION, AND METABOLISM

The three dietary methylxanthines are readily absorbed from the gastrointestinal tract and distributed throughout body water. They are extensively metabolized in the liver, primarily to uric acid derivatives that are, in turn, excreted in the urine. Females taking oral contraceptives have significantly slower rates of catabolism of caffeine than females not taking oral contraceptives and males (44). In addition, fluoroquinolones impair caffeine and theophylline metabolism, resulting in increased serum concentrations (46).

METHYLXANTHINE-CONTAINING FOODS

The methylxanthine content of foods and beverages has been widely studied via high-performance liquid chromatography (44, 47). Rough estimates of the quantities of the methylxanthines are given in Table 29.3. These values may fluctuate widely, depending on the variety of food and its preparation. For example, Robusta coffee blends yield higher caffeine content in general than Arabica blends (44). Furthermore, brewing times and methods can alter the caffeine content by 100% in certain teas and coffees (44).

ADVERSE EFFECTS OF CAFFEINE

As noted, caffeine exerts pharmacologic effects on a variety of organ systems. Consequently, adverse pharmacologic reactions to caffeine-containing foods and beverages are manifested in many ways.

Large quantities of coffee and tea are known to

Table 29.3
Methylxanthine Content of Foods and Beverages

	Theophylline	Caffeine	Theobromine
Coffee	100–150 mg/cup	—	—
Cola	40 mg/12 oz	—	—
Tea	30–40 mg/cup	3 mg/cup	0.3 mg/cup
Cocoa	4 mg/cup	60 mg/cup	—
Milk chocolate	6 mg/oz	60 mg/oz	—
Baking chocolate	35 mg/oz	350 mg/oz	—

produce clinical symptoms that mimic anxiety and panic disorders (48). In a placebo-controlled trial of caffeine consumption in patients diagnosed as having panic disorder or agoraphobia with panic attacks and in normal controls, caffeine produced significantly greater increases in subject-related anxiety, nervousness, fear, nausea, palpitations, restlessness, and tremors in patients compared with controls (49). Furthermore, these effects were correlated with plasma caffeine levels and were reported to resemble those experienced during panic attacks. The only somatic effect that differed significantly from baseline in the normal controls was an increase in tremors (49). In addition, caffeine abstention has been reported to reduce the frequency of panic attacks in this patient population (50). A central adenosine receptor dysfunction in patients with panic attacks has been proposed as an explanation for their increased sensitivity to caffeine (51).

Two cases of caffeine-induced urticaria reported in the literature were diagnosed by double-blind, placebo-controlled challenge (52, 53). Although the mechanism remains obscure, both cases were inhibited by pretreatment with terfenadine, suggesting mediator release and H_1 receptor stimulation in the pathogenesis of the reactions.

Withdrawal from caffeine often produces migraine headache in susceptible individuals. Other common effects described in normal healthy individuals and attributed to dietary caffeine include insomnia, palpitations, nausea, and diuresis.

Capsaicin

The genus *Capsicum* encompasses several species, including chili peppers, red peppers, paprika, tabasco pepper, and Louisiana long pepper. Capsicum has been used for centuries by cultures around the world to enhance the flavor of relatively bland foodstuffs, as well as for its medicinal and irritant properties. Although more than 100 volatile compounds are present in capsicum oleoresin, capsaicin represents the important biologically active compound and is used most frequently for its pharmacotherapeutic benefits (54). Approximately 70% of the irritant effect

of these foods that accounts for their "hot" sensation derives from their capsaicin content (55).

Capsaicin's initial irritant action is mediated by release of the neurosecretory compound substance P from nociceptive nerve fibers. Substance P depolarizes neurons to produce vascular dilation, smooth muscle stimulation, and pain. Repeated exposure to capsaicin results in blockage of substance P synthesis, diminishing the neuron's ability to transmit pain. This process provides the basis on which capsaicin creams are used for such painful conditions as rheumatoid arthritis, osteoarthritis, diabetic neuropathy, postherpetic neuralgia, postmastectomy pain syndrome, and reflex sympathetic dystrophy (54).

The most common (adverse) effect associated with capsaicin is the "burning" oral sensation associated with its ingestion. In this instance, capsaicin binds strongly through its lipophillic side chain to the lipoproteins of oral mucosal receptors. To hinder this strong interaction and "cool the burn," a lipophillic phosphoprotein such as casein (present in milk, nuts, chocolate, and some beans) is more effective than cold water (56). A case of plasma cell gingivitis has also been attributed to oral exposure to capsaicin (57).

Adverse pharmacologic effects associated with capsaicin have also been reported in several tissues following exposure by several routes. Gastric installation has been shown to result in significant increases in gastric acid and pepsin secretion, as well as mucosal microbleeding and exfoliation (58). Nausea, vomiting, abdominal pain, and perforated viscus with peritonitis have all been reported following ingestion of multiple peppers at a single sitting (59, 60). Inhalation has been reported to result in cough in occupationally exposed capsicum processing workers (61) and in laryngospasm (62). Involvement with the eyes causes pain, tearing, erythema, and blepharospasm; this effect leads to use of "pepper sprays" to ward off would-be attackers. Both acute and chronic dermatologic manifestations can also occur when handling capsicum. Possible acute effects include skin irritation, erythema, and burning pain without vesiculation. In chronic exposures, severe dermatitis with vesiculation can occur (63). A case of Sweet's syndrome in a pepper preserver has also been attributed to capsaicin (64).

Ethanol

Ethanol, the most widely abused pharmacologic substance in the world, exerts diverse effects on several body systems. The most prominent effects of ethanol consumed in moderate amounts act on the CNS. Ethanol can also act as a peripheral vasodilator and diuretic. It exerts its effects on the brain by dissolving in neuronal plasma membranes, thereby altering the movement of chloride and calcium ions involved in regulation of electrical signals and neurotransmitter release. Ethanol's diuretic effect is thought to relate to its ability to inhibit posterior pituitary secretion of antidiuretic hormone (65). Both the diuretic and CNS effects of ethanol are well known and not commonly mistaken for allergic reactions. The histamine-releasing ability of ethanol was discussed earlier. Consequently, this section will focus on other responses to ethanol dependent upon its peripheral vasodilatory properties that are sometimes mistaken for ethanol "allergy."

The mechanism of ethanol-induced peripheral vasodilation remains incompletely understood. Both direct effects—possibly mediated through increases in nitric oxide synthase activity (66, 67)—and centrally mediated effects (68) have been suggested. Both normal individuals and those with metabolic deficiencies can experience ethanol's vasodilatory effects. In normal subjects, nasal congestion with increases in upper airway resistance (69) and mild cutaneous flushing reactions have been noted within minutes of ethanol ingestion. Alcohol sensitivity refers to a symptom complex that can consist of cutaneous flushing, tachycardia, hypotension, somnolence, nausea, and vomiting. This response is thought to be mediated by increased levels of acetaldehyde resulting from inhibited enzymatic action of aldehyde dehydrogenase (ALDH). It can occur following ethanol interaction with disulfuram, metronidazole, griseofulvin, quinacrine, hypoglycemic sulfonylureas, phenothiazines, or phenylbutazone in normal individuals or in individuals deficient in one of the mitochondrial isoenzymes of ALDH designated ALDH$_2$.

ALDH$_2$ deficiency is common in certain Asian groups (affecting approximately 50% of Chinese, Japanese, and Koreans) and has been reported to be protective against development of alcoholism (70, 71). It appears only rarely among non-Mongolian ethnic groups. The inactive ALDH$_2$ allele appears dominant such that both homozygotes and heterozygotes exhibit ALDH$_2$ deficiency and alcohol sensitivity. Both heterozygotes and homozygotes for the inactive ALDH$_2$ allele experience symptoms to varying degrees within minutes of ingestion, responding with elevations in serum cortisol (72). Extreme cases of ethanol sensitivity presenting with coma have been reported (73). Treatment is supportive. A cutaneous ethanol patch test has been suggested as a more reliable indicator of the ALDH phenotype than self-reported ethanol-induced flushing (74).

Myristicin

The spice nutmeg is derived from the dried fruit of the nutmeg tree (Myristica fragrans). Taken in moderation as a flavoring for foods, nutmeg is innocuous. Large quantities can precipitate psychosis, however. The active ingredient in nutmeg thought to be responsible for this adverse effect is myristicin. Structurally, myristicin is similar to mescaline (75). It has been proposed that myristicin may be metabolized in vivo to an amphetamine-like compound with effects similar to those of lysergic acid diethylamide (76). It remains unclear whether myristicin or one or more metabolites accounts for its psychoactive properties, as synthetic myristicin does not always precipitate hallucination (77). Some investigators questioned nutmeg's psychoactive properties and have reviewed various medicinal uses of this spice (78). One tablespoon of grated nutmeg (roughly 7 g) contains about 2% myristicin by weight (79). Symptoms generally appear three to eight hours after ingesting more than one tablespoon. The most prominent effects involve the central nervous and cardiovascular systems. Apprehension, fear of impending death, anxiety, and visual hallucinations accompanied by regular tachycardia are common (80, 81). Patients may also experience palpitations, nausea, vomiting, and chest pressure. Because dry mouth, fever, cutaneous flushing, and blurred vision can occur, acute nutmeg intoxication is sometimes mistaken for anticholinergic intoxication. One differentiating physical examination feature is that myristicin usually (82)—

though not always (83)—causes miosis rather than mydriasis.

Treatment for acute nutmeg intoxication is supportive. Emesis induction of an unknown ingestion is controversial. Many patients ingesting a toxic quantity of nutmeg are nauseated and will vomit spontaneously. Activated charcoal with sorbitol may decrease the systemic absorption, thereby mitigating the duration and severity of symptoms. Various psychotropics have also been employed, including diazepam and haloperidol for anxious and hallucinogenic features (80, 81).

REFERENCES

1. Sapika N. Food pharmacology. Springfield, Illinois: Charles C. Thomas Publishers, 1969.
2. Metcalfe DD. Food hypersensitivity. J Allergy Clin Immunol 1984;73.749–762.
3. Irvine WT, Duthie HL, Watson NG. Urinary output of free histamine after a meat meal. Lancet 1959;1:1061–1064.
4. Hughes JM, Merson MH. Fish and shellfish poisoning. N Engl J Med 1976;295:1117–1120.
5. Geiger E. Role of histamine in poisoning with spoiled fish. Science 1955;121:865–866.
6. Blakesley ML. Scombroid poisoning: prompt resolution of symptoms with cimetidine. Ann Emer Med 1983;12:104–106.
7. Simon RA, Stevenson DD, Arrygave CM, Tan EM. The relationship of plasma histamine to the activity of bronchial asthma. J Allergy Clin Immunol 1977;60:312–316.
8. Ginsberg R, Bristow MR, Kantrowitz N, Baim DS, Harrison DC. Histamine provocation of clinical coronary artery spasm: implications concerning pathogenesis of variant angina pectoris. Am Heart J 1981;102:819–822.
9. Glaser D, De Tarnowsky GO. Cimetidine and red wine headaches. Ann Int Med 1983;98:413.
10. Motil KJ, Scrimshaw NS. The role of histamine in scombroid poisoning. Toxicology Lett 1979;3:219.
11. Morrow JD, Margolies GR, Rowland BS, Roberts LJ. Evidence that histamine is the causative toxin of scombroid-fish poisoning. N Engl J Med 1991;324:716–720.
12. Green JP, Prell' GD, Khandelwal JK, Blandina P. Aspects of histamine metabolism. Agents and Actions 1987;22:1–15.
13. Schayer RW. The metabolism of histamine in various species. Br J Pharmacol 1956;11:472–473.
14. Sjaastad O. Fate of histamine and N-acetylhistamine administration into the human gut. Acta Pharmacol 1966;24:189–202.
15. Kusche J, Schmidt J, Schmidt A, Lorenz W. Diamine oxidases in the small intestine of rabbits, dogs and pigs: separation from soluble monoamine oxidases and substrate specificity of the enzymes. Agents and Actions 1975;5:440–441.
16. Sattler J, Lorenz W. Intestinal diamine oxidases and enteral-induced histaminosis: studies on three prognostic variables in an epidemiological model. J Neural Transm Suppl 1990; 32:291–314.
17. Senanayake N, Vyravavathan S. Histamine reactions due to

18. Uragoda CG, Kottegoda SR. Adverse reactions to isoniazid on ingestion of fish with a high histamine content. Tubercle 1977;58:83–89.
19. Feldman JM. Histaminuria from histamine rich foods. Arch Intern Med 1983;143:2099–2102.
20. Malone MH, Metcalfe DD. Histamine in foods: its possible role in non-allergic adverse reactions to ingestants. N Engl Regional Allergy Proc 1986;7:241–245.
21. Chin KW, Garriga MM, Metcalfe DD. The histamine content of oriental foods. Food Chem Toxic 1989;27:283–287.
22. Gellert GA, Ralls J, Brown C, Huston J, Merryman R. Scombroid fish poisoning underreporting and prevention among noncommercial recreational fishers. West J Med 1992;157:645–647.
23. Food and Drug Administration. Defect action levels for histamine in tuna; availability of guide. Fed Regist 1982;47:487.
24. Hughes JM, Potter ME. Scombroid-fish poisoning: from pathogenesis to prevention. N Engl J Med 1991;324:766–768.
25. American Academy of Allergy and Immunology Committee on Adverse Reactions to Foods. U.S. Department of Health and Human Services. NIH Publication No. 84-2442, 1984.
26. Chander H, Batish VK, Babu S, Bhatia KL. Amine production by *Streptococcus lactis* under different growth conditions. Acta Microbiol Pol 1988;57:61–64.
27. Lan NC, Heinzman C, Gal A, Klisak I, Orth U, Lai E, Grimsby J, Sparkes RS, Mohandas T, Shih JC. Human monoamine oxidase A and B genes map to Xp11.23 and are deleted in a patient with Norrie disease. Genomics 1989;4:552–559.
28. Grimsby J, Chen K, Wang LJ, Lan NC, Shih JC. Human monoamine oxidase A and B genes exhibit identical exon-intron organization. Proc Nat Acad Sci USA 1991;88:3637–3641.
29. Kanazawa I. Short review on monoamine oxidase and its inhibitors. Eur Neurol 1994;34(suppl 3):36–39.
30. Marley E, Blackwell B. Interactions of monoamine oxidase inhibitors, amines, and foodstuffs. Adv Pharmacol Chemother 1970;8:185–239.
31. Food interacting with MAO inhibitors. Med Lett Drugs Ther 1989;31:11–12.
32. Da Prada M, Zucher G. Tyramine content of preserved and fermented foods or condiments of Far Eastern cuisine. Psychopharmacology 1992;106:s32–s34.
33. Raiteri M, Levi G. A reinterpretation of tyramine sympathomimetic effect and tachyphylaxis. J Neurosci Res 1986;16:439–441.
34. Smith I, Kellow AH, Hanington E. A clinical and biochemical correlation between tyramine and migraine headache. Headache 1970;10:43–51.
35. Moffett A, Swash M, Scott DF. Effect of tyramine in migraine: a double blind study. J Neurol Neurosurs Psychiatry 1972;35:496–499.
36. Ziegler DK, Stewart R. Failure of tyramine to induce migraine. Neurology 1977;27:725–726.
37. Chaytor JP, Crathorne B, Saxby MJ. The identification and significance of 2-phenylethylamine in foods. J Sci Fd Agric 1975;26:593–598.
38. Zeller EA, Mosnaim AD, Borison RL, Huprikar SV. Phenylethylamine: studies on the mechanism of its physiological action. Adv Biochem Psychopharmacol 1976;15:75–86.
39. Sabelli HC, Borison RL. 2-Phenylethylamine and other adren-

ingestion of tuna fish *(Thunnus arentivittatus)* in patients on anti-tuberculosis therapy. Toxicon 1980;19:184–185.

ergic modulators. Adv Biochem Psychopharmacol 1976;15:69–74.

40. Sandler M, Youdim MBH, Hanington E. A phenylethylamine oxidising defect in migraine. Nature 1974;250:335–337.
41. Feldman JM, Lee EM. Serotonin content of foods: effect on urinary excretion of 5-hydroxyindoleacetic acid. Am J Clin Nutr 1985;42:639–643.
42. Crout JR, Sjoerdsma A. The clinical and laboratory significance of serotonin and catecholamines in bananas. N Engl J Med 1959;261:23–26.
43. Ojo GO, Parratt JR. Urinary excretion of 5-hydroxyindoleacetic acid in Nigerians with endomyocardial fibrosis. Lancet 1966;1:854–856.
44. Spiller GA. The methylxanthine beverages and foods: chemistry, consumption and health effects. Prog Clin Biol Res 1984;158:1–413.
45. Craig CR, Stitzel RE. Modern pharmacology. Boston, MA: Little, Brown, 1994, 383–385.
46. Marchbanks CR. Drug–drug interactions with fluoroquinolones. Pharmacotherapy 1993;13(pt 2):23S–28S.
47. Terada H, Sakabe Y. High performance liquid chromatographic determination of theobromine, theophylline and caffeine in food products. J Chromatography 1984;291:453–459.
48. Greden JF. Anxiety or caffeinism—a diagnostic dilemma. Am J Psychiatry 1974;131:1089–1092.
49. Charney DS, Heninger GR, Jatlow PI. Increased anxiogenic effects of caffeine in panic disorders. Arch Gen Psychiatry 1985;42:233–243.
50. Bruce MS, Lader M. Caffeine abstention in the management of anxiety disorders. Psychological Med 1989;19:211–214.
51. Nutt D, Lawson C. Panic attacks: a neurochemical overview of models and mechanisms. Br J Psychiatry 1992;160:165–178.
52. Pola J, Subiza J, Armentia A, Zapata C, Hinojosa M, Losada E, Valdivieso R. Urticaria caused by caffeine. Ann Allergy 1988;60:207–208.
53. Gancedo SQ, Freire P, Rivas MF, Davila I, Losada E. Urticaria from caffeine. J Allergy Clin Immunology 1991;88:680–681.
54. Cordell GA, Araujo OE. Capsaicin: identification, nomenclature, and pharmacotherapy. Ann Pharmacother 1993;27:330–336.
55. Mack RB. Capsaicin annum: another revenge from Montezuma. N C Med J 1994;55:198–200.
56. Henkin R. Cooling the burn from hot peppers. JAMA 1991;266:2766.
57. Serio FG, Siegel MA, Slade BE. Plasma cell gingivitis of unusual origin. A case report. J Periodontol 1991;62:390–393.
58. Myers BM, Smith L, Graham DY. Effect of red pepper and black pepper on the stomach. Am J Gastroenterol 1987;82:211–214.
59. Bartholomew LG, Carlson HC. An unusual cause of acute gastroenteritis. Mayo Clin Proc 1994;69:675–676.
60. Landau O, Gutman H, Ganor A, Nudelman I, Rivlin E, Reiss R. Post-pepper pain, perforation and peritonitis. JAMA 1992;268:1686.
61. Blanc P, Liu D, Juarez C, Boushey HA. Cough in hot pepper workers. Chest 1991;99:27–33.
62. Rubin HR, Wu AW, Tunis S. Warning—inhaling tabasco products can be hazardous to your health. West J Med 1991;155:550.
63. Burnett JW. Capsicum pepper dermatitis. Cutis 1989;43:534.
64. Greer JM, Rosen T, Tschen JA. Sweet's syndrome with an exogenous cause. Cutis 1993;51:112–114.
65. Craig CR, Stitzel RE. Modern pharmacology. Boston, MA: Little, Brown, 1994, 451–457.
66. Greenberg SS, Xie J, Wang Y, Kolls J, Shellito J, Nelson S, Summer WR. Ethanol relaxes pulmonary artery by release of prostaglandin and nitric oxide. Alcohol 1993;10:21–29.
67. Davda RK, Chandler J, Crews FT, Guzman NJ. Ethanol enhances the endothelial nitric oxide synthase response to agonists. Hypertension 1993;21:939–943.
68. Malpas SC, Robinson BJ, Maling TJB. Mechanism of ethanol-induced vasodilation. J Appl Physiol 1990;68:731–734.
69. Robinson RW, White DP, Zwillich CW. Moderate alcohol ingestion increases upper airway resistance in normal subjects. Am Rev Respir Dis 1985;132:1238–1241.
70. Crabb DW, Dipple KM, Thomasson HR. Alcohol sensitivity, alcohol metabolism, risk of alcoholism and the role of alcohol and aldehyde dehydrogenase genotypes. J Lab Clin Med 1993;122:234–240.
71. Yoshida A. Genetic polymorphisms of alcohol metabolizing enzymes related to alcohol sensitivity and alcoholic diseases. Alcohol Alcoholism 1994;29:693–696.
72. Will TL, Nemeroff CB, Ritchie JC, Ehlers CL. Cortisol responses following placebo and alcohol in Asians with different ALDH2 genotypes. J Stud Alcohol 1994;55:207–213.
73. Lerman B, Bodony R. Ethanol sensitivity. Ann Emer Med 1991;20:1128–1130.
74. Yu PH, Fang CY, Dyck LE. Cutaneous vasomotor sensitivity to ethanol and aldehyde: subtypes of alcohol-flushing response among Chinese. Alcohol Clin Exp Res 1990;14:932–936.
75. Sapeika N. Pharmacodynamic action of natural food. Wld Rev Nutr Diet 1978;29:115–123.
76. Mack RB. Toxic encounters of the dangerous kind: the nutmeg connection. NC Med J 1982;43:439.
77. Framesworth NR. Nutmeg poisoning. Am J Psychiatry 1979;136:858–859.
78. Van Gils C, Cox PA. Ethnobotany of nutmeg in the spice islands. J Ethnopharmacol 1994;42:117–124.
79. Archer AW. Determination of safrole and myristicin in nutmeg and mace by high-performance liquid chromatography. J Chromatol 1988;438:117–121.
80. Abernathy MK, Becker LB. Acute nutmeg intoxication. Am J Emerg Med 1992;10:429–430.
81. Brenner N, Frank OS, Knight E. Chronic nutmeg psychosis. J Roy Soc Med 1993;86:179–180.
82. Payne RB. Nutmeg intoxication. N Engl J Med 1963;269:36–38.
83. Ahmed A, Thompson HS. Nutmeg mydriasis. JAMA 1975;234:3.

30

THE MANAGEMENT OF FOOD ALLERGY

Laurie J. Smith
Anne Muñoz-Furlong

Introduction

Allergic reactions to foods encompass a spectrum of symptoms ranging from trivial discomfort to life-threatening and fatal anaphylactic reactions. The relationship of a food to a reaction may be very clear, as in an acute IgE-mediated reaction following peanut ingestion. In such cases, elimination of the food should prevent the onset of symptoms. The overall contribution of a food to the production of eczema or eosinophilic gastroenteritis may be less well understood, however, and elimination of the offending antigen may not necessarily result in complete resolution of the disease.

The primary recommendation for prevention of an allergic reaction to a food allergen is avoidance of the offending food. Because 100% compliance with this strategy is rarely possible or even likely, instruction on emergency treatment is needed to dealing with accidental ingestion. Treatment of food allergy may include attempts to prevent sensitization, medications to prevent or palliate symptoms associated with ingestion of the antigen, the possibility of immunotherapy, and controversial approaches such as low-dose desensitization, challenge, and neutralization techniques.

Avoidance

The best strategic approach to the management of true food hypersensitivity is complete avoidance of

The opinions or assertions contained herein are the private views of the authors and are not to be construed as official or as reflecting the views of the Department of the Army or the Department of Defense.

the allergen. This categorical recommendation for avoidance assumes that the correct diagnosis has been made and that the specific allergen or allergens have been accurately identified as true culprits in disease causation. It is critical to provide adequate information about the allergen, including the types of food in which it may be found and the various terms that are used in ingredient lists to identify it. A discussion of possible pitfalls that can arise even with punctilious care is imperative.

ALLERGEN IDENTIFICATION

The foods most commonly implicated in food allergy are egg, peanut, milk, soy, wheat, fish, shellfish, and tree nuts (1). Literally any food has the potential to cause an allergic reaction, however. Some foods, such as eggs and peanuts, are allergenic in both cooked and raw form, while others, such as fruits and vegetables, may lose some or most of their allergenicity after being cooked.

Ostensibly, avoidance of the offending food with careful menu planning and label reading would appear reasonably possible. The literature is replete with reports of accidental exposures of food-sensitive individuals to the very antigen they are striving to avoid, however. Even minute quantities of an allergen may provoke serious reactions in extremely sensitive patients. The following discussion identifies potential problem areas and provides suggestions for heightening vigilance.

LABEL READING

Food-allergic individuals should be cautioned to read the ingredient label on all foods. This step should be repeated every time they shop, as ingredients may change without warning. Patients should also learn the scientific and technical names for foods that may appear on labels. The Food Allergy Network (10400 Eaton Place, Ste 107, Fairfax, VA 22030-2208, 800-929-4040) provides wallet-size laminated cards with terms used on labels that identify common food allergens. These "How to Read a Label" cards contain lists of synonyms and ciphers under which milk, egg, wheat, peanut, soy, shellfish, and tree nuts may masquerade. The cards are updated regularly, as new terms are identified.

Understanding kosher rules and markings can make label reading easier (2). A "D" indicates that a product contains dairy products, even if its presence is not disclosed on the ingredient statement. Products that list a "D" on the front but may not list milk on the ingredient statement include tuna, sliced bread and bread sticks, breakfast cereals, cookies, imitation butter flavor, pancake syrup, pretzels, fruit snacks, cake mixes, and frostings. In some cases, milk may be present in the natural flavors. A "D.E." (Dairy Equipment) on a label signifies that the product was manufactured on equipment also used to produce dairy-containing food. As a result, the product might possibly contain trace amounts of milk protein (2).

"Pareve" or "Parve" on a label indicates that a rabbinical agency has determined that this product does not contain dairy products and should be safe for people with milk allergy. Errors can occur, however. Anaphylaxis was reported in one milk-sensitive child after ingestion of pareve-labeled food (3). The cause of the reaction was traced to milk contamination during preparation of the product.

Under current food labeling laws, casein or caseinates are considered additives even though they are milk-derived proteins. Foods that contain these ingredients can be legally advertised as non-dairy products. Examples of foods listed as non-dairy that may contain milk include coffee whiteners, whipped toppings, and imitation cheeses.

Ingredients categorized as flavors are often used in small quantities in commercially processed foods. More than 2000 artificial flavoring chemicals are currently approved for food use. Many food manufacturers buy flavors from suppliers that consider the contents of their flavors to be a trade secret (4). Most

Table 30.1
Selected Terms That May Indicate the Hidden Presence of a Food Allergen

Milk Protein
Caramel color
Natural flavoring
Caramel flavoring
High protein flavor

Soy Protein
Vegetable broth
Vegetable starch
Vegetable gum

Wheat Protein
Gelatinized starch
Modified starch
Vegetable gum
Modified food starch
Vegetable starch
Starch

Corn Protein
Food starch
Vegetable gum
Modified food starch
Vegetable starch

flavors are not required to be listed individually on the label. Natural flavors are often derived from products including milk, wheat, and soy. The law now requires that the source of protein hydrolysates used as flavorings must be identified (5). Confusion may still exist given that "modified food starch" on the label may mean corn (the most common ingredient), or may refer to tapioca, potatoes, or rice (6). Thus, many ambiguous labeling practices persist that may camouflage the presence of an allergen (Table 30.1).

Some foods may appear to be so straightforward that the patient may not feel it necessary to scrutinize the label for hidden allergens. Alternatively, they may be so complex that the label is merely perused, or the food product is considered so unlikely to be allergenic that the label is never reviewed at all (Table 30.2).

CROSS-CONTAMINATION

Even with careful labeling, concealed allergens may still adulterate a food. One source of contamination results during the processing of foods. Although the

Table 30.2
Foods Whose Labels Contain Allergens, But the Food Is So Common That No Need Exists to Check the Label

Food	Ingredient
Worcestershire sauce	Anchovies, sardines
Barbecue sauce	Pecans
Imitation butter flavor	Milk proteins
Water-added ham	Milk and soy
Sweet and sour sauce	Wheat and soy
Egg substitutes	Egg white
Low fat peanut butter	Soy
Pet food*	Eggs, wheat, milk, and soy

*Toddlers may sample pet food off the floor.

production lines are cleaned thoroughly between each product run, mistakes can occur, placing some products at high risk for cross-contamination. It has been reported that some semi-sweet (non-dairy) chocolate may be manufactured on the same line as milk-containing products (e.g., milk chocolate), making contamination possible (7). Granola bars are often produced on the same line as products that contain peanuts or a variety of nuts, which could allow the granola bars to become contaminated with substances not listed on the label (4). Products that contain multiple ingredients can sometimes incorporate a stray ingredient from another product. In some cases, small pieces of peanuts or nuts have remained in the equipment after thorough cleaning, then become accidentally dislodged during the next production run (4). Various types of nut butter, including peanut butter, are commonly run on the same production line, allowing contamination of subsequent products (4). Ice cream containing nuts may be sieved to remove the nuts so that the base can be used for another flavor of ice cream. This policy may result in unsuspected contamination with nut allergen (8). Since 1992, pasta products have been required to label all contents. "Egg-free" pasta is usually processed in the same facility as egg-containing pasta—sometimes on shared processing equipment—and it is virtually impossible to guarantee that any pasta is always egg-free (9).

Bulk food bins rarely list the ingredients of the foods they contain, and shoppers may inadvertently transfer a scoop from one bin to another (4). Cheese is often sliced on the same equipment as deli meats,

making cross-contamination possible (4). It is common practice to place various types of doughnuts, croissants, and muffins together in display cases, where they are likely to contaminate one another.

EATING AWAY FROM HOME

When food not personally prepared and served in one's home is consumed, the risk of encountering a hidden allergen increases. A peanut-sensitive teenager made her own jam sandwich while on a camping trip (10). She was not aware that the knife had been used earlier to spread peanut butter and had been wiped but not washed. She died minutes after eating the sandwich. It is essential that food-allergic individuals develop a polite assertiveness while eating out. Particular care should be taken to make inquiries about ingredients as specific as possible. A peanut-sensitive teenager died after eating an egg roll at an oriental restaurant (11). He apparently had asked the waiter if any of the food was cooked in peanut oil, and was assured that the restaurant did not use any peanut oil. He may not have inquired about the use of peanuts, which the restaurant used in its egg rolls.

Many sources of hidden allergens may be encountered while eating out. For example, almonds may be used in dressings for chicken entrées, sauces used on fresh fruit, and in baked goods (4). Eggs have been used to create foam for milk toppings on specialty coffee drinks, as glue to hold meatballs together, and as a glaze on baked goods (4). Peanut butter has been used to thicken chili, Mexican salsa, spaghetti sauce, hot chocolate, and brown gravy (4). It has also been used as the "glue" to hold egg rolls and Rice Krispie treats together, to add crunch and texture to pie crusts and cheesecakes, and to add flavor to brownies.

Food preparation methods should always be questioned. For example, is the grill greased with butter? Is the cooking oil reused to fry a variety of foods? Fish-allergic individuals should avoid seafood restaurants even if they order a non-fish meal because the oil, grill, and other cooking areas are likely to contain small amounts of fish or shellfish protein that could contaminate the fish-free meal. Chinese, Thai, and Indian foods frequently contain nuts, fish, shellfish, or peanuts. In addition, family-style buffets can be a potential source of cross-contamination as the same spoon may be used for serving different foods. It is not prudent to assume that what is safe in one fast-food restaurant will necessarily remain safe in another. Although food preparation at chain restaurants is usually standardized, regional differences may exist in products served or ingredients used (12).

Nuts and other toppings are often accidentally dropped into containers of ice cream. Furthermore, the scoopers for the various flavors are often placed in a common tub of water, which may contain protein from all of the different flavors. Commercially prepared muffins frequently include chopped nuts. Even "plain" dishes may be prepared using shared equipment or utensils and may inadvertently become contaminated.

When traveling outside the United States, other problems may arise. In Europe, for example, product labels do not have to list all ingredients. A booklet entitled *Travel Guide: Tips for Traveling with Food Allergy* (The Food Allergy Network) includes information and advice for managing meals while traveling (13).

Some individuals are so sensitive to an antigen that simply breathing the cooking odor of a food can cause a severe or even fatal reaction. A bean-allergic child reportedly died after inhaling fumes released from a pressure cooker filled with garbanzo beans (14), while a shrimp-sensitive woman is said to have suffered fatal anaphylaxis within minutes after a waiter in a restaurant walked past her carrying a sizzling shrimp dish (15).

Treatment of a Food-Allergic Reaction

Because ingestion of a food allergen can occur even with stringent avoidance measures a treatment protocol must be prescribed that is immediately available in case of inadvertent ingestion of the offending allergen. The booklet *Just One Little Bite Can Hurt* (The Food Allergy Network) is a reference that can be recommended to patients to raise their own awareness, and that of their families, friends, and teachers, to the potential severity of food allergy (14).

TREATMENT OF A MILD REACTION

No clear clinical distinction is drawn in food allergy between mild and severe reactions analogous to the classification of generalized reactions to insect stings in children (16, 17). For the purposes of this discussion, a mild reaction might be considered urticaria only, with no other systemic symptoms appearing, in a patient who is not at high risk for serious anaphylaxis; alternatively, it might consist of mouth itching only, in a subject who has the oral allergy syndrome (18) and no risk factors. Risk factors for serious reactions to foods include asthma (19), peanut or nut as the food allergen (19–22), previous history of severe reaction to any food (23), extreme atopy (with elevated IgE and multiple positive skin tests, atopic dermatitis, food allergy, and asthma) (23–26), and use of beta-blocking medications (24) (Table 30.3).

For an individual with a history of a mild reaction to a food, with none of the risk factors listed above, who accidentally ingests that food, treatment may be limited to an antihistamine. It should be clearly understood that antihistamines possess no anti-anaphylactic activity and are never a substitute for epinephrine. Whether such a subject who has experienced a mild allergic reaction to a food should routinely carry epinephrine remains the subject of some debate (23–26). The following recommendations from recent sources should be taken into consideration: "all patients with IgE-mediated food allergy should be warned about the possibility of developing a severe anaphylactic reaction and should be educated in the appropriate treatment measures to be taken in case of an accidental ingestion" (21), and "persons experiencing generalized urticaria only, without other signs or symptoms, should receive epinephrine and be observed" (27), and "epinephrine should be prescribed and kept available for all children and adolescents with IgE-mediated food aller-

Table 30.3
Risk Factors for a Severe Allergic Reaction to a Food

Asthma
Extreme atopy
History of prior anaphylaxis to any food
Beta-blocker treatment
Peanut as the allergen

Table 30.4
Signs and Symptoms of Anaphylaxis

Organ System	Signs and Symptoms
Skin	Flushing
	Pruritus
	Urticaria
	Angioedema
	"Goose-bumps"
Respiratory	
Upper	Hoarseness
	Stridor
	"Lump in throat"
Lower	Chest tightness
	Dyspnea
	Wheezing
Cardiovascular	Dizziness
	Syncope
	Hypotension
	Loss of consciousness
Gastrointestinal	Abdominal cramping
	Nausea and vomiting
	Diarrhea
Genitourinary	Uterine cramping
	Uterine bleeding
Neurological	"Feeling of impending doom"
	Headache

gies . . ." (23). The mild reactor could keep epinephrine available for use, but reserve actual administration to occasions on which more severe symptoms develop. All individuals should be instructed in the signs and symptoms of anaphylaxis (Table 30.4) and warned to use epinephrine immediately and seek emergency care if this reaction occurs.

TREATMENT OF MODERATE TO SEVERE REACTION

Any individual who has a history of an IgE-mediated reaction to a food—especially if it was more severe than urticaria only, or mouth itching only as part of the oral allergy syndrome—and/or who has any of the risk factors listed above should be considered at risk for a more serious subsequent reaction. Some of the most severe reactions may not, in fact, have urticaria associated with the symptom complex (23, 28). The treatment of choice in such cases is epinephrine administered by injection (23, 26, 29, 30). The point at which to administer epinephrine remains controversial. Traditionally, administration was de-

layed until the onset of serious symptoms; evidence suggests, however, that it is poor policy to wait for severe symptoms to develop in high-risk subjects (23, 29, 31, 32). In any patient with a history of a severe reaction, epinephrine should be administered as soon as it is realized that the allergenic food has been ingested.

Epinephrine is available in premeasured doses from two sources. The EpiPen (Center Laboratories, Port Washington, New York) is a unit-dose device for use in adults and children weighing 25 kg or more (33). It delivers 0.3 mg of epinephrine as 0.3 mL of 1 : 1000 solution in an automatic syringe preloaded for intramuscular injection. The EpiPen Jr. (Center Laboratories, Port Washington, New York) is intended for smaller children; it delivers 0.15 mg epinephrine in 0.3 mL of 1 : 2000 dilution of epinephrine. In children weighing less than 15 kg, one may either administer the EpiPen Jr. or dispense a needle and syringe and vials of epinephrine for accurate dosing of smaller amounts. The usual dose of epinephrine is 0.01 mg/kg body weight up to a maximum of 0.3 mL, but larger doses may be well tolerated. The Ana-Kit and Ana-Guard (Miles Inc., Allergy Products, West Haven, Connecticut) both contain syringes with epinephrine 1 : 1000 capable of delivering two premeasured doses of 0.3 mL, either subcutaneously or intramuscularly. The syringe barrel has 0.1 mL graduations so that smaller doses can be delivered by discarding an aliquot before injecting the remainder.

Inhaled epinephrine delivered by metered-dose devices has been compared with injected epinephrine (34–36). Theoretically, this treatment could allow more rapid deposition of epinephrine at the site of laryngeal edema. Doses of 10 to 20 puffs of metered-dose inhaler-delivered epinephrine may produce serum levels of epinephrine comparable to those provided with the injection of 0.3 mL of 1 : 1000 epinephrine, although the duration of effect may be somewhat shorter. An extensive literature on this approach as a treatment for acute anaphylaxis does not exist (24, 37), but anecdotal reports of successful use of this treatment are known (25).

An antihistamine (H_1 antagonist) is often prescribed to treat an acute reaction to a food, especially when pruritus and urticaria occur (38, 39). The choice of the antihistamine dictates dosing. A nonsedating antihistamine, such as terfenadine or lorata-dine, may be appropriate. A single oral dose of astem-izole achieves effective therapeutic levels too slowly to be useful in acute treatment (40). Antihistamines should never be used as a substitute for epinephrine (27).

Corticosteroids provide no immediate effect, but they are usually recommended for use early in the treatment of moderate to severe anaphylaxis, in the hope that they will prevent or ameliorate a prolonged or biphasic reaction (41). Furthermore, they restore the responsiveness of beta receptors to their agonists. The usual physiologic response to shock is an increased production of adrenocortical hormones; with severe hypotension, however, this reaction may not occur. Patients who have severe anaphylaxis or who have received corticosteroid therapy during the previous 6 months should receive pharmacologic doses of corticosteroids (27, 42).

TREATMENT OF EXTREMELY SEVERE REACTIONS

Life-threatening anaphylaxis from food ingestion is known to occur (23, 29). Compromise of the upper and lower respiratory systems are the most common causes of severe or fatal anaphylaxis, although cardiovascular reactions, including shock, can develop (28, 43). In such cases, treatment should begin with an assessment of the patient's level of consciousness and vital signs and the establishment of an adequate airway. The treatment approach should be tailored to the condition of the patient (Table 30.5). If any question arises about the adequacy of cardiopulmonary function, the caregiver should administer supplemental oxygen, secure an intravenous line, and begin cardiac monitoring.

Hypotension

If the blood pressure is decreased, place the patient in a recumbent position with the legs elevated, unless this position would exacerbate extreme dyspnea from bronchospasm. The drug of choice is aqueous epinephrine 1:1000 (1 mg/mL) administered subcutaneously or intramuscularly at a dose of 0.01 mg/kg up to a dose of 0.3 mL, provided circulation is maintained. Additional doses may be necessary as

Table 30.5
Management of Anaphylaxis

Assessment
Check airway; secure if necessary
Assess level of consciousness
Obtain vital signs
Estimate body weight

Initial treatment
Epinephrine

Further treatment based on evaluation of clinical condition

General	Cardiovascular symptoms
H$_1$ antihistamines	Intravenous fluids
Corticosteroids	Colloid
O$_2$	Crystalloid
Trendelenburg position	H$_1$ and H$_2$ antihistamines
	Inotropic agents
Respiratory symptoms	Vasopressors
Nebulized beta agonist	Glucagon
Aminophylline	Assisted ventilation
Nebulized epinephrine	

dictated by the patient's clinical condition. Epinephrine's alpha-agonist properties increase total systemic vascular resistance and elevate diastolic pressure to improve coronary blood flow. Its vasoconstrictor effect may decrease angioedema and urticaria, while its beta-agonist actions facilitate bronchodilation and positive inotropic and chronotropic cardiac activity (42). If the patient is in shock, intravenous epinephrine may be given. If intravenous access is impossible, epinephrine can be administered via an endotracheal tube. The optimal dose is not known but should probably be at least 2 to 2.5 times the peripheral intravenous dose in a 1:10,000 concentration (44). For intravenous use, an initial bolus may be made from 0.1 mL of 1:1000 epinephrine added to 10 mL of saline, resulting in a 1:100,000 solution with a total of 100 μg of epinephrine. This solution should be infused slowly over 5 to 10 minutes (45). According to ACLS guidelines, to prepare epinephrine for continuous intravenous infusion, add 1 mg (1 mL) of 1:1000 dilution of epinephrine to 500 mL of 5% dextrose in water to give a 2 μg/mL concentration (44). Start the infusion at 1 μg/min and increase it gradually to a maximum of 10 μg/min as dictated by the clinical response. Intravenous infusion of epinephrine should be undertaken under monitored conditions with extreme caution. Complications from epinephrine treatment derive from the combination of excessive alpha-adrenergic activity and increased systolic and diastolic blood pressure, creating the risk of a hypertensive crisis; in addition, the treatment may lead to excessive beta-agonist activity that can produce cardiac ischemia and dysrhythmias (42).

In anaphylaxis, extensive third-space fluid loss and decreased peripheral resistance result in hypotension that may respond poorly to epinephrine alone. Rapid correction of hypovolemia should be initiated with colloid solutions, although crystalloid fluids have been successfully used as well. The volume and rate of fluid administration should be guided by arterial pressure, central venous pressure, heart rate, and hematocrit levels. It may be necessary to obtain pulmonary wedge pressure and cardiac index. Antishock garments have been used in refractory hypotension from anaphylaxis (46), although this strategy could further increase pulmonary congestion and should be avoided in patients with an elevated pulmonary wedge pressure (42). An inotropic agent such as dopamine may be necessary. Alpha-adrenergic agents such as norepinephrine and metaraminol should be administered only after fluid replacement, correction of acid–base balance, and inotropic agents have failed (42). If hypotension persists, elective assisted ventilation should be considered as a means of decreasing the work of breathing and preventing possible respiratory failure and arrest from inspiratory muscle fatigue.

In the hypotensive patient, the combination of H_1 and H_2 antihistamines may represent an additional treatment strategy. Studies suggest that this combination could protect against the decrease in diastolic blood pressure linked to histamine (47, 48). For example, 1 mg/kg diphenhydramine and 4 mg/kg cimetidine could be infused slowly (49). The effectiveness of this therapy as a prophylactic agent in preventing histamine-induced hypotension is generally accepted (38, 50). Its use in the treatment of acute anaphylaxis remains more controversial (27, 51–53).

In patients with refractory hypotension who have been receiving beta blockers, glucagon may provide increased myocardial contractility without affecting beta-adrenergic receptors (54), and thus be useful in the treatment of anaphylactic shock (55). Care should be taken with glucagon as its action to increase contractility may vary, it has gastrointestinal side effects, and its vasodilating effect may decrease blood pressure (42). The opiate antagonist naloxone has also been reported to aid in the treatment of shock (56), but its use remains experimental at this time (42). Future trends in treatment of cardiovascular collapse may include drugs that attenuate the excessive production of endothelin-derived relaxing factor by inhibiting the enzyme nitric oxide synthetase that produces it, and newer cyclic-AMP specific phosphodiesterase inhibitors and prostaglandin E_1 to promote pulmonary vasodilation (57).

Respiratory Symptoms

Food allergy has caused severe asthmatic attacks that have resulted in death or required mechanical ventilation (19, 23). The treatment approach to this bronchospasm should resemble that for any asthma attack, with the proviso that recurrent or prolonged severe obstruction may occur, necessitating that observation continue for at least 4 hours after a satisfactory response to treatment (23). A beta agonist such as albuterol, nebulized with oxygen, provides the basis of treatment. If upper airway edema appears, nebulized racemic epinephrine may be administered. In the face of severe bronchospasm, intravenous aminophylline may be used, although albuterol, aminophylline, and hypoxia carry some risk of additive cardiac toxicity (42). Intubation and assisted ventilation may be necessary (23, 28). Edema of the upper airway, a less common effect, may also occur (43). Intubation or cricothyroidotomy may be necessary.

ADVICE TO PATIENTS

All patients with food allergy should be instructed in avoidance of the incriminated food. They need to know the early warning symptoms of a reaction to a food. Even if they have previously had only mild reactions, they should be instructed in the manifestations of more severe allergic reactions. Each food-allergic subject must maintain constant scrutiny of his or her diet. All food-allergic subjects should receive information concerning emergency medical identification systems such as MedicAlert (Turlock, California). Some debate has arisen about which food-allergic patients should receive a prescription for epinephrine, although all agree that subjects at risk for a severe food allergic reaction should carry epinephrine (23, 25). The medical record should include documentation of patient instruction in the identification and treatment of an allergic reaction. The patient should be urged to carry epinephrine at all times and to use it early in the course of a reaction, as lack of epinephrine administration can prove catastrophic (19, 23). Patients should be warned that, while an H_1 antihistamine may ease symptoms of itching and urticaria, this medication is not a substitute for epinephrine.

MANAGEMENT OF FOOD ALLERGY AT SCHOOL

Food allergy in the school-age child presents special difficulties. Under the Public Law 93-112, The Rehabilitation Act of 1973, Section 504 (which defines disability), children with food allergies meet the criteria of being disabled (58). Such children are eligible for modifications in the school program even if they do not require special education. Modifications may include health services, such as administration of medication at school, and supplementary aids, such as menu information and ingredient substitution in school meal programs. The U.S. Department of Agriculture's nondiscrimination regulations (7 CFR 15b) and the regulations governing the National School Lunch Program and School Breakfast Program make it clear that substitutions to the regular meal pattern must be instituted for a child whose disability restricts his or her diet when supported by a medical statement signed by a licensed physician (58). The medical statement must identify the participant's disability and include an explanation of why the disability restricts the participant's diet, the major life activity affected by the disability, the food or foods to be omitted from the participant's diet, and the choice of foods from which substitutions can be selected. A food-allergic student cannot be excluded from field trips, eating in the cafeteria, or participation in class projects because of the food allergy. In addition, schools cannot require parents to sign a liability

waiver or come to the school themselves to administer emergency medications (59).

Special care must be taken to provide appropriate education for school personnel (32, 60, 61). A written emergency health care plan should be placed on file at the school. An example of such a plan is provided in Figure 30.1 (59). The school must keep epinephrine available for a child, be willing and able to administer it, and call the rescue squad, even if no school nurse is present on the premises (58, 62). The Food Allergy Network has prepared a School Food Allergy Program that contains a binder with information and a video for managing food allergy at school.

Prevention of Food Allergy

In addition to allergen avoidance, prevention of food allergy may include preventing sensitization to allergens by means of early allergen avoidance, administering drugs to allow ingestion of the food culprit, and altering established food sensitivity through immunological modification.

PREVENTION OF SENSITIZATION

Since 1936, when Grulee and Sanford reported that infants who were breast-fed developed less eczema than those who received cow's milk, the idea of manipulating the infant's diet to decrease the development of allergic disease has drawn great attention (63). This topic has been extensively reviewed by Zeiger (64). The picture that emerges does not present a strong argument for the success of this approach (65).

Carefully performed studies in Sweden have shown that neither avoidance nor ingestion of large amounts of cow's milk or egg during the third trimester of pregnancy affect the development of atopic disease from birth to 5 years of age (66–68). Many studies have found that dietary intervention after delivery may result in a lower incidence of food allergy and atopic dermatitis by age 12 to 24 months (66, 69–74). Such dietary intervention has included modalities such as strict breast feeding combined with avoidance of highly allergenic foods by the lactating mother, or the use of protein hydrolysate

Emergency Health Care Plan

ALLERGY TO: _____

Student's
Name: _____ D.O.B.: _____ Teacher: _____

Asthmatic Yes* ☐ No ☐ *High risk for severe reaction

Signs of an allergic reaction include:

Systems:	Symptoms:
•MOUTH	itching & swelling of the lips, tongue, or mouth
•THROAT*	itching and/or a sense of tightness in the throat, hoarseness, and hacking cough
•SKIN	hives, itchy rash, and/or swelling about the face or extremities
•GUT	nausea, abdominal cramps, vomiting, and/or diarrhea
•LUNG*	shortness of breath, repetitive coughing, and/or wheezing
•HEART*	"thready" pulse, "passing-out"

The severity of symptoms can quickly change. *All above symptoms can potentially progress to a life-threatening situation!

ACTION:

1. If ingestion is suspected, give _____
   medication/dose/route

   and _____ immediately!

2. CALL RESCUE SQUAD: _____

3. CALL: Mother _____ Father _____ or emergency contacts

4. CALL: Dr. _____ at _____

**DO NOT HESITATE TO ADMINISTER MEDICATION OR CALL RESCUE SQUAD
EVEN IF PARENTS OR DOCTOR CANNOT BE REACHED!**

_____ _____   _____ M.D. _____
Parent Signature   Date   Doctor's Signature   Date

EMERGENCY CONTACTS   TRAINED STAFF MEMBERS

1. _____   1. _____ Room ____

   Relation: _____ Phone: _____

2. _____   2. _____ Room ____

   Relation: _____ Phone: _____

3. _____   3. _____ Room ____

   Relation: _____ Phone: _____

For children with multiple food allergies, use one form for each food.

Figure 30.1
_____

Example of a written emergency health care plan.

439

formula instead of breast feeding and diet regulation. Zeiger *et al.* published an outcome study on 165 children aged 7 who were at high risk to develop atopic disease (75). These children had been followed since birth in a prospective randomized, controlled study of food allergen avoidance. In the prophylaxis group, the mother had avoided cow's milk, egg, and peanut in the last trimester of pregnancy and throughout lactation, and the infant had avoided cow's milk until age 1, eggs until age 2, and fish until age 3. The control infants followed standard infant feeding practices. Although a significant reduction in food allergy and atopic dermatitis was noted in the prophylaxis group by age 1, this effect had faded by age 2 and disappeared by age 4 (69, 76). By age 7, no difference was found in the development of food allergy or any other atopic disease in either group (75). Even in carefully designed studies, it appears that dietary manipulation might lessen the frequency of food allergy during infancy—a time when it may be quite troublesome—but it does not seem to affect the eventual outcome of food allergy, and has not resulted in any decrease in the frequency of respiratory allergic diseases (69–73, 76, 77). Prophylactic feeding with soy formula has not been found to be effective in preventing the development of food allergy (64).

DRUG TREATMENT

Although the major emphasis in preventing food allergy involves avoidance with instructions for treatment if accidental ingestion occurs, it is not always possible to avoid a food entity completely. It would be desirable to have a drug that could be taken either before deliberate ingestion of a food or on a regular basis to decrease reaction to an accidentally or episodically ingested food. The drugs that have received the most attention for this purpose are ketotifen and cromolyn.

Ketotifen

Ketotifen has both antihistaminic and anti-anaphylactic properties (39). One double-blind, placebo-controlled study did not find that ketotifen protected against fish-induced asthma, although oral cromoglycate had some protective effect (78). Other studies

have found limited protection against asthma, with some protection against skin and gastrointestinal manifestations (79), some protection against smaller amounts of food (80), and protective effect in atopic dermatitis (81–85). The extent of protection has proved difficult to evaluate as the studies have involved various formats, including term follow-up with elimination diets, regular diets, and food challenges with ketotifen administered for varying periods of time. In addition, the documentation of food allergy and the end points for symptom improvement have varied. Ketotifen may play a role in the management of some allergic disorders such as atopic dermatitis, but more studies are needed. At present, ketotifen is not available in the United States.

Sodium Cromoglycate

Sodium cromoglycate prevents mast cell mediator release in vitro if given before antigen challenge, and is frequently used in the management of allergic rhinitis and asthma. Its use in food allergy is more controversial and has been the subject of several reviews (39, 86–88) and more than 100 articles (bibliography provided by Fisons Pharmaceuticals, Rochester, New York 14603). As with ketotifen, the studies present challenges to interpretation. Many fail to document the presence of food allergy adequately in the study subjects or mix together a variety of food allergy manifestations or food intolerances. Some administer cromolyn in either open or blinded fashion with a variety of treatment doses, timing, and duration. Treatment outcome may be established by open provocation challenge, blinded challenge, open elimination diets, and open regular diets. Two studies will be reviewed below.

Buscinco *et al.* (89) performed a double-blind, crossover trial with oral cromolyn in aqueous solution, 30–50 mg/kg/day, in 31 children whose atopic dermatitis was shown to be exacerbated by foods. The children were divided into two groups: one underwent placebo treatment for 8 weeks followed by cromolyn for 8 weeks, while the other received cromolyn followed by placebo. A baseline of 2 weeks of strict elimination diet preceded the study phase. The first 4 weeks of each trial included elimination of the specific food allergen, while the second 4 weeks reintroduced the food. The children who received placebo followed by cromolyn experienced a significant decrease in symptom scores while on the cromolyn. The children who received cromolyn followed by placebo did not see a decline in scores. This variation was interpreted as a possible carry-over effect of the cromolyn when administered first. When one inspects the data, however, some problems emerge. The mean initial symptom score for all study children was 54. The children entered the drug study phase after a rigorous 2-week elimination diet with a mean symptom score of 23.5. The cromolyn and placebo scores were evaluated regardless of the treatment order: cromolyn plus elimination diet, 9.5; cromolyn plus challenge diet, 7.7; placebo plus elimination diet, 13.3; and placebo plus challenge diet, 22.5. The overall cromolyn plus challenge diet score was lower than the cromolyn plus elimination diet, and the placebo plus challenge diet was lower than the initial score for a strict elimination diet (93). Cromolyn apparently had some effect, but these changes were small compared with the impact of the elimination diet on baseline symptom scores and are difficult to interpret.

In the other study, Burks *et al.* (90) carried out a double-blind, crossover design with a challenge at the end of each treatment arm. Children with known food allergy received either placebo or oral cromolyn, 30–40 mg/kg/day, in four divided doses for 7 days and then were challenged in a double-blind fashion with a placebo-food and the food allergen on 2 separate days in a research unit. The challenges were separated by a 3 to 5 week washout period. Two of 10 subjects failed to respond to the food in either trial. The remainder of the subjects showed no differences in the amount of food antigen causing a reaction, time until reaction, or duration of symptoms provoked in either the cromolyn or placebo sessions.

Some investigators suggest that the preponderance of the evidence supports a role for the use of cromolyn in the treatment of some food-allergic patients (86–88), while others do not agree that it deserves a place in the current management of food allergy (91–93). Most studies of oral cromolyn have involved treatment of atopic dermatitis in which foods are not usually the sole cause of the condition, or in more ill-defined clinical situations with gastrointestinal or urticarial symptoms that are not solely related to food allergy. Some evidence suggests that both ketotifen (83) and cromolyn (94, 95) may prevent the increase in mucosal permeability after an allergen is ingested, but the significance of these findings is not known. No one is advocating the use of cromolyn to prevent anaphylaxis or to allow an individual with moderate to severe food allergy to deliberately ingest an allergenic food.

ALLERGEN IMMUNOTHERAPY

Allergen immunotherapy remains a time-honored treatment for allergy. Because of the severe and persistent nature of peanut allergy, it was hoped that a trial of immunotherapy could alter the natural course of this condition. Oppenheimer *et al.* reported the results of a double-blind, placebo-controlled study in three subjects with anaphylactic sensitivity to peanuts who underwent rush desensitization with peanut allergen (96). A follow-up study of this group 1 month after rush immunotherapy revealed a 10- to 100-fold reduction in prick skin test sensitivity and a 2- to 20-fold increase in antigen dose on double-blind, placebo-controlled challenge (97). Both rush and maintenance immunotherapy were associated with a significant frequency of generalized reactions. Although this modality may eventually represent a treatment for food sensitivity, it currently remains highly experimental (98).

A controversial therapy that purports to identify and treat food sensitivity involves using intradermal injection of suspected allergens to provoke a symptom and then injecting a different dose of this allergen to "neutralize" the reaction (99, 100). Several studies have evaluated this technique with negative results (101, 102), including a double-blind, placebo-controlled study conducted in 1990 (103). This group found that the provocation–neutralization technique "appears to lack scientific validity" and any previously reported success "appears to be the result of suggestion and chance" (103).

Summary

The management of food allergy requires identification of the allergen, detailed allergen avoidance instructions, and a treatment regimen for accidental ingestion. Even if a food allergen can be identified with certainty, avoidance maneuvers are fraught with difficulties. Written instructions, access to newsletters such as *The Food Allergy News* (published by The Food Allergy Network) warning jewelry (MedicAlert; Turlock, California), and careful planning are all essential in managing food allergy. At present, efforts to prevent sensitization to foods or to allow the deliberate ingestion of food allergens with drug pre-treatment remain at the experimental stage, as does the use of allergen immunotherapy to desensitize the food-allergic patient.

REFERENCES

1. James JM, Burks AW. Foods. Immunol Allergy Clin NA 1995;15:477–488.
2. Regenstein JM, Regenstein CE. Kosher foods and allergies. Food Allergy News 1994;1:7.
3. Gern JE, Yang E, Evrard HM, Sampson HA. Allergic reactions to milk-contaminated "nondairy" products. N Engl J Med 1991;324:976–979.
4. Taylor SL, Muñoz-Furlong A. Understanding food labels. Fairfax: Food Allergy Network, 1994, 16.
5. Segal M. What's in a food. FDA Consumer 1993; May (Special Report):46–50.
6. Koerner CB. Answers to diet dilemmas. Food Allergy News 1993;3:6.
7. Koerner CB. Diet dilemmas. Food Allergy News 1993;2:6.
8. Taylor SL. Choose your ice cream flavor wisely. Food Allergy News 1995;4:7.
9. Taylor SL. Eggs in pasta products. Food Allergy News 1993;2:3.
10. Duncanson J, Freed DA. Allergy to nuts kills teen on school trip. Toronto Star 1994 July 19:A1 and A11.
11. Hoffman S, Goforth C. Fatal allergy suspected; student reacts after egg roll. Cincinnati Enquirer Friday, March 7, 1995:C1,C4.
12. Muñoz-Furlong A. Dining tips and strategies. Food Allergy News 1993;2:7.
13. Muñoz-Furlong A. Travel guide. Fairfax: Food Allergy Network, 1994, 16.
14. Muñoz-Furlong A, Sampson HA. Just one little bite can hurt. Fairfax: The Food Allergy Network, 1992, 8.
15. Meff E. Hatfield woman's allergy reaction rare, but deadly. Reporter Thursday, December 15, 1994:A5.
16. Valentine MD, Schuberth KC, Kagey-Sobotka A, Graft DF, Kwiterovich KA, Szklo M, et al. The value of immunotherapy with venom in children with allergy to insect stings. N Engl J Med 1990;323:1601–1603.
17. Bierman CW. Venom immunotherapy: who should receive it? J Pediatr 1995;126:257–258.
18. Enberg RN. Food-induced oropharyngeal symptoms: the oral allergy syndrome. Immunol Allergy Clin NA 1991;11:767–772.
19. Settipane GA. Anaphylactic deaths in asthmatic patients. Allergy Proc 1989;10:271–274.
20. Sampson HA. Peanut anaphylaxis. J Allergy Clin Immunol 1990;86:1–3.
21. Yunginger JW, Squillace DL, Jones RT, Helm RM. Fatal anaphylactic reactions induced by peanuts. Allergy Proc 1989;10:249–253.
22. Boyd GK. Fatal nut anaphylaxis in a 16-year-old male: case report. Allergy Proc 1989;10:255–257.
23. Sampson HA, Mendelson L, Rosen JP. Fatal and near-fatal anaphylactic reactions to food in children and adolescents. N Engl J Med 1992;327:380–384.
24. Patel L, Radivan FS, David TJ. Management of anaphylactic reactions to food. Arch Dis Childhood 1995;71:370–375.
25. Hourihane JO'B, Warner JO. Management of anaphylactic reaction to food (letter to editor). Arch Dis Childhood 1995;72:274.
26. Sampson HA, Metcalfe DD. Immediate reactions to foods. In: Metcalfe DD, Sampson HA, Simon RA, eds. Food allergy adverse reactions to foods and food additives. 1st ed. Boston: Blackwell Scientific Publications, 1991, 99–112.
27. Yunginger JW. Anaphylaxis. Ann Allergy 1992;69:87–96.
28. Smith PL, Kagey-Sobotka A, Bleecker ER, Traystman R, Kaplan AP, Gralnick H, et al. Physiologic manifestations of human anaphylaxis. J Clin Invest 1980;66:1072–1080.
29. Yunginger JW, Sweeney KG, Sturner WQ, Giannandrea LA, Teigland JD, Bray M, et al. Fatal food-induced anaphylaxis. JAMA 1988;260:1450–1452.
30. AAAI Board of Directors. The use of epinephrine in the treatment of anaphylaxis. Position statement. J Allergy Clin Immunol 1994;94:666–668.
31. Yunginger JW. Lethal food allergy in children. N Engl J Med 1992;327:380–384.
32. American Academy of Pediatrics, Section on Allergy and Immunology, ad hoc Committee on Anaphylaxis in School. Anaphylaxis at school: etiologic factors, prevalence, and treatment. Pediatrics 1993;91:316.
33. Saryan JA, O'Loughlin JM. Anaphylaxis in children. Ped Annals 1992;21:590–598.
34. Dahlöf C, Mellstrand T, Svedmyr N. Systemic absorption of adrenaline after aerosol, eye-drom and subcutaneous administration to healthy volunteers. Allergy 1987;42:215–221.
35. Warren JB, Doble N, Dalton N, Ewan PW. Systemic absorption of inhaled epinephrine. Clin Pharmacol Ther 1986;40:673–678.
36. Heilborn H, Hjemdahl P, Daleskog M, Adamsson U. Comparison of subcutaneous injection and high-dose inhalation of epinephrine—implications for self-treatment to prevent anaphylaxis. J Allergy Clin Immunol 1986;78:1174–1179.
37. Allergy Section, Canadian Paediatric Society. Fatal anaphylactic reactions to food in children. Can Med Assoc J 1994;150:337–339.
38. Lieberman P. The use of antihistamines in the prevention and treatment of anaphylaxis and anaphylactoid reactions. J Allergy Clin Immunol 1990;86:684–686.
39. Sogn D. Medications and their use in the treatment of adverse reactions to foods. J Allergy Clin Immunol 1986;78:238–243.
40. Richards DM, Brogden RN, Heel RC, Speight TM, Avery GS. Astemizole: a review of its pharmacodynamic properties and therapeutic efficacy. Drugs 1984;28:38–61.
41. Stark BJ, Sullivan TJ. Biphasic and protracted anaphylaxis. J Allergy Clin Immunol 1986;78:76–83.
42. Perkin RM, Anas NG. Mechanisms and management of anaphylactic shock not responding to traditional therapy. Ann Allergy 1985;54:202–208.
43. Delage C, Irey NS. Anaphylactic deaths: a clinico-pathologic study of 43 cases. J Forensic Med 1972;17:527–540.

44. Cummins RO, ed. Textbook of advanced cardiac life support. American Heart Association, Washington, DC, 1994, 7–14.

45. Barach EM, Nowak RM, Lee TG, Tomlanovich MC. Epinephrine for treatment of anaphylactic shock. JAMA 1984; 251:2118–2122.

46. Bickell WH, Dice WH. Military antishock trousers in a patient with adrenergic-resistant anaphylaxis. Ann Emerg Med 1994; 13:189–190.

47. Kaliner M, Sigler R, Summers R, Shellhamer JH. The effects of infused histamine: analysis of the effects of H-1 and H-2 histamine receptor antagonists upon cardiovascular and pulmonary responses. J Allergy Clin Immunol 1981;68:365–371.

48. Kaliner M, Shellhamer JH, Ottesen EA. Effects of infused histamine: correlations of plasma histamine levels and symptoms. J Allergy Clin Immunol 1982;69:283–289.

49. Marquardt DL, Wasserman SI. Anaphylaxis. In: Middleton E Jr, Reed CE, Ellis EF, Adkinson NF Jr, Yuninger JW, Busse WW, eds. Allergy principles and practice. 4th ed. St. Louis: Mosby, 1993;1525–1536.

50. Ring J, Behrendt H. H$_1$- and H$_2$-antagonists in allergic and pseudoallergic diseases. Clin Exp Allergy 1990;20:43–49.

51. Fisher M McD. Clinical observations on the pathophysiology and treatment of anaphylactic cardiovascular collapse. Anaesth Intens Care 1986;14:17–21.

52. De Soto H, Turk P. Cimetidine in anaphylactic shock refractory to standard therapy. Anesth Analg 1989;69:264–265.

53. Kelly JS, Prielipp RC. Is cimetidine indicated in the treatment of acute anaphylactic shock? Anesth Analg 1990;71:104–105.

54. Farah AE. Glucagon and the circulation. Pharmacol Rev 1983;35:181–217.

55. Zaloga GP, Wm D, Holmboe E, Chernow B. Glucagon reversal of hypotension in a case of anaphylactoid shock. Ann Int Med 1986;105:65–66.

56. Gullo A, Romano E. Naloxone and anaphylactic shock. Lancet 1983;1:819.

57. Levy JH. New concepts in the treatment of anaphylactoid reactions in anesthesia. Ann Fr Anesth Réanim 1993;12:223–227.

58. Muñoz-Furlong A, Goldberg E. Students with food allergies: what do the laws say? Fairfax: The Food Allergy Network, 1994, 19.

59. Muñoz-Furlong A. The school food allergy program. Fairfax: The Food Allergy Network, 1995.

60. Hay GH, Harper TB III, Courson FH. Preparing school personnel to assist students with life-threatening food allergies. J School Health 1994;64:119–121.

61. American Academy of Pediatrics, Committee on School Health. Guidelines for urgent care in school. Pediatrics 1990;86:999–1000.

62. Ordover EL, Boundy KB. Educational rights of children with disabilities. Cambridge, MA: Center for Law and Education, 1991, 120.

63. Grulee CG, Sanford HN. The influence of breast and artificial feeding on infantile eczema. J Pediatr 1936;9:223–225.

64. Zeiger RS. Development and prevention of allergic disease in childhood. In: Middleton E Jr, Reed CE, Ellis EF, Adkinson NF Jr, Yuninger JW, Busse WW, eds. Allergy: principles and practice. 4th ed. St. Louis: Mosby, 1993, 1137–1171.

65. Hill DJ, Hosking CS. Preventing childhood allergy. Med J Austr 1993;158:367–369.

66. Lilja G, Dannaeus D, Foucard T, Graff-Lonnevig V, Johansson SGO, Öman H. Effects of maternal diet during late pregnancy and lactation on the development of atopic diseases in infants up to 18 months of age—in vivo results. Clin Exp Allergy 1989;19:473–479.

67. Lilja G, Dannaeus A, Falth-Magnusson K, Graff-Lonnevig V, Johansson SG, Kjellman NI, et al. Immune response of the atopic woman and fetus: effects of high- and low-dose food allergen intake during pregnancy. Clin Allergy 1988;18:131–142.

68. Falth-Magnusson K, Kjellman NIM. Allergy prevention by maternal elimination diet during pregnancy: a 5-year follow-up study. J Allergy Clin Immunol 1992;89:709–713.

69. Zeiger RS, Heller S, Mellon MH, Forsythe AB, O'Connor RD, Hamburger RN, et al. Effect of combined maternal and infant food-allergen avoidance on development of atopy in early infancy: a randomized study. J Allergy Clin Immunol 1989; 84:72–89.

70. Chandra RK, Puri S, Suraiya C, Cheema PS. Influence of maternal diet during lactation and use of formula feeds on development of atopic eczema in high risk infants. Br Med J 1989;299:228–230.

71. Chandra RK, Hamed A. Cumulative incidence of atopic disorders in high risk infants fed whey hydrolysate, soy, and conventional cows milk formulas. Ann Allergy 1991;67:129–132.

72. Halken S, Host A, Hansen LG, Osterballe O. Preventive effect of feeding high-risk infants a casein hydrolysate formula or an ultrafiltrated whey hydrolysate formula. A prospective, randomized, comparative clinical study. Pediatr Allergy Immunol 1993;4:173–181.

73. Businco L, Dreborg S, Einarsson R, Giampietro PG, Host A, Keller KM, et al. Hydrolysed cow's milk formulae. Allergenicity and use in treatment and prevention. Pediatr Allergy Immunol 1993;4:101–111.

74. Arshad SH, Matthews S, Gant C, Hide DW. Effect of allergen avoidance on development of allergic disorders in infancy. Lancet 1992;339:1493–1497.

75. Zeiger RS, Heller S. The development and prediction of atopy in high-risk children: follow-up at age seven years in a prospective randomized study of combined maternal and infant food allergen avoidance. J Allergy Clin Immunol 1995;95:1179–1190.

76. Zeiger RS, Heller S, Mellon MH, Halsey JF, Hamburger RN, Sampson HA. Genetic and environmental factors affecting the development of atopy through age 4 in children of atopic parents: a prospective randomized study of food allergen avoidance. Pediatr Allergy Immunol 1992;3:110–127.

77. Sigurs N, Hattevig G, Kjellman B. Maternal avoidance of eggs, cow's milk, and fish during lactation: effect on allergic manifestations, skin-prick tests, and specific IgE antibodies in children at age 4 years. Pediatrics 1992;89:735–739.

78. Ellul-Micallef R. Effect of oral sodium cromoglycate and ketotifen in fish-induced bronchial asthma. Thorax 1983;38:527–530.

79. Neffen H, Oehling A, Subira ML. A study of the protective effect of ketotifen in food allergy. Allergol Immunopathol 1980;8:97–104.

80. Zanussi C, Ortolani C, Pastorello E. Dietary and pharmacologic management of food intolerance in adults. Ann Allergy 1983;51:307–310.

81. Cipandi G, Scordamaglia A, Ruffoni S, Pizzorno G, Canonica GW. Ketotifen treatment of adverse reactions to foods: clinical

and immunological effects. Curr Med Res Opin 1986;10:346–350.

82. Osvath P, Kelenhegyi K, Micskey E. Comparison of ketotifen and DSCG in treatment of food allergy in children. Allergol et Immunopathol 1986;14:515–518.

83. Molkhous P, Dupont C. Ketotifen treatment of atopic dermatitis and other food allergy diseases. Allergy 1989;44(suppl 9):117–123.

84. Molkhous P, Dupont C. Ketotifen in prevention and therapy of food allergy. Ann Allergy 1987;59(part II):187–193.

85. Boner AL, Richelli C, Antolini I, Vibelli C, Andri L. The efficacy of ketotifen in a control double-blind challenge study in patients with food allergy. Ann Allergy 1986;67:61–64.

86. Businco L, Cantani A. Food allergy in children: diagnosis and treatment with sodium cromoglycate. Allergol et Immunopathol 1990;18:339–348.

87. Businco L, Cantani A. Oral sodium cromoglycate in the management of atopic dermatitis in children. Allergy Proc 1991;12:333–338.

88. Edwards AM. Oral sodium cromoglycate: its use in the management of food allergy. Clin Exp Allergy 1995;25(suppl 1):31–33.

89. Businco L, Benincori N, Cantani A, Nini G, Businco E, et al. Double-blind crossover trial with oral sodium cromoglycate in children with atopic dermatitis due to food allergy. Ann Allergy 1986;57:433–438.

90. Burks AW, Sampson HA. Double-blind placebo-controlled trial of oral cromolyn in children with atopic dermatitis and documented food hypersensitivity. J Allergy Clin Immunol 1988;81:417–423.

91. James JM, Sampson HA. An overview of food hypersensitivity. Pediatr Allergy Immunol 1992;3:67–78.

92. Burks AW, Sampson H. Food allergies in children. Curr Prob Pediatr 1993;23:230–252.

93. James JM, Burks AW. Food hypersensitivity in children. Curr Opin Pediatr 1994;6:661–667.

94. André C, André F, Colin L. Effect of allergen ingestion challenge with and without cromoglycate cover on intestinal permeability in atopic dermatitis, urticaria and other symptoms of food allergy. Allergy 1989;44(suppl 9):47–51.

95. Van Elburg RM, Heymans HSA, De Monchy JGR. Effect of disodiumcromoglycate on intestinal permeability changes and clinical response during cow's milk challenge. Pediatr Allergy Immunol 1993;4:79–85.

96. Oppenheimer JJ, Nelson HS, Bock A, Christensen F, Leung DY. Treatment of peanut allergy with rush immunotherapy. J Allergy Clin Immunol 1992;90:256–262.

97. Nelson HS, Conkling C, Areson J, Sampson HA, Bock A, Leung DYM. Treatment of patients anaphylactically sensitive to peanuts with injections of peanut extract. J Allergy Clin Immunol 1994;93:211.

98. Sampson HA. Food allergy and the role of immunotherapy. J Allergy Clin Immunol 1992;90:151–152.

99. Lee CH, Williams RI, Binkley EL Jr. Provocative testing and treatment for foods. Arch Otolaryngol 1969;90:87–94.

100. Rinkel HJ, Lee CH, Brown DW Jr, Willoughby JW, Williams JM. The diagnosis of food allergy. Arch Otolaryngol 1964;79:71–79.

101. Crawford LV, Lieberman P, Harfi HA, et al. A double-blind study of subcutaneous food testing sponsored by the Food Committee of the American Academy of Allergy. J Allergy Clin Immunol 1976;57:236 (abstract).

102. Bronsky EA, Burkley DP, Ellis EF. Evaluation of the provocative food skin test technique. J Allergy 1971;47:104 (abstract).

103. Jewett DL, Fein G, Greenberg MH. A double-blind study of symptom provocation to determine food sensitivity. N Engl J Med 1990;323:429–433.

31

NATURAL HISTORY AND PREVENTION OF FOOD HYPERSENSITIVITY

N.-I. Max Kjellman
Bengt Björkstén

Introduction

Food hypersensitivity is a commonly encountered condition, especially in infancy and early childhood (1–3). The highest prevalence occurs between 1.5 and 3 years of age, when in this age group as many as 25% have been reported to have adverse reactions to food. Only a minority of these reactions depend on immunologic mechanisms (i.e., allergy). Allergy prevalence is influenced by family history, exposure to food allergens, and factors acting as adjuvants for sensitization (4). Food hypersensitivity—especially of the immediate type—is linked to the atopic state (5). The major food allergens in infants and young children are hen's egg, cow's milk, cereals, peanuts, and tree nuts. Allergy to vegetables and fruits dominates in children older than 10 years of age and in adolescents (includes oral allergy syndrome) (2, 6). No proof exists of an increase in the prevalence of milk allergy during the last few decades, although it may be reasonable to suspect that pollen-associated food allergies, such as those against peaches and celery, may have increased as a consequence of the increasing incidence of hayfever (7). The prevalence of adverse reactions to food additives is much lower, and was found in one study to represent 1% of school children (8). Furthermore, positive oral provocation tests with preservatives and food colors were restricted to children with concomitant allergic manifestations to food allergens.

Food hypersensitivity may be a transient phenomenon, but in many subjects immediate-type food allergy provides the first evidence of a genetic predis-position toward development of atopic disease (9–11), predicting allergic manifestations that appear later in the respiratory tract (12–14). In such atopic children, food allergens (egg, nuts, peanuts, and milk) dominate as to sensitizing agents during the first 2 to 3 years of life. In older children, sensitization occurs mostly against inhalant allergens (15).

This chapter deals with the natural history of food sensitization (IgE antibody production) and symptoms and signs of food hypersensitivity. It also summarizes attempts to prevent the development of food allergy and other atopic manifestations (Fig. 31.1)—that is, primary prevention.

The etiology of food allergy and atopic disease is multifactorial and based on genetic factors. Often, an interaction occurs between several risk factors that leads to sensitization and symptoms of allergy in the genetically predisposed subject (Table 31.1; see Fig. 31.1). Ongoing inflammation enhances further sensitization. The age and previous immunologic experiences of the subject have important implications for the outcome of ingestion of foods or inhalation of allergens. Infants are particularly susceptible to sensitization. In early infancy, the response of the infant is influenced by maternal immunity (16)—for example, by transplacental transfer of immunoglobulins and by various components of breast milk.

Genetic Factors

A family history of atopic disease increases the risk for food hypersensitivity during the first six years of

Table 31.1.
Factors of Importance for the Development of Allergy/Atopic Disease

Factor	Reference
Family history (parents and siblings)	
Frequency of disease	(126, 127)
Type of disease	(126)
Age at onset	(4)
S-IgE level	(1, 128)
IgE antibodies to allergens	(62, 128)
Pregnancy	
Smoking habits	(38)
Drug use	(16, 40)
Delivery	
Use of opiates	(129)
Instrumental	(16)
Time of the year	(41, 130–132)
Neonatal period	
Invasive procedures	(133)
Formula feeding	(44, 45)
Infancy	
Country of birth	(134)
Type of feeding	(37, 76)
Maternal food intake/lactation period	(29, 87, 135)
Early weaning	(56, 66, 76, 136)
Exposure to tobacco smoke	(38, 66, 137)
Exposure to inhalant allergens	
Animals	(66, 114, 131, 137, 138)
Pollens	(71, 139)
Plants	(140, 141)
Mites	(114, 142, 143)
Infections	(64, 66, 77, 144)
Indoor climate	(114, 145)
Outdoor pollution	
Factories	(145)
Diesel exhausts	(146)
Socioeconomic factors	(137)

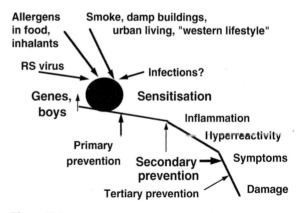

Figure 31.1

Factors of importance for the progress of allergy and for various levels of prevention.

life (4). Thus, 13% of young children with no parental history of atopic disease have demonstrated a history of food hypersensitivity, compared with 29% of those with an unilateral family history and 58% of children with a bilateral family history of atopic disease. Breast feeding appears to represent an especially important factor for delaying manifestations of allergy in children with a family history of atopic disease (17) or with other indications of a high risk for allergy (18, 19).

In a large prospective Danish study, cow's milk hypersensitivity, as proved by provocation tests, occurred in 2.2% of all infants and in 16% of those with two atopic parents (20). The risk for cow's milk allergy (CMA) in subsequent children when a child in the family already had CMA was estimated to be even higher (1 in 3) (21). In another study in infants with a family history of allergy, 3% developed CMA and 8% egg allergy (22). Sensitization was even more common, with 4% sensitized to cow's milk and 16% to egg. In a British study, sensitization to egg was confirmed in 30% of infants with at least one atopic parent (23).

Exposure to Food Allergens

SENSITIZATION BEFORE BIRTH

Little evidence exists to prove transfer of food allergens from mother to fetus through the placenta, and only a few cases have verified food sensitization in utero (24–27). Studies in newborn infants with a high genetic predisposition for allergy (Table 31.2) have failed to find IgE antibodies to foods (1, 28, 29). Recent studies indicate, however, that T cells of neonates may be primed in utero, as they may respond to food and inhalant allergens (30–32).

Maternal food intake during pregnancy appears to have little effect on subsequent allergy. In one randomized study of pregnancies at high allergy risk, all products containing cow's milk and egg were

Table 31.2
Indications for Considering Special Preventive Measures

Verified allergy/atopic disease in both parents or one parent and a sibling
Severe atopic disease in one family member
Elevated cord blood IgE (i.e., >0.5 kU/L)
Sensitization to any allergen during infancy (10, 147)
Food allergy or atopic dermatitis appearing in infancy

avoided during the last trimester of pregnancy, but not after birth. The avoidance diet did not influence the development of IgE antibodies to foods in the children, nor did it affect the incidence or prevalence of food allergy and atopic disease in children younger than 5 years of age (22, 28, 33, 34). The only discernible effect related to maternal diet involved lower levels of IgG antibodies to foods in the maternal sera. Similarly, the administration of high amounts of milk and egg during the last trimester resulted in increased maternal serum IgG antibodies to milk and egg (28, 35), but no significant effect was observed on the development of allergy/atopic disease during infancy. Thus, 24% in the high-maternal-intake group developed allergy prior to 18 months of age, as compared with 19% in the control group.

Despite these results, maternal elimination of highly allergenic foods during pregnancy—either completely or partially—has been utilized in high-allergy-risk pregnancies in some studies (36, 37). In these reports the maternal diet period continued after birth and several other allergy-preventive measures were taken with the infants, including environmental control measures in the study group but not in the control group. Consequently, conclusions cannot be drawn from these studies regarding the importance of an elimination diet during pregnancy. In summary, maternal dietary manipulation during pregnancy does not seem to be warranted. Such a practice may even prove harmful, as nutrition may be suboptimal unless the maternal diet is carefully monitored, preferably by a dietitian (22).

Maternal smoking during pregnancy and infancy increases the risk for allergic manifestations in the child [summarized in (38)]. It is also associated with wheezing during the first three years of life and reduced lung function in children younger than six years of age (39). Furthermore, smoking during pregnancy is associated with low birth weight and perinatal complications (38), which may, in turn, increase the likelihood of pulmonary disease in childhood. Smoking in young women should, therefore, be strongly discouraged, and it should be completely avoided during pregnancy, particularly if the fetus carries a high genetic risk for allergy. Similarly, beta-blocking agents like metoprolol should probably be avoided during pregnancy (40).

SENSITIZATION AFTER BIRTH

The season of birth appears to be important, not only for sensitization to inhalant allergens like pollens, house dust mites, and pets, but also for sensitization to foods. In a Dutch study, the highest risk for egg and cow's milk sensitization was found in babies born during November and January (41). The authors have made similar observations (Björkstén and Kjellman, unpublished). The reasons behind a seasonal effect on sensitization to foods remain unknown, but possible explanations include adjuvant effects from an indoor climate, tobacco smoke, and infections. Food allergens, inhaled with indoor airborne dust during the winter, could also possibly contribute (42, 43), as infants typically spend 95% of their time indoors.

Neonates may also be more prone to food sensitization than older infants (e.g., to cow's milk) (44, 45). As a consequence, most recommend that even occasional cow's milk formula feeds should be avoided in the maternity ward. If supplementary feeding of babies becomes necessary, then only glucose or a truly hypoallergenic formula should be given as a substitute until breast milk amounts are sufficient. On the other hand, in one study cow's milk formula given repeatedly and in large amounts in the maternity ward before breast milk became available was associated with a reduced risk for allergic disease in infants having a family history of allergy (46). A follow-up investigation when the children were 4 to 6 years of age, however, revealed no significant remaining effect (47). In the absence of supporting evidence from a randomized and blind study, however, intentional early introduction of highly allergenic foods should be regarded as experimental and, therefore, avoided.

Food sensitization may also occur via antigen

present in breast milk as the result of maternal food intake (45, 48–51). This possibility may explain why some infants manifest allergic symptoms when they ingest a certain food for the first time (48). Increased macromolecular uptake from the gut may occur during the first weeks of life, especially in preterm babies, which could partly explain the increased risk for sensitization early in life (52). Sensitization in extensively breast-fed infants may even be associated with a higher risk for a subsequent severe allergy than sensitization later during infancy (53), possibly because these infants are the most susceptible.

Introduction of cow's milk into the diet of infants during—as compared with after the first six months of age—may increase the risk for milk sensitization by a factor of three (54) and double the risk for milk hypersensitivity (55). In one study, late introduction of all allergenic foods, in addition to breast feeding for 6 months or more, delayed the onset of food allergy and atopic eczema (56). Intake of four or more solid foods before the child reached 4 months of age significantly increased early development of atopic dermatitis and led to a nearly threefold increase in the occurrence of chronic and recurrent atopic dermatitis before the age of 10 years (57). Introducing solid foods before 12 weeks of age significantly increased the risk for atopic dermatitis before 2 years of age (58). Furthermore, wheeze and prolonged cough were more often reported in babies who were younger than 8 weeks of age when solid foods were introduced (58). In a well-designed Finnish study, however, it was reported that children introduced to fish and citrus fruit after 12 months of age had almost the same frequency of food allergy at 3 years of age (2.3% to fish) as did control children (3.3%) who began eating such food items between 3 and 6 months of age (59).

Several studies have indicated that transient sensitization to food is a common event in a large proportion of normal infants (10, 11, 60, 61). Thus, low concentrations of IgE antibodies to foods can appear during a short period in infancy in approximately 25% of apparently healthy children with no previous, present, or subsequent food allergies or atopic diseases. The mechanism behind the development of tolerance in most children remains unclear, and a simple relationship between dose of ingested

allergen and either sensitization or induction of tolerance has not been outlined.

Subjects with a genetic predisposition for atopic sensitization tend to produce high concentrations of antibodies to foods, often before the development of obvious food allergy—that is, as a predictor of subsequent atopic disease (11). Infants with a genetic predisposition for allergy also appear to experience difficulties in limiting ongoing IgE production, and they may produce IgE antibodies to foods over a prolonged time, even in the absence of symptoms of allergy to the specific food. Sensitization to egg, peanut, or cow's milk in infancy, however, is associated with a high risk for various other allergic manifestations at the age of 7 years (11, 62).

Infection and Sensitization

The most important allergy-preventive effects of breast milk may be mediated via protection against infection (63). The importance of infection during early infancy for the development of allergy continues to inspire debate. For many years, it was assumed that infection, especially those of a respiratory nature, increased the risk for sensitization (64). This assumption is now being questioned in light of data gleaned from recent animal studies and epidemiological surveys (65). On the one hand, children younger than 5 years of age who were admitted to a hospital for asthmatic symptoms were reported to have had more respiratory tract infections before the age of 18 months than controls (66), and severe respiratory syncytial (RS) virus bronchiolitis appears to significantly increase the risk for subsequent asthma and sensitization to common allergens (67). A low occurrence of RS virus infections and severe gastrointestinal infections among breast-fed babies may indirectly reduce the risk for allergy and tissue hyperreactivity (63, 66, 68).

On the other hand, infants today seem to experience less severe and also fewer episodes of gastroenteritis in industrialized countries. Despite this trend, the prevalence of allergy is increasing. It has been suggested that the lower incidence of early infection may delay maturation of the immune system, thereby contributing to the increase in allergic diseases (65).

This idea is supported by several epidemiological studies (69–71). The lower incidence of allergic rhinitis and sensitization to common allergens in school children in Estonia as compared with children in Sweden has been attributed to "domestic crowding," and a higher number of infections during infancy and early childhood in Estonia than in Sweden (70). An inverse relationship also appears to exist between atopy and the number of siblings (69), particularly older siblings (71). Possibly, infection early in life enhances suppression of IgE antibody formation, while it undoubtedly triggers and aggravates respiratory symptoms in the already-sensitized individual.

Breast Feeding

Breast feeding provides many advantages over formula feeding, including optimal nutrition, low cost, and nearness between the baby and the mother. Furthermore, breast milk contains components from the mother's humoral and cellular immune systems and protects the baby against infection in the respiratory and gastrointestinal tracts (63, 72, 73). Undoubtedly, breast milk is the best infant food for the first months of life. The presence of small amounts of mercury and pesticides in breast milk does not change this value.

Breast feeding has also been recommended for the prevention of food allergy and other atopic diseases, especially in infants with a genetic predisposition for development of allergy and atopic diseases (74). Some studies support the protective effect of breast feeding in infants who are predisposed to allergy (75, 76). No general agreement has been reached regarding approach, however, as a protective effect was not confirmed in other studies (77, 78). Sensitization to food is common in young infants even during the period of exclusive breast feeding (12, 22). Several possible explanations exist for different results in various studies (Table 31.3).

Grulee and Sanford demonstrated as early as 1936 an incidence of atopic eczema that was seven times higher in infants fed cow's milk than in breastfed infants (74). Such large differences have not been confirmed by other investigators, and several more recent studies have failed to demonstrate a clear

Table 31.3
Flaws in the Design of Several
Studies of Allergy Prevention

Samples too small (statistician and/or epidemiologist not consulted in advance), resulting in low numbers and poor handling of data, rendering conclusions and recommendations invalid
Study population selected from the general population rather than genetically susceptible infants
Randomization not performed (self-selection infers bias)
Definitions of disease and allergy not stated in advance or definitions variable in multicenter trials
Objective parameters missing
Accuracy of tests and questionnaires not evaluated
Unrealistic, complex programs resulting in high drop-out rates or hidden noncompliance
No accounting for drop-outs
Poor supervision of compliance to program
Evaluation not blinded
Follow-up period often too short for disease to develop (i.e., bronchial asthma, which normally is not established by 18 months of age)

benefit from exclusive breast feeding (79). This advantage may relate to today's use of less allergenic heat-treated, milk-based formula instead of natural cow's milk. Unknown environmental factors may also possibly have such strong impact on the development of allergy as to obscure a modest protective effect from breast feeding.

Johnstone and Dutton compared children in an allergy-prevention program, where a soy formula was given at weaning, to a control group on cow's milk formula (80). They found no difference in the incidence of atopic eczema or milk allergy but did report an almost threefold lower cumulative incidence of allergic respiratory disease (bronchial asthma, hayfever, and perennial allergic rhinitis) prior to 10 years of age in the study group, as compared with the controls. Saarinen reported a reduced incidence of atopic symptoms and otitis media in infants fed breast milk for at least 6 months who received no supplementary food before 6 months of age, as compared with a control group that followed routine feeding recommendations (56). A more recent prospective study with a follow-up period lasting until subjects reached 17 years of age by Saarinen indicated that the protective effects of breast feeding are particularly obvious for respiratory manifestations (81).

In one open, uncontrolled study, vigorous efforts were made to reduce allergen exposure in infants at high risk of allergy (54). Although fewer symptoms were observed compared with those expected from the family history, many children became sensitized and experienced symptoms of food allergy despite the prevention program. A threefold lower incidence of symptoms was found in infants who apparently had not ingested cow's milk during the first 12 months of life as compared with infants who indicated indirect evidence of milk exposure. Compliance with the diet, elimination of pets, smoking habits, and other factors were disappointingly low, however (about 50%).

If breast feeding provides a protective effect against asthma and food allergy, how can it be explained? Breast feeding for more than a few weeks is associated with a postponed introduction of foreign foods. It is also linked to less maternal smoking.

Factors present in human milk that influence the immune system of the infant, including secretory IgA and immune cells, may play an important role in the enhancement of immunity and tolerance in the neonate (72, 73). IgE-suppressing factors have also been demonstrated in vitro in human colostrum (82). Breast milk is not nonallergenic, as it contains small quantities of native food allergens. At the same time, however, it contains antibodies directed toward foods. Lack of such antibodies has been associated with a higher incidence of allergy symptoms (83). Human milk contains very low levels of IgE antibodies, metachromatically staining cells, and eosinophils (84). The roles played by these components remain unknown.

The effect of maternal avoidance of highly allergenic foods (cow's milk, egg, and peanuts) during late pregnancy and throughout lactation, combined with late introduction of milk, egg, fish, citrus fruits, and peanuts into an infant's diet, was examined in a randomized study in 288 high-allergy-risk families (62, 85, 86). A highly hydrolyzed casein formula (Nutramigen) was given as a substitute for breast milk when necessary. The control group had an unrestricted diet. The cumulative prevalence of atopic disease was more than 50% lower in the prophylaxis group at 12 months of age, but no significant difference in period prevalence appeared at 24 months of age or later. A threefold reduction in food-associated atopic dermatitis, hives, and/or gastrointestinal disease was observed in the first 12 months in the

prophylaxis group, and the cumulative prevalence of food allergy (definite + probable) declined by a factor of three at 12 and 24 months of age. Positive prick skin tests were also found more often in the control group (29%) than in the prophylaxis group (17%). The difference was due primarily to a higher prevalence of sensitization to cow's milk (12% versus 1%). The effects were only temporary, however. No differences were seen at 4 and 7 years regarding current food allergy, atopic dermatitis, allergic rhinitis, asthma, lung function, or food or aeroallergen sensitization (62, 86). Many practical problems were encountered during the study period. No significant reduction in wheezing, asthma, or allergic rhinitis occurred. The researchers concluded that the effects of food restrictions were limited to the first year of life and to dermatitis.

Allergens present in breast milk are regarded as important sensitizing agents. A maternal elimination diet during the first three months of lactation (complete avoidance of all cow's milk, egg, and fish) reduced the occurrence of early food sensitization and food-allergic symptoms (29). Atopic eczema was significantly less frequently observed in the first 6 months after birth. When eczema developed, it was significantly less severe in the infants of mothers who followed an elimination diet as compared with the control group. Only highly devoted mothers were included in the study. The conclusion was that mothers who want to make special efforts to delay the onset of allergy could be recommended to follow a strict elimination diet during lactation, provided that they receive support and their dietary intake is surveyed by a dietitian. One follow-up study at 4 years revealed a lower cumulative prevalence and period prevalence of atopic dermatitis in the diet group as compared with the control group (87). Such results are interesting but need to be confirmed in a truly randomized and blindly evaluated study.

Infant Formulas for Allergy Protection

The choice of formula when breast feeding proves inadequate, or when the mother prefers early weaning, has attracted interest. Soy formula has been recommended by some based on the studies by Glaser and Johnstone (36). Further, sensitization is less often induced by soy than with cow's milk in animal experiments (88). Soy sensitization is frequently seen in subjects hypersensitive to cow's milk. Many of these patients can tolerate soy, as judged from provocation tests (89).

The possible allergy-preventive effect of soy formulae remains an open question. In one study (90), no allergy-preventive effect was seen when soy formula was compared with cow's milk formula at weaning in babies of two atopic parents.

In another study, the use of soy for allergy prevention was recommended, even though a case of soy anaphylaxis occurred (91). Soy allergy tends to be more prolonged than cow's milk allergy. It also seems more difficult for soy-allergic subjects to avoid soy than for cow's milk-allergic subjects to avoid milk. Hence, soy formula is not routinely recommended for preventive purposes in high-risk babies (92).

Arshad and Hide in a complex protocol assessed the effects of dietary and environmental measures in a randomized study of 120 high-allergy-risk babies (93). The intervention group received a hydrolyzed soy formula, in addition to breast milk from mothers who strictly avoided egg, cow's milk, wheat, and nuts. The babies avoided cow's milk to 9 months of age, and were fed wheat from 10 months and egg from 11 months of age. The intervention group also slept on polyvinyl-covered mattresses, and an acaricide was applied to carpets and upholstered furniture to reduce dust mite exposure. The control group followed standard feeding recommendations, and no environmental measures were suggested. At 12 months of age, the intervention group had less allergic problems (13% versus 40%; OR 6.3, 95% CI 2.0–20.1). The prevalences of eczema and asthma at 12 months of age were also significantly lower in the intervention group as compared with the control group. At 2 years of age, the children in the intervention group still had a lower prevalence of allergy (29% versus 58%; p < 0.005) (94) and positive prick skin tests were less common than in the control group (p < 0.005), both for house dust mites and other allergens (p < 0.05). A nonsignificant trend was found toward a lower prevalence of food intolerance, eczema, and

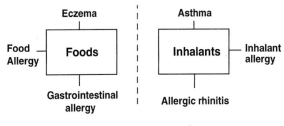

Figure 31.2

Factors affected by elimination of allergens and adjuvants among foods and inhalants.

asthma in the intervention group at 2 years of age. Further follow-up will reveal if this complex approach to allergy prevention is more successful than isolated dietary measures (Fig. 31.2).

Highly hydrolyzed casein preparations like Nutramigen and Alimentum only rarely elicit anaphylactic reactions in milk-allergic subjects (95–97). A similar hydrolysate, Pregestimil, which is recommended for use up to 4 months of life in babies with a family history of allergy, was associated with a reduced occurrence of atopic eczema at 4 years. It had no effect on the prevalence of asthma (98). Highly hydrolyzed casein preparations fulfilling the criteria for hypoallergenicity are currently recommended not only for children with proven cow's milk hypersensitivity, but also for allergy prevention in high-allergy-risk infants when a substitute for breast milk is needed (37, 92, 99–101). A highly hydrolyzed whey product (Profylac) is also recommended for preventive purposes. Its efficacy appears to be similar to that of Nutramigen (102).

Because of their high costs and the poor taste of highly hydrolyzed milk based products, less hydrolyzed products based on various cow's milk proteins have been developed. The allergenicity of these products varies (103), and severe reactions have been noted in children who were fed a partially hydrolyzed whey protein formula (104–106). The products contain some beta-lactoglobulin. Because animal experiments have shown that low doses of allergen may be particularly sensitizing while high doses tend to induce tolerance (107, 108), these hydrolysates are questionable for preventive purposes (Table 31.4) (92). New products should be properly evaluated in ran-

Table 31.4
Requirements for a "Hypoallergenic Formula"

Nutritionally adequate and safe
Provides a feeling of satisfaction to the baby
Acceptable regarding taste and smell
Acceptable regarding cost and availability
Hypoallergenic and virtually non-immunogenic as confirmed by
the following tests:
- Immunization tests in animals
- Prick skin tests in children allergic to the raw material of the formula
- Histamine release from cells of children allergic to the raw material
- Crossed radioimmunoelectrophoresis, immunoblot, or sensitive assays with serum samples from subjects allergic to the raw material
- Oral provocation tests in children allergic to the raw material

domized, blind, controlled studies performed by independent scientists, focusing on high-allergy-risk infants. Results should be compared with those for the best available hypoallergenic formula and with a normal cow's milk formula as "placebo."

Factors Influencing the Prognosis of Food Hypersensitivity

Many allergies to food tend to disappear with age (13–15). Differences in disappearance rates depend on the allergen and on individual factors in the person subject to the allergy. Preschool children with food allergy appear to have a more than twofold higher chance to outgrow their food allergy than school children (13). The mean duration of food allergy after establishing a diagnosis of food allergy was 71% after 3 years, 50% after 6 years, and 28% after 9 years (15).

Most children with cow's milk allergy can tolerate at least small amounts of cow's milk before 3 years of age. In a population-based prospective provocation study ($n = 1749$), cow's milk allergy was diagnosed in 2.2% of infants (20). Clinical tolerance was achieved in 56% by 12 months, in 77% at 2 years, and in 87% at 3 years. The presence of IgE antibodies to cow's milk indicated a poorer prognosis regarding recovery as well as a greater risk for the appearance of IgE antibodies to inhalants and for atopic disease

after the age of 3 years (20). Other investigators have reported that a low level of milk-specific serum IgE and a diminishing prick skin test wheal to cow's milk indicate a favorable prognosis (109, 110). A low IgE to IgG antibody ratio was also found to be favorable (110).

Egg allergy usually subsides before 7 years of age, while allergy to fish, soy, and nuts tends to persist for a considerably longer time (13–15). The prognosis for the disappearance of egg allergy was poor in children with early onset of egg allergy and in children who experienced more than one atopic manifestation (14). A favorable prognosis was associated with a decreasing prick skin test wheal to egg, a short duration of symptoms, and the absence of respiratory symptoms and angioedema (14).

Preventive Measures

GENERAL RECOMMENDATIONS

Allergy preventive measures have, for the most part, been recommended for and tested in babies with a high risk for allergy (i.e., babies with a bilateral family history of allergy or a unilateral family history combined with a high serum IgE concentration in cord blood). A valid family history is not always easily obtained, however, and a neonatal IgE determination is not ideal for allergy risk screening because of its low sensitivity (111). There is also no other clinically suitable test for the prediction of allergy in the baby, although combinations of tests may be used to select candidates for clinical studies (19).

Focusing on only high-risk neonates will have a limited effect on childhood health in general, as high-risk babies represent only 5% of neonates (1). By 11 years of age, about 60% of high-risk babies will have suffered from obvious atopic disease at some point (112). Many of them have a history of multiple diseases or severe disease. Such patients constitute 10% of all children who have exhibited any atopic disease up to 11 years of age. Therefore, to reduce the overall incidence of childhood allergy, general recommendations to families of intermediate- and low-risk neonates are also desirable. Unfortunately, the effects of allergy preventive measures have not been assessed in these groups. Pending the outcome of such studies, some general recommendations based on results of epidemiologic studies are suggested.

The effect of passive exposure to tobacco smoke is well established. Hence, a nonsmoking environment for all children should be encouraged by education and, if necessary, reinforced by law. Children should be encouraged never to take up smoking. In addition, smokers should obtain support to break the habit. Smoking during pregnancy and in the homes of infants should be strongly discouraged. Environmental tobacco smoke pollution in public places should also be regarded as a major health hazard. Maternal smoking during pregnancy represents a major health problem, and is associated with numerous risks for the fetus, including growth retardation, perinatal complications, and childhood allergy.

Breast feeding should be actively promoted. The WHO recommendation of breast feeding is for at least 6 months, if feasible. This strategy may prove advantageous also in the context of allergy prevention.

"Modern living" includes several factors that, when alone or taken together, may affect the risk for development of allergy and atopic diseases. Diversity of early infant feeding may pose a problem. Furthermore, the thorough insulation and tightness of modern houses may lead to considerable problems with high indoor humidity, even in areas with a dry and cold climate (113). Mite allergen levels increase with rising humidity, greater age of a building, and certain building characteristics (e.g., concrete slab on the ground) (114, 115). Higher levels of mite antigen are found in older mattresses and in dust from carpeted floors. Building materials are often selected for their practicality, with little attention paid to their possible health effects. "Sick buildings" (116) may emit numerous chemical compounds with unknown effects. Ventilation is often insufficient in modern buildings and may add to indoor pollution. Humidity and indoor mold growth constitute considerable health problems (117). Thus, authorities should define appropriate construction and maintenance standards. Everyone could be encouraged to ventilate homes and to reduce shower times to minimize the water load of the home.

The ubiquitous presence of allergens from furred pets—for example, in homes (even those without pets), public places, day-care centers, and schools (42, 118–120)—also presents a risk for the development of allergy and for eliciting symptoms. The levels of animal antigens in many schools and day-care centers are high enough to induce airway inflammation and bronchial hyperreactivity in sensitized asthmatics (121) and to trigger sensitization of nonasthmatics (122). Cleaning procedures should be improved, although they will not entirely eliminate pet allergens (123). Indirect contacts with pet allergens should be reduced. Pet owners must learn how to reduce contamination of their clothing with pet allergens.

Education of medical personnel, teachers, social welfare personnel, and others regarding allergy and atopic disease should be improved to make life easier for subjects with allergic problems. Such education might potentially reduce the risk for development of allergy and atopic diseases in the general population.

PREVENTION IN GENETICALLY SUSCEPTIBLE INFANTS

High-allergy-risk families (Table 31.2) should have access to information on available preventive measures (Table 31.5). In addition, recommendations should be made known to relevant authorities to improve the indoor and outdoor environment. Preventive measures should be put in perspective, however, and the families must be aware of what can be achieved by dietary manipulations—namely, a delay in the onset of symptoms rather than prevention of disease. This delay may well make it worth the effort, however.

Presently, there is no test capable of identifying high-allergy-risk families. If a carefully obtained history of allergy in the parents and any siblings reveals disease in the immediate family, however, then pet ownership should be discouraged. It has also been suggested that families with a history of allergy should not have babies immediately before or during the peak pollen season (122, 123). Not enough data exist, however, to support such advice that would interfere with family life and planning.

Expectant mothers should avoid foods they cannot tolerate, but no evidence suggests that eliminating certain allergenic foods would reduce the risk for

Table 31.5
Recommendations for Families of Infants with a
High Risk for Allergy and Atopic Disease

Before pregnancy
No smoking
Home sanitation; remove pets and wall-to-wall carpets; check
    quality of air conditioning (risk of microbial growth) and venti-
    lation
Acaracides not recommended

During pregnancy
No smoking
Home sanitation; no pets, wall-to-wall carpets, or damage due to
    dampness
Promote breast feeding; instructions and information to both
    parents*

At maternity ward
No smoking
No cow's milk formula—not even occasionally at night
Promote breast feeding
Inform about alternative breast milk substitutes with proven
    hypoallergenicity

At home
Sanitation
No smoking
Promote breast feeding for at least 4 to 6 months; instructions
    and information to both parents
Inform about a really hypoallergenic alternative to breast milk
Avoid other foods before 4 months of age
Highly allergenic foods (egg, fish, nuts, peanuts) introduced only
    after 1 year of age
Late start when possible at day-care centers (i.e., after 18 months)

*Dietary restrictions should always be supported by a dietitian.

allergy in their babies. Immunotherapy (hyposensitization) should not be begun during pregnancy given
the risk of reactions. Ongoing immunotherapy can,
however, be continued. Asthma medication should
be optimized to reduce the risk for premature birth
and the need for instrumental delivery. Damage due
to dampness in the home should be corrected, and
mite growth kept at a minimum.

After birth, breast feeding should be encouraged
and a safe alternative—i.e., a truly hypoallergenic
formula—should be recommended. Partially hydrolyzed infant formulas, although often aggressively
marketed, should not be considered reliable for allergy prevention. Occasional feedings of cow's milk
formula at the maternity ward should be eliminated
and efforts made to prevent the administration of
such formula during the night.

Breast feeding should be recommended for the
first 6 months, and if possible without the introduction of any additional food. Introduction of egg, fish,
citrus fruits, nuts, and peanuts should be avoided for
the first 12 months of life. New food items should be
introduced one at a time, in at least weekly intervals.
This procedure allows any sensitivity to be more
easily recognized. Indoor pets should also be avoided,
at least during the first 2 years of life. If at this age
the child is healthy and has no history of allergy or
symptoms and signs of atopic disease, having a pet
appears to pose no high allergy risk.

Day-care centers often have a poor indoor climate (124) and the levels of cat and dog allergen
found there may be high (120). Infants and young
children at day-care centers also have a greater number of respiratory tract infections (125). Postponing
the start of this type of day care until after infancy is
recommended in some prevention programs (76).

No elimination diet for the mother or thorough
home sanitation program should be recommended
unless the family is highly motivated. The dietary
intake of mother and child must be supervised and
family members supported through the period of
preventive measures. Otherwise, a risk exists for negative effects on the well-being and the economy of the
family (Table 31.6).

Research should focus on immune mechanisms,
the importance of adjuvants for sensitization, and the
development of tolerance. Well-conducted, randomized, blind trials in large numbers of high-allergy-risk
infants should compare the various allergy preventive
programs, including the effect of avoidance of allergenic foods and adjuvants for sensitization in com-

Table 31.6
Risks Associated with Allergy Preventive Measures

Malnutrition
High cost for family and society
Anxiety in the family
Overprotection of the child
Disturbed family interaction
Social isolation of the family
Disappointment/anger when symptoms develop
Poor compliance (e.g., intermittent cow's milk formula intake) is
    probably worse than regular intake

parison with early continuous exposure to high doses of food allergens, to determine the best way to prevent the development of atopic diseases.

Conclusion

Food allergy in infancy and early childhood often represents the first manifestation of atopic disease. Thus, although the prognosis with regard to food allergy is usually good, allergic diseases of the respiratory tract remain common some years later. Few simple and documented allergy preventive measures are currently available. One of these approaches involves strict avoidance of exposure to tobacco smoke. Other reasonable measures include promotion of breast feeding, preferably for six months. Only hypoallergic infant formulas may be considered for prevention, while various partially hydrolyzed preparations and soy formulas are not routinely recommended for this purpose. A combination of measures to optimize indoor air (i.e., to keep humidity and indoor allergen levels low) is necessary to reduce the risk for later respiratory allergy in high-risk babies.

Acknowledgments

Financial support by the Swedish Medical Research Council (grant number 7510), the National Organization for the Prevention of Asthma and Allergy, and the National Institute of Public Health, Stockholm, is gratefully acknowledged.

REFERENCES

1. Croner S, Kjellman N-IM, Eriksson B, Roth A. IgE screening in 1701 newborn infants and the development of atopic disease during infancy. Arch Dis Child 1982;57:364–368.
2. Kajosaari M. Food allergy in Finnish children aged 1–6 years. Acta Paediatr Scand 1982;71:815–819.
3. Anderson J, Sogn D, eds. Adverse reactions to foods. Bethesda, MD: National Institutes of Public Health, 1984, 1–220.
4. Kjellman N-IM. Development and prediction of atopic allergy in childhood. In: Boström H, Ljungstedt N, eds. Skandia International Symposia: Theoretical and clinical aspects of allergic diseases. Stockholm: Almqvist & Wicksell, 1983, 55–73.
5. Van Asperen P, Kemp A, Mellis C. A prospective study of the clinical manifestations of atopic disease in infancy. Acta Paediatr Scand 1984;73:80–85.
6. Kivity S, Dunner K, Marian Y. The pattern of food hypersensitivity in patients with onset after 10 years of age. Clin Exp Allergy 1994;24:19–22.
7. Åberg N, Hesselmar B, Åberg B, Eriksson B. Increase of asthma, allergic rhinitis and eczema in Swedish schoolchildren between 1979 and 1991. Clin Exp Allergy 1995;25:815–819.
8. Fuglsang G, Madsen C, Saval P, Østerballe O. Prevalence of intolerance to food additives among Danish school children. Pediatr Allergy Immunol 1993;4:123–129.
9. Dannaeus A, Johansson S, Foucard T. Clinical and immunological aspects of food allergy in childhood. II. Development of allergic symptoms and humoral immune response to foods in infants of atopic mothers during the first 24 months of life. Acta Paediatr Scand 1978;67:497–504.
10. Hattevig G, Kjellman B, Johansson SGO, Björkstén B. Clinical symptoms and IgE responses to common food proteins in atopic and healthy children. Clin Allergy 1984;14:551–559.
11. Hattevig G, Kjellman B, Björkstén B. Clinical symptoms and IgE responses to common food proteins and inhalants in the first 7 years of life. Clin Allergy 1987;17:571–578.
12. Bock SS. The natural history of food sensitivity. J Allergy Clin Immunol 1982;69:173–177.
13. Ford PK, Taylor B. Natural history of egg hypersensitivity. Arch Dis Child 1982;57:649–652.
14. Esteban MM, Pascual C, Madero R, Diaz Pena JM, Ojeda JA. Natural history of immediate food allergy in children. In: Businco L, Ruggieri F, eds. Proceedings of the first Latin food allergy workshop. Rome: Fisons SpA, 1985, 27–30.
15. Sigurs N, Hildebrand H, Hultquist C, et al. Sensitization in childhood atopic disease identified by Phadebas RAST, serum IgE and Phadiatop. Pediatr Allergy Immunol 1990;1:74–78.
16. Björkstén B, Kjellman N-IM. Perinatal factors influencing the development of allergy. Clin Rev Allergy 1987;5:339–347.
17. Björkstén B. Does breast feeding prevent the development of allergy? Immunol Today 1983;4:215–217.
18. Juto P, Möller C, Engberg S, Björkstén B. Influence of type of feeding on lymphocyte function and development of infantile allergy. Clin Allergy 1982;12:409–416.
19. Odelram H, Kjellman N-IM, Björkstén B. Predictors of atopy in newborn babies. Allergy 1995;50:585–52.
20. Høst A, Halken S. A prospective study of cow milk allergy in Danish infants during the first 3 years of life. Allergy 1990;45:587–596.
21. Gerrard JW, MacKenzie JWA, Goluboff N, Garson JZ, Maningas CS. Cow's milk allergy: prevalence and manifestations in an unselected series of newborns. Acta Paediatr Scand 1973;273(suppl):1–21.
22. Fälth-Magnusson K, Kjellman N-IM. Development of atopic disease in babies whose mothers were on exclusion diet during pregnancy—a randomized study. J Allergy Clin Immunol 1987;80:968–975.
23. Rowntree S, Cogswell J, Platts-Mills T, Mitchell E. Development of IgE and IgG antibodies to food and inhalant allergens in children at risk of allergic disease. Arch Dis Child 1985;60:727–735.
24. Michel FB, Bousquet J, Greiller P, Robinet-Levy M, Coulomb

Y. Comparison of cord blood immunoglobulin E concentrations and maternal allergy for the prediction of atopic disease in infancy. J Allergy Clin Immunol 1980;65:422–430.

25. Businco L, Marchetti F, Pellegrini G, Perlini R. Predictive value of cord blood IgE levels in "at risk" newborn babies and influence of type of feeding. Clin Allergy 1983;13:503–508.

26. Delespesse G, Sarfati M, Lang G, Sehon A. Prenatal and neonatal synthesis of IgE. Monogr Allergy 1983;18:83–95.

27. Høst A, Husby S, Gjesing B, Larsen J, Løwenstein H. Prospective estimation of IgG, IgG subclass and IgE antibodies to dietary proteins in infants with cow milk allergy. Allergy 1992;47:218–229.

28. Lilja G, Dannaeus A, Fälth-Magnusson K, et al. Immune response of the atopic woman and foetus; effects of high- and low-dose food allergen intake during late pregnancy. Clin Allergy 1988;18:131–142.

29. Hattevig G, Kjellman B, Sigurs N, Björkstén B, Kjellman N-IM. Effect of maternal avoidance of eggs, cow's milk and fish during lactation upon allergic manifestations in infants. Clin Exp Allergy 1989;19:27–32.

30. Kondo N, Kobayashi Y, Shinoda S, et al. Cord blood lymphocyte responses to food antigens for the prediction of allergic disorders. Arch Dis Child 1992;67:1003–1007.

31. Piccini M-P, Mecacci F, Sampognaro S, et al. Aeroallergen sensitization can occur during fetal life. Int Arch Allergy Appl Immunol 1993;102:301–303.

32. Warner J, Miles E, Jones A, Warner J. Is deficiency of interferon gamma production by allergen triggered cord blood cells a predictor of atopic eczema? Clin Exper Allergy 1994;24:423–430.

33. Fälth-Magnusson K, Kjellman N-IM, Magnusson K. Antibodies IgG, IgA and IgM to food antigens during the first 18 months of life in relation to feeding and atopic disease. J Allergy Clin Immunol 1988;81:868–875.

34. Fälth-Magnusson K, Kjellman N-IM. Allergy prevention by maternal elimination diet during late pregnancy—a 5-year follow-up of a randomized study. J Allergy Clin Immunol 1992;89:709–713.

35. Lilja G, Dannaeus A, Foucard T, Graff-Lonnevig V, Johansson S, Öman H. Effects of maternal diet during late pregnancy and lactation on the development of atopic diseases in infants up to eighteen months of age—in vivo results. Clin Exp Allergy 1989;19:473–479.

36. Glaser J, Johnstone D. Prophylaxis of allergic disease in the newborn. J Am Med Assoc 1953;153:620–622.

37. Zeiger R, Heller S, Mellon M, O'Connor R, Hamburger R. Effectiveness of dietary manipulation in the prevention of food allergy in infants. J Allergy Clin Immunol 1986;78:224–238.

38. Halken S, Høst A, Nilsson L, Taudorf E. Passive smoking as a risk factor for development of obstructive respiratory disease and allergic sensitization. Allergy 1995;50:97–105.

39. Martinez F, Wright A, Taussig L, et al. Asthma and wheezing in the first six years of life. N Engl J Med 1995;332:133–138.

40. Björkstén B, Finnström O, Wichman K. Intrauterine exposure to the beta-adrenergic receptor-blocking agent metoprolol and allergy. Int Arch Allergy Appl Immunol 1988;87:59–62.

41. Aalberse RC, Nieuwenhuys EJ, Hey M, Stapel SO. "Horoscope effect" not only for seasonal but also for non-seasonal allergens. Clin Exp Allergy 1992;22:1003–1006.

42. Dybendal T, Elsayed S. Dust from carpeted and smooth floors. V. Cat (Fel d I) and mite (Der p I and Der f I) allergen levels

in school dust. Demonstration of the basofil histamine release induced by dust from classrooms. Clin Exp Allergy 1992;22:1100–1106.

43. Crespo J, Pascual C, Dominguez C, Ojeda I, Muñoz F, Esteban M. Allergic reactions associated with airborne fish particles in IgE-mediated fish hypersensitive patients. Allergy 1995;50:257–261.

44. Stinzing G, Zetterström R. Cow's milk allergy, incidence and pathogenetic role of early exposure to cow's milk formula. Acta Paediatr Scand 1979;68:383–387.

45. Høst A, Husby S, Østerballe O. A prospective study of cow's milk allergy in exclusively breast-fed infants. Acta Paediatr Scand 1988;77:663–670.

46. Lindfors A, Enocksson E. Development of atopic disease after early administration of cow milk formula. Allergy 1988;43:11–16.

47. Lindfors A, Danielsson L, Enocksson E, Johansson S, Westin S. Allergic symptoms up to 4–6 years of age in children given cow milk neonatally. A prospective study. Allergy 1992;47:207–211.

48. Gerrard J. Allergy in breast fed babies to ingredients in breast milk. Ann Allergy 1979;42:69–71.

49. Cant A, Marsden R, Kilshaw P. Egg and cow's milk hypersensitivity in exclusively breast fed infants with eczema, and detection of egg protein in breast milk. Br Med J 1985;291:932–935.

50. Jakobsson I, Lindberg T, Benediktsson B, Hansson B. Dietary bovine betalactoglobulin is transferred to human milk. Acta Paediatr Scand 1985;74:342–345.

51. Cavagni G, Paganelli R, Caffarelli C, et al. Passage of food antigens into circulation of breast-fed infants with atopic dermatitis. Ann Allergy 1988;61:361–365.

52. Eastham E, Lichauco T, Grady M, Walker A. Antigenicity of infant formulas: role of immature intestine on protein permeability. J Pediatrics 1978;93:561–564.

53. Cantani A, Ragno V, Businco L. Natural history of IgE-mediated food allergy in fully breast-fed babies. Report of 21 cases with follow up to 19 years. Pediatr Allergy Immunol 1992;2:131–134.

54. Hamburger R, Casilas R, Johnson R, Mellon M, O'Connor R, Zeiger, R. Long-term studies in prevention of food allergy: patterns of IgG anti cow's milk antibody responses. Ann Allergy 1987;59:175–178.

55. Halpern S, Sellars W, Johnson R, Anderson D, Saperstein S, Reisch J. Development of childhood allergy in infants fed breast, soy or cow milk. J Allergy Clin Immunol 1973;51:139–151.

56. Saarinen UM. Prophylaxis for atopic disease: role of infant feeding. Clin Rev Allergy 1984;2:151–167.

57. Fergusson D, Horwood L, Shannon F. Early solid feeding and recurrent childhood eczema, a 10-year longitudinal study. Pediatrics 1990;86:541–546.

58. Forsyth J, Ogston S, Clark A, Florey C, Howie P. Relation between early introduction of solid food to infants and their weight and illnesses during the first two years of life. Br Med J 1993;306:1572–1576.

59. Saarinen U, Kajosaari M. Does dietary elimination in infancy prevent or only postpone a food allergy? Lancet 1980;i:166–167.

60. Foucard T. A follow up study of children with asthmatoid bronchitis. Acta Pædiatr Scand 1973;62:633–644.

61. Hattevig G, Kjellman B, Björkstén B. Appearance of IgE antibodies to ingested and inhaled allergens during first 12 years of life in atopic and non-atopic children. Pediatr Allergy Immunol 1993;4:182–186.

62. Zeiger R, Heller S. The development and prediction of atopy in high risk children: follow-up at age seven years in a prospective randomized study of combined maternal and infant food allergen avoidance. J Allergy Clin Immunol 1995;95:1179–1190.

63. Pullan C, Tooms G, Martin A, Gardner P, Webb J, Appleton D. Breast-feeding and respiratory syncytial virus infection. Br Med J 1980;281:1034–1036.

64. Frick O, German D. Development of allergy in children. Association with virus infection. J Allergy Clin Immunol 1979;63:228–241.

65. Holt P. Environmental factors and primary T-cell sensitisation to inhalant allergens in infancy: reappraisal of the role of infections and air pollution. Pediatr Allergy Immunol 1995;6:1–10.

66. Rylander E, Pershagen G, Eriksson M, Nordvall L. Parental smoking and other risk factors for wheezing bronchitis in children. Eur J Epidemiol 1993;9:517–526.

67. Sigurs N, Bjarnason R, Sigurbergsson F, Kjellman B, Björkstén B. Asthma and immunoglobulin E antibodies after respiratory syncytial virus bronchiolitis: a prospective cohort study with matched controls. Pediatrics 1995;95:500–505.

68. Soothill J. Prevention of atopic allergic disease. Ann Allergy 1983;51:229–232.

69. Von Mutius E, Martinez FD, Fritzsch C, Nicolai T, Reitmeir P, Thiemann HH. Skin test reactivity and number of siblings. Br Med J 1994;308:692–695.

70. Bråbäck L, Breborowicz A, Julge K, et al. Risk factors for respiratory symptoms and atopic sensitization in the Baltic area. Arch Dis Child 1995;72:487–493.

71. Strachan D. Epidemiology of hay fever: towards a community diagnosis. Clin Exp Allergy 1995;25:296–303.

72. Pittard W, Bill K. Immunoregulation by breast milk cells. Cell Immunol 1979;42:437–441.

73. Prentice A. Breast feeding increases concentrations of IgA in infants' urine. Arch Dis Child 1987;62:792–795.

74. Grulee C, Sanford H. The influence of breast and artificial feeding on infantile eczema. J Pediatr 1936;9:223–225.

75. Vandenplas Y, Sacre L. Influences of neonatal serum IgE concentration, family history and diet on the incidence of cow's milk allergy. Eur J Pediatr 1986;145:493–495.

76. Businco L, Cantani A, Meglio P, Bruno G. Prevention of atopy: results of a long-term (7 months to 8 years) follow-up. Ann Allergy 1987;59(part II):183–186.

77. Cogswell JJ, Mitchell EB, Alexander J. Parental smoking, breast feeding and respiratory infection in development of allergic disease. Arch Dis Child 1987;62:338–344.

78. Björkstén B, Kjellman N-IM. Does breast-feeding prevent food allergy? Allergy Proc 1991;12:233–237.

79. Van Asperen P, Kemp A, Mellis C. Relationship of diet in the development of atopy in infancy. Clin Allergy 1984;14:525–532.

80. Johnstone D, Dutton A. Dietary prophylaxis of allergic disease in children. N Engl J Med 1966;274:715–719.

81. Saarinen UL. Breastfeeding as prophylaxis against atopic disease: prospective follow-up study until 17 years old. Lancet 1995;346:1065–1069.

82. Sarfati M, Vanderbeeken Y, Rubio-Trujillo M, Duncan D, Delespesse, G. Presence of IgE suppressor factors in human colostrum. Eur J Immunol 1986;16:1005–1008.

83. Machtinger S, Moss R. Cow's milk allergy in breast-fed infants: the role of allergen and maternal secretory IgA antibody. J Allergy Clin Immunol 1986;77:341–347.

84. Vassella C, Hjälle L, Björkstén B. Basophils and eosinophils in human milk in relation to maternal allergy. Ped Allergy Immunol 1992;3:184–189.

85. Zeiger R, Heller S, Mellon M, et al. Effect of combined maternal and infant food allergen-avoidance on development of atopy in early infancy: a randomized study. J Allergy Clin Immunol 1989;84:72–89.

86. Zeiger RS, Heller S, Mellon MH, Halsey JF, Hamburger RN, Sampson HA. Genetic and environmental factors affecting the development of atopy through age 4 in children of atopic parents: a prospective randomized study of food allergen avoidance. Pediatr Allergy Immunol 1992;3:110–127.

87. Sigurs N, Hattevig G, Kjellman B. Maternal avoidance of eggs, cow's milk and fish during lactation: effect on allergic manifestations, skin-prick tests and specific IgE antibodies in children at age 4 years. Pediatrics 1992;89:735–739.

88. Piacentini G, Benedetti M, Spezia E, Boner A, Bellanti J. Anaphylactic sensitizing power of selected infant formulas. Ann Allergy 1991;67:400–402.

89. Giampietro P, Ragno V, Daniele S, Cantani A, Ferrara M, Businco L. Soy hypersensitivity in children with food allergy. Ann Allergy 1992;69:143–146.

90. Kjellman N-IM, Johansson S. Soy versus cow's milk in infants with a biparental history of atopic disease: development of atopic disease and immunoglobulins from birth to 4 years of age. Clin Allergy 1979;9:347–358.

91. Bardare M, Vaccari A, Allievi E, et al. Influence of dietary manipulation on incidence of atopic disease in infants at risk. Ann Allergy 1993;71:366–371.

92. Bruijnzeel-Koomen C, Ortolani C, Aas K, et al. Position paper: adverse reactions to food. Allergy 1995;50:623–635.

93. Arshad S, Matthews S, Gant C, Hide D. Effect of allergen avoidance on development of allergic disorders in infancy. Lancet 1992;339:1493–1497.

94. Hide DW, Matthews S, Matthews L, et al. Effect of allergen avoidance in infancy on allergic manifestations at age two years. J Allergy Clin Immunol 1994;93:842–846.

95. Bock SA. Probable allergic reaction to casein hydrolysate. J Allergy Clin Immunol 1989;84:272.

96. Saylor JD, Bahna SL. Anaphylaxis to casein hydrolysate formula. J Pediatr 1991;118:71–74.

97. Oldaeus G, Björkstén B, Einarsson R, Kjellman N-IM. Antigenicity and allergenicity of cow milk hydrolysates intended for infant feeding. Pediatr Allergy Immunol 1991;4:156–164.

98. Mallet E, Henocq A. Long-term prevention of allergic diseases by using protein hydrolysate formula in at-risk infants. J Pediatr 1992;121:S95–S100.

99. Kjellman N-IM. Food allergy—treatment and prevention. Ann Allergy 1987;59:168–174.

100. Committee on Nutrition of the American Academy of Pediatrics. Hypoallergenic formulas. Pediatrics 1989;83:1068–1069.

101. Businco L, Dreborg S, et al. ESPACI position paper: hydrolysed cow's milk formulae. Allergenicity and use for treatment and prevention. Pediatr Allergy Immunol 1993;4:101–111.

102. Halken S, Høst A, Hansen L, Østerballe O. Preventive effect of feeding high-risk infants a casein hydrolysate formula or an ultrafiltrated whey hydrolysate formula. A prospective, randomized, comparative clinical study. Pediatr Allergy Immunol 1993;4:173–181.

103. Oldaeus G, Bradley CK, Björkstén B, Kjellman N-IM. Allergenicity screening of "hypoallergenic" milk-based formulas. J Allergy Clin Immunol 1992;90:133–135.

104. Ellis M, Short J, Heiner D. Anaphylaxis after ingestion of a recently introduced hydrolyzed whey protein formula. J Pediatr 1991;110.74–77.

105. Ragno V, Giampietro P, Bruno G, Businco L. Allergenicity of milk protein hydrolysate formulae in children with cow's milk allergy. Eur J Pediatr 1993;152:760–762.

106. Businco L, Lucenti P, Arcese G, Ziruolo G, Cantani A. Immunogenicity of so-called hypoallergenic formula in at-risk babies: two case reports. Clin Exp Allergy 1994;24:42–45.

107. Jarrett E, Hall E. The development of IgE-suppressive immunocompetence in young animals: influence of exposure to antigen in the presence and absence of maternal immunity. Immunology 1984;53:365–373.

108. Ahlstedt S, Björkstén B. Specific antibody responses in rats and mice after daily immunization without adjuvant. Int Arch Allergy Appl Immunol 1983;71:293 299.

109. Hill DJ, Firer MA, Ball G, Hosking CS. Natural history of cow's milk allergy in children: immunological outcome over 2 years. Clin Exp Allergy 1993;23:124–131.

110. James JM, Sampson HA. Immunologic changes associated with the development of tolerance in children with cow milk allergy. J Pediatr 1992;121:371–377.

111. Kjellman N-IM. IgE in neonates is not suitable for general allergy risk screening. Pediatric Allergy Immunol 1994;5:1–4.

112. Croner S, Kjellman N-IM. Development of atopic disease in relation to family history and cord blood IgE levels. Eleven-year follow-up in 1654 children. Pediatr Allergy Immunol 1990;1:14–20.

113. Munir A, Björkstén B, Einarsson R, et al. Mite allergens in relation to home conditions and sensitization of asthmatic children from three climatic regions. Allergy 1995;50:55–64.

114. Wickman M, Nordvall SL, Pershagen G. Risk factors in early childhood for sensitization to airborne allergens. Pediatr Allergy Immunol 1992;3:128–133.

115. Van Strien R, Verhoeff A, Brunekreef B, Van Wijnen J. Mite allergen in house dust: relationship with different housing characteristics in the Netherlands. Clin Exp Allergy 1994;24:843–853.

116. Finnegan M, Pickering C. Building related illness. Clin Allergy 1986;16:389–405.

117. Platt S, Martin C, Hunt S, Lewis C. Damp housing, mould growth, and symptomatic health state. Br Med J 1989;298:1673–1678.

118. Enberg R, Shamie S, McCullough J, Ownby D. Ubiquitous presence of cat allergen in cat-free buildings: probable dispersal from human clothing. Ann Allergy 1993;70:471–474.

119. Custovic A, Taggart S, Woodcock A. House dust mite and cat allergen in different indoor environments. Clin Exp Allergy 1994;24:1164–1168.

120. Munir A, Einarsson R, Dreborg S. Mite (*Der p* I, *Der f* I), cat (*Fel d* I) and dog (*Can f* I) allergens in dust from Swedish day-care centres. Clin Exp Allergy 1995;25:119–126.

121. Ihre E, Zetterström O. Increase in non-specific bronchial responsiveness after repeated inhalation of low doses of allergen. Clin Exp Allergy 1993;23:298–305.

122. Munir A, Einarsson R, Schou C, Dreborg S. Allergens in school dust. I. The amount of the major cat and dog allergens in dust from Swedish schools is high enough to probably cause perennial symptoms in most asthmatic school children sensitized to cat and dog. J Allergy Clin Immunol 1993;91:1067–1074.

123. Munir A, Einarsson R, Dreborg S. Indirect contact with pets can confound the effect of cleaning procedures for reduction of animal allergen levels in house dust. Pediatr Allergy Immunol 1994;5:32–39.

124. Bakke J, Levy F. Indoor air quality in kindergartens—relation to health effects. Indoor Air '90 1990;1:3–8.

125. Harsten G, Prellner K, Heldrup J, Kalm O, Kornfält R. Acute respiratory tract infections in children. Acta Paediatr Scand 1990;79:402–409.

126. Kjellman N-IM. Atopic disease in seven-year-old children. Acta Paediatr Scand 1977;66:465–471.

127. Åberg N. Familial occurrence of atopic disease: genetic versus environmental factors. Clin Exp Allergy 1993;23:829–834.

128. Marsh D, Bias W, Ishizaka K. Genetic control of basal serum immunoglobulin E level and its effect on specific reaginic sensitivity. Proc Nat Acad Sci 1974;71:3588–3592.

129. Golding J, Peters TJ. The epidemiology of childhood eczema: a population based study of associations. Paediatr Perinat Epid 1987;1:67–94.

130. Morrison Smith J, Springett VH. Atopic disease and month of birth. Clin Allergy 1979;9:153–157.

131. Suoniemi I, Björkstén F, Haahtela T. Dependence of immediate hypersensitivity in the adolescent period on factors encountered in infancy. Allergy 1981;36:263–268.

132. Croner S, Kjellman N-IM. Predictors of atopic disease: cord blood IgE and month of birth. Allergy 1986;41:68–70.

133. Johnstone D, Roghmann K, Pless I. Factors associated with the development of asthma and hay fever in children: the possible risks of hospitalization, surgery and anesthesia. Pediatrics 1975;56:398–403.

134. Morrison Smith J. Skin test and atopic allergy in children. Clin Allergy 1973;3:269–275.

135. Gerrard J, Perelmutter L. IgE-mediated allergy to peanut, cow's milk and egg in children with special reference to maternal diet. Ann Allergy 1986;56:351–354.

136. Kajosaari M, Saarinen UM. Prophylaxis of atopic disease by six months total solid food elimination. Acta Paediatr Scand 1983;72:411–414.

137. Arshad S, Hide D. Effect of environmental factors on the development of allergic disorders in infancy. J Allergy Clin Immunol 1992;90:235–241.

138. Rugtveit J. Environmental factors in the first months of life and the possible relationship to later development of hypersensitivity. Allergy 1990;45:154–156.

139. Björkstén F, Suoniemi I. Time and intensity of first pollen contacts and risk of subsequent pollen allergies. Acta Med Scand 1981;209:299–303.

140. Axelsson I, Johansson S, Zetterström O. A new indoor allergen from a common non-flowering plant. Allergy 1987;42:604–611.

141. Axelsson I. Allergy to *Ficus benjamina* (weeping fig) in non-atopic subjects. Allergy 1995;50:284–285.

142. Sporik R, Holgate S, Platts-Mills T, Cogswell J. Exposure to house-dust mite allergen (*Der p* I) and the development of asthma in childhood. N Engl J Med 1990;8:502–507.

143. Kuehr J, Frischer T, Meinert R, *et al.* Mite allergen exposure is a risk for the incidence of specific sensitization. J Allergy Clin Immunol 1994;94:44–52.

144. Strannegård Ö, Strannegård I, Rystedt I. Viral infections in atopic dermatitis. Acta Derm Venereol 1985;114(suppl):121–124.

145. Andrae S, Axelson O, Björkstén B, Kjellman N-IM. Symptoms of bronchial hyperreactivity and asthma in relation to environmental factors. Arch Dis Child 1988;63:473–478.

146. Ishizaki T, Koizumi K, Ikemori R, Ishiyama Y, Kishibiki E. Studies of prevalence of Japanese cedar pollinosis among residents in a densely cultivated area. Ann Allergy 1987; 58:265–270.

147. Sigurs N, Hattevig G, Kjellman B, Kjellman N-IM, Nilsson L, Björkstén B. Appearance of atopic disease in relation to serum IgE antibodies in children followed up from birth for 4 to 15 years. J Allergy Clin Immunol 1994;94:757–763.

32

DIETS AND NUTRITION

Celide Barnes Koerner
Hugh A. Sampson

Over the past several decades, a variety of desensitization routines and medications have been reported as being useful in the treatment of food hypersensitivity. A recent study in patients with a history of peanut-induced anaphylaxis suggested that rush immunotherapy was efficacious in diminishing the severity of the reactions to peanut following an oral food challenge (1). The high rate of side effects associated with this form of immunotherapy make it unlikely that it will be utilized in any general clinical setting, however. Other claims of therapeutic modalities have not been substantiated in patients with challenge-documented food allergy utilizing appropriately controlled trials. Consequently, strict elimination of the offending food antigen remains the only proven therapy for food hypersensitivity. It is best accomplished by teaching patients and parents to limit use of commercially prepared foods, to read food labels, and to watch for unsuspected sources of food antigens (e.g., peanut butter may be used in chili sauce, egg rolls, and other foods). In the United States, food manufacturers are required by law to list all ingredients of the food product, except if it is an incidental additive, "flavoring" (e.g. casein), or spice, which constitutes 2% or less of the total protein (requirements vary throughout the world, but are generally less stringent). Thus, patients (or their parents) must contact manufacturers to inquire about these ingredients. Complete elimination diets have been shown to lead to the loss of clinical reactivity to many foods (development of clinical tolerance) in about one-third of children and adults after one to two years (2, 3).

Instituting a food elimination diet should be considered comparable to prescribing a medication, which always carries a definite risk–benefit ratio.

Consequently, appropriate diagnostic measures must be undertaken before special diets are implemented. Unfortunately, broadly restricted diets have all too frequently been prescribed on the basis of history, standard allergy tests (e.g., skin tests, RASTs), or unsubstantiated tests (e.g., cytotoxic tests, food immune complexes, food-specific IgG or IgG4) and have resulted in severe malnutrition (4–6) or delayed diagnosis of severe underlying disorders (7, 8).

As specialists in the diagnosis and management of adverse food reactions, allergists and other health care professionals must recognize the enormous task and emotional burden placed on patients and families by the prescription of elimination diets. The time required to purchase groceries and prepare these special meals is drastically increased, eating at restaurants becomes difficult and in some cases impossible, and eating at friends' homes or at school often needs to be curtailed. Consequently, social isolation and eating disorders may result from implementation of food restrictions.

Although it is often helpful to think of foods in certain botanical families, no clinical evidence supports consistent broad intra-botanical or intra-species cross-reactivity (9–11). In addition, most patients are allergic to only one or two foods; widespread dietary restrictions, therefore, are rarely necessary (12, 13). Every effort must be made to diagnose food allergies correctly and to educate patients in proper elimination diets. Inappropriate parental obsession with food allergies is only reinforced when physicians fail to validate historical claims or laboratory studies. In extreme cases, this obsession may present as Munchausen by proxy, which should be considered a form of child abuse (14).

461

Basic Nutritional Requirements

Calorie and protein requirements for children are based on their age and weight (13):

Age	kcal/kg/day	g protein/kg/day
Infants < 1 year of age	90–100	1.6–2.2
Children 1 to 3 years	102	1.2
Children 4 to 10 years	70–90	1.0–1.1
Preadolescent and adolescents	40–55	0.8–1.0

A child's rate of growth is typically used to assess the adequacy of calories and protein in their diets. Any change in his or her growth pattern may indicate either a deficiency or an excess of these nutrients.

Vitamin and mineral requirements are based on the Recommended Dietary Allowances (RDA) established by the National Academy of Sciences. When assessing children's diets, 100% of the RDAs is considered optimal for all vitamins and minerals. Typically, supplementation is recommended when a child's intake of a nutrient represents less than two-thirds of the RDA, and attempts at increasing intake by dietary modification have proved unsuccessful. The vitamin and mineral supplement should be chosen based on the needs of the child. Very large doses of supplements are unnecessary as no evidence supports intake in excess of the RDAs (15).

Children's diets should contain a wide variety of foods, as no "perfect" foods exist. The macro-nutrient breakdown of a child's diet is generally 15% to 20% protein, 45% to 55% carbohydrates, and 30% to 35% fat. Approximately 65% to 70% of the child's protein requirements should be in the form of high-quality protein—i.e., animal products or complimentary proteins that provide all of the essential amino acids (16). The carbohydrate intake should emphasize complex carbohydrates because their nutrient contribution is preferable to that of simple sugars. Fats in the diet should be varied so that the child's intake consists of an equivalent blend of saturated, monounsaturated and polyunsaturated fats. Typically, the diet of a child who consumes animal products includes adequate amounts of saturated fats. Consequently, added fats should take the form of vegetable oils and margarines that would provide mono- and polyunsaturated fats.

Assessing Nutritional Status

Strict elimination diets may produce deficiency disorders in individuals of any age. Because a growing child is the most susceptible to dietary deficiency from restricted diets, however, the emphasis of this section will be placed on assessment of the pediatric patient. Before one can ascertain whether a restricted diet has affected a child's growth, expected growth for the child must be defined. A child is generally expected to maintain or improve his or her growth rate consistent with previously established growth patterns. Table 32.1 defines normal growth rates for height and weight based on NCHS/CDC statistics at the 50th percentile. If a child varies significantly from these growth channels, further investigation of his or her growth is warranted.

Waterlow has developed a classification system that defines both stunting and wasting (17). "Height for age" is utilized as a measure of "stunting." Stunting is classified as being "mild," "moderate," or "severe." Increments of 5% are used because they represent approximately two standard deviations around the mean for "height for age." "Weight for height" is utilized as a measure of "wasting"; like stunting, it is classified as "mild," "moderate," or "severe." In this case, increments of 10% are used because they represent approximately one standard deviation around the mean. Table 32.2 provides Waterlow's classification of stunting and wasting.

To determine how the Waterlow classification is utilized, consider the following example. A 4-year-old boy whose height is 96 cm and whose weight is 13.5 kg would have the following plot (see Example A, Figs. 32.1 and 32.2):

Height—96 cm; 5–10th percentile for age
(based on NCHS/CDC)
Weight—13.5 kg; 3–5th percentile for age

$$\frac{\text{"Height for age"} = \text{actual height}}{\text{Height for age at 50th percentile}} \times 100$$

or

$$\frac{96 \text{ cm}}{102.9 \text{ cm}} \times 100 = 93\%$$

$$\frac{\text{"Weight for height"} = \text{actual weight}}{\text{Weight for height at 50th percentile}} \times 100$$

Table 32.1
Median Height and Weight Gains.

	Height Expected Change		Weight Expected Change	
	Boy	*Girl*	*Boy*	*Girl*
0–6 mo	17.3 cm	16.0 cm	4.5 kg	4.0 kg
6 mo–12 mo	8.3 cm	8.4 cm	2.4 kg	2.3 kg
12 mo–18 mo	6.3 cm	6.6 cm	1.3 kg	1.3 kg
18 mo–24 mo	5.2 cm	5.6 cm	1.1 kg	1.1 kg
24 mo–30 mo	4.8 cm	4.3 cm	1.2 kg	1.2 kg
30 mo–3 yr	4.5 cm	4.1 cm	1.1 kg	1.1 kg
3 yr–3 6/12 yr	4.2 cm	3.8 cm	1.1 kg	1.0 kg
3 6/12 yr–4 yr	3.8 cm	3.7 cm	1.0 kg	0.9 kg
4 yr–4 6/12 yr	3.7 cm	3.4 cm	1.0 kg	0.8 kg
4 6/12 yr–5 yr	3.3 cm	3.4 cm	1.0 kg	0.9 kg
5 yr–5 6/12 yr	3.2 cm	3.2 cm	1.0 kg	0.9 kg
5 6/12 yr–6 yr	3.0 cm	3.0 cm	1.0 kg	0.9 kg
6 yr–6 6/12 yr	2.9 cm	3.0 cm	1.0 kg	1.1 kg
6 6/12 yr–7 yr	2.7 cm	3.0 cm	1.2 kg	1.2 kg
7 yr–7 6/12 yr	2.7 cm	2.9 cm	1.1 kg	1.5 kg
7 6/12 yr–8 yr	2.6 cm	2.9 cm	1.3 kg	1.5 kg
8 yr–8 6/12 yr	2.6 cm	2.9 cm	1.4 kg	1.8 kg
8 6/12 yr–9 yr	2.6 cm	2.9 cm	1.4 kg	1.9 kg
9 yr–9 6/12 yr	2.6 cm	3.0 cm	1.6 kg	2.0 kg
9 6/12 yr–10 yr	2.7 cm	3.1 cm	1.7 kg	2.0 kg
10 yr–10 6/12 yr	2.8 cm	3.2 cm	1.9 kg	2.2 kg
10 6/12 yr–11 yr	3.0 cm	3.3 cm	2.0 kg	2.3 kg
11 yr–11 6/12 yr	3.1 cm	3.4 cm	2.2 kg	2.2 kg
11 6/12 yr–12 yr	3.3 cm	3.3 cm	2.3 kg	2.3 kg
12 yr–12 6/12 yr	3.3 cm	3.1 cm	2.5 kg	2.3 kg
12 6/12 yr–13 yr	3.5 cm	2.5 cm	2.7 kg	2.3 kg
13 yr–13 6/12 yr	3.4 cm	1.9 cm	2.8 kg	2.2 kg
13 6/12 yr–14 yr	3.2 cm	1.4 cm	3.0 kg	2.0 kg
14 yr–14 6/12 yr	3.1 cm	0.8 cm	3.0 kg	1.8 kg
14 6/12 yr–15 yr	2.8 cm	0.6 cm	2.9 kg	1.6 kg
15 yr–15 6/12 yr	2.5 cm	0.3 cm	2.8 kg	1.3 kg
15 6/12 yr–16 yr	2.0 cm	0.3 cm	2.6 kg	0.9 kg
16 yr–16 6/12 yr	1.7 cm	0.3 cm	2.3 kg	0.5 kg
16 6/12 yr–17 yr	1.0 cm	0.4 cm	1.9 kg	0.3 kg
17 yr–17 6/12 yr	0.5 cm	0.3 cm	1.5 kg	0
17 6/12 yr–18 yr	0.1 cm	0.3 cm	1.1 kg	0

(Modified from: Hamill PVV, Drizd TA, Johnson CL, Reed RB, Roche AF, Moore WM. Physical growth: National Center for Health Statistics percentiles. Am J Clin Nutr 1979;32:607–629.)

or

$$\frac{13.5 \text{ kg}}{13.9 \text{ kg}} \times 100 = 97\%$$

His growth would be considered as being mildly stunted, but showing no signs of wasting. This condition may indicate an acute nutritional insult—i.e., one that could occur when a severely restricted diet

Table 32.2
Waterlow Classification of Wasting or Stunting. Percentage of height for age and weight for height based on the 50th percentile of the Boston growth standard.

	Normal	Mild	Moderate	Severe
Stunting (low weight for age)	>95%	90%–95%	85%–90%	<85%
Wasting (low weight for height)	>90%	80%–90%	70%–80%	<70%

(Waterlow JC. Classification and definition of protein-energy malnutrition. In: Beaton GH, Bengoa JM, eds. Nutrition in preventive medicine. Geneva: WHO 1976, 530–555.)

is implemented for an extended period of time. This degree of undernutrition could eventually evolve into wasting if dietary modification is not initiated.

If a change in growth rate occurs in a child on a restricted diet, the first area of dietary intake to evaluate is the average daily caloric intake. For children who are attempting to maintain normal growth, the RDA may be used as the yardstick with which to measure their intake (Table 32.3).

For example, a 4-year-old boy who is at the 50th percentile for height for age would be approximately 103 cm tall and should weigh 16.5 kg to be at the 50th percentile for weight for height (see Example B, Figs. 32.1 and 32.2). His average daily caloric intake should be 1485 calories based on his weight multiplied by the RDA for calories (16.5 kg × 90 kcal/kg).

These same standards can be utilized to determine caloric needs for a child who is wasted or stunted. For a wasted child who is 103 cm tall, but who weighs only 14 kg, the following equation would be used to determine caloric requirements for catch-up weight gain (see Example C, Figs. 32.1 and 32.2):

$$\frac{\text{Weight for height at the 50th percentile}}{\text{Actual body weight}} \times 90$$
(calories for age)

or

$$\frac{16.5 \text{ kg}}{14 \text{ kg}} \times 90 = 106 \text{ cal/kg for catch-up weight gain}$$

This child would, therefore, require 1485 calories (106 cal/kg × 14 kg) for catch-up growth.

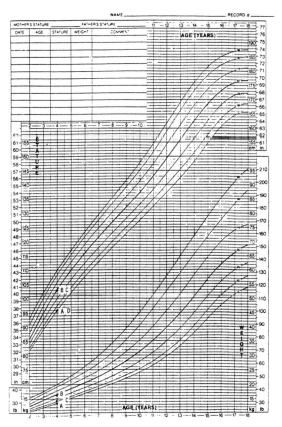

Figure 32.1

Height for age and weight for age. Reprinted with permission of Ross Laboratories, Columbus, OH 43216, from NCHS Growth Charts, © 1986 Ross Laboratories.

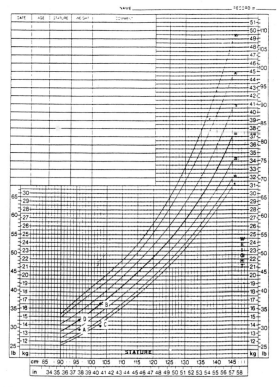

Figure 32.2

Weight for height. Reprinted with permission of Ross Laboratories, Columbus, OH 43216, from NCHS Growth Charts, © 1986 Ross Laboratories.

For the stunted child (e.g., a 4-year-old whose height is 96 cm), the following equation can be used to determine calories for catch-up growth (see Example D, Figs. 32.1 and 32.2):

Weight for actual height at 50th percentile
        × calories for age = calories for catch-up growth

or

$$14.6 \text{ kg} \times 90 \text{ cal/kg} = 1314 \text{ cal}$$

If the child's average caloric intake matches this level, it should be increased to satisfy the caloric requirements for a child who is at the 50th percentile for both height for age and weight for height.

Caloric requirements for catch-up growth can also be calculated by utilizing the child's estimated basal metabolic rate for his or her actual weight. Caloric requirements are estimated to be two times the basal metabolic rate (BMR). For a 14-kg child, the BMR would be 680 calories and 1360 calories would be required per day for catch-up growth. (See Table 32.4 for basal metabolic rates.)

Protein requirements are the second area of dietary intake that should be evaluated. Basically, 65% to 70% of a child's protein requirements should consist of high-quality protein, or protein of high biological value (16). A high-biological-value protein comes from an animal source. Thus, one or more of the following foods should be included in the child's diet: eggs, milk products, poultry, meat, or fish. An

Table 32.3
Recommended Dietary Allowances.

Age (Years)	Calories per Kilogram Ideal Weight	Protein per Kilogram Body Weight
0–0.5	108	2.2
0.5–1	98	1.6
1–3	102	1.2
4–6	90	1.1
7 10	70	1.0
11–14 Males	55	1.0
15–18 Males	45	0.9
19–22 Males	40	0.8
11–14 Females	47	1.0
15–18 Females	40	0.8
19–24 Females	38	0.8

Modified from Subcommittee on the Tenth Edition of the RDAs, Food and Nutrition Board Commission on Life Sciences National Research Council. Recommended Dietary Allowances, 10th ed. Washington, DC: National Academy Press, 1989, 33.

Table 32.4
Standard Basal Calories Based on Patient's Weight. (Vaughan VC, McKay RJ, Nelson WE, eds. Parenteral Fluid Therapy in Nelson Textbook of Pediatrics 1975. Philadelphia: WB Saunders Company, 1975, 251.)

Weight in Kilograms	Calories per 24 Hours Both Sexes
3	140
5	270
7	400
9	500
11	600
13	650
15	710
17	780
19	830
21	880

Weight in Kilograms	Male	Female
25	1020	960
29	1120	1040
33	1210	1120
37	1300	1190
41	1350	1260
45	1410	1320
49	1470	1380
53	1530	1440
57	1590	1500
61	1640	1560

exception should be made if the child is following a "vegan" vegetarian diet (which excludes all animal products, even milk and eggs). In such a case, the diet must be analyzed to ensure that it includes complimentary proteins that would provide adequate amounts of all essential amino acids. The remaining portion of dietary protein can be provided via plant proteins, which are called low-biological-value proteins. The National Academy of Sciences has established recommended daily dietary allowances for protein (18). Protein requirements are based on age and determined by body weight; for example, a 4-year-old requires 1.1 of protein per kilogram of body weight. Thus, a 4-year-old boy weighing 16.5 kg should consume a minimum of 18 g of protein per day, of which approximately 12.0 g should consist of high-biological-value protein (19). (See Table 32.3 for recommended protein intakes.)

The final area of the diet that should be evaluated involves the child's intake of vitamins and minerals. This intake should be compared with the RDAs for vitamins and minerals and the estimated safe and adequate daily dietary intake of other vitamins and minerals [see RDAs (15)] (Tables 32.5 and 32.6). The RDAs include a safety factor in their recommended levels to accommodate variation in bioavailability and individual requirements (20). If a patient's intake of a nutrient falls below 65% of the established standards, it may be considered to be deficient. The patient (or the patient's family) should be provided with a list of foods that represent good sources of the deficient nutrient or nutrients. If these foods cannot be incorporated into the child's diet, then a multivitamin and mineral supplement should be prescribed.

To undertake this type of dietary evaluation, an allergist generally requires the assistance of a registered dietitian. The patient or parents of a child should be instructed on the proper recording of dietary intake, and asked to keep a record for a period of 3 to 7 days. The completed dietary record may then be analyzed by one of the many available computer programs. The Food and Nutrition Information Center (FNIC) provides a complete listing of available nutrient analysis software that is updated quarterly and made available via the Internet (fnic@nalusda.gov) or the World Wide Web (http://www.nalusda.gov/fnic.html). The patient's average daily intake can

Table 32.5
RDAs for Vitamins and Minerals. Food and Nutrition Board, National Academy of Sciences—National Research Council. Recommended Dietary Allowances,[a] Revised 1989 Designed for the maintenance of good nutrition of practically all healthy people in the United States.

Category	Age (years) or Condition	Weight[b] (kg)	Weight[b] (lb)	Height[b] (cm)	Height[b] (in.)	Protein (g)	Fat-Soluble Vitamins Vitamin A (μg RE)[c]	Vitamin D (μg)[d]	Vitamin E (mg α-TE)[c]	Vitamin K (μg)
Infants	0.0–0.5	6	13	60	24	13	375	7.5	3	5
	0.5–1.0	9	20	71	28	14	375	10	4	10
Children	1–3	13	29	90	35	16	400	10	6	15
	4–6	20	44	112	44	24	500	10	7	20
	7–10	28	62	132	52	28	700	10	7	30
Males	11–14	45	99	157	62	45	1,000	10	10	45
	15–18	66	145	176	69	59	1,000	10	10	65
	19–24	72	160	177	70	58	1,000	10	10	70
	25–50	79	174	176	70	63	1,000	5	10	80
	51+	77	170	173	68	63	1,000	5	10	80
Females	11–14	46	101	157	62	46	800	10	8	45
	15–18	55	120	163	64	44	800	10	8	55
	19–24	58	128	164	65	46	800	10	8	60
	25–50	63	138	163	64	50	800	5	8	65
	51+	65	143	160	63	50	800	5	8	65
Pregnant						60	800	10	10	65
Lactating	1st 6 months					65	1,300	10	12	65
	2nd 6 months					62	1,200	10	11	65

[a] The allowances, expressed as average daily intakes over time, are intended to provide for individual variations among most normal persons as they live in the United States under usual environmental stresses. Diets should be based on a variety of common foods in order to provide other nutrients for which human requirements have been less well defined. See text for detailed discussion of allowances and of nutrients not tabulated.
[b] Weights and heights of Reference Adults are actual medians for the U.S. population of the designated age, as reported by NHANES II. The median weights and heights of those under 19 years of age were taken from Hamill *et al.* (1979) (see pages 16–17). The use of these figures does not imply that the height-to-weight ratios are ideal.
[c] Retinol equivalents, 1 retinol equivalent = 1 μg retinol or 6 μg β-carotene. See text for calculation of vitamin A activity of diets as retinol equivalents.
[d] As cholecalciferol, 10 μg cholecalciferol = 400 IU of vitamin D.
[e] α-Tocopherol equivalents, 1 mg d-α tocopherol = 1 α-TE. See text for variation in allowances and calculation of vitamin E activity of the diet as α-tocopherol equivalents.
[f] 1 NE (niacin equivalent) is equal to 1 mg of niacin or 60 mg of dietary tryptophan.

be compared with the standards described above for calories, protein, vitamins, and minerals, and a nutritional intervention program established.

Modifying Diet for Diagnosis

Double-blind, placebo-controlled food challenges represent the "gold standard" by which to diagnose food allergy. In the early stages of the diagnostic work-up, however, elimination diets are often utilized. If a limited number of foods are suspected, they may be totally eliminated from the diet for as long as two weeks prior to anticipated challenge. When food allergy is suspected but no specific foods are implicated, highly restrictive diets are sometimes employed. Such diets might include the following provisions:

Infants < 4 months: casein hydrolysate or amino acid formula (e.g., Neocate)
4–8 months: infant diet + rice cereal + pears
9–24 months: 4–8 months diet + rice + squash + lamb

| Water-Soluble Vitamins | | | | | | | Minerals | | | | | | |
Vitamin C (mg)	Thiamin (mg)	Ribo-flavin (mg)	Niacin b (mg NE)	Vitamin B$_6$ (mg)	Folate (μg)	Vitamin B$_{11}$ (μg)	Calcium (mg)	Phos-phorus (mg)	Mag-nesium (mg)	Iron (mg)	Zinc (mg)	Iodine (μg)	Sele-nium (μg)
30	0.3	0.4	5	0.3	25	0.3	400	300	40	6	5	40	10
35	0.4	0.5	6	0.6	35	0.5	600	500	60	10	5	50	15
40	0.7	0.8	9	1.0	50	0.7	800	800	80	10	10	70	20
45	0.9	1.1	12	1.1	75	1.0	800	800	120	10	10	90	20
45	1.0	1.2	13	1.4	100	1.4	800	800	170	10	10	120	30
50	1.3	1.5	17	1.7	150	2.0	1,200	1,200	270	12	15	150	40
60	1.5	1.8	20	2.0	200	2.0	1,200	1,200	400	12	15	150	50
60	1.5	1.7	19	2.0	200	2.0	1,200	1,200	350	10	15	150	70
60	1.5	1.7	19	2.0	200	2.0	800	800	350	10	15	150	70
60	1.2	1.4	15	2.0	200	2.0	800	800	350	10	15	150	70
50	1.1	1.3	15	1.4	150	2.0	1,200	1,200	280	15	12	150	45
60	1.1	1.3	15	1.5	180	2.0	1,200	1,200	300	15	12	150	50
60	1.1	1.3	15	1.6	180	2.0	1,200	1,200	280	15	12	150	55
60	1.1	1.3	15	1.6	180	2.0	800	800	280	15	12	150	55
60	1.0	1.2	13	1.6	180	2.0	800	800	280	10	12	150	55
70	1.5	1.6	17	2.2	400	2.2	1,200	1,200	320	30	15	175	65
95	1.6	1.8	20	2.1	280	2.6	1,200	1,200	355	15	19	200	75
90	1.6	1.7	20	2.1	260	2.6	1,200	1,200	340	15	16	200	75

Reprinted with permission from RECOMMENDED DIETARY ALLOWANCES: 10th edition, National Academy Press, 1989.

> 24 months: 9–24 months diet + fresh lettuce + potato + safflower oil + tea + sugar

or

Amino acid formula (e.g., Neocate One +)

Restricted diets are not without risk, and if prolonged, can lead to malnutrition and growth retardation. A restricted diet that has been implemented without confirmation by a double-blind, placebo-controlled food challenge should be instituted for only a brief (1–6 weeks) period. With IgE-mediated disorders, symptomatic improvement should appear within 1 to 2 weeks; in contrast, with several of the non–IgE-mediated gastrointestinal hypersensitivities (e.g., food-induced enteropathy or allergic eosinophilic gastroenteritis), significant symptomatic improvement may not be seen for 4 to 6 weeks. No evidence exists that more prolonged restrictive diets are necessary for any of the well-substantiated food hypersensitivities.

When only one or two foods are "suspect," the patient or parents of a child may eliminate these foods while including other foods from similar food categories. For example, if eggs and wheat are the "suspect" foods, the diet can be supplemented with other sources of animal protein and other grains to replace the nutrients contributed from eggs and wheat. A common mistake is to eliminate foods from the diet without replacing them with alternative nutrient sources. For example, a child who is egg- and wheat-restricted and consumes no breads or other baked goods may have a diet that is deficient in certain B vitamins and iron, as fortified breads and baked goods contribute significant amounts of these nutrients. Milk presents a more difficult nutritional restriction. Attempts should be made to replace milk with a soy (Isomil, Prosobee, Nursoy, or Soyalac) or a protein hydrolysate (Alimentum, Nutramigen, or Pregestimil; but *not* Good Start, which is a partial whey hydrolysate) or an amino acid formula (Neocate, Neocate One +, EO 28, or Tolorex), which will

Table 32.6
Estimated Safe and Adequate Daily Dietary Intakes of Other
Vitamins or Minerals[a] (Trace or Ultra-Trace Minerals)

Category	Age (years)	Vitamins	
		Biotin (μg)	Pantothenic Acid (mg)
Infants	0–0.5	10	2
	0.5 1	15	3
Children and adolescents	1–3	20	3
	4–6	25	3–4
	7–10	30	4–5
	11 +	30–100	4–7
Adults		30–100	4–7

Category	Age (years)	Trace Elements[b]				
		Copper (mg)	Manganese (mg)	Fluoride (mg)	Chromium (μg)	Molybdenum (μg)
Infants	0–0.5	0.4–0.6	0.3–0.6	0.1–0.5	10–40	15–30
	0.5–1	0,6–0.7	0.6–1.0	0.2–1.0	20–60	20–40
Children and adolescents	1–3	0.7–1.0	1.0–1.5	0.5–1.5	20–80	25–50
	4–6	1.0–1.5	1.5–2.0	1.0–2.5	30–120	30–75
	7–10	1.0–2.0	2.0–3.0	1.5–2.5	50–200	50–150
	11 +	1.5–2.5	2.0–5.0	1.5–2.5	50–200	75–250
Adults		1.5–3.0	2.0–5.0	1.5–4.0	50–200	75–250

[a] Because there is less information on which to base allowances, these figures are not given in the main table of RDA and are provided here in the form of ranges of recommended intakes.
[b] Since the toxic levels for many trace elements may be only several times usual intakes, the upper levels for the trace elements given in this table should not be habitually exceeded.

provide the nutrients typically found in milk and milk products.

If a strict elimination diet is instituted, one should attempt to provide a nutritionally complete diet. Table 32.7 provides sample meal patterns that would meet greater than 75% of a 4-year-old child's RDAs. The enriched rice milk provides calcium and vitamin D at levels found in milk. If enriched rice milk is unavailable, the diet would need to be supplemented for these two nutrients. (Table 32.8 lists types of calcium supplements.)

A highly restricted diet is monotonous and should be "opened" with the introduction of one previously restricted food every four to five days. Symptom records should be maintained during both periods of complete elimination and reintroduction. Long-term dietary restriction of various foods re-

quires confirmation of hypersensitivity by double-blind, placebo-controlled food challenges, as sole reliance on an elimination diet can lead to an erroneous diagnosis of food allergy. An excessive number of foods are often eliminated because environmental factors confound the evaluation, resulting in an erroneous diagnosis of hypersensitivity. Equally likely is that key food allergies will be missed because the patient maintains the same level of disease activity throughout the trial period and the patient (or his or her parents) is unable to detect any significant changes.

Infrequently formula-only diets are instituted. If a child can tolerate a protein hydrolysate formula (such as Nutramigen, Pregestimil, or Alimentum), it should be used rather than an amino acid formula, such as Neocate. A protein hydrolysate formula is

Table 32.7
Sample Meal Patterns

Sample Meal Pattern 1

Breakfast
1 cup enriched rice milk
1 cup grits, enriched
2 homemade pork sausage patties
2 egg-, milk-, wheat-free banana rice muffins

Lunch
1 broiled lamb chop
1 serving french-fried potatoes
½ cup cooked carrots
1 cup enriched rice milk

Dinner
1 broiled pork chop
1 boiled potato
½ cup cooked squash
1 serving canned pears
1 cup enriched rice milk

Vegetable oils or unsalted, milk-free margarine can be used to provide additional calories.

Sample Meal Pattern 2

Breakfast
1 cup enriched rice milk
1 cup puffed rice cereal
2 ounce grilled fresh ham slice
2 rice pancakes with pure maple syrup

Lunch
3 ounce ground lamb patty
2 slices egg-, milk-, and wheat-free bread
1 ounce potato chips
½ cup applesauce
1 cup enriched rice milk

Dinner
1 broiled pork chop
1 cup white rice
1 serving cooked spinach
1 serving canned pineapple
1 cup enriched rice milk

Vegetable oils or unsalted, milk-free margarine can be used to provide additional calories.

Sample Meal Pattern 3

Breakfast
1 cup enriched rice milk
1 cup cream of rice cereal
4 slices bacon
2 egg-, milk-, wheat-free corn muffins

Lunch
2 slices fresh ham
2 slices of egg-, milk-, and wheat-free bread
1 ounce potato chips
1 banana
1 cup enriched rice milk

Table 32.7 (Continued)

Dinner
1 boiled lamp chop
1 baked potato
1 serving cooked broccoli
1 serving canned peaches
1 cup enriched rice milk

Vegetable oils or unsalted, milk-free margarine can be used to provide additional calories.

preferable because amino acid formulas are very costly and should be utilized only in documented cases of failure on protein hydrolysate formulas. If an amino acid formula becomes necessary, products are available for various age groups, from infants through adults. (Table 32.9 contains a chart comparing these products.) Amino acid formulas should be analyzed for their protein, essential fatty acids, vitamin, and mineral content, and modified as needed.

Table 32.8
Calcium-Fortified Foods and Supplements

Fortified Food	Elemental Calcium (mg)
6 fl oz Minute Maid Calcium Fortified Orange Juice	200
6 fl oz Gerber Graduate Juices	200
6 fl oz Hawaiian Punch Double C	110
6 fl oz Sunny Delight Calcium Orange Drink	250
8 fl oz Enriched Rice Dream Rice Milk	300
1 oz Total cereal	200

Supplement	Elemental Calcium (mg/tablet)
Alka-Mints Chewable	340
Calci-Mix	500 mg/capsule
Cal Quik	400 mg/tsp
Neo-calglucon syrup	115 mg/tsp
Rolaids	220
Extra Strength Rolaids	400
Titralac Regular Chewable tablets	168
Titralac Extra Strength tablets	300
Tums	200
Tums E-X	300

Table 32.9
Comparison of Nutrient Content of Elemental
Formulas (per 1000 kilocalories)

Nutrients	Neocate	Neocate One + pwd	Tolerex
Energy, kcal/g of powder	4.21	4.00	3.75
Protein equivalent, g	31	25	21
Fat, g	45	35	1.5
Carbohydrate, g	117	146	230
Calcium, mg	1240	620	560
Phosphorus, mg	931	620	560
Magnesium, mg	124	90	220
Iron, mg	18.5	7.7	10
Zinc, mg	16.6	7.7	8.3
Manganese, mg	0.9	1.0	1.6
Copper, mg	1.24	1.0	1.1
Iodine, mcg	154	60	83
Sodium, mg	373	200	460
Potassium, mg	1551	930	1200
Chloride, mg	772	350	955
Selenium, mcg	37.3	15.4	83
Chromium, mcg	35.6	30	28
Molybdenum, mcg	47.5	35	83
Vitamin A, mcg RE	1227	350	833
Vitamin D, mcg	21.75	7.8	5.5
Vitamin E, mg α-TE	7.65	5.5	11.4
Vitamin K, mcg	87.9	15	37
Vitamin C, mg	92.6	31	33
Thiamine, mg	0.926	0.5	0.8
Riboflavin, mg	1.378	0.65	0.9
Vitamin B_6, mg	1.235	0.8	1.1
Vitamin B_{12}, mcg	1.70	0.7	3.3
Niacin, mg	15.44	9.0	11
Folic acid, mcg	102	60	220
Pantothenic acid, mg	6.2	2.4	5.6
Biotin, mcg	31	20	170
Osmolality at std dilution (mg mOsms/kg)	342	610	550

Management of Food-Allergic Patients

A few foods are responsible for the majority of allergic reactions (21). In adults, these foods include nuts, peanuts, fish, and shellfish. In children, the main culprits include egg, milk, peanuts, soy, wheat, and fish. The elimination of each of these foods and the potential nutritional consequences will be addressed separately.

MILK

Once a patient has been diagnosed as milk-allergic, milk must be completely removed from the diet. No milk or milk by-products are allowed—not even in small amounts. Table 32.10 lists words found on food product labels that would indicate the presence of milk proteins (i.e., "milk words"). Any product that contains one or more of these words on its label ingredient list should not be consumed on a milk-restricted diet. In addition, patients should be instructed to contact food manufacturers regarding ingredients such as caramel, brown sugar and natural flavors, margarine, chocolate, and high-protein flours that may contain milk or milk by-products. Simplesse is a fat substitute made from either egg or milk protein; it should be avoided by individuals sensitive to either milk or egg. In addition, deli meats may suffer cross-contamination resulting from slicing cheese products or other meat products containing milk. Processed meats—including hot dogs, sausages, and luncheon meats—may contain milk proteins, particularly the low- and reduced-fat product varieties. In some products, milk proteins may be labeled as "natural flavoring." In these cases, kosher labeling may help indicate whether the product contains milk proteins. Other hidden sources of milk products may include "carryover contamination" during processing of the food product [e.g., non–milk-based desserts, fruit juices, and drinks in single serving tetra packs (vacuum-sealed cardboard boxes)].

A child on a milk-restricted diet may not be consuming adequate amounts of the following nutrients: vitamin D, vitamin B_{12}, riboflavin, pantothenic acid, calcium, and phosphorus. Milk is a nutrient-"dense" food and a primary source of calcium and vitamin D. To emphasize the importance of milk as a source of nutrients for a growing child's diet, consider the following example. A child of 4 to 6 years of age who typically consumes three 8-ounce glasses of milk per day receives the following nutrients from the milk intake alone: 100% of the vitamin B_{12}, riboflavin, and calcium requirements; 75% to 85% of the vitamin D and phosphorus requirements; and 55% to 60% of his pantothenic acid requirements. Alternative sources of these nutrients may be pro-

Table 32.10
Label Ingredients That Indicate the Presence
of Milk Protein

Artificial butter flavor
Butter, butter fat
Buttermilk and buttermilk solids
Casein
Caseinates (ammonium, calcium, magnesium, potassium,
    sodium)
Cheese, cottage cheese, curds
Cream
Custard, pudding
Ghee
Half and Half
Hydrolysates (casein, milk protein, protein, whey, whey protein)
Lactalbumin, lactalbumin phosphate
Lactoglobulin
Lactose
Milk (derivative, protein, solids, malted, condensed, evaporated,
    dry, whole, low-fat, nonfat, skim)
Nougat
Rennet casein
Sour cream and sour cream solids
Whey (delactosed, demineralized, protein concentrate)
Yogurt

Label Ingredients That *May* Indicate the Presence of Milk Protein

Brown sugar flavoring	Margarine
Caramel flavoring	Natural flavoring
Chocolate	Simplesse
High-protein flour	

vided in milk-free formula preparations such as casein hydrolysates and soy formulas. Children currently on "infant" milk-free formulas should continue on these formulas as long as they remain acceptable to the child. Such formulas need not be discontinued based on the child's age. If a formula has been discontinued, attempts should be made to reintroduce milk-free formulas or enriched soy or rice milk beverages into children's diets to provide a good source of calcium, phosphorus, vitamin A, and vitamin D. A child on a milk-restricted diet who does not receive a milk substitute will require calcium and vitamin D supplementation.

Alternative sources of the other major nutrients found in milk include meats, legumes, nuts, and whole grains. Children who are milk-allergic may sometimes react to one or more of these alternative nutrient sources as well, which makes balancing their nutritional intake more difficult. Obtaining regular dietary intake records for patients can assist in identifying possible nutrient deficiencies. Nutrient intake is considered inadequate when the patient consumes less than two-thirds of the various RDAs as based on a minimum of a three-day diet record average. Supplementation should be provided either by dietary modification, vitamin and mineral supplementation, or provision of a nutritionally complete milk-free formula.

EGG

A patient who has been diagnosed as having a food hypersensitivity to eggs must avoid all forms of eggs. Table 32.11 lists words that indicate the presence of egg protein. Any product whose label contains one or more of these words in the ingredient list should not be consumed by a patient on an egg-restricted diet.

Eggs are not an essential food in the diet of an adult or child. They represent a dietary source of vitamin B_{12}, pantothenic acid, folacin, riboflavin, selenium, and biotin. One egg provides between 10% and 20% of a 4- to 6-year-old child's requirements for these nutrients. Typically, these nutrients can easily be supplied by other foods in the patient's diet, however.

Eggs are incorporated in a wide variety of products because of their excellent physical properties in food processing (e.g., coagulation, stabilization, emulsification). They may be used to form the custard

Table 32.11
Label Ingredients That Indicate the
Presence of Egg Proteins

Albumin
Dried egg
Egg, egg white, egg yolk
Egg powder, egg solids, egg substitutes
Eggnog
Globulin
Livetin
Lysozyme
Mayonnaise
Meringue
Ovalbumin
Ovomucin, ovomucoid, ovovitellin
Simplesse

base of ice creams and yogurts. Egg whites may be used to give pretzels, bagels, and other baked goods a shiny outer finish. (Labels may not indicate the presence of an egg glaze on some bakery products, such as breads and rolls.) Because eggs are used in coating batters for fried foods, the egg-allergic patient should avoid buying fried foods from vendors who do not maintain separate vats for frying each type of food sold because of the possibility of food protein carryover. Egg whites or shells may be used as clarifying agents in soup stocks, consommes, bouillons, and coffees. In addition, eggs have been used in imitation shellfish and institutional pureed foods to improve texture and appearance.

For each egg required in cooking, the following substitutions can be made:

1. Mix 1 packet of unflavored gelatin with 1 cup boiling water. Substitute 3 tablespoons of this liquid for each egg. Refrigerate the remainder for as long as 1 week, and microwave it to liquefy it for reuse. Use this mixture in recipes with another source of leavening (i.e., baking powder or baking soda).
2. 1½ tablespoons water plus 1½ tablespoons oil plus 1 teaspoon baking powder.
3. 1 teaspoon baking powder plus 1 tablespoon water plus 1 tablespoon vinegar (add vinegar separately at the end for rising).
4. 1 teaspoon yeast dissolved in ¼ cup warm water.
5. 1 tablespoon apricot puree (works as a binder, not a leavening agent).

One problem that may occur on an egg-restricted diet is the unintentional limitation of grain products, as many such foods contain egg. A child's diet that is limited in eggs and grain is apt to be inadequate in some of the B vitamins and possibly iron. Thus, it is important to teach families how to prepare foods without eggs.

PEANUTS

Peanut sensitivity is fairly common in both children and adults, but somewhat easier to manage than sensitivity to its legume relative, soybeans. The majority of individuals who are allergic to peanuts are not generally affected adversely by tree nuts such as pecans, walnuts, or almonds. In such a situation, other nuts can be substituted for peanuts, either in baked goods or as homemade nut butter spreads. Peanut protein (especially peanut butter) is used in a variety of different foods; some foods known to contain peanuts or peanut products include marzipan, chili, spaghetti sauces, shish kabobs, egg rolls, ethnic dishes, cereals, crackers, soups, baked goods, frozen desserts, and candy. Foods that contain peanut or peanut products may be labeled with the following "peanut words": peanut, peanut butter; peanut extracts; peanut flour; cold pressed, expressed, or expelled peanut oil; ground nuts; and mixed nuts. Hydrolyzed plant and vegetable protein is typically derived from soybean in food from the United States, but imported foods frequently use peanuts as a source for this ingredient. The term "natural flavoring" should also be regarded with caution, as this generic term encompasses any food component added to impart a particular flavor and can include any of the major allergenic foods.

An important issue that remains unresolved is the quantity of peanut antigen necessary to provoke an allergic response. In a study reported by Walzer, the investigator induced a wheal-and-flare reaction at a passively sensitized skin site with an intravenous injection of the protein nitrogen equivalent of 1/44,000 of one peanut kernel (22). In the Johns Hopkins series, allergic reactions (both cutaneous and gastrointestinal) have developed after children contacted residual peanut butter on counters or tables wiped-clean of visible material. Two patients developed wheezing and urticaria after a jar of peanut butter was opened in front of them, similar to a case reported by Fries (23). Utilizing double-blind, placebo-controlled food challenges, 50 mg to 100 mg of peanut flour has elicited allergic symptoms in some children. It should be remembered, however, that the most sensitive patients—those experiencing life-threatening anaphylaxis—were not challenged. Although occasional reports of allergic reactions to peanut oil have surfaced, a study of 10 peanut allergic adults failed to demonstrate any reactivity (24). Some of the alleged reactions to peanut oil probably relate to the presence of other food protein in oil used for frying (e.g., fish and other seafood). Some caution may still be necessary. To be 95% certain that 95% of peanut-allergic patients will not react to peanut oil, 58 peanut-allergic individuals would have to receive a peanut oil challenge with no untoward reactions (i.e., to satisfy table of confidence bounds for population failure rate).

Peanuts provide the following nutrients: niacin, magnesium, vitamin E, manganese, and chromium in significant amounts and smaller amounts of potassium, vitamin B_6, folacin, phosphorus, copper, and biotin. Fortunately, many other foods, including other nuts, can provide these same nutrients. Thus, a peanut restriction alone would not negatively affect a growing child's diet.

TREE NUTS

A variety of nuts have been implicated as the cause of severe anaphylactic reactions: almond, Brazil nut, cashew, chestnut, filbert, hazelnut, hickory, macadamia, pecan, pine nut, pistachio, and walnut. Tree nuts are being added to an increasing variety of foods such as barbecue sauces, cereals, crackers, and frozen desserts. Ethnic foods, commercially prepared baked goods, and candy can be cross-contaminated with nuts as they are frequently used in some varieties of foods. Foods that list natural flavors must be checked for the possible use of nuts as a flavoring agent. Table 32.12 provides a list of tree nuts and ingredients that contain tree nuts. Absent from this list are coconut, water chestnut, nutmeg, and mace, which are not restricted on a diet that eliminates tree nuts.

Although reports of nut sensitivity would indicate that it is one of the most common food hypersensitivities in adults, little information is available regarding actual prevalence. Patients suffering from an anaphylactic reaction to one nut are often told to avoid other nuts because of potential cross-reactivity, although little information exists to validate this belief. Not infrequently, patients allergic to peanuts (a legume) mistakenly avoid nuts as well. In one study of peanut-allergic children, 19 of 32 challenge-positive children were skin-tested to nuts (25); 12 of 19 had a positive skin test to one or more nuts (walnut, 11; filbert, 10; cashew, 9; almond, 6; pecan, 6; and pistachio, 6). None of these children experienced a positive double-blind challenge to a nut. Although

Table 32.12
Label Ingredients That Indicate the Presence of Tree Nuts

Almonds
Brazil nut
Cashew
Chestnut
Filbert/hazelnut
Gianduja (a creamy mixture of chocolate and chopped toasted nuts found in premium or imported chocolate)
Hickory nut
Macadamia nut
Marzipan/almond paste
Nougat
Nut butters, nut oil, nut paste
Pecan
Pine nut (Pignolia, Pinion)
Pistachio
Walnut

immunologic cross-reactivity (or multiple asymptomatic sensitivity) may be common, it is unlikely that a nut-allergic patient will react to a variety of different nuts. Until this subject has been carefully addressed with double-blind challenge studies, however, caution must be exercised in recommending the ingestion of different nuts in nut-allergic patients.

SOYBEAN

Soybean hypersensitivity is much less common than peanut sensitivity, but avoidance of soy products can prove much more difficult. Soybeans constitute a major component of processed food products in the United States and other parts of the world. Both soybeans and soybean products are incorporated in infant formulas, baked goods, canned tuna, cereals, crackers, soups, and sauces. Table 32.13 lists "soy words" denoting foods that may contain soy protein. In addition, soy is often utilized as a carrier protein for flavorings as it is relatively flavorless and readily absorbs the flavors of other foods. Individuals on soy exclusion diets should contact the manufacturers of foods containing natural flavors or flavorings to ensure that the product does not contain soy protein.

The processing of most soybean oils removes the protein portion. A study conducted in seven soy-allergic individuals found no reactions to soy oil when the subjects were challenged blindly with soy

Table 32.13
Label Ingredients That Indicate the
Presence of Soy Protein

Miso
Shoyo sauce
Soy flour, soy grits, soy milk, soy nuts, soy sprouts
Soy protein concentrate, soy protein isolate
Soy sauce
Tempeh
Textured vegetable protein (TVP)
Tofu

Label Ingredients That *May* Indicate the Presence of Soy Protein

Flavorings
Hydrolyzed plant protein
Hydrolyzed soy protein
Hydrolyzed vegetable protein
Natural flavoring
Vegetable broth, vegetable gum, vegetable starch

oil (26). As in the blinded challenge study to peanut oil, patient numbers were insufficient to state unequivocally that soy oil is safe in all highly sensitive soy patients. Currently, children with soybean sensitivity are allowed to consume soybean oil and soy lecithin. If a child's allergic symptoms continue or show signs of reexacerbation, however, all soybean products should be eliminated during a trial period.

Soybeans contribute the following nutrients to a patient's diet: thiamin, riboflavin, vitamin B_6, folacin, calcium, phosphorus, magnesium, iron, and zinc. Like the foods previously discussed, soybeans alone do not make major contributions to overall nutrition, but the exclusion of foods that contain soybean proteins may have a dramatic dietary impact.

The classification of foods by botanical family has inspired considerable confusion about the importance of intra-botanical cross-reactivity, especially in relation to legumes. A study in challenge-proven legume-allergic patients demonstrated that symptomatic reactivity to multiple members of the legume family is rare, despite evidence for broad antibody cross-reactivity provided by prick skin tests or RAST results (9, 27). This study reported that, among 69 patients who had one or more positive prick skin tests to legumes, 41 patients (59%) had legume sensitivity documented via blinded challenge or convincing history of severe anaphylaxis. Of the 41 legume-sensitive

patients, only 2 (5%) exhibited symptomatic reactivity to more than one legume. Both of these individuals had a history of severe anaphylaxis following peanut ingestion and a positive challenge to soybeans. When they were maintained on a peanut- and soybean-restricted diet both lost their symptomatic soybean reactivity within one to three years of the initial challenge. Both patients were able to consume other legumes without any problems. This study indicates that a symptomatic reactivity to one legume does not necessitate the elimination of the entire legume food family unless a clinical hypersensitivity to each legume is individually confirmed by blinded oral challenges.

FISH

Fish is reported to be one of the most common causes of food allergic reactions in adults, and one of the most common causes of food allergy for individuals of all ages in countries where large quantities of fish are consumed. *Gad c* 1, a parvalbumin, has been well characterized, and is believed similar in many species of fish (28). Consequently, it is generally recommended that fish-allergic individuals avoid all species of fish. In a study of fish-allergic patients undergoing double-blind challenges to a number of different fish species, most patients allergic to one species of fish could safely ingest a different species (10). Results of skin tests and RASTs indicate extensive cross-reactivity among fish species and do not help determine which fish can be ingested safely (29). One should assume extensive cross-reactivity among fish and eliminate all fish from the diet of fish-allergic patients unless blinded challenges are conducted to determine which fish species may be eaten safely. If a fish-allergic patient can tolerate certain fish species, he or she must be very careful when eating at restaurants to ensure that the fish species ordered is not substituted with another species.

A food allergy to fish may be welcomed by some children in the United States, for whom fish is typically not a favorite food. Fish can provide some key nutrients to a child's diet, however, in addition to providing an alternative source of high-biological-value protein. A 3.5 ounce serving of fish provides significant amounts of niacin, vitamin B$_6$, vitamin B$_{12}$, vitamin E, phosphorus, and selenium. To a somewhat lesser degree, it also serves as a dietary source of potassium, magnesium, and iron.

Typically fish is not a hidden ingredient in foods. Foods that may contain unsuspected fish or fish products include worcestershire sauce (if it contains anchovy), caesar salad, caviar, and roe. In addition, fish is sometimes flavored and sold as imitation lobster or other shellfish.

SHELLFISH

Allergic reactions to various shellfish, crustacea (shrimp, crabs, lobster, and crawfish), and mollusks (clams, oysters, and scallops) reportedly are common in adults. Extensive work is focusing on the characterization of various crustacean and mollusk antigens. In practice, individuals allergic to one shellfish are told to avoid other shellfish because skin testing or RASTs commonly demonstrate cross-reactivity. Little data are available to support or refute this practice, so caution must continue to be exercised in recommending consumption of other seafood in shellfish-allergic patients. Shellfish are generally not "hidden" in foods, but occasionally different shellfish may be included in dishes unbeknownst to a waiter in a restaurant.

WHEAT

Because wheat is a predominant food product in the United States and other countries, wheat elimination diets are particularly difficult for a patient and his or her family to maintain. Children on wheat-restricted diets are severely limited in their selection of foods. Cereals, breads, pastas, crackers, and cookies are obviously limited, as are some sauces, lunch meats, snack foods, and candy. Families complying with this restriction generally can utilize products made from oats, rice, rye, barley, or corn that may be available in grocery or health food stores. One study indicates that as many as 20% of wheat-allergic children will react to another cereal grain (11). Additionally, caution is advised with the use of two products: Kamut, an ancient wheat grain, and Triticale, a hybrid of wheat and rye. These foods have not yet been clini-

cally evaluated in wheat-sensitive individuals. In addition, wheat-allergic patients may use specialty food products intended primarily for people with gluten-sensitive enteropathy (celiac disease), who must avoid all gluten-containing grains (i.e., wheat, oats, barley, and rye). These foods may be found in special dietary shops or ordered via mail-order companies. Finally, a large number of wheat-free recipes are available from which to prepare a variety of baked goods, thereby permitting greater variety in the diet and improved nutrient density.

A child who must follow a wheat elimination diet should avoid all types of wheat products. Table 32.14 lists foods that may or do contain wheat products. Any food item that includes one of these ingredients should not be consumed on a wheat exclusion diet. A child on a wheat avoidance diet faces a risk related to insufficient intake of the following nutrients: thiamin, riboflavin, niacin, iron, selenium,

Table 32.14
Label Ingredients That Indicate the Presence of Wheat Proteins

Bread crumbs
Bran
Bulgar
Cereal extract
Couscous
Cracker meal
Durum wheat
Enriched flour
Farina
Gluten
Graham flour
High-gluten flour, high-protein flour
Semolina wheat
Spelt
Vital gluten
Wheat bran, wheat germ, wheat gluten, wheat malt, wheat starch
Whole wheat flour

Label Ingredients That *May* Indicate the Presence of Wheat Protein

Gelatinized starch
Hydrolyzed vegetable protein
Kamut
Modified food starch, modified starch
Natural flavoring
Soy sauce
Starch
Triticale
Vegetable gum, vegetable starch

and chromium. Four servings of wheat products will provide 20% to 40% of the requirements for these nutrients in a 4- to 6-year-old child's diet. The thiamin, riboflavin, niacin, or iron in baked goods derives from the fortification of wheat flours to levels found in whole grains. Wheat products also contribute to a patient's intake of magnesium, folacin, phosphorus, and molybdenum. Given that wheat contributes several important nutrients, a child on a wheat elimination diet should have his or her intake evaluated for possible nutritional inadequacies.

RICE

Rice allergy is much less common than wheat allergy. Because rice is not a principal food in the typical U.S. diet, it is considerably easier to avoid than either wheat or corn. A rice exclusion diet alone should not cause any dietary problems. If rice avoidance is combined with elimination of another cereal grain, however, evaluation of nutrient intake may be more important. Rice contributes thiamin, riboflavin, niacin, and iron, primarily via fortification of these nutrients. "Rice words" found on food labels that may indicate its presence as an ingredient include rice flour, rice starch, rice noodles, and rice bran. Foods that contain these items should be avoided on a rice elimination diet.

CORN

Fortunately, a true allergy to corn is very rare. Corn elimination diets are very difficult to manage because corn and corn products constitute ingredients in a majority of processed food products, primarily in the form of corn sweeteners or cornstarch. Table 32.15 lists words that may indicate the presence of corn protein in the product (i.e., "corn words") and thus must be avoided on a corn exclusion diet. Corn oil is not listed as a food to avoid. Because the allergenic portion (protein) is removed in the processing of corn oil, it is considered safe for corn-sensitive patients. A small study challenging documented corn-allergic patients with corn oil, corn sugar, and corn syrup provoked no reactions, whereas blinded challenge with cornstarch did provoke one reaction (30). In the

Table 32.15
Label Ingredients That Indicate the Presence of Corn Proteins

Baking powder
Caramel flavoring
Corn, corn alcohol, corn flour, cornstarch, cornmeal
Corn sweetener, corn syrup solids
Dextrates, dextrins
Grits
Hominy
Maize
Maltodextrins
Marshmallow
Powdered sugar

Label Ingredients That *May* Indicate the Presence of Corn Proteins

Food starch
Modified food starch
Vegetable gum
Vegetable starch

Johns Hopkins series, one corn-allergic patient also reacted to cornstarch on blinded challenge.

As can be seen from the list of "corn words," a corn elimination diet would restrict consumption of a variety of foods, including baked goods, beverages, candy, canned fruits, cereals, cookies, jams, jellies, lunch meats, snack foods, and syrups. A patient on a corn elimination diet must rely on alternative sweeteners, thickeners, and leavening agents, such as fruit juices, beet or cane sugar, maple syrup, honey, aspartame, wheat starch, potato starch, rice starch, tapioca, baking soda, and cream of tartar. As with a wheat exclusion diet, many commonly available convenience items must be avoided. The patient may, however, be able to find some convenience foods that have either eliminated sugar from the food or substituted a sweetener such as natural fruit juices or honey. Health food stores typically carry a variety of baked goods and some candies that are made with safe ingredients. The family may also use homemade foods.

Corn elimination affects nutrient intake primarily through the exclusion of other food products containing corn protein, rather than because of the nutrient contribution of corn alone. Corn contributes thiamin, riboflavin, niacin, and iron, via fortification of corn products; it also provides chromium. These nutrients are found in similar amounts in other grain products such as wheat or rice, so any other fortified grain could be substituted for corn. A child who is being strictly maintained on a corn elimination diet may benefit from a dietary evaluation, as the nutritional adequacy of his or her diet would depend on the family's ability to provide varied alternative foods.

OTHER GRAINS

The remaining grains—i.e., oats, barley, and rye—will not be discussed individually because they provoke food sensitivities less commonly than most of the foods discussed earlier. It should be noted, however, that most "all purpose flours" contain barley, and should, therefore, be taken into consideration in patients with suspected wheat sensitivity. Information on gluten-free diets may be obtained from the Celiac Sprue Association USA, P.O. Box 700, Omaha, Nebraska 68131-0700 [telephone (402) 558-0600] or Ener-G Foods, Inc., P.O. Box 84487, Seattle, Washington 98124 [telephone (206) 767-6660].

Conclusion

In caring for the patient with adverse food reactions, specific food hypersensitivities should be appropriately identified and an elimination diet instituted that not only restricts the offending allergens, but also provides the patient with a sound nutritional basis. Fortunately, most patients are allergic to only one or two foods, so prescribed diets are not too restrictive. When multiple food sensitivities are identified, however, the patient is at risk for nutritional inadequacies and it is imperative to enlist the assistance of a dietitian to formulate an appropriate diet. In addition, the dietitian can provide a variety of recipes (such as those listed in the appendix of this chapter) that will allow patients with multiple food sensitivities to maintain some variety in their diet.

The key to a food elimination diet is the avoidance of known allergens at all times. For this reason, it is recommended that patients use "allowed" fresh fruits, vegetables, meats, poultry, and whole grains to prepare homemade foods. When commercially prepared foods are used, the patient (or the patient's

parents) must read the labels and contact the manufacturer to ascertain whether certain allergens are present. Patients must be reminded to recheck labels constantly because the ingredients in various products (especially store brands) may change over time as the food manufacturer obtains new suppliers. In some cases, regional differences have been reported in product ingredients of national brands. Many questions will arise regarding specific food allergies for which no definite answers exist: for example, whether various vegetable oils (e.g., soy, peanut, corn) are safe for all highly sensitized patients, or whether soy lecithin or corn syrup solids are safe for soy- or corn-allergic patients. In cases of inadequate information, the severity of the patient's allergic history must be considered when selecting the dietary restrictions. For example, some caution in the use of peanut oil may be recommended in a patient who experiences life-threatening anaphylaxis, whereas products with soy lecithin would not be restricted in a soy-allergic patient with mild abdominal complaints.

Patients with severe food hypersensitivities must be taught to self-administer emergency medications. In addition, they must be reminded to carry emergency medications (e.g., Epi-Pen, AnaGuard, or ANA Kit) for use in case they accidentally ingest a food to which they are allergic. In two instances of fatal anaphylactic reactions secondary to food allergen ingestion, all victims knew they were allergic to the allergen they unknowingly ingested, but failed to take adequate emergency treatment measures (31, 32).

Another problem that is becoming increasingly recognized involves "cross-contaminants" in processed foods. For example, most tofu ice creams are manufactured in dairy plants where machinery is supposed to be carefully cleaned. Nevertheless, several cases of milk-sensitive children experiencing allergic reactions after ingesting tofu ice creams have been reported in which the tofu ice creams were found to contain significant levels of cow's milk proteins (33). Similarly, a child experienced an anaphylactic reaction after ingesting a small amount of a popsicle that came off the same line used to make creamsicles. Sensitive assays for detecting small concentrations of food proteins now being developed in several laboratories may eventually prove useful in screening ostensibly "safe" foods to which patients react. If patients react to a food that should not cause an allergic reaction, they should be instructed to save a portion of the food so that it may be analyzed by a laboratory capable of measuring small quantities of contaminating food proteins.

Restaurants and other public eating places continue to represent a high-risk environment for many food-allergic patients. Patients must be counseled to be very aggressive and precise about their specific food allergies when questioning the wait staff about the contents of various dishes. For example, a peanut-allergic patient should ask whether a dish contains any peanut, peanut butter, or peanut oil—not just whether it includes peanut oil. He or she should explain the seriousness of the allergy and, if uncomfortable about the response given by the server, insist on speaking to the chef. If some doubt remains, the best strategy is to not order the dish in question.

With the use of the double-blind, placebo-controlled food challenge to establish a firm diagnosis of food hypersensitivity and the careful monitoring of the dietary content and nutritional requirements, food-allergic patients can thrive and maintain a normal lifestyle.

Appendix

The following recipes have been contributed by the Food Allergy Network and patient families. The Food Allergy Network provides an extensive resource of educational materials for both individuals with food allergies and caregivers for people with food allergies. For a detailed listing of available information, contact the network at (800) 929-4040 or through the Internet (http://www.food allergy.org/). All recipes are free of milk, egg, peanut, nut, fish, and shellfish. In addition, some recipes will also be free of other allergens as noted.

M, E, P, S, N, Free

Deep Dish Pizza

2 pkg Quick Rise dry yeast
2 cup warm water (90°)
½ cup vegetable oil
4 tblsp olive oil
½ cup cornmeal
5½ cup flour

In a food processor or heavy duty mixer, dissolve yeast in water. Add oils, cornmeal, and 3 cups flour. Beat 10 minutes. Attach dough hook and add the remaining 2½ cups flour. Knead for several minutes with the machine. Let rise until doubled in bulk, and then punch down. Let rise again and punch down.

Using olive oil, oil large (10 inch) round cake pans. Place dough in the center of the pan, use your finger to push dough out to the edge and up the sides of the pan. Dough should be about ⅛ inch thick.

Place cheese or meat on the bottom of the pie. Next, add tomatoes or tomato sauce and other toppings as desired.

Bake at 475° for 20 to 40 minutes, checking frequently.

Makes crust for 2–3 pizzas.

M, E, P, S, N, Free

Wacky Cake

1½ cup flour
1 cup sugar
½ tsp salt
3 tblsp cocoa
1 tsp baking soda
1 tsp vanilla extract
1 tblsp vinegar
5 tblsp oil
1 cup cold water
confectioner's sugar

Preheat oven to 350°. Sift dry ingredients into mixing bowl. Add vanilla, vinegar, oil, and water. Blend well, pour into ungreased 9-inch square pan. Bake at 350° for 25 to 30 minutes. Sprinkle with confectioner's sugar.

Alternate: Omit cocoa powder, and add one mashed banana after adding water.

M, E, P, S, N, Free

Gingersnaps

¾ cup milk-free margarine
1 cup brown sugar
¼ cup molasses
2 tblsp orange juice
2¼ cup flour
2 tsp baking soda
½ tsp salt
1 tsp ground ginger
1 tsp ground cinnamon
½ tsp ground cloves

Cream the margarine, brown sugar, molasses, and orange juice. Sift together in a separate bowl the flour, baking soda, salt, ground ginger, ground cinnamon, and ground cloves. Stir the dry ingredients into the molasses mixture.

Form into small balls. Roll in granulated sugar; place 2 inches apart on greased cookie sheet. Bake in moderate oven (375°) for 12 minutes. Makes about 5 dozen cookies.

M, E, P, N, W, Free

Brett Derek's Lasagna

Ingredients/Preparation

3 cup Italian style tomato sauce
3 lb firm tofu blended thoroughly

Mix tofu with

½ cup fresh lemon juice
4 tsp honey or sugar
6 tblsp oil
4 tsp basil
1 tsp garlic powder or
    minced garlic
2 tsp salt (optional)
2 medium eggplants
        or
5 Japanese eggplants
(sweeter)

Cut into ¼ inch thick slices and soak in salt water for 5 minutes; rinse the salt off. Dredge the eggplant slices in rice flour mixture.

Mix together

1¼ cup rice flour
½ cup cornmeal
1 tsp oregano
2 medium cloves garlic
    crushed
dash of pepper
½ tsp salt (optional)

Oven-brown eggplant. Lay on cookie sheet with light oil and bake at 350° until brown. Turn.

Layer in 9 × 13 pan

1 cup of sauce
1 layer of eggplant
1 thick layer of tofu mix
1 layer of eggplant
2 cup of sauce
remainder of tofu

Bake at 350° for 35 minutes. Remove, set, cut, and serve.

M, E, P, S, N, W, Free

Pumpkin Bread

½ cup milk-free margarine
1 cup sugar
2 tsp baking powder
4 tblsp water
1 cup canned pumpkin
¼ cup water
1 tsp vanilla
½ tsp cinnamon
½ tsp nutmeg
¼ tsp ginger
1¾ cup barley flour
1 tsp baking soda
½ tsp salt
½ cup raisins (optional)

Cream margarine, then add sugar, and set aside. Sift together cinnamon, nutmeg, ginger, flour, baking soda, and salt. Add baking powder dissolved in 4 tablespoons of water into sugar/margarine mixture. Alternatively, add dry ingredients with pumpkin and ¼ cup water mixtures. Blend well. Add raisins. Pour into 9 × 5 × 3 greased loaf pan. Bake at 350° for 1 hour.

M, E, P, S, N, W, Free

Banana Muffins

2 mashed bananas
⅓ cup sugar
¼ cup corn oil
2 tsp baking powder
½ tsp vanilla
1¼ cup rice flour
½ tsp baking soda

Preheat oven to 325°. Grease muffin tins.

Mix the bananas, sugar, and oil together well. Add the baking powder, vanilla, rice flour, and baking soda to the banana mixture. Mix well.

Pour into the muffin tins and bake for 25 minutes until done.

M, E, P, S, N, W, Free

Oatmeal Cake

1 cup milk-free margarine
1 cup brown sugar
4 cup quick oats
1 tblsp baking powder
1 tblsp vanilla
½ cup hot water

Mix all ingredients together. Flatten into ungreased 9 × 13 pan and let stand for 10 minutes.

Bake at 350° for 60 minutes. Cut into squares and cool.

M, E, P, S, N, W, Free

Brett's Gingerbread Men

¼ cup milk-free margarine
½ cup sugar
½ cup molasses
1¼ cup rye flour
1¼ cup cornstarch
1 tsp baking soda
¼ tsp ground cloves
¾ tsp ground cinnamon
¼ tsp ginger
½ tsp salt
½ cup hot water

Preheat oven to 350°. Grease cookie sheets.

Cream margarine. Add sugar and then molasses. Sift dry ingredients and add alternately with water. If dough is too gummy, add rye flour.

Roll dough to ¼ inch thickness on floured board. Cut out and decorate. Bake for 8 minutes.

M, E, P, S, N, W, Free

Oatmeal Cookies

1 cup milk-free margarine
1 cup brown sugar
1 cup granulated sugar
4 cup quick oats
½ tblsp baking powder
½ tblsp baking soda
1 tblsp vanilla
¼ cup hot water
1 tsp cinnamon
1 cup raisins (optional)

Preheat oven to 350°. Mix all ingredients together. Drop onto ungreased cookie sheet. Bake for 25 to 30 minutes, until golden brown.

Cool, then remove from baking sheet. The cookies must be cool before they can be removed or they tend to crumble.

M, E, P, S, N, W, Free

Puffed Rice Treats

½ stick milk-free margarine
40 regular size marshmallows

5 cup puffed rice cereal
milk-free margarine (to grease pan)

Grease an 8 × 8 × 2 baking dish. Melt the margarine in a large pot over low heat. Add marshmallows and stir until completely melted. Remove from heat and add puffed rice. Stir until mixture is well-coated. Pour into baking dish, then flatten with a spoon. Let cool before cutting into bars.

M, E, P, S, N, W, Free

Playdough

1 cup cornstarch
1 tsp baking soda
1¼ cup water and food coloring, little oil

Cook until mealy. Put on a plate. Cover with a damp cloth. Allow to cool. Knead.

Note: Doesn't keep very well, but is fun for someone who can't use wheat-based dough.

M, E, P, S, N, Free

Home-Style Pancakes

2 cup flour
4 tsp baking powder
½ tsp. salt
2 tblsp sugar
2 cup water
3 tblsp oil
¼ tsp vanilla extract

Sift dry ingredients together. Add remaining ingredients and beat together.

Pour the batter to form circles approximately 4 inches in diameter onto a hot, lightly greased griddle or heavy skillet. Cook for 2 to 3 minutes or until pancakes have a bubbly surface and slightly dry edges. Turn pancakes; cook for 2 to 3 minutes more or until golden brown.

Suggestions: For a special treat, pour this batter onto a hot griddle and form into a teddy bear, Mickey Mouse, or bunny shape.
Add banana slices, blueberries, or other fruit to batter for variety.

Note: This batter can be used to make waffles.

M, E, P, S, N, Free

English Muffin Bread

6 cup flour
2 pkg active dry yeast
1 tblsp sugar

2 tsp salt
¼ tsp baking soda
2½ cup water
cornmeal

Grease two 8½ × 4½ pans and sprinkle with cornmeal. Combine 3 cup flour, yeast, sugar, salt, and baking soda; set aside. Heat water until very warm (120° to 130°). Add to dry mixture; beat well. Stir in rest of flour to make a stiff batter. Divide between two loaf pans. Sprinkle tops with cornmeal. Cover and let rise in warm place for 45 minutes.

Preheat oven to 400°. Bake for 25 minutes. Remove from pans immediately and cool on wire racks. Slice and toast bread. This bread freezes well.

M, E, P, S, N, Free

Blueberry Muffins

½ cup milk-free, soy-free
    margarine at room
    temperature
1 cup plus 2 tblsp sugar
3 tblsp water, 3 tblsp oil, 2
    tsp baking powder,
    mixed together
1 tsp vanilla extract
2 tsp baking powder
¼ tsp salt
2 cup flour
½ cup water
2½ cup blueberries
1 tblsp sugar mixed with
    ¼ tsp ground nutmeg

Preheat oven to 375°. Line 12-muffin tin with paper liners. In a medium-size bowl, beat margarine until creamy. Beat in the sugar until pale and fluffy. Beat in water, oil, and baking powder. Add vanilla, remaining baking powder, and salt.

Fold in half of the flour with a spatula and half of the water. Add remaining flour and water. Fold in blueberries. Scoop batter into muffin cups. Sprinkle with nutmeg sugar. Bake 25 to 30 minutes or until golden brown. Let muffins cool slightly before serving.

M, E, W, P, S, N, G, Free

Corn Muffins

⅓ cup shortening
¼ cup sugar
1 cup Cream of Rice cereal

1 tblsp baking powder
⅔ cup warm water
¼ tsp salt
1 tsp vanilla extract
1 tsp grated lemon rind
⅔ cup cornmeal

Preheat oven to 375°. Line muffin tins with paper liners. Cream shortening and sugar. Mix rice cereal and baking powder in warm water. Combine with sugar and shortening mixture. Mix in remaining ingredients. Spoon into muffin cups (small muffins have a better texture). Bake 25 minutes. Makes 8 muffins.

Note: These muffins hold together better if you let them cool a few hours or overnight.

M, E, P, S, N, Free

Sweet Potato Muffins

1 cup flour, sifted
1 tsp baking powder
¼ tsp baking soda
½ tsp salt
½ tsp ground cinnamon
½ tsp ground nutmeg (optional)
¼ cup sugar
¼ cup water
½ cup cooked mashed
    sweet potatoes (about
    1 large potato)
1½ tblsp water, 1½ tblsp
    oil, 1 tsp baking pow-
    der, mixed together
2 tblsp milk-free, soy-free
    margarine, melted

Preheat oven to 350°. Line muffin tins with paper liners. In medium bowl, sift together flour, baking powder, baking soda, salt, cinnamon, and nutmeg. Set aside. Combine sugar, water, sweet potatoes, water, oil, and baking powder mixture, and margarine in mixing bowl. Add to flour mixture. Stir until well moistened. Fill prepared muffin tins two-thirds full. Bake 25 minutes.

M, E, P, S, N, Free

Zucchini Bread

3 cup flour
½ tsp baking powder
1 tsp salt
2 tsp cinnamon

1 tsp baking soda
2 cup grated zucchini
    (about 3 medium-size
    zucchinis)
4½ tblsp water, 4½ tblsp
    oil, 3 tsp baking pow-
    der, mixed together
1 cup oil
3 tsp vanilla extract
2 cup sugar

Preheat oven to 350°. Sift together first 5 ingredients. Add the remaining ingredients and mix well. Pour into loaf pans. Bake 55 minutes. Makes 3 loaves.

Note: This recipe freezes well.

M, E, P, S, N, Free

Doughnut Holes

½ cup plus 2 tblsp milk-free, soy-free margarine, softened
1 cup sugar
3 tblsp water, 3 tblsp oil, 2 tsp baking powder, mixed together
3 cup flour
4½ tsp baking powder
½ tsp salt
½ tsp nutmeg
1 cup apple juice
(or water)

Preheat oven to 350°. Line mini-size muffin tins with paper liners. Blend margarine with sugar. Add the water, oil, and baking powder mixture. Mix well and then set aside. Sift together flour, baking powder, salt, and nutmeg. Add to the margarine and sugar mixture. Blend in the apple juice and mix together thoroughly. Fill muffin tins two-thirds full. Bake 15 minutes or until doughnut holes are golden brown.

Suggestions: Combine ½ cup sugar with ½ tsp cinnamon; set aside. Melt 6 tblsp margarine. While doughnuts are still warm, roll them in the margarine, and then in cinnamon sugar.

M, E, W, P, S, N, Free

Potato Stuffing

6 medium potatoes
⅔ cup finely chopped
    onion
6 tblsp finely chopped
    fresh parsley

4 tblsp milk-free, soy-free
    margarine
salt
pepper

Peel and boil the potatoes in salted water. Drain, dice them, and set aside. In a large frying pan, gently fry the onion and parsley in margarine. Add potatoes. Stir to coat the potatoes evenly. Season to taste. Place potato stuffing in poultry and roast.

M, E, P, S, N, Free

Snacking Cake

1½ cup flour
1 tsp baking soda
1 tsp cinnamon
½ tsp nutmeg
½ tsp salt
3 tblsp oil, 3 tblsp water, 2
    tsp baking powder,
    mixed together
½ cup oil
½ cup brown sugar, firmly
    packed
½ cup white sugar
1½ cup finely grated car-
    rots (4 large)
1 (8-oz) can crushed pine-
    apple, packed in its
    own juice, undrained

Preheat oven to 350°. Grease a 9-inch square or 7 × 11 inch pan. In a large bowl, mix together flour, baking soda, cinnamon, nutmeg, and salt. Set aside. In another bowl, combine oil, water, and baking powder mixture with the oil. Add sugars. Stir well and then set aside. In a third bowl, combine the carrots and pineapple with its juice. Set aside.

Stir the oil, water, and baking powder mixture into the dry ingredients. Stir in the carrot–pineapple mixture. Spoon batter into the prepared pan. Bake 30 to 40 minutes or until a cake tester inserted in the center comes out clean.

Suggestions: This cake is delicious! Top with confectioner's sugar poured over a doily to dress it up for dessert or a party.

M, E, P, S, N, Free

Cinnamon Crunch Cookies

1⅓ cup flour
1 tsp cream of tartar

½ tsp baking soda
⅛ tsp salt
½ cup milk-free, soy-free
    margarine, softened
¾ cup sugar
½ tsp vanilla extract
1½ tblsp water, 1½ tblsp
    oil, 1 tsp baking pow-
    der, mixed together
2 tsp ground cinnamon
    mixed with ¼ cup
    sugar

Preheat oven to 400°. Grease cookie sheets. Stir together flour, cream of tartar, baking soda, and salt; set aside. In mixer bowl, combine margarine and sugar; beat until fluffy. Blend in vanilla. Beat in water, oil, and baking powder mixture. Gradually add to flour mixture, beating until just combined.

Drop by rounded teaspoons into the cinnamon sugar mixture. Roll cookies to coat well, shaping them into balls as you roll. Arrange balls about 1½ inches apart on greased baking sheets. Bake until edges are golden brown (8 to 10 minutes). Transfer to wire racks to cool. Makes about 3 dozen cookies.

Note: This cookie mixture can go from freezer to oven.

M, E, W, P, N, Free

Coffee Can Vanilla Ice Cream

1 1-lb coffee can and lid,
    emptied and cleaned
1 3-lb coffee can and lid,
    emptied and cleaned
1 cup milk-free, nondairy
    creamer
1 cup soy milk
½ cup sugar
½ tsp vanilla extract
1 cup rock salt, divided
crushed ice

Put all ingredients except rock salt and ice in the smaller can. Cover with lid. Place smaller can inside the 3-lb can. Pack crushed ice around outside of small can. Pour at least ¾ cup rock salt evenly over ice. Cover the can and tape lid securely.

Roll back and forth on a table for 15 minutes. Open outer can and remove inner can. Remove lid. Scrape the ice cream off the sides of the can and stir the mixture to an even consistency. Replace lid. Drain ice water from larger can.

Insert smaller can and pack with more ice and salt. Roll back and forth for 15 minutes or until can frosts over. Stir and serve. Immediately freeze unused ice cream.

Suggestions: Fruit, crushed cookies, or a bit of coconut milk can be added for variety.

M, E, W, P, S, N, Free

Coconut Rice Pudding

6 cup coconut water
1 cup uncooked medium-
    grain rice
½ cup sugar
¼ tsp salt
2 tsp vanilla extract

Combine coconut water, rice, sugar, and salt in medium saucepan. Over medium heat, stir frequently until bubbles form around the edge. Reduce heat to low. Cover and simmer about 1 hour, or until rice is tender. Stir occasionally. Stir in vanilla extract. Cover and refrigerate until well chilled, about 3 hours.

Note: Excess coconut water can be kept in the refrigerator for later use or can be used as a refreshing coconut drink.

Coconut Water

1 (15-oz) can Coco Lopez
    Cream of Coconut
5 cans water

Before opening Coco Lopez, shake can well. Pour contents into a large pitcher. Add water. Stir well.

REFERENCES

1. Oppenheimer JJ, Nelson HS, Bock SA, Christensen F, Leung DYM. Treatment of peanut allergy with rush immunotherapy. J Allergy Clin Immunol 1992;90:256–262.
2. Sampson HA, Scanlon SM. Natural history of food hypersensitivity in children with atopic dermatitis. J Pediatr 1989;115:23–27.
3. Pastorello EA, Stocchi L, Pravettoni V, et al. Role of elimination diet in adults with food allergy. J Allergy Clin Immunol 1989;84:475–483.
4. Bierman CW, Shapiro GC, Christie DL, et al. Eczema, rickets, and food allergy. J Allergy Clin Immunol 1978;61:119–127.
5. Lloyd-Still JD. Chronic diarrhea of childhood and the misuse of elimination diets. J Pediatr 1979;95:10–13.
6. David TJ, Waddington E, Stanton RHJ. Nutritional hazards of elimination diets in children. Arch Dis Child 1984;59:323–325.
7. Robertson DA, Ayres RC, Smith CL, Wright R. Adverse consequences arising from misdiagnosis of food allergy. Br Med J 1988;297:719–720.

8. Labib M, Gama R, Wright J, *et al.* Dietary maladvice as a cause of hypothyroidism and short stature. Br Med J 1989;298:232–233.

9. Bernhisel-Broadbent J, Sampson HA. Cross-allergenicity in the legume botanical family in children with food hypersensitivity. J Allergy Clin Immunol 1989;83:435–440.

10. Bernhisel-Broadbent J, Scanlon SM, Sampson HA. Fish hypersensitivity. I. In vitro and oral challenge results in fish-allergic patients. J Allergy Clin Immunol 1992;89:730–737.

11. Jones SM, Magnolfi CF, Cooke SK, Sampson HA. Immunologic cross-reactivity among cereal grains and grasses in children with food hypersensitivity. J Allergy Clin Immunol 1995;96: 341–351.

12. Sampson HA, McCaskill CM. Food hypersensitivity in atopic dermatitis: evaluation of 113 patients. J Pediatr 1985;107:669– 675.

13. Bock SA, Atkins FM. Patterns of food hypersensitivity during sixteen years of double-blind placebo-controlled food challenges. J Pediatr 1990;117:561–567.

14. Warner JO, Hathaway MJ. Allergic form of Meadow's syndrome (Munchausen by proxy). Arch Dis Child 1984;59:151– 153.

15. Subcommittee on the Tenth Edition of the RDAs, Food and Nutrition Board, Commission on Life Sciences, National Research Council. Recommended dietary allowances, 10th ed. Washington, DC: National Academy Press, 1989, 33, 66.

16. Ibid. 65.

17. Waterlow JC. Classification and definition of protein-energy malnutrition. In: Beaton GH, Bengoa JM, eds. Nutrition in preventive medicine. Geneva: WHO, 1976, 530–555.

18. Subcommittee on the Tenth Edition of the RDAs, Food and Nutrition Board, Commission on Life Sciences, National Research Council. Recommended dietary allowances, 10th ed. Washington, DC: National Academy Press, 1989, 66.

19. Ibid. 65–66.

20. Ibid. 2.

21. Sampson HA. Food allergy. J Allergy Clin Immunol 1989;84:1062–1067.

22. Walzer M. Absorption of allergens. J Allergy 1942;13:554–562.

23. Fries JH. Peanuts: allergic and other untoward reactions. Ann Allergy 1982;48:220–226.

24. Taylor SL, Busse WW, Sachs MI, Parker JL, Yuninger JW. Peanut oil is not allergenic to peanut-sensitive individuals. J Allergy Clin Immunol 1981;68:372–375.

25. Bock SA, Atkins FM. The natural history of peanut allergy. J Allergy Clin Immunol 1989;83:900–904.

26. Bush RK, Taylor SL, Nordlee JA, Busse WW. Soybean oil is not allergenic to soybean-sensitive individuals. J Allergy Clin Immunol 1985;76:242–245.

27. Bernhisel-Broadbent J, Taylor S, Sampson HA. Cross-allergenicity in the legume botanical family in children with food hypersensitivity. II. Laboratory correlates. J Allergy Clin Immunol 1989;84:701–709.

28. Elsayed S, Aas K, Sletten K, Johansson SGO. Tryptic cleavage of a homogeneous cod fish allergen and isolation of two active polypeptide fragments. Immunochem 1972;9:647–661.

29. Bernhisel-Broadbent J, Sampson HA. Oral challenge and in vitro study results in fish hypersensitive patients. J Allergy Clin Immunol 1990;85:270.

30. Loveless MH. Allergy for corn and its derivatives: experiments with a masked ingestion test for its diagnosis. J Allergy 1950;21:500–511.

31. Yuninger JW, Sweeney KG, Sturner WQ, Giannandrea LA, *et al.* Fatal food-induced anaphylaxis. JAMA 1988;260:1450–1452.

32. Sampson HA, Mendelson L, Rosen JP. Fatal and near-fatal food-induced anaphylaxis in children. N Engl J Med 1992;327:380–384.

33. Gern JA, Yang E, Evrard HM, Sampson HA. Allergic reactions to milk-contaminated "Non-Dairy" products. N Engl J Med 1991;324:976–979.

33

FOOD TOXICOLOGY

Steve L. Taylor

*F*ood toxicology could be defined as the science that establishes the basis for judgments about the safety of foodborne chemicals. The central axiom of toxicology, as set forth by Paracelsus in the 1500s, states: "Everything is poison. Only the dose makes a thing not a poison." Thus, all chemicals in foods—whether natural or synthetic, inherent, adventitious, or added—are potentially toxic. The vast majority of foodborne chemicals are not hazardous because the amounts of each foodborne chemical in the typical diet are insufficient to cause injury. Because all chemicals have a toxic potential, the degree of risk posed by exposure to any specific chemical is determined by the dose, duration, and frequency of exposure (and especially in the case of allergies, the degree of the individual's sensitivity). The age-old practice of eating moderate amounts of a varied diet protects most consumers from any harm. Unusual diets can sometimes result in intoxications from chemicals that would normally be considered safe and desirable. For example, the intake of large amounts of vitamin A proved hazardous to polar explorers who consumed large amounts of polar bear liver (1).

Acute adverse reactions to foods occur through many mechanisms, including infections (viral, bacterial, parasitic), various intoxications, and allergies and intolerances. Food allergies are the major focus of this book. Other medical conditions, including some food intoxications, cause symptoms resembling food allergies; these other conditions must be considered and ruled out before reaching any diagnosis of food allergy.

Food intoxications encompass all food-associated illnesses that are caused by chemicals in food, although foodborne chemicals vary greatly in their toxicity. All consumers are susceptible to most food intoxications. Food allergy can be viewed as a cate-gory of food intoxication that affects only certain individuals in the population. Other categories of food intoxications, such as metabolic food disorders, also affect only certain individuals. This chapter will focus on the more common types of acute foodborne intoxications, including the most common metabolic food disorders.

Intoxications Caused by Synthetic Chemicals in Foods

Most of the synthetic chemicals in foods (e.g., food additives, agricultural chemical residues, and chemicals migrating from packaging materials) have been rigorously tested for toxicity. These synthetic chemicals remain safe under normal circumstances of exposure, although adverse reactions can occur from misuse, whether intentional or accidental. Other chapters in this book cover adverse reactions to food additives, so we will focus on a few additional food additives, agricultural chemical residues, packaging migrants, and other man-made chemicals that can occur in foods at concentrations sufficient to cause concern.

OTHER FOOD ADDITIVES

Niacin

Excessive consumption of niacin (also known as nicotinic acid), which is part of the B vitamin complex, can cause acute onset of flushing, pruritus, rash, and burning or warmth in the skin, especially on the face and upper trunk (2). Some patients experience gastrointestinal discomfort (3). Outbreaks have occurred from the excessive enrichment of flour used to make pumpernickel bagels (3) or cornmeal (4) as the result of inaccurate or inadequate labeling of food ingredient containers. Such episodes occur only rarely because the amount of niacin required to elicit such symptoms is at least 50 times the recommended dietary allowance (3, 4). The symptoms of niacin intoxication are self-limited and without sequelae.

Sorbitol and Other Polyhydric Alcohols

Sugar alcohols, such as sorbitol, are widely used as sweeteners in dietetic food products. They are especially common in candy and chewing gum because of their non-cariogenic properties. Diarrhea can result from the excessive consumption of sugar alcohols (5). Sorbitol and the other sugar alcohols are not as easily absorbed as sugar. Because of their slow absorption, ingestion of excessive amounts of these sweeteners cause an osmotic-type diarrhea. In several reported cases, consumers ingested more than 20 g of these sweeteners per day, although infants appeared more susceptible to the osmotic effects than adults (5). In one representative case, the ingestion of 12 pieces of hard candy over a short period of time provided 36 g of sorbitol and resulted in diarrhea (6). The illness is self-limited.

Toxic Oil Poisoning

In 1981 and 1982, an epidemic occurred in Spain linked to the ingestion of unlabeled, illegally marketed cooking oils (7, 8). A total of 19,828 cases and 315 deaths were recorded in this epidemic (9). The tainted cooking oil contained oils from both plant and animal sources, but some of the oils were denatured and intended for industrial uses. The causative toxin in the oils remains unknown, although fatty acid anilides resulting from the denaturation process are suspected to be at least partially responsible (9, 10).

The clinical manifestations of this illness involved multiple organ systems (9, 10). In the first few days after ingestion of the oil, patients experienced fever, chills, headache, tachycardia, cough, chest pain, and pruritus. Physical examinations revealed various skin exanthema, splenomegaly, and generalized adenopathy. Pulmonary infiltrates were noted in 84% of patients, probably as the result of increased capillary permeability. The intermediate phase of the illness

tended to begin in the second week and persist through the eighth week post-ingestion. Gastrointestinal symptoms—primarily abdominal pain, nausea, and diarrhea—predominated. Clinical examination revealed marked eosinophilia in 42% of patients, high IgE levels, thrombocytopenia, abnormal coagulation patterns, and evidence of hepatic dysfunction with abnormal enzymes. Some patients became jaundiced, and many had hepatomegaly. The late phase of the illness developed in 23% of cases, emerging after two months of illness. This phase was characterized initially by neuromuscular and joint involvement. Later, patients developed vasculitis and a scleroderma-like syndrome. Patients complained of intense muscular pain, edema, and progressive muscular weakness. In addition, muscular atrophy became apparent in some patients. Neurological involvement included depressed deep tendon reflexes, anesthesia, and dysesthesia. Neuromuscular weakness led to respiratory problems that eventually progressed to pulmonary hypertension and thromboembolic phenomena. The scleroderma-like symptoms included Raynaud's phenomenon, sicca syndrome, dysphagia, and contractures attributable to thickening collagen in the skin. Vascular lesions were noted in all organs, apparently resulting from endothelial proliferation and thrombosis. All patients in the late-phase group had antinuclear antibody, and many generated antibodies against smooth muscle and skeletal muscle (11). The pathological and clinical features are consistent with an autoimmune mechanism for this illness. Because the precise causative agent and its mechanism have not been delineated, a recurrence is not impossible (9). If present in small amounts in other foods, the toxin may also produce or aggravate other clinical conditions (9).

AGRICULTURAL CHEMICALS

A wide variety of chemicals are used in modern agricultural practices. Residues of these chemicals can linger in raw and processed foods, although federal regulatory agencies evaluate the safety of such chemicals and regulate and monitor their use on food products (5). The major categories of agricultural chemicals include insecticides, herbicides, fungicides, fertilizers, and veterinary drugs, including antibiotics.

Insecticides

Insecticides are added to foods to control the extent of insect contamination. The major categories of insecticides include organochlorine compounds (DDT, chlordane, and others—many of which are now banned), organophosphate compounds (e.g., parathion and malathion), carbamate compounds (e.g., carbaryl and aldicarb), botanical compounds (e.g., nicotine and pyrethrum), and inorganic compounds (e.g., arsenicals).

The exceedingly low residue levels of insecticides found in most foods do not pose a particular hazard, especially on an acute basis. Large doses of insecticides can prove toxic to humans, however. For example, the organophosphates and carbamates are cholinesterase inhibitors that act as neurotoxins by blocking synaptic nerve transmission. Several factors explain the low degree of hazard associated with insecticide residues in foods: (1) the level of exposure is very low; (2) some insecticides are not very toxic to humans; (3) some insecticides decompose rapidly in the environment; and (4) many different insecticides are used, which limits exposure to any specific insecticide.

No food poisoning incidents have ever been attributed to the proper use of insecticides on foods. Problems have occasionally arisen from the inappropriate use of certain insecticides, however (12). An outbreak of aldicarb intoxication from watermelons occurred on the U.S. West Coast in 1985 (13). Aldicarb use on watermelons is prohibited because excessive levels of aldicarb become concentrated in the edible portion of the melon. In this episode, several farmers used aldicarb illegally, resulting in consumer illnesses and the recall and destruction of thousands of watermelons. A total of 1373 illness reports were received in this outbreak, with 78% classified as probable or possible aldicarb poisoning cases (13, 14). This episode represents the largest known outbreak of pesticide poisoning in North America (13, 14). Aldicarb has also been involved in several food poisoning outbreaks associated with ingestion of hydroponically grown cucumbers (14, 15). The symptoms of aldicarb intoxication include nausea, vomiting, diarrhea, and mild neurological manifestations such as dizziness, headache, blurred vision, and loss of balance (13–15). Many other episodes of pesticide intoxications have resulted from the misuse of pesticides, including contamination of foods during storage and transport, use of pesticides in food preparation after they were mistakenly identified as common food ingredients such as sugar and salt, and misuse of pesticides in agricultural practice as noted above (12).

Herbicides

Herbicides are applied to control the growth of weeds. Among the more important herbicides are chlorophenoxy compounds (e.g., 2,4-D), dinitrophenols (e.g., dinitroorthocresol), bipyridyl compounds (e.g., paraquat), substituted ureas (e.g., monuron), carbamates (e.g., propham), and triazines (e.g., simazine).

Generally, herbicide residues in foods do not represent a hazard to consumers. No food poisoning incidents have ever resulted from the proper use of herbicides on food crops. The lack of hazard from herbicide residues derives from the low level of exposure, their low degree of toxicity to humans and selective toxicity toward plants, and the use of many different herbicides, which limits exposure to any specific herbicide.

Because most herbicides are selectively toxic to plants, they pose little risk to humans. The bipyridyl compounds are an exception. These nonselective herbicides are toxic to humans, affecting the function of the lung (16). No food poisoning incidents have ever been attributed to inappropriate use of the bipyridyl compounds, however.

Fungicides

Fungicides prevent the growth of molds on food crops. Important fungicides include captan, folpet, dithiocarbamates, pentachlorophenol, and the mercurials. The hazards from foodborne fungicides are minuscule because exposure is quite low, most fungicides do not accumulate in the environment, and fungicides are typically not very toxic.

The mercurial compounds and hexachlorobenzene represent exceptions to this statement. The mercurials are often used to treat seed grains to prevent mold growth during storage. Although these seed grains are usually colored pink and are clearly intended for planting rather than consumption, consumers have occasionally eaten these treated seed grains and developed mercury poisoning (12). Although deaths have resulted in several severe episodes, mild cases of mercury intoxication can be manifested in gastrointestinal symptoms such as abdominal cramps, nausea, vomiting, and diarrhea and dermal symptoms such as acrodynia and itching (12). Hexachlorobenzene caused one of the most massive outbreaks of pesticide poisoning in recorded history, affecting more than 3000 individuals in Turkey from 1955 to 1959 (17). This fungicide was used to treat seed grain that was consumed rather than planted. The symptoms were quite severe, including a 10% mortality rate, porphyria cutanea tarda, ulcerated skin lesions, alopecia, porphyrinuria, hepatomegaly, and thyroid enlargement (17).

Fertilizers

The most commonly used fertilizers incorporate combinations of nitrogen and phosphorus compounds. Nitrogen fertilizers are oxidized to nitrate and nitrite in the soil, both of which are hazardous to humans if ingested in large amounts. Infants are particularly susceptible to nitrate and nitrite intoxication. Some plants, such as spinach, can accumulate nitrate to hazardous levels if allowed to grow on overfertilized fields. Because nitrite is more toxic than nitrate, a more serious situation results if nitrate-reducing bacteria are allowed to proliferate on these foods.

Acute nitrite intoxications have occurred. In low doses, the symptoms include flushing of the face and extremities, gastrointestinal discomfort, and headache. In larger doses, cyanosis, methemoglobinemia, nausea, vomiting, abdominal pain, collapse, and death can occur (18). The lethal dose of nitrite is approximately 1 g in adults (18). Several intoxications have occurred from ingestion of overfertilized spinach (19). The problem arises from consumption of nitrate-rich, unprocessed spinach, where conversion to nitrite has occurred before ingestion, probably as the result of bacterial action (18). Improper storage of carrot juice has allowed nitrate-reducing bacteria to proliferate, resulting in the accumulation of hazardous levels of nitrite in the product (20).

Veterinary Drugs and Antibiotics

Food-producing animals are often treated with a variety of veterinary drugs, especially antibiotics. Residues in foods typically remain quite low. Acute food poisoning incidents have not occurred as a result of properly used veterinary drugs and antibiotics. Penicillin probably represents the most important concern because of the potential for allergic reactions to penicillin residues. The likelihood of allergic reactions to the very low levels of penicillin residues found in foods is quite remote, however (21).

CHEMICALS MIGRATING FROM PACKAGING MATERIALS AND CONTAINERS

Chemicals migrating from packaging materials into foods and beverages do not represent a significant source of chemical exposure. A variety of chemicals, including plastic monomers, plasticizers, stabilizers, printing inks, and others, do migrate at extremely low levels into foods. These chemicals do not often create hazards for consumers. Lead and tin are perhaps the main concerns associated with packaging materials. The storage of acidic foods in inappropriate containers can result in the leaching of toxic heavy metals, such as zinc, into the food. Contact of acidic beverages with copper may also cause the release of potentially hazardous levels of copper into the beverage. Cadmium and iron are also occasionally implicated in heavy metal intoxications associated with foods (22).

Lead

Lead exposure from foods has always represented a comparatively moderate contributor to overall environmental lead exposure. The migration of lead from Pb-soldered cans previously inspired concern. In the United States, Pb-soldered cans have been phased out of use. The main issue with lead contamination remains the occasional use of lead-based glazes on pottery or paint on glassware that may come in contact with acidic foods or beverages. Lead is a well-known toxicant that can affect the nervous system, the kidney, and the bone.

Tin

Tin plate is commonly used in the construction of metal cans for foods. The inner surfaces of these cans are lined with a lacquer material when cans are used for acidic foods or beverages. Acute tin intoxication has occurred from the inappropriate placement of tomato juice or fruit cocktail in unlined cans (22, 23). Because tin is poorly absorbed, patients experience the primary symptoms of bloating, nausea, abdominal cramps, vomiting, diarrhea, and headache occurring 30 minutes to 2 hours after consumption of the acidic product (23).

Copper

Copper poisoning, which is characterized primarily by nausea and vomiting, most commonly occurs from faulty check valves in soft-drink vending machines (5). The check valves prevent contact between the acidic, carbonated beverage and the copper tubing that delivers water or ice in the machine. Several outbreaks of copper poisoning have resulted from flaws in such machines (24).

Zinc

Zinc intoxication typically results from the storage of acidic foods or beverages in galvanized containers (22, 25). Episodes have involved fruit punch and tomato juice (22). Zinc is a potent emetic, and symptoms of intoxication from this metal include irritation of the mouth, throat, and abdomen, nausea, vomiting, dizziness, and collapse.

INDUSTRIAL CHEMICALS

Industrial and/or environmental pollutants often migrate into foods in small amounts. On rare occasions, hazardous levels of such chemicals enter the food supply, often with devastating consequences.

Polychlorinated Biphenyls (PCBs) and Polybrominated Biphenyls (PBBs)

On several occasions, foods have been contaminated with PCBs and PBBs (5). PCBs and PBBs, which persist in the environment, are considered to be toxic pollutants generated by industrial practices. PBBs are commonly used as fire retardants, while PCBs are frequently used in transformer fluid. PCBs and PBBs are not worrisome acute toxicants in foods. Because they are lipid-soluble, however, the chronic effects of exposure to these contaminants in foods create a concern. The most infamous incident involved the accidental contamination of dairy feed in Michigan with PBBs, which resulted in the destruction of many cows and their milk. Leaking transformers have contributed to the contamination of feeds with PCBs, which in turn led to the destruction of chickens, eggs, and egg-containing food products. Pollution of Lake Michigan with PCBs has reached such sufficient levels in recent years that commercial fishing on Lake Michigan has ceased.

Mercury

Minamata disease due to mercury intoxication remains the classic example of the contamination of foods by industrial pollutants. An industrial firm located on the shores of Minamata Bay in Japan dumped mercury-containing wastes into the bay, where bacteria converted the inorganic mercury into highly toxic methylmercury. More than 1200 cases of mercury intoxication occurred among consumers of Minamata Bay fish that became contaminated with the methylmercury (26). Symptoms included tremors and other neurotoxic effects and kidney failure.

Intoxications Caused by Naturally Occurring Chemicals in Foods

The naturally occurring chemicals in foods are less frequently tested for their potential toxic effects than synthetic chemicals. While the vast majority of naturally occurring chemicals in foods are safe under the normal circumstances of exposure, some potentially hazardous situations do exist. Naturally occurring chemicals with significant pharmacological activity (e.g., the vasoactive amines, methylxanthines, ethanol, and myristicin) are covered elsewhere in this book. Such chemicals can, however, elicit a wide variety of adverse reactions, including both acute and chronic intoxications. Naturally occurring toxicants could be defined as those naturally occurring chemicals in foods that might pose a hazard under typical circumstances of exposure; they are more likely to be hazardous under such circumstances than are synthetic chemicals. Although chronic illnesses (e.g., cancer) are undeniably important, this chapter will focus exclusively on acute intoxications caused by natural, foodborne toxicants.

NATURALLY OCCURRING CONTAMINANTS

Naturally occurring contaminants can be produced in foods as the result of contamination by bacteria, molds, algae, and insects. The chemicals produced from these biological sources can linger in foods even after the living organism has been removed or destroyed. Naturally occurring contaminants are not always present in foods and can be avoided with the prevention of contamination. Such contaminants represent the most important and potentially hazardous chemicals of natural origin existing in foods. The bacterial and insect toxins will not be discussed in any detail. The bacterial toxins cause familiar diseases such as staphylococcal food poisoning and botulism (27, 28). The insect toxins have not been studied to any extent, and their impact on human health remains uncertain.

Ciguatera Poisoning

Ciguatera poisoning, which results from the ingestion of fish that have fed on toxic dinoflagellate algae, is the most common cause of acute foodborne disease of chemical etiology reported to the U.S. Centers for Disease Control. This foodborne illness is common throughout the Caribbean and much of the Pacific, but is now encountered around the world due to the improved distribution of fish (29, 30). In the United States, the illness occurs most frequently in Florida, Hawaii, and the Virgin Islands (30–32). The fish most commonly implicated in cases of ciguatera poisoning are grouper, red snapper, barracuda, amberjack, kingfish, Spanish mackerel, mahi-mahi, sea bass, surgeon fish, and eels, although many different fish species may be involved (31, 33, 34). These fishes, which are all reef and shore species, acquire the toxic agents by feeding on smaller fishes that consume the toxin in

the form of poisonous planktonic algae (34). Several species of dinoflagellate algae can produce toxins of the type associated with ciguatera poisoning (30); *Gambierdiscus toxicus* is one of the most prominent (30, 34, 35). Although several toxins may be involved, the major toxin is a lipid-soluble, polyether compound with a molecular weight of 1112, known as ciguatoxin (33). Ciguatoxin has ionophoric properties (30, 33). The toxins accumulate in the liver and viscera of the fish, but enough can enter the muscle tissues to cause ciguatera poisoning among humans ingesting these fish (34). The toxins are heat-stable and remain unaffected by processing or cooking practices (34).

The symptoms of ciguatera poisoning tend to vary, perhaps confirming the role of several different dinoflagellate algae and several different toxins in this syndrome (33). The predominant symptoms associated with ciguatera poisoning include gastrointestinal and neurological manifestations (30, 33), although the gastrointestinal symptoms predominate in some cases, while the neurological symptoms predominate in other instances (30). Gastrointestinal symptoms include nausea, vomiting, diarrhea, and abdominal cramps. Neurological symptoms include dyesthesia, paresthesia (especially in the perioral region and extremities), pruritus, vertigo, muscle weakness, malaise, headache, and myalgia. A peculiar reversal of hot and cold sensations occurs in approximately 65% of patients (30). In severe cases, the neurological manifestations can progress to delirium, pruritus, dyspnea, prostration, brachycardia, and coma (30). Many patients recover within a few days or weeks, although treatment is difficult and some deaths from cardiovascular collapse have occurred (34).

Paralytic Shellfish Poisoning

Paralytic shellfish poisoning results from the ingestion of mollusks, such as clams, mussels, cockles, and scallops, that have become poisonous by feeding on toxic dinoflagellate algae (34). Paralytic shellfish poisoning occurs worldwide but is commonly encountered along the Pacific and North Atlantic coasts of North America, the coastal areas of Japan, and the southern coast of Chile (34). Several species of toxic dinoflagellate algae have been implicated in paralytic shellfish poisoning; *Gonyaulax catanella* and *G. ta-*

marensis are two of the most common culprits (34, 36). The blooms of the toxic dinoflagellates are quite sporadic, so most shellfish will be hazardous only during the times of the blooms (37). While most shellfish species clear the toxins from their system within a few weeks after the end of the dinoflagellate bloom, a few species, such as the Alaskan butter clam, appear to retain the toxin for long periods (34). The neurotoxins involved in paralytic shellfish poisoning, known as saxitoxins (34, 36, 38), bind to and block the sodium channels in nerve membranes (36). Because the saxitoxins are heat-stable, processing and cooking have no effect on the toxicity of the shellfish (34).

By blocking nerve transmission, the saxitoxins act as very potent neurotoxins. The symptoms of paralytic shellfish poisoning include a tingling sensation and numbness of the lips, tongue, and fingertips, followed by numbness in the legs, arms, and neck, ataxia, giddiness, staggering, drowsiness, incoherent speech progressing to aphasia, rash, fever, and respiratory and muscular paralysis (39). Death from respiratory failure occurs frequently—usually within 2–12 hours, depending upon the dose ingested. No antidotes are known, although prognosis is good if the victim survives the first 24 hours of the illness (34).

Amnesic Shellfish Poisoning

Amnesic shellfish poisoning was first recognized following an outbreak in Canada in 1987 (40). Amnesic shellfish poisoning associated with the ingestion of mussels from Prince Edward Island resulted in more than 100 cases and at least 4 deaths (40, 41). The source of the toxin was a planktonic algae, *Nitzchia pungens,* which was blooming in an isolated area of Prince Edward Island at the time of the outbreak (42). The toxin itself was identified as domoic acid, a neuroexcitatory amino acid (43).

Amnesic shellfish poisoning is characterized by gastrointestinal symptoms and unusual neurological abnormalities (40). The gastrointestinal symptoms, which occur within the first 24 hours, include vomiting, abdominal cramps, and diarrhea. The neurological symptoms, which appear within 48 hours, encompass severe incapacitating headaches, confusion, loss of short-term memory, and, in a few cases, seizures and coma. Severely affected patients who

did not die in the Canadian outbreak experienced prolonged neurologic sequelae, including memory deficits and motor or sensorimotor neuronopathy or axonopathy (41).

Diarrhetic Shellfish Poisoning

Diarrhetic shellfish poisoning is primarily associated with the ingestion of clams that have become toxic through ingestion of toxic dinoflagellate algae of the genus *Dinophysis* (44). Only one known outbreak has occurred in North America, although more frequent outbreaks have occurred in Japan, Europe, and Chile (44). The toxins responsible for diarrhetic shellfish poisoning are polyether compounds: okadaic acid, dinophysistoxins, and pectenotoxins (45). Symptoms include diarrhea, nausea, vomiting, and abdominal cramps (44).

Pufferfish Poisoning

Pufferfish poisoning occurs primarily in Japan and China, the only parts of the world where pufferfish are regularly consumed. Of the 30 species of pufferfish found worldwide, most are not toxic (34). The most hazardous pufferfish belong to the *Fugu* genus, which are considered delicacies in Japan and China. These pufferfish contain a potent neurotoxin called tetrodotoxin (34). For many years, the toxin was thought to be produced by the fish, but some evidence now exists that marine bacteria may represent the original source of the toxin (46). Tetrodotoxin is heat-stable and, like saxitoxin, acts by blocking the sodium channels in nerve cell membranes. The symptoms of tetrodotoxin poisoning usually begin with a tingling sensation of the fingers, toes, lips, and tongue, followed by nausea, vomiting, diarrhea, and epigastric pain (34, 47). Twitching, tremors, ataxia, paralysis, and death often ensue (47). The fatality rate is approximately 60% in untreated cases (47). Most of the tetrodotoxin accumulates in the liver, viscera, and roe of the pufferfish. Careful cleaning of the fish, prior to ingestion of the edible muscle is required to safeguard against tetrodotoxin intoxication (34).

MYCOTOXINS

Mycotoxins are produced by a wide variety of molds that can grow and produce toxins on numerous types of foods (48). Most of the known mycotoxins have been recognized through the toxic effects they produce in domestic animals fed moldy feed grains. A few mycotoxins are noteworthy because they are known hazards for humans.

Ergotism

Ergotism was the first recognized mycotoxin-associated illness (48). The responsible mold is *Claviceps purpurea*, which can infect the grains of rye, wheat, barley, and oats. The last recorded outbreak of ergotism occurred in Europe in 1951. Ergotism, which is caused by a group of toxins known as the ergot alkaloids, is manifested in two forms: gangrenous ergotism and convulsive ergotism. Gangrenous ergotism (also known as St. Anthony's fire) is characterized by a burning sensation in the feet and hands, followed by progressive restriction of blood flow to the hands and feet that ultimately results in gangrene and loss of limbs. Convulsive ergotism is characterized by hallucinations that lead to convulsive seizures and sometimes death. Modern agricultural practices and grain milling procedures have virtually eliminated ergotism as a concern.

Alimentary Toxic Aleukia

Alimentary toxic aleukia (ALA) was first observed in Russia during World War II, when it was associated with the consumption of overwintered millet that contained trichothecene mycotoxins (48). Trichothecenes are a group of mycotoxins produced by molds of the genus *Fusarium*. ALA occurs in four stages. In the first stage, affected individuals experience burning sensations in the mouth, throat, and esophagus, followed 1 to 3 days later by diarrhea, nausea, and vomiting. The gastrointestinal symptoms cease after about 9 days. The second stage of ALA begins during the second week and lasts through the second month. It involves bone marrow destruction, agranulocytosis, anemia, and loss of platelets. Small hemorrhages begin to appear at the end of this stage. The third stage of ALA, which lasts for 5 to 20 days, involves total loss of bone marrow with necrotic angina, sepsis, agranulocytosis, moderate fever, larger hemorrhages on the skin, and necrotic skin lesions. Bronchial pneumonia usually develops along with abscesses and hemorrhages in the lungs. The fourth stage of ALA

is death, which occurs in approximately 80% of cases within three months of the onset of symptoms. In the Russian cases, the exact species of *Fusarium* and the trichothecenes responsible for ALA were not identified, nor were the level of contamination of the millet with trichothecenes determined.

Fusarium molds are very common on grain crops worldwide. Trichothecene mycotoxins continue to occur at low levels in many cereal foods. No acute illnesses in humans (including ALA) have been attributed to trichothecene intoxication since the original outbreak, however. The effects of ingestion of low levels of toxic trichothecenes on humans remain uncertain.

NATURALLY OCCURRING CONSTITUENTS

Many fungi, some plants, and a few animals contain hazardous levels of naturally occurring toxicants. Such fungi, plants, and animals should not be eaten, but are sometimes accidentally or intentionally consumed, resulting in foodborne illness. Furthermore, many plants and animals contain levels of naturally occurring toxicants that are probably not hazardous to humans ingesting typical amounts of these foods. The ingestion of abnormally large quantities of such foods is, however, potentially hazardous. In addition, some naturally occurring toxicants are inactivated or removed during processing or preparation of foods prior to consumption; the failure to adhere to such processing and preparation practices can result in foodborne illness.

Poisonous Animals

Very few animal species are poisonous, although several species of poisonous fish and other marine animals have been identified (47, 49). Pufferfish (described earlier) is the best-known example, although the toxin in pufferfish may actually emanate from bacteria (46).

Animal tissues and products contain very few naturally occurring toxicants that could cause adverse reactions if ingested in abnormally large quantities. The best example of such a toxicant is vitamin A (1). The ingestion of polar bear livers and fish livers in large quantities has led to vitamin A intoxication (1). Cases of vitamin A intoxication have also occurred in infants resulting from feeding diets rich in vitamin A (e.g., chicken livers and fortified milk) and carotenoids (e.g., pureed carrots), while also administering daily vitamin supplements (50).

Poisonous Plants

Many poisonous plants exist in nature (51). Classic examples include water hemlock and nightshade, which were historically used to poison one's enemies. While consumers purchasing foods from commercial sources usually avoid the ingestion of poisonous plants, intoxications occur each year in individuals who have harvested their own foods in the wild (52). As an example, an elderly couple succumbed after mistaking foxglove for comfrey while harvesting herbs for tea; foxglove contains digitalis (53). In another example, a team member in a desert survival course died after eating a salad prepared in part from a *Datura* species, jimsonweed (52). Jimsonweed contains tropane alkaloids, including atropine. While atropine is a useful pharmaceutical agent, its ingestion from natural sources in uncontrolled doses can prove fatal. Atropine has potent anticholinergic properties, and individuals ingesting jimsonweed and other plants containing tropane alkaloids can suffer neurotoxic effects.

More rarely, intoxications from poisonous plants may occur with products purchased from commercial sources (54). In one well-investigated outbreak, a commercial herbal tea was contaminated with *Senecio longilobis*, a well-known poisonous plant (54). The herbal tea, called gordolobo yerba, was sold within the Mexican–American community in Arizona, where it was promoted as a cure for colic, viral infections, and nasal congestion in infants. Several infants died from the ingestion of this contaminated herbal tea. *Senecio* and many other plants contain a group of chemicals known as pyrrolizidine alkaloids, which can cause both acute and chronic symptoms. Chronic low doses produce liver cancer and cirrhosis (34). Acute symptoms associated with the contaminated herbal tea included ascites, hepatomegaly, veno-occlusive liver disease, abdominal pain, nausea, vomiting, headache, and diarrhea (54). Death resulted from liver failure.

Occasionally, intoxications from poisonous plants occur from the intentional addition of such materials to foods. The intentional inclusion of marijuana in bakery items represents the most common example.

Many plant-derived foods contain naturally occurring toxicants at doses that are not hazardous, at least on an acute basis, unless large quantities of the food are eaten. Examples include solanine and chaconine in potatoes, oxalates in spinach and rhubarb, furan compounds in mold-damaged sweet potatoes, and cyanogenic glycosides in lima beans, cassava, and many fruit pits (55). The cyanogenic glycosides (34, 55), for example, can release cyanide from enzymatic action occurring during the storage and processing of the foods or on contact with stomach acid. Commercial varieties of lima beans contain minimal amounts of these cyanogenic glycosides, with an HCN yield of 10 mg per 100 g of lima beans (wet weight) noted. Because the lethal oral dose of cyanide for humans is 0.5 mg/kg body weight, a 70 kg adult would need to ingest 35 mg of cyanide, which would require consumption of at least 350 g of lima beans. Such levels of consumption are quite unlikely, and human illnesses from cyanide intoxication from lima bean ingestion have not been identified. Wild varieties of lima beans contain much higher levels of the cyanogenic glycosides (as much as 300 mg HCN/100 g), however, and would likely be hazardous to consume. Cyanide intoxications have occurred in Africa and South America from consumption of cassava, which is sometimes ingested in large quantities when other foods are lacking (34, 55). Cyanide intoxication has also occurred from the ingestion of fruit pits (34), including the grinding of pits with the fruit in food processors during the preparation of jams and wines. Symptoms of cyanide intoxication include a rapid onset of peripheral numbness and dizziness, mental confusion, stupor, cyanosis, twitching, convulsions, coma, and death (34).

Many toxic constituents of plants are inactivated or removed during food processing and preparation. For example, raw soybeans contain trypsin inhibitors, lectins, amylase inhibitors, saponins, and various antivitamins (34). Fortunately, these toxicants become inactivated during the heating and fermentation processes used with soybeans. Failure to remove or inactivate these toxicants can result in foodborne illness.

For example, raw kidney beans contain lectins that are typically inactivated during cooking. In the United Kingdom, immigrants who did not thoroughly cook kidney beans have experienced nausea, vomiting, abdominal pain, and bloody diarrhea from ingestion of the lectins (34).

Poisonous Mushrooms

Many species of mushrooms are poisonous. The harvesting of mushrooms in the wild can be a hazardous practice. In the United States, numerous intoxications occur each year from the ingestion of poisonous mushrooms (22). Poisonous mushrooms contain a variety of naturally occurring toxicants that can be classified into Groups I–VI (34, 56).

The Group I toxins, which are the most hazardous, include amatoxin and phallotoxin. Amatoxin is produced by *Amanita phalloides,* the death cap mushroom. Amatoxin poisoning occurs in three stages. In the first stage, abdominal pain, nausea, vomiting, diarrhea, and hyperglycemia begin 6 to 24 hours after ingestion of the mushrooms. A short period of remission then occurs. The third—and often fatal—stage involves severe liver and kidney dysfunction, hypoglycemia, convulsions, coma, and death. Death resulting from hypoglycemic shock occurs 4 to 7 days after the onset of symptoms.

The Group II toxins are hydrazines, of which gyromitrin is the best-known example. Gyromitrin is produced by *Gyromitra esculenta,* or false morel mushrooms. The symptoms associated with ingestion of these mushrooms include a bloated feeling, nausea, vomiting, watery or bloody diarrhea, abdominal pain, muscle cramps, faintness, and ataxia occurring with a 6 to 12 hour onset time.

The Group III toxins are characterized by muscarine and affect the autonomic nervous system. Muscarine is found in fly agaric *(Amanita muscarina),* sometimes in association with the Group I toxins. Symptoms include perspiration, salivation, lacrimation with blurred vision, abdominal cramps, watery diarrhea, constriction of the pupils, hypotension, and a slowed pulse; these symptoms follow rapidly on the heels of ingestion of the poisonous mushrooms.

The Group IV toxins cause symptoms only when ingested with alcoholic beverages. Coprine, which is produced by *Coprinus atramentarius,* is the best ex-

ample of a Group IV toxin. Symptoms include flushing of the neck and face, distension of the veins in the neck, swelling and tingling of the hands, metallic taste, tachycardia, and hypotension progressing to nausea and vomiting. Symptoms appear within 30 minutes of ingestion of the mushrooms and can last for as long as 5 days.

The Group V and VI toxins act primarily on the central nervous system, causing hallucinations. The Group V toxins, which include ibotenic acid and muscimol, cause dizziness, drowsiness followed by hyperkinetic activity, confusion, delirium, incoordination, staggering, muscular spasms, partial amnesia, a coma-like sleep, and hallucinations beginning 30 minutes to 2 hours after ingestion. Fly agaric is a prime source of the Group V toxins.

The Group VI toxins include psilocybin and psilocin. The symptoms of the Group VI toxins include pleasant or aggressive mood, anxiety, unmotivated laughter and hilarity, compulsive movements, muscle weakness, drowsiness, hallucinations, and sleep. The Group VI toxins are found in Mexican mushrooms, *Psilocybe mexicana.* Symptoms usually begin 30 to 60 minutes after ingestion of the mushrooms, and recovery often occurs spontaneously in 5 to 10 hours. When the dose of the Group VI toxins is high, prolonged and severe sequelae—even death—can occur.

Metabolic Food Disorders

Like food allergies, metabolic food disorders affect only certain individuals within the overall population. These individuals display increased sensitivity to certain chemicals in foods because they lack an enzyme necessary to metabolize that particular chemical or because they have a genetic abnormality that renders them especially susceptible to the toxic effects of a specific foodborne chemical. The best examples of metabolic food disorders are lactose intolerance and favism.

LACTOSE INTOLERANCE

Lactose intolerance is associated with an inherited deficiency in the amount of the enzyme β-galactosidase in the small intestine (57, 58). β-Galactosidase is necessary for the hydrolysis of the milk disaccharide, lactose, into its constituent monosaccharides, glucose and galactose. While glucose and galactose can be absorbed and used for metabolic energy, lactose cannot be absorbed without prior hydrolysis. If β-galactosidase activity is insufficient, incomplete hydrolysis of the lactose from milk or dairy products occurs. Undigested lactose passes into the colon, where the large numbers of bacteria will convert it to CO_2, H_2, and H_2O. Symptoms associated with lactose intolerance include abdominal cramps, flatulence, and frothy diarrhea.

Almost all individuals are born with sufficient levels of β-galactosidase activity. With increasing age, however, the levels of enzyme activity diminish. At some point, the levels of β-galactosidase activity may become insufficient to handle the load of lactose ingested in the diet. Symptoms of lactose intolerance can begin to appear in the early teenage years and often worsen with advancing age (59). Many lactose-intolerant individuals can tolerate some lactose in their diets—often as much as the amount found in an 8-oz glass of milk (60). The degree of tolerance may lessen with advancing age, however.

Lactose intolerance is an inherited trait. It affects only 6% to 12% of all Caucasians, but ultimately affects 60% to 90% of some ethnic groups, including African Americans, Native Americans, Hispanics, Asians, Jews, and Arabs (57, 58).

Treatment involves dairy product avoidance diets, although some dairy products can usually be ingested without ill effects. Lactose-intolerant individuals can often safely consume yogurt if it contains live bacterial cultures with β-galactosidase (61). Lactose-hydrolyzed milk is also available in many markets.

FAVISM

Favism is caused by the ingestion of fava beans or the inhalation of pollen from the *Vicia faba* plant by individuals with a deficiency of the enzyme glucose-6-phosphate dehydrogenase (G6PDH) in their erythrocytes (62). Erythrocyte G6PDH deficiency is the most common enzyme deficiency in the world, affecting perhaps 100 million individuals. It is most prevalent among Oriental Jewish communities in Israel, Sardinians, Cypriot Greeks, African Americans, and some African populations (62). This deficiency is virtually unknown in northern Europeans, North American Indians, and Eskimos (62). The G6PDH enzyme is essential for maintaining adequate levels of the reduced form of glutathione (GSH) and nicotinamide dinucleotide phosphate (NADPH) in erythrocytes. GSH and NADPH protect the erythrocyte membrane from oxidation. Fava beans contain two potent, naturally occurring oxidants: vicine and convicine. These oxidants can damage the erythrocyte membranes in G6PDH-deficient individuals, but not in normal persons. Exposure to fava beans in sensitive individuals results in acute hemolytic anemia (62). The typical symptoms include pallor, fatigue, dyspnea, nausea, abdominal and/or back pain, fever, and chills. In a few severe cases, hemoglobinuria, jaundice, and renal failure may occur.

Favism is not a common malady in the United States, as fava beans are rarely ingested there. Instead, it occurs primarily in the Mediterranean area, the Middle East, China, and Bulgaria, where the genetic trait is fairly prevalent and fava beans are consumed more frequently.

REFERENCES

1. DiPalma JR, Ritchie DM. Vitamin toxicity. Ann Rev Pharmacol Toxicol 1977;17:133–148.
2. Press E, Yeager L. Food "poisoning" due to sodium nicotinate—report of an outbreak and a review of the literature. Am J Public Health 1962;52:1720–1728.
3. Campana L, Redmond S, Nitzkin JL, et al. Niacin intoxication from pumpernickel bagels—New York. J Am Med Assoc 1983;250:160.
4. Burkhalter J, Shore M, Wollstadt L, et al. Illness associated with high levels of niacin in cornmeal—Illinois. CDC Morbidity Mortality Wkly Rpts 1981;30:11–12.
5. Taylor SL. Chemical intoxications. In: Cliver DO, ed. Food-borne diseases. San Diego: Academic Press, 1990, 171–182.
6. Taylor SL, Byron B. Probable case of sorbitol-induced diarrhea. J Food Prot 1984;47:249.
7. Kilbourne EM, Rigau-Perez JG, Heath CW Jr, et al. Clinical epidemiology of toxic oil syndrome: manifestations of a new illness. N Engl J Med 1983;309:1408–1414.
8. Noriega AR, Gomez-Reino J, Lopez-Encuentra AL. Toxic epidemic syndrome, Spain 1981. Lancet 1982;2:697–702.
9. Condemi JJ. Unusual presentations. In: Chiaramonte LT, Schneider AT, Lifshitz F, eds. Food allergy—a practical approach to diagnosis and management. New York: Marcel Dekker, 1988, 231–254.
10. World Health Organization. Toxic oil syndrome—current

knowledge and future perspectives. Copenhagen: WHO Regional Publications, European Series no. 42, 1992.

11. Rodriguez M, Nogura AE, Del Villaras S, et al. Toxic synovitis from denatured rapeseed oil. Arthritis Rheum 1982;25:1477–1480.

12. Ferrer A, Cabral R. Toxic epidemics caused by alimentary exposure to pesticides. Food Additives Contaminants 1991;8:755–776.

13. Green MA, Heumann MA, Wehr HM, et al. An outbreak of watermelon-borne pesticide toxicity. Am J Publ Health 1907;77.1431–1434.

14. Goldman LR, Beller M, Jackson RL. Aldicarb food poisonings in California, 1985–1988; toxicity estimates for humans. Arch Environ Health 1990;45:141–147.

15. Goes EA, Savage EP, Gibbons G, Aaronson M, Ford SA, Wheeler HW. Suspected foodborne carbamate pesticide intoxication associated with ingestion of hydroponic cucumbers. Am J Epidemiol 1980;111:254–260.

16. Taylor SL, Nordlee JA, Kapels LM. Foodborne toxicants affecting the lung. Pediatr Allergy Immunol 1992;3:180–187.

17. Schmid R. Cutaneous porphyria in Turkey. N Engl J Med 1960;268:397–398.

18. Fassett DW. Nitrates and nitrites. In: Committee on Food Protection. Toxicants occurring naturally in foods, 2nd ed. Washington, DC: National Academy of Sciences, 1973, 7–25.

19. Sinios A. Methemoglobinemia von nitrat gehalt in spinat. Munch Med Wochenschr 1964;1180–1182.

20. Keating JP, Lell ME, Straus AW, Zarkowsky H, Smith GE. Infantile methemoglobinemia caused by carrot juice. N Engl J Med 1973;288:825–826.

21. Dewdney JM, Edwards RG. Penicillin hypersensitivity—is milk a significant hazard?: a review. J Royal Soc Med 1984;77:866–877.

22. Hughes JM, Horwitz MA, Merson MH, Barker WH Jr, Gangarosa EJ. Foodborne disease outbreaks of chemical etiology in the United States, 1970–1974. Am J Epidemiol 1977;105:233–244.

23. Barker WH Jr, Runte V. Tomato juice associated gastroenteritis, Washington and Oregon, 1969. Am J Epidemiol 1972;96:219–226.

24. Hamel AJ, Drawbaugh R, McBean AM, Watson WN, Witherell PE. Outbreak of acute gastroenteritis due to copper poisoning—Vermont. CDC Morbidity Mortality Wkly Rpis 1977;26:218.

25. Brown MA, Thom JV, Orth GL, et al. Food poisoning involving zinc contamination. Arch Environ Health 1964;8:657–660.

26. Kurland LT, Faro SN, Siedler H. Minamata disease. World Neurol 1960;1:370–395.

27. Bergdoll MS. Staphylococcal food poisoning. In: Cliver DO, ed. Foodborne diseases. San Diego: Academic Press, 1990, 85–106.

28. Sugiyama H. Botulism. In: Cliver DO, ed. Foodborne diseases. San Diego: Academic Press, 1990, 107–125.

29. Bagnis R, Kuberski T, Laugier S. Clinical observations on 3,009 cases of ciguatera (fish poisoning) in the South Pacific. Am J Trop Med Hyg 1979;28:1067–1073.

30. Russell FE, Egen NB. Ciguatoxic fishes, ciguatoxin (CTX) and ciguatera poisoning. J Toxicol Toxin Rev 1991;10:37–62.

31. Lawrence DN, Enriquez MB, Lumish RM, Maceo A. Ciguatera fish poisoning in Miami. J Am Med Assoc 1980;244:254–258.

32. Morris JG Jr, Lewin P, Hargrett NT, Smith W, Blake PA, Schneider R. Clinical features of ciguatera fish poisoning—a

study of the disease in the US Virgin Islands. Arch Int Med 1982;142:1090–1092.

33. Hokama Y, Miyahara JT. Ciguatera poisoning: clinical and immunological aspects. J Toxicol Toxin Rev 1986;5:25–53.

34. Taylor SL, Schantz EJ. Naturally occurring toxicants. In: Cliver DO, ed. Foodborne diseases. San Diego: Academic Press, 1990, 67–84.

35. Bagnis R, Chanteau S, Chungue E, Hurtel JM, Yasumoto T, Inoue A. Origins of ciguatera fish poisoning: a new dinoflagellate, Gambierdiscus toxicus Adachi and Fukuyo, definitely involved as a causal agent. Toxicon 1980;18:199–208.

36. Shimizu Y. The chemistry of paralytic shellfish toxins. In: Tu AT, ed. Handbook of natural toxins. vol. 3. Marine toxins and venoms. New York: Marcel Dekker, 1988, 63–85.

37. Taylor SL. Marine toxins of microbial origin. Food Technol 1988;42:94–98.

38. Hall S, Reichardt PB. Cryptic paralytic shellfish toxins. In: Ragelis EP, ed. Seafood toxins. Washington, DC: Am Chem Soc, 1984, 113–124.

39. Schantz EJ. Seafood toxicants. In: Committee on Food Protection. Toxicants occurring naturally in foods, 2nd ed. Washington, DC: National Academy of Sciences, 1973, 424–447.

40. Perl TM, Bedard L, Kosatsky T, Hockin JC, Todd ECD, Remis RS. An outbreak of toxic encephalopathy caused by eating mussels contaminated with domoic acid. N Engl J Med 1990;322:1775–1780.

41. Teitelbaum JS, Zatorre RJ, Carpenter S, et al. Neurologic sequelae of domoic acid intoxication due to the ingestion of contaminated mussels. N Engl J Med 1990;322:1781–1787.

42. Bates SS, Bird CJ, DeFreitas ASW, et al. Pennate diatom Nitzchia pungens as the primary source of domoic acid, a toxin in shellfish from eastern Prince Edward Island, Canada. Can J Fish Aquatic Sci 1989;46:1203–1215.

43. Wright JLC, Boyd RK, DeFreitas ASW, et al. Identification of domoic acid, a neuroexcitatory amino acid, in toxic mussels from eastern Prince Edward Island. Can J Chem 1989;67:481–490.

44. Yasumoto T, Murata M, Oshima Y, Matsumoto GK, Clardy J. Diarrhetic shellfish poisoning. In: Ragelis EP, ed. Seafood toxins. Washington, DC: Am Chem Soc, 1984, 207–216.

45. Yasumoto T, Murata M. Polyether toxins involved in seafood poisoning. In: Hall S, Stricharty G, eds. Marine toxins—origin, structure and molecular pharmacology. Washington, DC: Am Chem Soc, 1990, 120–132.

46. Yasumoto T, Yasumura D, Yotsu M, Michishita T, Endo A, Kotaki Y. Bacterial production of tetrodotoxin and anhydrotetrodotoxin. Agr Biol Chem 1986;50:793–795.

47. Halstead BW. Fish toxins. In: Hui YH, Gorham JR, Murrell KD, Cliver DO, eds. Foodborne disease handbook. vol. 3. Diseases caused by hazardous substances. New York: Marcel Dekker, 1994, 4463–4496.

48. Marth EH. Mycotoxins. In: Cliver DO, ed. Foodborne diseases. San Diego: Academic Press, 1990, 137–157.

49. Halstead BW. Other poisonous marine animals. In: Hui YH, Gorham JR, Murrell KD, Cliver DO, eds. Foodborne disease handbook. vol. 3. Diseases caused by hazardous substances. New York: Marcel Dekker, 1994, 497–528.

50. Hayes KC, Hegsted DM. Toxicity of the vitamins. In: Committee on Food Protection. Toxicants occurring naturally in foods, 2nd ed. Washington, DC: National Academy of Sciences, 1973, 235–253.

51. Smith RA. Poisonous plants. In: Hui YH, Gorham JR, Murrell

KD, Cliver DO, eds. Foodborne disease handbook. vol. 3. Diseases caused by hazardous substances. New York: Marcel Dekker, 1994, 187–226.

52. Huxtable RJ. Herbal teas and toxins: novel aspects of pyrrolizidine poisoning in the United States. Perspect Biol Med 1980;24:1–14.

53. Cooper L, Grunenfelder G, Blackmon J, Fretwell M, Raey J, Allard J, Bartleson B. Poisoning associated with herbal teas— Washington. CDC Morbid Mortal Wkly Rpt 1977;26:257–259.

54. Stillman AE, Huxtable R, Consroe P, Kohnen P, Smith S. Hepatic veno-occlusive disease due to pyrrolizidine poisoning in Arizona. Gastroenterology 1977;73:349–353.

55. Beier RC, Nigg HN. Toxicology of naturally occurring chemicals in foods. In: Hui YH, Gorham JR, Murrell KD, Cliver DO, eds. Foodborne disease handbook. vol. 3. Diseases caused by hazardous substances. New York: Marcel Dekker, 1994, 1–186.

56. Spoerke DG Jr. Mushrooms: epidemiology and medical management. In: Hui YH, Gorham JR, Murrell KD, Cliver DO,

eds. Foodborne disease handbook. vol. 3. Diseases caused by hazardous substances. New York: Marcel Dekker, 1994, 433–462.

57. Kocian J. Lactose intolerance. Int J Biochem 1988;20:1–5.

58. Lemke PJ, Taylor SL. Allergic reactions and food intolerances. In: Kotsonis FN, Mackey M, Hjelle J, eds. Nutritional toxicology. New York: Raven Press, 1994, 117–137.

59. Taylor SL. Allergic and sensitivity reactions to food components. In: Hathcock JN, ed. Nutritional toxicology. vol. II. New York: Academic Press, 1987, 173–198.

60. Lisker R, Aguilas L. Double blind study of milk lactose intolerance. Gastroenterology 1978;74:1283–1285.

61. Gallagher CR, Molleson AL, Caldwell JH. Lactose intolerance and fermented dairy products. Cult Dairy Prod J 1977;10:22, 24.

62. Mager J, Chevion M, Glaser G. Favism. In: Liener IE, ed. Toxic constituents of plant foodstuffs, 2nd ed. New York: Academic Press, 1980, 265–294.

34

NEUROLOGIC REACTIONS TO FOODS AND FOOD ADDITIVES

Richard W. Weber

T. Ray Vaughan

*T*he impact of foods or food additives on neurological functioning has received varying levels of attention, ranging from case reports to double-blind, placebo-controlled challenges. Signs and symptoms range from those that are purely subjective to those that may be validated by objective findings. This chapter will deal with syndromes such as food-induced migraine and epilepsy. Other chapters address issues of behavior and psychologic functioning.

Migraine Headache

Migraine headache is a common affliction occurring in 5% to 30% of the general population, with a familial predisposition in 60% to 80% of cases, and affecting females three times more often than males. A recent survey of 20,468 individuals revealed that 5.7% of males and 17.6% of females suffered one or more migraines per year (1). The prevalence was highest between 35 and 45 years of age. Based on this study, it was estimated that, in the U.S. population, 8.7 million females and 2.6 million males suffer moderate to severe disability from migraine. In 1962, the Ad Hoc Committee on the Classification of Headache defined migraine as "recurrent attacks of headache, widely varied in intensity, frequency, and duration. The attacks are commonly unilateral in onset; are usually associated with anorexia and, sometimes, with nausea and vomiting; some are preceded by, or associated with, conspicuous sensory, motor, and mood disturbances; and are often familial" (2). Migraine may be divided into several clinical syndromes.

"Classic migraine" presents with an "aura" or prodrome, frequently visual in nature, that precedes onset of the headache by 5 to 30 minutes. The visual disturbance typically involves "scintillating scotomata"—multicolored saw-toothed arcs—that may move across the visual field. "Common migraine" lacks a prodrome before the headache. "Complicated migraine" indicates the association of more significant neurologic dysfunction such as hemiplegia; symptoms may persist beyond the duration of the headache but usually resolve spontaneously.

Precipitating factors of migraine are varied, and include stress, bright lights or loud sounds, physical exertion, fasting, menses or oral contraception use (although migraine frequently improves during pregnancy), and foods. No definitive laboratory tests exist to confirm the diagnosis. Electroencephalogram abnormalities have been noted but are minimal and more common in childhood migraine. The diagnosis of migraine is based primarily on history and the exclusion of other medical conditions that may mimic migraine, such as aneurysm, temporal arteritis, carcinoid tumor, pheochromocytoma, brain tumor, arteriovenous malformation, glaucoma, mastocytosis, or carotid or vertebrobasilar vascular insufficiency.

THEORIES OF MIGRAINE ETIOLOGY

Despite its description centuries ago, no firm consensus has been reached on the etiology of migraine. The frequently pulsatile nature of the headache suggested a vascular theory in which the aura represents an initial phase of regional intracerebral vasoconstriction, followed by vasodilatation, with inflammation explaining the headache. This theory was supported by evidence of slowed intracerebral blood flow in patients with classic migraine, although patients with common migraine show no similar changes. A recent report of spontaneous migraine during a positron-emission tomography study in a patient with common migraine revealed bilateral cerebral hypoperfusion spreading anteriorly from the occipital lobes to the temporal and parietal lobes (3).

The neurogenic theory suggested that the basic defect centered on neuronal response to certain neurotransmitters and that vascular changes took a secondary place to neuronal impulses and the vasoactive properties of such neurotransmitters as substance P (4). Abnormalities in serotonin metabolism have been described in the platelets of patients with migraine, but it remains unclear whether these changes represent primary defects or epiphenomena from drug effects (4, 5). It has proved difficult to reconcile these theories with the actions of a variety of agents that have been found empirically to either provoke or relieve migraine.

One review, however, reinforces the idea that migraine headache may have several levels of pathophysiologic triggering and potentiating factors that consolidate neurogenic and vasogenic elements (6). This hypothesis proposes that ionic and metabolic cortical mechanisms release nociceptive substances that stimulate trigeminovascular sensory fibers. These impulses cause pain and release vasoactive neuropeptides such as substance P and neurokinin A, inducing vasodilatation and protein extravasation, and thereby causing further nociceptive substance release and sensory nerve-ending sensitization. Receptors for 5-hydroxytryptamine on sensory nerve endings and vascular smooth muscle are central to this cascade. The large numbers of dural mast cells have also been implicated as participating in this process (6). Given the complexity of the initiating and potentiating elements of the migraine reaction, a great variety of therapeutic modalities may be possible.

DIET MANIPULATION IN MIGRAINE

Diets may play a role in determining migraine severity by limiting precursor availability for generation of vasoactive mediators or nociceptor transmitters. Car-

bohydrate-rich, protein-tryptophan-low diets have been attempted to modify migraine headaches (7). If platelet serotonin is actually a precipitator of the vasoconstrictory phase of migraine, the restricted dietary intake of serotonin and the serotonin precursor tryptophan could potentially lower levels within platelets, thereby alleviating migraine headaches. It has also been suggested that increased brain serotonin levels may improve migraine through the anti-nociceptive system. Insulin release following consumption of carbohydrate-rich meals would increase tryptophan availability to the brain, with subsequent increased serotonin synthesis. Hasselmark and coworkers tried such a diet for 50 days (after a 30-day routine diet) in 10 migraine patients (7). Three patients dropped out, leaving four with classic migraine and three with common migraine. Three of four with classic migraine experienced a marked improvement in headache frequency, while none of the common migraineurs noted a benefit from the diet. No differences in platelet serotonin uptake were found. The authors felt that the beneficial effect could be due to either a decrease in the ingestion of migraine-precipitating foods or an increase in brain serotonin levels.

ASSOCIATION OF FOOD ALLERGY AND MIGRAINE

Allergy to food is self-reported more commonly by migraine patients than by individuals with non-migrainous headache or without headache (8). As pointed out by Pinnas and Vanselow in their review of the relationship between allergy and migraine (9), the association between these two conditions is more than 100 years old. In 1885, Trousseau included periodic headache in the allergic diathesis; in 1918, Tileston likened migraine to asthma; and in 1919, Pagniez considered migraine as a manifestation of anaphylaxis (9). Several later reports identified food allergy as the cause of migraine, but methodological issues made these reports less than compelling. A series of reports also linked attacks to specific foods such as milk, egg, fish, beef, pork, and chocolate (10). In 1927, Vaughan reported that 10 of 33 migraine patients studied showed specific food triggers (11). These foods were identified by skin testing, followed by elimination and subsequent rechallenge with the incriminated foods. With the exception of a solitary blinded challenge, the challenges were conducted in an open fashion. Shortly thereafter, Eyermann reported that 69% of headache patients improved on an elimination diet (12). Forty-four subjects had headaches with suspected foods, beginning 3 to 6 hours after ingestion. The components of the diet were based on the results of skin tests; of the subjects who did not respond to the diet, 53% had positive tests. This finding suggests overinterpretation of the skin test responses. In addition, many of the patients did not have accepted criteria for migraine headache. Balyeat and Rinkel stated that of 202 migraine patients managed with food skin testing and elimination diets, 120 had 60% or greater improvement, with only 12% of the patients demonstrating little or no improvement (13). In 1932, DeGowin reported results with 60 migraine patients who had positive prick or intradermal skin tests to foods (14). Elimination diets in 42 patients brought complete relief in 33% of subjects and partial relief in another 45%; incidence of headache following reintroduction of foods was not reported.

These early studies suggested that food allergy, as demonstrated by immediate positive results of a skin test, was a significant cause of migraine headache. They were flawed, however, by being open studies that were susceptible to expectation bias and placebo effect. Subsequently, the mainstream of migraine opinion moved away from the causative role of allergy. Nonetheless, in 1952 Unger and Unger published a paper entitled "Migraine Is an Allergic Disease" (15). Curiously, the preceding article in that issue of the *Journal of Allergy*, by Schwartz, was entitled "Is Migraine an Allergic Disease?" (16). Schwartz's report detailed aspects of his extensive epidemiologic work in Denmark, involving 241 asthmatics, 200 nonallergic controls, and their 3815 relatives spanning four generations. He found no difference in the frequency of migraine in relatives of asthmatics and normal controls. He attributed this finding to the commonness of migraine, which meant that it was not unexpected to find it occurring in allergic kindreds.

Unger and Unger investigated 55 patients with skin tests, elimination diets, food diaries, and a "feeding test" to identify migraine-provoking foods (15). All foods ingested for 24 hours before the onset of migraine were recorded. The patients were challenged with the suspected food after 2 weeks on an elimination diet. If no reaction occurred within 1 hour, a second portion was given, and the patients recorded all symptoms for the next 24 hours. Using this protocol, 35 of the 55 patients achieved complete relief of migraine symptoms, 9 had 75% or greater relief, and another 2 had 50% to 65% improvement. In 9 patients, no benefit was determined. Food skin testing in this study was not helpful, identifying a provoking food only five times. This study was reminiscent of earlier open studies, but certain findings repeatedly appeared. A substantial number of migraineurs showed marked improvement on elimination diets. Recurrence of headache coincided with the reintroduction of certain foods, and the onset of the headache could be delayed 3 to 6 hours after ingestion of the provoking agent. Food skin tests varied in their ability to help in defining diets.

A scattering of open studies over the next 25 years supported the value of elimination diets in migraine but offered little insight into their mechanisms of action. In 1979, Grant reported remarkable results in 60 patients placed on a strict lamb-and-pear elimination diet (17). Of an initial group of 126 migraineurs, 35 discontinued the diet, and data were reported on only 60 patients. After 5 days of the diet, foods were reintroduced singly, with symptoms and pulse rate monitored for 1.5 hours. This technique led to improvement in all of the patients, and complete resolution in 51 subjects (85%). The number of foods found to provoke symptoms for each patient ranged from 1 to 30, with a mean of 10. No blinded challenges were performed, and these results no doubt reflect a substantial placebo effect. Likewise, the use of the pulse test has no documented validity and could lead to the unnecessary elimination of numerous foods. Finally, the 31 patients who continued the diet but were not included in the data analysis presumably exhibited less striking results.

Monro and coworkers reported 47 migraine patients managed with elimination and rotation diets (18). Twenty-three of the 36 patients completing the diet phase were able to identify provoking foods. Subsequently, conduct of the radioallergosorbent test (RAST) to a battery of foods found migraine-provoking foods to have higher RAST titers than foods not producing headaches. In a further report, these workers presented 9 migraine patients with reproducible food sensitivity documented by elimination diets with open challenges (19). Administration of high-dose oral cromolyn blocked headache in 5 patients, unlike placebo. The benefits of a strict milk-protein-free diet for classic migraine was reported in 1983 (20). Of 26 patients, 18 improved on the diet; all of these patients had documented lactase deficiency. One additional lactase-deficient patient did not improve on the diet; the remainder of the subjects were not lactose-intolerant. When Hughes and colleagues placed 21 migraine patients on a "semi-elemental" diet for a week, 19 had a marked reduction of headache severity during the week of observation (21). These unblinded studies suggested that a large percentage of migraineurs would benefit from the elimination of specific foods, and that more stringent diets would more likely produce success.

Double-blind, placebo-controlled (DBPC) challenges are necessary to clarify issues in an area where cause and effect are assessed by subjective symptomatology such as headache. Only a small number of such studies have been conducted. A preliminary report by Vaughan and colleagues in 1983, however, linked the value of food skin tests and DBPC food capsule challenges in adult migraine patients (22). In that same year, Egger and associates studied 99 children who suffered from at least one migraine per week for a minimum of six months (23). They were maintained for three to four weeks on an "oligoantigenic" diet: one meat, lamb or chicken; one carbohydrate, rice or potato; one fruit, apple or banana; one vegetable, brassica; and water and vitamin supplements. If no benefit was derived (more than one headache per week in the final two weeks of the diet), the alternative foods were tried. Patients who improved on the diet were then reintroduced to foods in normal portions daily for one week. Those who could identify a provoking food entered the DBPC challenge phase. Eighty-eight completed the diet, 78 recovered fully, 4 were greatly improved, and 6 received no benefit with the diet. Of the 82 who improved, 74 had migraines with one or more foods, with median onset of headache being two days after reintroduction of the responsible food. DBPC food challenges were performed with 40 children. Twenty-six responded to the active agent alone, 2 to the

placebo, 4 to both, and 8 to neither (p < 0.001). Prick skin testing was not helpful: the testing would have identified all of the precipitants in only 3 patients. Eighty-nine percent of the children completing the diet phase recovered completely; in 29.5% of those children, at least one provocative food was verified via DBPC challenge.

A DBPC study reported by Atkins and coworkers was negative, however (24). They studied 36 children by taking a history, conducting a physical examination, and carrying out a battery of 20 food prick skin tests. Sixteen suspected a food or additive; in 2 of these subjects, the skin test was positive. Foods suggested by the patients were studied with a total of 19 DBPC challenges, but none provoked a migrainous attack. Twenty patients could not identify any precipitants, and of these only 5 experienced more than two headaches per week. After these 5 subjects were placed on an elimination diet, 2 became headache-free. Headaches did not recur on resumption of a normal diet, however. The differences between the outcomes of these two studies may be explained by differences in protocol and patient selection. Egger placed all of his patients on the elimination diet, probably dealt with a more severely affected group, and challenged subjects with larger amounts of foods over several days. The prolonged challenge might lead to more false positives because of the recurring nature of spontaneous migraine. Because headache may be delayed several hours in onset, patients may not identify the culpable agents, and testing only history-suspected items would falsely lower the response rate.

Mansfield, Vaughan, and coworkers published data on 43 migraine adult patients referred from a neurology clinic (25). Prick skin testing was performed with a battery of 83 foods. Foods that resulted in positive skin tests were eliminated from the diet for one month, and patients with negative skin tests were placed on a wheat, corn, milk, and egg elimination diet. Patients experiencing at least a two-thirds reduction in headache frequency underwent a series of single-blind challenges with capsules containing a total of 8 g of desiccated food or a similar number of placebo capsules. Those with positive challenges returned for DBPC challenges. Thirteen of 43 (30%) met the two-thirds reduction criteria while on the diet. Of 7 who underwent DBPC challenges, no patient responded to placebo, 5 had migraine with the active challenge, and 2 did not experience headache in either challenge.

With a different population of patients, Vaughan and associates performed a study of 104 adult migraine subjects in another DBPC protocol (26–28). All patients had migraine verified by a neurologist and documented headache frequency of at least three per month on a regular diet using a symptom-food diary. Food skin tests were performed with 83 foods. All foods suggested by skin tests and history, as well as wheat, corn, milk, and egg, were eliminated for one month. Patients with a greater than 50% reduction in headache frequency underwent further study. Foods were reintroduced in an open fashion and eaten three times daily. Patients who felt that they could identify at least one provoking food entered into the DBPC phase. Foods were given in capsule form three times daily, with the challenge sequence taking four days, comprising two placebo (P) and two active days (A). The order was randomized with the caveat that the two active days were always together: A-A-P-P; P-A-A-P; or P-P-A-A. [Egger had reported than some patients reacted only with larger amounts of the incriminated food, on a second day of challenge (23).] A positive challenge was defined as headache occurring on both days or on the second challenge day, and any response to placebo was considered a negative challenge.

Forty of the 104 patients (38.5%) had a greater than 50% reduction in migraine frequency, with only 8 becoming headache-free. Twenty-seven of 36 undergoing open challenges could identify at least one precipitant, with a range of one to four foods noted. Of 24 patients with DBPC challenges, 15 had migraine on both active days and 2 on the second day only. Three reported headache on placebo, and 4 had no migraine at all. Thus, more than one-third of the 104 adult migraine patients had improvement on an elimination diet, and 17 of 104 (16%) had reproducible DBPC demonstration of food-induced migraine. In contrast to the impression given by Vaughan's earlier study, but in agreement with the Egger study, food skin testing was not uniformly helpful (22, 23). Skin tests were positive for less than half of the documented food triggers (Table 34.1). The skin test neither consistently identified migraine provoking

Table 34.1
Value of Double-Blind Food Challenges and Skin Tests in Migraineurs (26–28)

Patient #	Positive Open Challenges	Skin Test Results	Positive Double-Blind Challenges
1	Egg	1+	Egg
	Milk	0	
	Wheat	1+	
2	Coffee	2+	Coffee
	Maple syrup	ND	
3	Wheat	3+	Wheat
4	Black-eyed peas	4+	Black-eyed peas
	Pinto beans	3+	
5	Egg	1+	Egg
	Chocolate	0	
6	Egg	0	Egg
	Milk	0	
7	Wheat	0	Wheat
	Cheese	0	
8	Wheat	0	Wheat
9	Wheat	0	Wheat
	Chocolate	0	
10	Milk	0	Milk
	Wheat	0	
	Chocolate	0	
	Cheese	0	
11	Cheese	0	Cheese
	Chocolate	0	
12	Corn	0	Corn
	Wheat	0	
13	Coffee	0	Coffee
14	Cheese	0	Cheese
	Chocolate	0	
15	Corn	0	Corn
	Soy	0	
16	Wheat	0	Wheat
	Egg	0	.

foods nor identified migraineurs more likely to benefit from dietary manipulation.

PHARMACOLOGIC TRIGGERING AGENTS

In 1925, Curtis-Brown had proposed that defective protein metabolism was responsible for migraine headache, leading to "protein poisoning" by certain foods such as chocolate, eggs, fruit, tomatoes, mushrooms, and meats (29). Migraine could, therefore, occur on the first exposure to the specific food, and patients would improve on restrictive diets. Although no support ultimately emerged for this theory, it did introduce the concept that food intolerance in migraine patients could be due to some pharmacologic action of a constituent.

In the 1960s, a syndrome of severe pounding headache was described in patients taking monoamine oxidase inhibitors when they ingested certain foods containing tyramine. Hanington noted that such foods were also frequently incriminated by migraine sufferers as causing their headaches (30). A double-blind challenge showed an 80% response of headache to 125 mg of tyramine, and an 8% response to placebo in 45 migraine patients (31). Other studies that followed confirmed tyramine sensitivity in migraineurs. On the other hand, a series of papers appeared that could not demonstrate a significant role for tyramine. In a double-blind, placebo-controlled (DBPC) trial, Moffett and coworkers studied 8 migraine patients who believed tyramine precipitated their symptoms, another 10 migraineurs without this history, and 7 patients with both migraine and epilepsy (32). The patients with presumed tyramine headache had symptoms as often with placebo as with tyramine, 1 patient with epilepsy had a tyramine-induced headache, and none of the other migraineurs had headache. Forsythe and Redmond found that 12 of 61 children reacted to a blinded challenge using 100 mg tyramine; a second group of 38 children included only five that reacted to tyramine (33). Ziegler and Stewart reported results in 80 patients using a higher dose of 200 mg of tyramine (34). Forty-nine patients had symptoms with neither tyramine nor placebo, 12 with both substances, 11 with placebo alone, and only 8 with tyramine alone. Additionally, tyramine-free diets have failed to affect headache frequency (35).

Traditional provokers of migraine such as chocolate, cheeses, and red wine may not contain tyramine, but appreciable quantities of phenylethylamine (36). This vasoactive amine crosses the blood–brain barrier and can significantly disrupt cerebral blood flow. Five of six patients with histories of chocolate-induced migraine developed headaches within eight hours of an open challenge of 100 g of chocolate (37). Sandler and associates studied 36 patients who believed that chocolate precipitated headache (38). The subjects received either 3 mg phenylethylamine or placebo in a single-blinded fashion. Eighteen patients reported headache with the amine, whereas 6 reported headache with placebo, a statistically significant difference. When Schweitzer and coworkers analyzed a number of chocolate varieties, however, they found about 150-fold less phenylethylamine in these preparations than in those preparations tested by Sandler (39). These authors postulated that either chocolate-induced migraine was not due to phenylethylamine or migraine sufferers were sensitive to extremely low levels of this substance. Another DBPC study examined 25 patients with a history of chocolate- or cocoa-induced migraine (40). Eight patients reported headache with only chocolate, 5 with only placebo, 1 with both substances, and 11 with neither. Fifteen patients underwent repeat challenges with different chocolate and placebo preparations, and 5 had migraine with chocolate alone—only 2 of whom had produced the same result in the first trial. The authors therefore concluded that chocolate on its own rarely precipitated migraine.

Another study reported symptom improvement in 28 patients with chronic headache following the institution of a histamine-free diet (41). The patients adhered to a diet that eliminated alcoholic beverages, fish, cheeses, sausages, and pickled cabbage for months. After four weeks, 4 lost their headaches, 15 had greater than 50% improvement, and 9 had no change; after 1 year, 8 of 9 patients continued to see improvement. Salfield and coworkers reported a trial of 39 children with migraine that used high-fiber diets, with half of the children randomly allocated to a diet also low in dietary vasoactive amines (42). Dietary vasoamines had no influence as both groups improved equally, with significant decreases in headache; this study reinforces the need for double-blind studies. Although some patients probably are sensitive to substances such as tyramine and phenylethylamine, it is difficult to demonstrate appreciable numbers of reactors in controlled settings. Lai and associates performed clinical assessments and electroencephalograms (EEG) on 38 patients with diet-induced migraine (43). After a control day, the patients were challenged with a combination of red wine, chocolate, and sharp cheddar cheese; 16 developed headache, including 4 with scotomata. Abnormalities in the EEG appeared but generally did not serve to separate headache responders from nonresponders. All of the patients with headache showed photic driving of the

EEG compared with only 64% of the nonresponders (p < 0.01); the significance of this finding is uncertain.

A number of people experience headache after the ingestion of hot dogs or cured meats. The incriminated vehicles in these instances are nitrites, which serve as coloring agents in the meats. High concentrations of nitrites are found in hot dogs, bacon, ham luncheon meats, smoked fish, and some imported cheeses; it is not uncommon to find levels much higher than the FDA-recommended levels of 200 ppm. The headache usually begins within minutes or hours after ingestion, is bitemporal or bifrontal, and is pulsatile approximately 50% of the time (44). The mechanism involved remains unclear.

Alcohol is commonly identified by migraineurs as a precipitant. Headache usually appears within 30 to 45 minutes after consumption, similar to the timing necessary to achieve cutaneous vasodilatation. Alcohol has little to no effect on cerebral blood flow, however, so intracerebral vasodilatation cannot be the mechanism by which alcohol causes headache. Depression of brain serotonin turnover by high levels of alcohol may play a role, given the influence of serotonin metabolism postulated in migraine (4, 5, 36). Red wine is incriminated more often than other forms of alcohol. Littlewood and associates assembled 19 migraineurs who believed that red wine—but not other forms of alcohol—provoked headache (45). Chilled red wine and vodka were consumed in a blinded fashion, and the incidence of headache compared. The alcohol content of the two preparations was similar, and the tyramine content of the wine was 2 mg/L. Less than 1 mg of tyramine was ingested. The wine produced significantly more headaches than the vodka. The authors believed that alcohol and tyramine were not responsible for the migraine headaches, instead suggesting other ingredients such as phenolic flavanoids (found in higher quantities in red than white wine) as possible triggers.

The "Chinese restaurant syndrome" induced by monosodium glutamate (MSG) comprises headache, facial tightness, warmth across the shoulders, and (less often) dizziness, nausea, and abdominal cramps (36). Approximately 30% of people ingesting oriental food experience such symptoms, which usually begin about 20 minutes after ingestion. Thresholds vary from 1.5 to 12 g, but are commonly below 3 g, the amount found in a portion of wonton soup. Symptoms are presumed to be due to central nervous system neuroexcitatory effects.

Since its introduction in 1981, the artificial sweetener aspartame has provoked numerous reports of adverse reactions. A large number of these reports included headache or were of a neurologic or behavioral nature (46). In 1987, a DBPC crossover study in 40 subjects reporting aspartame-induced headaches showed no differences in headache induction between the sweetener and placebo (47). The following year, another study demonstrated differing results (48). Twenty-five subjects began a 13-week study, although only 11 ultimately completed the protocol. A 4-week baseline period was followed by randomized sequential 4-week periods with either aspartame 300 mg q.i.d. or placebo, with the crossover periods separated by a 1-week washout. Headaches occurred twice as frequently on aspartame as on placebo or during the baseline period (p < 0.02). The differences were derived from a marked increase of headaches in 4 of the 11 subjects.

MEDIATORS AND IMMUNOLOGIC MECHANISMS IN MIGRAINE

Immunologic studies have generally proved unrewarding in migraine. Medina and Diamond reported no differences in total IgE between migraineurs and the normal population (35). Merrett and colleagues examined IgE levels in 74 adults with dietary migraine, 45 with nondietary migraine, 29 with cluster headache, and 60 normal controls (49). They found no differences in specific and total IgE in the groups with the exception of a higher total IgE in the cluster headache patients, which they attributed to a higher percentage being smokers. Specific IgE for cheese, milk, and chocolate showed no difference between dietary and nondietary migraine. Pradalier and coworkers performed duodenal biopsies for immunocyte enumeration in patients with common migraine (50). Twenty migraine patients—11 with food-induced migraine and 9 without—had mid-duodenal biopsies examined for lamina propria IgE, IgG, IgA, or IgM containing plasmocytes. No differences were observed between the two groups in terms of histologic appearance, total plasmocytes, or subsets. Ratner and associates have linked dietary migraine with lactase deficiency, presenting data on elevated IgM in 11 such migraine patients (51). Martelletti and coworkers, using a C1q binding assay, showed an increased incidence of circulating immune complexes in 21 patients with food-induced migraine (29% versus 10% in the control group) (52, 53). Activated T cells increased 4 hours after challenge, then decreased at 72 hours post-challenge. The authors speculated on the role of IL-2 receptors in food-induced migraine.

Three studies have examined mediator release in dietary migraine. Three patients in the Mansfield adult migraine study returned for repeat challenges and measurement of histamine plasma levels (25). Headache was provoked only with the active challenge and was associated with increases in histamine levels coinciding with or preceding the onset of the headache. Placebo challenge of two patients revealed little or no change in histamine.

Steinberg and colleagues reported an extensively evaluated single case of beef-induced migraine in a young woman (54). A threefold increase in histamine was noted as well as an increase of a PGF2α metabolite coinciding with the onset of the migraine following ingestion of the beef. Increased intracerebral blood flow was demonstrated with Xenon computerized tomography and Doppler ultrasonography. Prick skin test and RAST to beef gave negative results.

Olson and colleagues reported serial histamine and PGD levels during DBPC challenges in five patients with food-induced migraine (55). Placebo challenges produced no changes; with active challenge, all five subjects had a 3- to 38-fold increase in plasma histamine as well as increases in PGD$_2$ before or coinciding with the onset of symptoms. A second increase in the PGD$_2$ was noted 4 to 6 hours after ingestion; a similar increase did not appear in histamine. This discordance suggests the late recruitment of non-basophil inflammatory cells. Skin tests in this group all proved negative.

SUMMARY

A wealth of clinical data supports the contention that dietary migraine is a bonafide entity, with both pharmacologic and immunologic mechanisms involved in subsets of migraineurs (Table 34.2). Certainly, these conditions are not mutually exclusive, and both may operate in the same patient. The exact pathophysiology of these reactions remains unclear, although reproducible release of immediate hypersensitivity mediators has been convincingly demonstrated. The variable results of immediate skin testing suggest that, while some reactions may be IgE-mediated, many are probably pseudoallergic (i.e., akin to radiocontrast media reactions). Why release of these mediators causes migraine in susceptible persons and not more traditional allergic manifestations is unclear.

The exact frequency of dietary migraine in migraineurs as a whole is also not settled. Studies suggest that 15% may have reproducible triggers under controlled situations, but that twice that number may benefit from dietary restriction. While the majority of headache patients believe that connections exist between food intake and their headaches, fewer than half address this relationship with the assistance of their physicians, and fewer modify their dietary practices (56). The evaluation of such patients should begin with the appropriate history and physical examination and the exclusion of migraine-mimicking conditions. Once a diagnosis of migraine has been established and pharmacologic control achieved, it is reasonable to pursue possible dietary triggers. The global dietary restrictions suggested by some authors are probably not indicated. Although history may identify a number of triggers, some patients with reproducible headaches on DBPC challenges could

Table 34.2
Incriminated Agents in Dietary Migraine

Presumed Pharmacologic Action
Tyramine
Phenylethylamine
Phenolic flavanoids
Ethanol
Nitrites
Caffeine
Monosodium glutamate
Aspartame
Immunologic or Uncertain Action
Food proteins

not separate the causative agents during a normal diet.

Food skin testing is likely to present both false positives and false negatives, and should not be used as the sole diagnostic measure. RAST also offers little value. This restriction leaves the prospect of food diaries and elimination diets. For patients with infrequent migraines, a diary listing foods ingested in the previous 48 hours to a headache may prove useful. A diet eliminating wheat, corn, milk, and egg may be helpful for a period of two to four weeks. Patients benefiting from such a diet should reintroduce foods singly over three consecutive days. Foods not provoking symptoms should be returned freely to the diet. Suspect foods should be temporarily eliminated and then rechallenged. In patients with numerous suspected positives, challenges should be performed under blinded conditions to remove expectation or anxiety as confounding factors, and to avoid unnecessarily restricting the diet. Consulting with a nutritionist may be warranted for the rare patient who has multiple documented dietary triggers.

Epilepsy

Earlier in this century, epilepsy was compared with the similarly episodic syndromes of anaphylaxis and atopic disorders. Schwartz, in his monumental epidemiologic study of asthma and atopy in 4256 probands and relatives in Denmark, also collected data on migraine (as mentioned previously) and epilepsy (57). He found very few cases of epilepsy in these subjects, and no evidence for any genetic correlation between epilepsy and the atopic disorders. Nonetheless, a number of reports have linked allergy (frequently food-induced) and epilepsy. In 1927, Ward and Patterson skin-tested 1000 epileptics and 100 controls with various foods, finding reactivity between 37% and 67% in the patients, and 8% positivity in the controls (58).

In 1951, Dees and Lowenbach reported on 37 children with epilepsy who were treated with antiallergic therapy, environmental avoidance measures, elimination diets, and anticonvulsant therapy (59). Of these children, 22 met criteria for "allergic epilepsy": personal and family history of allergy, blood eosino-

philia, positive skin tests, and no organic disease of the central nervous system. The remainder had possible allergic disease, but did not meet all criteria; half had eosinophilia. Twenty of the "allergic" group and 13 of the "nonallergic" group had positive food skin tests. The predominant EEG finding was occipital dysrhythmia (73% of both groups), a rhythm that was also present in some allergic children without an overt seizure disorder. Thirteen of the allergic group were treated with allergen immunotherapy as well as the dietary and medical manipulations. Convulsions were controlled in 18 of 22 allergic children and 6 of 15 "nonallergic" children; anticonvulsant therapy was eventually phased out in 13 of the former subjects and 1 of the latter group. The authors suggested that epilepsy could have an allergic basis in certain cases, and could, therefore, conceivably be controlled with appropriate antiallergic therapy. They did not, however, provide any indication of how many epileptic children were surveyed to arrive at their study group. Thus, it is difficult to place this interesting observation in proper perspective.

In their assessment of food factors in migraine, Egger and colleagues reported several patients who had epilepsy and/or behavioral problems that also appeared to respond to the oligoantigenic diet (23). In a further study, they investigated children who either had epilepsy alone or in association with migraine, all of whom had difficult-to-control symptoms (60). None of the 18 patients with epilepsy alone improved on the oligoantigenic diet, while 40 of 45 patients with both epilepsy and migraine reported improvement of one or more symptoms. In followup ranging from seven months to three years, 25 patients had gained complete control of their epilepsy. Thirty-two patients had seizure during reintroduction of incriminated foods. In double-blind challenges of 16 children, 7 reacted to the suspected food only, none to placebo only, and one to both substances.

In a variant of reflex epilepsy, the food ingested does not precipitate the seizure, but rather the act of eating itself. This entity is called "eating epilepsy" and, while quite rare, appears to be more common in families in Sri Lanka and the Indian subcontinent (61–63). The seizure type is usually complex partial, does not occur with all meals, and usually happens at home. Many episodes are linked to the ingestion of rice, but since this food is a staple of the diet in these geographic areas, it is likely that this sensitivity is not truly specific (61). It has been postulated that stimulation of areas of the brain that receive sensory input during eating may lower the seizure threshold (64).

DIET MANIPULATION IN EPILEPSY

Seventy-five years ago, it was observed that many epilepsy patients remained free of seizures while fasting, and the benefit persisted after a return to a normal diet. This effect was suggested to be due to ketonemia, and a "ketogenic" high-fat, low-carbohydrate diet was proposed as treatment. Such a diet is rigid, requiring strict nutritional supervision, and is perceived as unpalatable and difficult to maintain (65, 66). It appeared useful in epilepsy, however, especially in younger-age children and those with seizures not responsive to antiepileptic medications. A report by Kinsman and associates showed benefit from the diet in 58 epileptic children requiring multiple medications (66). Seizure control improved in 67% of patients, with reduced medication in 64%, greater alertness in 36%, and improved behavior in 23%. Seventy-five percent of these improved patients were able to maintain the diet at least 18 months. A medium-chain triglyceride diet was found to be more ketogenic than the fat in the traditional diet, and felt to be more palatable; Sills and colleagues reported on their success with such a diet in 50 epileptic children (65). Eight achieved complete control of seizures (4 without medication), 4 had seizures reduced by 90%, and 10 by 50% to 90%. Extra dosing of the medium-chain triglycerides at bedtime proved useful in controlling nocturnal seizures. The mechanisms behind the diet's effectiveness remain unclear. Possibilities include alterations in acid–base balance, water and electrolyte distribution, or lipid concentrations, and direct action of ketone bodies (66).

EPILEPSY AND MIGRAINE

The link between migraine and epilepsy is apparent, especially given the work of Egger and colleagues, but the nature of the relationship remains unclear. In an editorial, Wilson addressed several overlapping issues (67). If attacks and auras are brief—especially if the attacks are stereotyped—a diagnosis of epilepsy is preferred; if attacks with prodrome have a longer duration, and if the impact on consciousness is primarily confusion, migraine may be more likely. Therapeutic trials of migraine prophylaxis and antiepileptic drugs may clarify the diagnosis. Several migraine–epilepsy syndromes have been identified: seizures with typical migraine prodrome; migraine with later development of epilepsy; and alternating hemiplegic migraine. In the first case, impairment of cerebral blood flow associated with migraine may precipitate the seizure. In the second condition, repeated ischemic insult may lead to an epileptogenic focus. Despite such cases, the relationship between epilepsy and migraine remains obscure. Can one condition trigger the other in a dually susceptible individual, or does epilepsy represent an epiphenomenon in a vascular disease (67)? Both mechanisms may occur in different patients.

SUMMARY

While food plays an important role in provoking attacks of migraine, less is known concerning dietary factors in epilepsy. The efficacy of ketogenic diets is well established, but the manner in which they operate remains uncertain. That allergic reactions or anaphylactoid reactions could trigger convulsions in susceptible patients appears likely, but DBPC studies are sparse, and would assist in validating the clinical observations made to date. In addition, studies investigating mediator release are needed.

Vertigo

In 1976, Dunn and Snyder reported their experience with 33 pediatric cases of benign paroxysmal vertigo, a syndrome of sporadic brief episodes of disequilibrium, nystagmus, and/or vomiting (68). During infancy, this condition is often manifested in the form of paroxysmal torticollis. While food allergy was considered in all cases, it was deemed likely in only four cases. Three children had histories suggestive of milk allergy; their attacks were eliminated by removing milk from the diet, with vertigo reappearing with milk challenges. Chocolate was suspected in another child, but could not be confirmed by challenge. The authors do not state whether these challenges were open or blinded. Therefore, at best, one-tenth of the cases had evidence for a food etiology.

A food cause for adult vertigo or Meniere's syndrome has been postulated. In 1923, Duke reported that five cases of Meniere's syndrome improved on elimination diets (69). Unfortunately, no well-performed, double-blind studies have been conducted. Reports are limited to the nonreproducible technique of provocation–neutralization. Substantiation of a role for food will require further study.

Hemiplegia

Several case reports exist of transient neurological deficits following presumed allergic reactions to foods. Cooke reported transient third cranial nerve palsy associated with hemiparesis, followed by an episode of contralateral blindness and paresthesia in a food-allergic patient (70). Symptoms resolved with avoidance of beef and pork, and challenges were not performed. In 1951, Staffieri and colleagues reported a case of right-sided hemiplegia immediately following after a meal; it was associated with angioedema, urticaria, purpura, and peripheral eosinophilia ranging from 34% to 40% (71). A wheat elimination diet was followed by resolution of the symptoms within a few days. To rule out coincidence, a total of four wheat challenges (apparently single-blinded) were performed over the ensuing four months, resulting initially in headache, followed by purpura and angioedema, and ultimately in skin manifestations alone. Passive transfer of skin-sensitizing antibodies was not successful. Such reports are fascinating, but probably indicate that anaphylactic reactions may be attended by edema almost anywhere, including the central and peripheral nervous systems.

REFERENCES

1. Stewart WF, Lipton RB, Celentano DD, Reed ML. Prevalence of migraine headache in the United States: relation to age, income, race, and other sociodemographic factors. JAMA 1992;267:64–69.
2. Ad Hoc Committee on the Classification of Headache. Classification of headache. Arch Neurol 1962;6:173–176.
3. Woods RP, Iacoboni M, Mazziotta JC. Brief report: bilateral spreading cerebral hypoperfusion during spontaneous migraine headache. N Engl J Med 1994;331:1689–1692.
4. Zeigler DK, Murrow RW. Headache. In: Joynt RJ, ed. Clinical neurology. Vol. 2, rev. ed. Philadelphia: JB Lippincott, 1988, 1–49.
5. D'Andrea G, Welch KMA, Grunfeld S, Levine SR, Nagel-Leiby S, Joseph R. Reduced platelet turnover of serotonin in diet restricted migraine patients. Cephalalgia 1987;7:141s–143s.
6. Moskowitz MA, Macfarlane R. Neurovascular and molecular mechanisms in migraine headaches. Cerebrovasc Brain Metab Rev 1993;5:159–177.
7. Hasselmark L, Malmgren R, Hannerz J. Effect of a carbohydrate-rich diet, low in protein-tryptophan, in classic and common migraine. Cephalalgia 1987;7:87–92.
8. Schéle R, Ahlborg B, Ekbom K. Physical characteristics and allergic history in young men with migraine and other headaches. Headache 1978;18:80–86.
9. Pinnas JL, Vanselow NA. Relationship of allergy to headache. Res Clin Stud Headache 1976;4:85–95.
10. Brown TR. Role of diet in etiology and treatment of migraine and other types of headache. JAMA 1921;77:1396–1400.
11. Vaughan WT. Allergic migraine. JAMA 1927;88:1383–1386.
12. Eyermann CH. Allergic headache. J Allergy 1930;2:106–112.
13. Balyeat RM, Rinkel HJ. Further studies in allergic migraine: based on a series of two hundred and two consecutive cases. Ann Intern Med 1931;5:713–728.
14. DeGowin EL. Allergic migraine: a review of sixty cases. J Allergy 1932;3:557–566.
15. Unger AH, Unger L. Migraine is an allergic disease. J Allergy 1952;23:429–440.
16. Schwartz M. Is migraine an allergic disease? J Allergy 1952;23:426–428.
17. Grant EC. Food allergies and migraine. Lancet 1979;1:966–969.
18. Monro J, Carini C, Brostoff J. Food allergy in migraine: study of dietary exclusion and RAST. Lancet 1980;2:1–4.
19. Monro J, Carini C, Brostoff J. Migraine is a food allergic disease. Lancet 1984;2:719–721.
20. Ratner D, Shoshani E, Dubnov B. Milk protein-free diet for nonseasonal asthma and migraine in lactose-deficient patients. Isr J Med Sci 1983;19:806–809.
21. Hughes EC, Gott PS, Weinstein RC, Binggeli R. Migraine: a diagnostic test for etiology of food sensitivity by a nutritionally supported fast and confirmed by long term report. Ann Allergy 1985;55:28–32.
22. Vaughan TR, Mansfield LE, Haverly RW, Chamberlin WM, Waller SF. The value of cutaneous testing for food allergy in the diagnostic evaluation of migraine headache. Ann Allergy 1983;50:362 (abstract).
23. Egger J, Wilson J, Carter CM, Turner MW. Is migraine food allergy? A double-blind controlled trial of oligoantigenic diet treatment. Lancet 1983;2:865–868.
24. Atkins FM, Ball BD, Bock A. The relationship between the ingestion of specific foods and the development of migraine headaches in children. J Allergy Clin Immunol 1988;81:185 (abstract).
25. Mansfield LE, Vaughan TR, Waller SF, Haverly RW, Ting S. Food allergy and adult migraine: double blind and mediator confirmation of an allergic etiology. Ann Allergy 1985;55:126–129.
26. Vaughan TR, Stafford WW, Miller BT, Weber RW, Tipton WR,

Nelson HS. Food and migraine headache (MIG): a controlled study. Ann Allergy 1986;56:522 (abstract).

27. Weber RW, Vaughan TR. Food and migraine headache. Immunol Allergy Clin N Am 1991;11:831–841.

28. Vaughan TR. The role of food in the pathogenesis of migraine headache. Clin Rev Allergy 1994;12:167–180.

29. Curtis-Brown R. Protein poison theory: its application to treatment of headache and especially migraine. Br Med J 1925;1:155–157.

30. Hanington E. Preliminary report on tyramine headache. Br Med J 1967;2:550–551.

31. Smith I, Kellow AH, Hanington E. A clinical and biochemical correlation between tyramine and migraine headache. Headache 1970;10:43–51.

32. Moffett A, Swash M, Scott DF. Effect of tyramine in migraine: a double-blind study. J Neurol Neurosurg Psychiatry 1972;35:496–499.

33. Forsythe WI, Redmond A. Two controlled trials of tyramine in children with migraine. Dev Med Child Neurol 1974;16:794–799.

34. Zeigler DK, Stewart R. Failure of tyramine to induce migraine. Neurol 1977;27:725–726.

35. Medina JL, Diamond S. The role of diet in migraine. Headache 1978;18:31–34.

36. Raskin NH. Chemical headaches. Ann Rev Med 1981;32:63–71.

37. Peatfield RC, Hampton KK, Grant PJ. Plasma vasopressin levels in induced migraine attacks. Cephalalgia 1988;8:55–57.

38. Sandler M, Youdim MBH, Hanington E. A phenylethylamine oxidising defect in migraine. Nature 1974;250:335–337.

39. Schweitzer JW, Friedhoff AJ, Schwartz R. Chocolate, beta-phenylethylamine and migraine re-examined. Nature 1975;257:256.

40. Moffett AM, Swash M, Scott DF. Effect of chocolate in migraine: a double-blind study. J Neurol Neurosurg Psychiatry 1974;37:445–448.

41. Wantke F, Götz M, Jarisch R. Histamine-free diet: treatment of choice for histamine-induced food intolerance and supporting treatment for chronical headaches. Clin Exp Allergy 1993;23:982–985.

42. Salfield SAW, Wardley BL, Houlsby WT, et al. Controlled study of exclusion of dietary vasoactive amines in migraine. Arch Dis Child 1987;62:458–460.

43. Lai C-W, Dean P, Ziegler DK, Hassanein RS. Clinical and electrophysiological responses to dietary challenge in migraineurs. Headache 1989;29:180–186.

44. Henderson WR, Raskin NH. "Hot-dog" headache: individual susceptibility to nitrite. Lancet 1972;2:1162–1163.

45. Littlewood JT, Glover V, Davies PTG, Gibb C, Sandler M, Rose FC. Red wine as a cause of migraine. Lancet 1988;1:558–559.

46. Evaluation of consumer complaints related to aspartame use. MMWR 1984;33:605–607.

47. Schiffman SS, Buckley CE III, Sampson HA, et al. Aspartame and susceptibility to headache. N Engl J Med 1987;317:1181–1185.

48. Koehler SM, Glaros A. The effect of aspartame on migraine headache. Headache 1988;28:10–14.

49. Merrett J, Peatfield RC, Rose FC, Merrett TG. Food related antibodies in headache patients. J Neurol Neurosurg Psychiatry 1983;46:738–742.

50. Pradalier A, De Saint Maur P, Lamy F, Launay JM. Immunocyte enumeration in duodenal biopsies of migraine without aura patients with or without food-induced migraine. Cephalalgia 1994;14:365–367.

51. Ratner D, Eshel E, Shneyour A, Teitler A. Elevated IgM in dietary migraine with lactase deficiency. Isr J Med Sci 1984;20:717–719.

52. Martelletti P, Sutherland J, Anastasi E, Di Mario U, Giacovazzo M. Evidence for an immune-mediated mechanism in food-induced migraine from a study on activated T-cells, IgG$_4$ subclass, anti-IgG antibodies and circulating immune complexes. Headache 1989;29:664–670.

53. Martelletti P. T cells expressing IL-2 receptor in migraine. Acta Neurol 1991;13:448–456.

54. Steinberg M, Page R, Wolfson S, Friday G, Fireman P. Food induced late phase headache. J Allergy Clin Immunol 1988;81:185 (abstract).

55. Olson GC, Vaughan TR, Ledoux R, et al. Food induced migraine: search for immunologic mechanisms. J Allergy Clin Immunol 1989;83:238 (abstract).

56. Guarnieri P, Radnitz C, Blanchard EB. Assessment of dietary risk factors in chronic headache. Biofeedback Self-Regulation 1990;15:15–25.

57. Schwartz M. Heredity in bronchial asthma: a clinical and genetic study of 191 asthma probands and 50 probands with baker's asthma. Acta Allergol 1952;5:14s–268s.

58. Ward RF, Patterson HA. Protein sensitization in epilepsy: a study of one thousand cases and one hundred normal controls. Arch Neurol Psychiatry 1927;17:427–443.

59. Dees SC, Lowenbach H. Allergic epilepsy. Ann Allergy 1951;9:446–458.

60. Egger J, Cater CM, Soothill JF, Wilson J. Oligoantigenic diet treatment of children with epilepsy and migraine. J Pediatr 1989;114:51–58.

61. Ahuja GK, Pauranik A, Behari M, Prasad K. Eating epilepsy. J Neurol 1988;235:444–447.

62. Senanayake N. Familial eating epilepsy. J Neurol 1990;237:388–391.

63. Senanayake N. "Eating epilepsy"—a reappraisal. Epilepsy Res 1990;5:74–79.

64. Fiol ME, Leppik IE, Pretzel K. Eating epilepsy: EEG and clinical study. Epilepsia 1986;27:441–446.

65. Sills MA, Forsythe WI, Haidukewych D, Macdonald A, Robinson M. The medium chain triglyceride diet and intractable epilepsy. Arch Dis Child 1986;61:1168–1172.

66. Kinsman SL, Vining EPG, Quaskey SA, Mellits D, Freeman JM. Efficacy of the ketogenic diet for intractable seizure disorders: review of 58 cases. Epilepsia 1992;33:1132–1136.

67. Wilson J. Migraine and epilepsy. Develop Med Child Neurol 1992;34:645–647.

68. Dunn DW, Snyder CH. Benign paroxysmal vertigo of childhood. Am J Dis Child 1976;130:1099–1100.

69. Duke WW. Meniere's syndrome caused by allergy. JAMA 1923;81:2179–2181.

70. Cooke RA. Allergic neuropathies. In: Cooke RA, ed. Allergy in theory and practice. Philadelphia: WB Saunders, 1947, 325–336.

71. Staffieri D, Bentolila L, Levit L. Hemiplegia and allergic symptoms following ingestion of certain foods. Ann Allergy 1951;10:38–39.

35

BEHAVIOR AND ADVERSE FOOD REACTIONS

John O. Warner

Introduction

In the last three decades, the immunopathology of allergic diseases has been unraveled, facilitating improvement in both diagnosis and treatment. Furthermore, the application of a rigorous scientific approach has aided the identification of foods as a cause of acute allergic disorders ranging from catastrophic anaphylaxis, angioedema, and urticaria, to chronic disorders such as atopic dermatitis and enteropathies. The scientific evidence supporting a role for foods in many allergic disorders is compelling enough to convince even the most skeptical clinician. Difficulties remain where no underlying mechanism can be found to explain the association between exposure to food and the reaction. As a result, no objective diagnostic test exists beyond dietary exclusion and double-blind, placebo-controlled food challenge. The latter procedure is well established and can reliably identify individuals with food intolerance as a cause of a range of physical disorders (1). The concept becomes strained, however, when the reaction to food cannot be measured as a change in function or physical symptoms but merely as a change in behavior.

Unsubstantiated claims primarily made in the lay media (rather than scientific channels) about "debilitating and chronic symptoms of ill health coming from an intolerance to certain foods" (2) have tended to polarize medical opinion against the idea that foods might affect behavior. The danger is that the profession's rejection of such claims will provide no help for individual patients and ignores the fact that some proven associations exist between food and aberrations in behavior.

Food and Behavior

Interest in the possibility that dietary variation might modify behavior is not a new concept. Indeed, this idea is fundamental to the practice of ayevedic medicine. Early scientific publications described so-called cerebral allergy (3) and food-induced tension-fatigue syndrome (4). At that time, the scientific basis of allergy had not been determined, and, not surprisingly, associations between exposure to food and changes in behavior were lumped into the all-embracing description of food allergy. Nevertheless, some early investigators did recognize that other factors might be relevant. Behavior was clearly affected on some occasions by the discomfort caused by primary allergic reactions such as urticaria, atopic dermatitis, or gastrointestinal reactions to food. Indeed, a survey of allergists in North America conducted in 1950 indicated that more than half had noticed changes in personality when patients known to be allergic were exposed to a provoking food (5). Consequently, elimination of the food was often associated with a dramatic improvement in affect. A tired, withdrawn child who has stayed awake most of the night with pruritus due to eczema will often become happy and friendly after major allergens have been eliminated and sleep is restored. Indeed, my own practice has provided the opportunity to observe a wide range of behavioral responses in children during double-blind challenge procedures. Sometimes the underlying physical reaction has not been detected by the parents. Thus, children with urticaria occurring on only the torso in response to a food challenge are sometimes observed by their parents to become extremely irritable and naughty (6). Meticulous challenge procedures combined with careful, thorough examination of the patients can validate such associations. When no physical abnormality is evident, it becomes more difficult to measure behavior change objectively using reproducible methods over short periods of time and thereby document responses to food challenge. Until such techniques are developed, controversy will continue to swirl about associations between isolated behavior disorder and reactions to food.

Pharmacological Effects of Food

CAFFEINE

It is self-evident that certain foods contain pharmacologically active substances that can affect behavior in all individuals to a greater or lesser extent. Caffeine in coffee and soft drinks has provided the most obvious example, as it exhibits potent pharmacological properties by directly activating the cerebral cortex to maintain wakefulness and improve concentration. Individual variation exists in sensitivity to the stimulant effects of caffeine, with some individuals becoming intensely anxious after exposure to high doses. Furthermore, regular moderate dosing with caffeine can lead to physical dependence, and withdrawal produces a range of symptoms, including depression, anxiety, fatigue, listlessness, sleepiness, decreased alertness, and headaches (7). Whether these concepts of variations in sensitivity and dependence can be extended to other pharmacologically active ingredients in foods has proved more difficult to establish. Some researchers have suggested, without any objective evidence, that this issue represents one of the greatest health problems of the age (8).

CHOCOLATE

Chocolate has often been regarded as another food containing pharmacologically active substances, including a range of vasoactive amines such as histamine, tryptophan, and serotonin, as well as methylxanthine and theobromine. Individuals claim "addiction" to chocolate in which abstinence produces symptoms of withdrawal, but these reports are very inconsistent. Milk chocolate apparently contains less of the pharmacologically active substances such

as methylxanthine, but appears to be the variety that is most frequently consumed by so-called chocoholics (9).

OTHER FOODS

Clearly, certain foods contain high levels of vasoactive substances, such as tyramine in cheese and histamine in various fermented foods and poorly stored scromboid fish (10). Individuals predisposed to irritable or difficult behavior may tend to show a greater degree of response to similar quantities of such substances in foods than relatively placid individuals. Furthermore, peptides in milk and wheat contain exorthine-like activity, which might be predicted to affect behavior (11).

VASOACTIVE MEDIATORS

Amino acids such as tryptophan (a precursor for serotonin) may be predicted to affect behavior, mood, and appetite if administered to individuals in high concentrations (12). It has even been suggested that the amount of carbohydrate-rich foods consumed affects the production of serotonin, which, in turn, influences the degree of hunger for carbohydrates (13). This hypothesis has led to a very tenuous line of argument about relationships between ingestion of food, changes in behavior, and the development of dependence and addiction to the food (8).

Some foods have been hypothesized to induce changes in brain perfusion that can mimic the abnormalities reportedly found in individuals with developmental learning difficulties (14). Varying the intake of precursors of vasoactive mediators might accentuate abnormalities in individuals with preexisting brain disorders that affect behavior.

HISTAMINE-RELEASING FOODS

High doses of the food coloring agent, tartrazine, can have a direct effect on basophil histamine release (15). It is, therefore, not surprising that a large dose of tartrazine administered in a double-blind food challenge can produce an increase in circulating histamine. Such challenges might potentially accentuate hyperactive behavior transiently by a direct pharmacological mechanism (16). Similar effects may occur with strawberries, tomato, pineapple, and alcohol (17).

Where a pharmacological effect of food is implicated, only high doses of the putative food will likely cause a significant problem. Thus, the concept of total dietary exclusion appears inappropriate. Furthermore, diagnosis is unlikely to be achieved by any standard tests for allergy.

Other Mechanisms

REACTIVE HYPOGLYCEMIA

It has been suggested that individuals with a high sugar intake develop reactive hypoglycemia several hours after ingestion, which, in turn, produces an aberration in behavior and cognitive performance (18). Diabetologists are only too familiar with the wide range of behavior disturbances that occur in individuals who become hypoglycemic. This observation has led to the claim that reactive hypoglycemia commonly causes neuropathologies ranging from schizophrenia to criminal behavior (19). The most widely publicized use of this diagnosis was in a court of law. An argument was put forward by the defense that the defendant, who was accused of murder, had diminished mental capacity as a result of overconsumption of sugar-containing "junk foods." The conviction was eventually for manslaughter, rather than first degree murder (7). No compelling evidence has subsequently been generated that would support this concept. Indeed, some well-conducted challenge studies have failed to find any association between dietary sucrose or aspartame and effects on childhood behavior or cognitive function (20–22).

SQUASH DRINKING SYNDROME

One possible alternative explanation is more credible and certainly requires further investigation. A survey of the drinking habits of 2- to 7-year-old children determined that few now drink water. Three-fourths of preschool children never drink water. Squash was by far the most frequently consumed drink; in some preschool children, it constituted as much as 50% of recommended daily energy intake (23). A group of eight children were described who were referred for a range of problems, including poor appetite, behavioral problems, poor weight gain, and loose stools. The subjects received a high percentage of their daily energy requirement in the form of high-energy drinks. The authors hypothesized that the children's appetites had been poor at mealtimes, which affected behavior during meals, as a consequence of the high-energy drinks they consumed during the day. Decrease in the energy ingested in drinks as a fraction of their diet resulted in an increased dietary intake of a range of other foods that, in turn, decreased stool frequency and improved all other symptoms, including behavior. They suggested that the features of the condition were sufficiently well characterized to be accepted as a clinical entity, to be called "Squash drinking syndrome" (24).

AMINO ACIDS AND IMMUNE RESPONSES

An intriguing study investigated the health and immune status of normal control subjects consuming diets free of tyrosine and phenylalanine. This regimen decreased the plasma tyrosine levels significantly and was associated with a decrease in platelet aggregation in response to adenosine diphosphate and platelet-activating factor. Natural killer, T-helper, and T-cytotoxic suppressor lymphocyte numbers increased proportionately relative to neutrophils (25). This investigation sought to delineate why diets limiting tyrosine and phenylalanine intake were sometimes associated with decrease in tumor size and metastases. They proposed that the increase in natural killer cell activity and decrease in platelet aggregation may provide the explanation. These alterations in immune competence might also have an impact on allergic phenomena.

Hyperkinetic Syndromes

Hyperactivity, hyperkinesis, or attention deficit hyperactivity disorder is characterized by a short attention span, impulsive behavior, and a range of other problems, including aggressiveness, disinhibition, and sudden mood changes. The behavior may become apparent at home, in school, or in other social situations or it may be pervasive in all environments. In school, these syndromes typically lead to under-achievement, and the disruptive behavior of the children often results in their exclusion from conventional schooling. The definitions, terminology, and diagnostic criteria for these conditions vary in different countries (26). In the United States, their prevalence is estimated as approximately 3%, whereas in Europe, the figure is 30-fold lower at 0.1%. This discrepancy creates great difficulty in comparing studies that have investigated the association between food and hyperkinetic syndrome. Even using standardized criteria for diagnosis, considerable variability occurs depending on the assessor (e.g., doctors, teachers, or parents). The disorder is more common in boys than girls. The prognosis has variously been described as being good, with resolution after a few years, or as persisting into adult life with antisocial behavior and alcoholism (27).

In the United Kingdom, where hyperkinetic syndrome (known there as hyperactivity) is considered to be a rare phenomenon that is often associated with other neurological deficits, the alternative label of "conduct disorder" is used more commonly to describe children with antisocial or disruptive behavior. This distinction is supported by a study that showed that antisocial and disruptive behavior in these children was independent of the classic features of hyperkinetic syndrome (28). Recent studies have suggested that a major determinant of hyperkinetic syndrome comprises a delay aversion. Such children have a self-imposed limitation on presentation time that makes them more likely to reduce overall delay levels during tasks to achieve frequent small rewards rather than to opt for large delayed rewards (29). This tendency has facilitated the development of a computerized system for recording delay aversion and might provide one of the first truly objective criteria by which to monitor food challenges. Trials of this technique are awaited with great interest.

THE FEINGOLD HYPOTHESIS

Feingold devised a diet excluding artificial food colors and flavors and naturally occurring salicylates that he claimed led to improvement in behavior disturbances in as many as 50% of both normal and neurologically damaged children. He proposed a pharmacological—rather than allergic—mechanism (30). The diet was enthusiastically embraced by organizations representing the interests of families with hyperactive children as well. The rationale for the natural salicylate exclusion has been shown to lack foundation, with many excluded foods containing no salicylate and some foods remaining in the diet including significant quantities (31). Attempts to confirm or refute the concept have encountered major difficulties. Most of the studies were not truly double-blind, and questions have been raised about diagnosis, case mix, type of elimination diet, timing and dose of challenge, lack of acknowledgment of carryover effect, and objectivity of the ratings of behavior change (27, 32).

The most commonly used rating system was devised by Conners, who has performed a number of meticulously conducted double-blind, crossover challenges (33). The results obtained from these studies have conflicted, however, showing either no difference between placebo and active challenge, or significant worsening of behavior during challenge periods (33–36). Two excellent studies by Harley and colleagues could not confirm any dramatic changes with diet, although small differences were suggested in relation to elimination of additives (37, 38). In 1983, the NIH Consensus Development Panel concluded that a limited positive association existed between the use of diet and decreased hyperactivity, but only a small proportion of children definitely responded (39). The panel also accepted that hyperactivity increased in a few children when challenged with artificial food colors but not placebo. On the other hand, it was very critical of many of the diet behavior studies.

Further attempts have been made to elaborate on this problem. Egger and colleagues recruited 76 children from a special clinic for hyperactive children who had high Conners' scores (40). An unusually high proportion had other associated allergic problems and neurological disabilities. Sixty-two of the children appeared to improve on a so-called oligoantigenic diet and 28 of these patients subsequently participated in a double-blind, placebo-controlled, single-crossover challenge. The challenge included various foods and very high doses of tartrazine and benzoic acid. The symptoms appeared worse in the active challenge period than in the placebo period, but a considerable order effect was observed and the significance of difference between the single active and placebo challenge was not great. Reactions mostly involved the artificial colors and preservatives, which provides some consistency with previous studies. The same group has repeated this study with a very similar outcome (41). The authors admit, however, that a high proportion of children had physical symptoms and their parents exhibited a particular interest in following a dietary approach, just as in their previous study. The findings cannot, therefore, be extrapolated to all children with behavior disorders.

The author's group conducted a study on 39 children referred to an allergy clinic with behavior problems supposedly associated with food colorings (16). The patients exhibited poor concentration, excessive fidgeting, and poor school performance. The parents asserted that even small doses of food colorings immediately exacerbated problems. Of the 39 children, only 19 completed a double-blind, placebo-controlled challenge with a mixture of 125 mg of various food colors or placebo in a seven-week challenge protocol, with two of the weeks randomized to daily active challenge. Significantly higher mean daily behavioral scores based on a 10-item Conners' checklist were determined in the active weeks compared with the placebo weeks, whereas somatic symptoms did not differ significantly between the two periods. Furthermore, the small changes in behavior scores had no relationship to changes in somatic symptoms or to atopic status in the children. Only two parents were able to identify all of the challenge weeks correctly. The majority could not detect any change in behavior during the course of the challenge. The high dropout rate leaves the study open to criticism, however, but reflects the nature of the problem. Several of the dropouts occurred within the first few days of challenge, with parents asserting severe reactions that were equally distributed between active and placebo periods. The other criticism of this study claimed that the Conners' scores were relatively low and, therefore, would not have normally been included as a diagnosis of true hyperkinetic syndrome (27). Nevertheless, these children do reflect the experience that might be expected in a general pediatric or allergy clinic rather than in a psychiatric setting.

One published study has investigated the value of so-called hyposensitization for children with apparent—albeit not objectively substantiated—food-induced hyperkinetic syndrome. The enzyme-potentiated vaccine contained 45 foods and 10 colorants; because it was prepared by one of the authors, the vaccine would be impossible to replicate. The significant improvement on active treatment remains difficult to explain and clearly requires further controlled study by independent groups. It is, however, salutary to note the authors' closing sentence in the paper, which stated that "restricted diets are socially disruptive, expensive and because of nutritional inadequacy may be dangerous. . . ." (42)

A recent publication described a well-constructed, blinded, placebo-controlled challenge with various doses of tartrazine or placebo in 34 children with behavior problems and 20 controls. Twenty-four of the index cases showed a response to tartrazine that appeared to be dose-related (43).

My conclusion from study of the literature on this topic remains the same as that of the NIH Consensus Development Panel. Evidence certainly exists to suggest that high doses of artificial food colors can produce adverse effects in a few children with behavior disorders, whether they have true hyperkinetic syndrome or conduct disorder. The effect is small. Little, if any, evidence supports the particular involvement of a range of other foods. It might seem reasonable to recommend a reduction in the intake of foods containing a high level of artificial colorings, irrespective of the mechanisms by which these additives might produce a problem. This lack of knowledge should not detract from the children receiving other therapy that may well prove more effective. Nevertheless, only one study has attempted to compare standard pharmacotherapy with dietary modification. The effect of stimulant medication was statistically significant, but the dietary effects appeared variable (44).

Food Aversion

Food aversion is a common phenomenon. Indeed, food phobias are probably universal. Psychologically based food intolerance occurs where a conditioned response is elicited by the recognition, appearance, smell, or taste of a particular food. It can arise following an unpleasant genuine reaction—for instance, an episode associated with gastroenteritis or even a previous genuine food intolerance. Such a reaction cannot be reproduced when the food is disguised in a double-blind challenge. At its most severe level, food aversion is associated with anorexia nervosa and the bulimic syndrome (45). In pediatric practice, it may appear as part of the so-called Munchausen by proxy syndrome. Parents (usually mothers) present children with multiple problems, leading to inappropriate extensive investigation and treatment. Allergy figures very prominently among the supposed problems, and the children are often following highly abnormal diets. The symptoms are fabricated apparently to fulfill a psychological need in the parent. Not only are the diets nutritionally inadequate, but the children also become socially isolated and learn a disease model from an early age that may persist throughout life (46). Some of these children are eventually submitted to worse forms of abuse (47).

It is imperative that food aversion be distinguished from genuine intolerance. Unfortunately, many clinicians will assert that it is impractical to carry out double-blind food challenges. Few clinicians feel they have enough experience or time to devote to such meticulous diagnostic procedures, which creates opportunities for practitioners of "fringe medicine" to capitalize on the failure of conventional medicine in dealing with a common and significant problem. Therefore, double-blind challenges should be performed not only for research, but also as an objective evaluation of the need for a continuing diet. Formal challenge may highlight a real underlying problem. If the challenge result is negative, it may still facilitate the introduction of more appropriate treatment.

In this respect, a recent publication has highlighted the consequences of failure to address the problem. A retrospective study of 11 children who were failing to thrive as a consequence of parental beliefs about multiple food allergies were identified from a sample of 700 children referred for evaluation (48). Skin tests were negative in 7 of the 11 children,

and double-blind food challenge was also negative in 9 of the 11 subjects. Two children reacted to foods— 1 to milk, and 1 to both milk and eggs. Both of these patients had more than 12 other foods excluded from their diets as well. Thus, the parental beliefs about food allergy in these children had resulted in significant failure to thrive that could have major long-term consequences. It is, therefore, imperative that professionals should not collude with such beliefs, but should carry out formal evaluation.

Where inappropriate diagnoses of food intolerance are established by dubious techniques, which in turn lead to major complications such as nutritional deficiencies, it is perfectly understandable that conventional medicine should aggressively highlight the problem (49). Patients and their parents might become dissatisfied with medical care if their beliefs are not sensitively addressed, however. One report of patients attending an allergy clinic noted that those in whom food hypersensitivity could not be confirmed by appropriate investigation had high levels of neurotic symptoms and low levels of classic atopic problems (50). Individuals with such "pseudo allergy" suffer from a range of underlying psychiatric problems, but present with an initially confusing array of symptoms involving many organ symptoms and ostensibly associated with exposure to foods (51). Successful treatment depends on recognition, sensitive handling, and demonstration by appropriate double-blind challenge that food is not the primary cause of the problem (52).

In infancy, this misperception occurs particularly frequently. Normal changes in an infant's stool character and frequency, or activity and sleep cycles, may be wrongly considered abnormal and attributed to changes in diet. Parental conviction is reinforced by not only media publicity but also the medical profession's inability to handle such concerns appropriately. It is often easier for medical staff to collude with the parents' belief, setting the scene for an escalation of dietary avoidance for any subsequent problem that the child may suffer (53). Indeed, one clinician has commented that "Not since mesmerism and phrenology were in vogue in the 19th century, has the public appeared so gullible and so vulnerable to fashionable nostrums" (54).

Conclusions

An excellent review on food sensitivity in the nervous system noted that ". . . there is, indeed, scientifically sound evidence to support an association between foods and abnormal behaviour in children. However, the frequency of this is less than that claimed by some psychologists, psychiatrists and allergists" (27). Notably, the conclusions of this detailed study of the literature do not support the concept of foods affecting adult behavior. The most compelling association links a transient effect of high doses of artificial food colorings to hyperkinetic syndrome. More work is required to elaborate on whether associations with other foods or additives are genuine and appropriately treated by dietary modification. Where patients have genuine food-associated behavior problems, additional underlying atopic diseases such as eczema, urticaria, and asthma are typically identified. More commonly, behavior disturbances have a psychosocial cause and, therefore, require psychosocial solutions. Continued preoccupation with diet will only detract from the principal cause of the problem and its resolution.

REFERENCES

1. Bock SA, Sampson HA, Atkins FM, *et al.* Double-blind placebo controlled food challenge as an office procedure: a manual. J Allergy Clin Immunol 1988;82:986–997.
2. Gamlin C. Cooking up a storm. New Scientist 8 July 1989:45–49.
3. Davison HM. The relation of allergy to character problems in children. Ann Allergy 1950;8:175.
4. Shannon WR. Neuropathic manifestations in infants and children as a result of anaphylactic reaction to foods contained in their diet. Am J Dis Child 1922;24:89–94.
5. Clarke TW. The relation of allergy to character problems in children. Ann Allergy 1950;8:175.
6. Supramaniam G, Warner JO. Artificial food additive intolerance in patients with angio oedema and urticaria. Lancet 1986;2:907–909.
7. Kanarek RB, Marks-Kaufman R. Nutrition and behaviour: new perspectives. New York: Van-Nostrand Reinhold, 1991.
8. Randolph TG, Moss RW. Allergies: your hidden enemy. 4th ed. Wellingborough: Thorsons Publishing Group, 1986.
9. Max B. This and that: chocolate addiction, the dual pharmacogenetics of asparagus eaters and the arithmetic of freedom. Trends Pharmacol Sci 1989;10:390–393.
10. Royal College of Physicians/British Nutrition Foundation. Food intolerance and food aversion. J Roy Coll Phys 1984;18:83–122.
11. Zioadron C, Streaty RA, Klee WA. Opioid peptides derived from food proteins. The exorphins. J Biol Chem 1979;254:2446–2449.
12. Finn R. Food allergy—fact or fiction: a review. J Roy Soc Med 1992;85:560–564.
13. Wurtman JJ. The carbohydrate cravers diet. Boston: Houghton-Mifflin, 1983.
14. Lou HC, Henriksen L, Bruhn P. Focal cerebral dysfunction in developmental learning difficulties. Lancet 1990;335:8–11.
15. Murdoch RD, Lessof MH, Pollock I, Young E. Effects of food additives on leukocyte histamine release in normal and urticarial subjects. J Roy Coll Phys 1987;21:251–256.
16. Pollock I, Warner JO. The effect of artificial food colours on childhood behaviour. Arch Dis Child 1990;65:74–77.
17. Moneret-Vautrin DA. False food allergies: non-specific reaction to foodstuffs. In: Lessof MA, ed. Clinical reactions to food. New York: John Wiley, 1983, 135–154.
18. Milich R, Wolraich M, Lundgren S. Sugar and hyperactivity: a critical review of empirical findings. Clin Psychol Rev 1986;6:493–513.
19. Pfeiffer CC. Mental and elemental nutrients: a physician's guide to nutrition and health care. New Canaan, CT: Keats Publishing, 1975.
20. Behar D, Rapoport JL, Adams AJ, *et al.* Sugar challenge testing with children considered behaviorally "sugar reactive." Nutr Behav 1984;1:277.
21. Wolraich ML, Lindgren SD, Sturnbo PJ, *et al.* Effects of diets high in sucrose or aspartame on the behaviour and cognitive performance of children. New Engl J Med 1994;330:301–307.
22. Shaywitz BA, Sullivan CM, Anderson GM, *et al.* Aspartame; behaviour and cognitive function in children with attention deficit disorder. Pediatrics 1994;93:70–75.
23. Petter LPM, Hourihane JO'B, Rolles CR. Is water out of vogue? A survey of the drinking habits of 2–7 year olds. Arch Dis Child 1995;72:137–140.
24. Hourihane JO'B, Rolles CR. Morbidity from excessive intake of high energy fluids: the "Squash drinking syndrome." Arch Dis Child 1995;72:141–143.
25. Norris JR, Meadows GG, Massey LK, *et al.* Tyrosine and phenylalanine-restricted formula diet augments immunocompetence in healthy humans. Am J Clin Nutr 1990;51:188–196.
26. Prendergast M, Taylor E, Rapoport JL, *et al.* The diagnosis of childhood hyperactivity: a US–UK cross national study of DSM-111 and ICD-9. J Child Psychol Psychiat 1988;29:289–300.
27. Robinson J, Ferguson A. Food sensitivity and the nervous system: hyperactivity, addiction and criminal behaviour. Nutrition Research Reviews 1992;5:203–223.
28. Taylor EA, Schachar R, Thorley G, Wieselberg M. Conduct disorder and hyperactivity. I. Separation of hyperactivity and antisocial conduct in British child psychiatric patients. Brit J Psychiat 1986;149:760–767.
29. Sonuga-Barke EJS, Taylor E, Sembi G, Smith J. Hyperactivity and delay aversion—I. The effect of delay on choice. J Child Psychol Psychiat 1992;33:387–398.
30. Feingold BF. Hyperkinesis and learning disabilities linked to artificial food flavours and colours. Am J Nursing 1975;75:797–803.
31. Swain AR, Dutton SP, Truswell AS. Salicylates in foods. J Am Diet Assoc 1985;85:950–960.
32. National Advisory Committee on Hyperkinesis and Food Addi-

tives. Final report to the Nutrition Foundation. New York, 1980.

33. Conners CK, Goyette CH, Southwick DA, *et al.* Food additives and hyperkinesis—controlled double blind experiment. Pedatrics 1976;58:154–166.

34. Goyette CH, Conners CK, Patti TA, Curtis LE. Effects of artificial colours on hyperactive children: a double blind challenge study. Psychopharmacol Bull 1978;14:39–40.

35. Conners CK, Goyette CH, Newman EB. Doze-time effect of artificial colours in hyperactive children. J Learning Difficulties 1980;13:512 516.

36. Conners CK. Artificial colours in the diet and disruptive behaviour: current status of research. In: Miller SA, ed. Nutrition and behaviour. Philadelphia: Franklin Institute Press, 137–143.

37. Harley JP, Ray RS, Tomasi L, *et al.* Hyperkinesis and food additives: testing the Feingold hypothesis. Pediatrics 1978;61: 818–828.

38. Harley JP, Matthews CG, Eichman P. Synthetic food colours and hyperreactivity in children: a double blind challenge experiment. Pediatrics 1978;62:975–980.

39. National Institutes of Health Consensus Development Panel. Conference statement: defined diets and hyperactivity. Am J Clin Nutrition 1983;37:161–165.

40. Egger J, Carter CM, Graham PJ, Gumley D, Soothill JF. A controlled trial of oligo-antigenic diet treatment in the hyperkinetic syndrome. Lancet 1985;1:940–945.

41. Carter CM, Urbanowicz M, Hemsley R, *et al.* Effect of a few-food diet in attention deficit disorder. Arch Dis Child 1993;69:564–568.

42. Egger J, Stolla A, McEwen LM. Controlled trial of hyposensitization in children with food induced hyperkinetic syndrome. Lancet 1992;331:1150–1153.

43. Rowe KS, Rowe KJ. Synthetic food colouring and behaviour: a dose response effect in a double blind placebo controlled repeated-measures study. J Pediatr 1994;125:691–698.

44. Williams JI, Cram DM, Tausig FT, Webster E. Relative effects of drugs and diet on hyperactive behaviours: an experimental study. Pediatrics 1978;61:811–817.

45. Joint Report of the Royal College of Physicians and the British Nutrition Foundation. Food intolerance and food aversion. J Roy Coll Phys 1984;18:83–122.

46. Warner JO, Hathaway MJ. Allergic form of Meadows syndrome (Munchausen by proxy). Arch Dis Child 1984;59:151–156.

47. Meadow R. Suffocation, recurrent apnoea and sudden infant death. J Pediatr 1990;117:351–357.

48. Roesler TA, Barry PC, Bock SA. Factitious food allergy and failure to thrive. Arch Pediatr Adolesc Med 1994;148:1150–1155.

49. David T. The overworked or fraudulent diagnosis of food allergy and food intolerance in children. J Roy Soc Med 1985;78(suppl. 5):21–31.

50. Pearson DJ, Rix KJB, Bentley SJ. Food allergy: how much in the mind? Lancet 1983;1:1259–1261.

51. Rix KJB, Pearson DJ, Bentley SJ. A psychiatric study of patients with supposed food allergy. Brit J Psychiatry 1984;145:121–126.

52. Pearson DJ. Pseudo food allergy. Brit Med J 1986;292:221–222.

53. Warner JO. Food and behaviour (allergy, intolerance or aversion). Pediatr Allergy Immunol 1993;4:112–116.

54. Lessof MH. Total allergy—the passing of a fashion. Resp Dis Pract 1986;1:4–6.

36

FOOD ALLERGY: PSYCHOLOGICAL CONSIDERATIONS

John C. Selner
Herman Staudenmayer

*O*ne vexing problem for allergists is the question of food-related psychosocial dysfunction. The many social aspects of eating are readily identified. They reflect cultural expectations and directives as assuredly as chemoreceptors perceive odor and exquisitely distinct olfactory signals help fashion the desire to eat. It is clear that satiation depends on complex neurologic mechanisms. Early neuroanatomic, glucostatic, thermostatic, and lipostatic theories that attempted to explain questions of hunger and satiety recognized the role of regulatory hormones (i.e., insulin, growth hormone, and serotonin) on gluco- and lipo receptors. This knowledge ultimately led to recognition of neuroreceptor and endocrine receptor activity, which regulates food response on a cellular level (1). The effects of amino acids like tyrosine and tryptophan fed to adults (2) and newborns (3) sharpen the focus on dietary regulation of brain catecholamines and peripheral sympathetic regulatory activity. These considerations have led to investigations of the role of amino acids and proteins as precursors of neurotransmitters (4) as well as the potential for neuropeptides to interact with organ systems that have seemingly different implications for homeostasis. The recognition of intracellular communication and the evidence for common evolutionary origins for neuropeptide, hormonal, and immunologic receptors (5) has given credence to observations linking psychological stress to opioid production and immune regulation (6). The further recognition that the metabolites of essential amino acids have the potential for significant pharmacologic properties (7), along with the current understanding that cold water

fish oils can alter the production of eicosapentaenoic acid in cell phospholipids (8), broadens the venue for interjecting food "allergy" into clinical practice. In this context, the word *allergy* reverts to its historical origins—altered reactivity or response—without the necessity for an immunologic implication. Current accepted nomenclature would refer to this condition as intolerance and reserve the term *allergy* for specific hypersensitivity involving an identifiable immune reaction occurring independent of any physiologic effect of the food or attendant food additives (9). Within this context, we have attempted to identify areas of potential confusion regarding food and the psychological manifestations alleged to be related to food intolerance.

Attention Deficit Disorders

Perhaps the most frequent psychological encounters for the practicing allergist involve attention deficit disorders, which in the 1970s were linked by some clinicians to salicylate and additives in foods (10). Symptoms of hyperactivity, in addition to impulsive, disruptive, and often destructive behavior and poor concentration with a limited attention span, have characterized hyperactivity as a syndrome. The consensus reached in the 1980s on this matter holds that the salicylate–additive relationship suggested by Feingold was not established on a scientific basis and could not be proved by controlled studies, albeit that these studies were not perfect (11). Furthermore, in most study groups, a subpopulation of children (1%–

3%) could be identified who appeared to have consistent social (behavior) or cognitive patterns when exposed to certain food additives (12). Whether similar observations could be made in controlled studies on adults is uncertain. The question of whether much larger doses than those used in reported studies would alter the results remains unanswered (13, 14). Animal experiments suggest that we should be slow to formulate judgments on this issue (15). The clinician should remain open to the identification of patients with intolerance to specific food additives. In addition, the use of double-blind ingestion challenges, followed by increasing quantities of the suspected food or additive over a period of days, may be necessary to exclude this possibility in any given case. The experience with wheat challenges, in which the development of signs and symptoms of dermatitis herpetiformis may take weeks to develop, should serve as a caution to the clinical investigator in this matter. Convenience and economic limitations often dictate the terms under which such challenges are done. It seems likely that cost-containment pressures will increase the likelihood of definitive conclusions being drawn from incomplete clinical testing.

Sugar

Certain sugars, especially sucrose, have been incriminated in the production of behavioral aberrations and cognitive dysfunction. This finding has led some to refer to sugar as a toxin (16). No consistent evidence to support adverse reactions to sugar has been published. Sugar evaluations are problematic and, of necessity, involve multivariant factors that confound attempts at precise conclusions. Nonetheless, results of such studies suggest that when sugar is compared with placebos, no significant impairment of social activity or learning is observed (17–21).

Hypoglycemia

All of the symptoms ascribed to attention deficit disorders and sugar-related behavioral aberrations have been attributed by one author or another to hypoglycemia. Physiologic experience with low blood sugar demonstrates clouded sensorium, fatigue, aggressive behavior, anxiety, irritability, palpitations, and tremoring, which are all ascribable to low blood sugar (22). Little argument exists in scientific circles that hypoglycemia does not occur with the frequency suggested by lay publications of the recent past. Furthermore, alcohol-related reactive hypoglycemia in normal subjects ingesting carbohydrates is common (23). Postprandial irritability or somnolence is frequent in individuals with very high carbohydrate intake. Dumping syndromes—either postsurgical or in patients with vast appetites—produce somnolence that is interpreted by some patients and clinicians as a sign of hypoglycemia and, at times, is extended to imply psychological importance. These observations have readily explainable metabolic origins and rarely have more than social implications.

Amino Acids

Amino acids have been identified as precursors to neurotransmitters required for normal brain function. Although progress has been made in understanding the competition between amino acids and carbohydrates for membrane transport and production of neurotransmitters, information on this subject is far from complete. Whether neurotransmitter quantity, quality, and function will be significantly altered by such competition remains to be clarified (24). The orthomolecular practice of providing patients with scores of dietary supplements including amino acids, based on a perceived need established by analysis of hair or body fluids, is used by some practitioners. We encountered a patient who manipulated more than 100 supplements per day by consulting the rotation axis of a crystal. This activity could be ascribed to certain readily identifiable needs of this patient. What was difficult to rationalize was the institution of this program, apparently without recognition of the important psychopathology of which it was a symptom. Opioids derived from the enzymatic hydrolysis of milk and wheat have been incriminated in mental changes, and studies have demonstrated food-derived opioid alterations in sleep induction and sleep patterning (25). This finding raises the question of whether gastric absorption of specific exorphin-like materials may account for some neuropsychological observations.

Tension–Fatigue Syndrome

First described in the early 1900s, this phenomenological presentation was subsequently described by Rowe (26) and Randolph (27) and extended by Speer to include underactivity and overactivity (28). For some clinicians, this syndrome became synonymous with the allergic child and involved fatigue, irritability, brain "fog," allergic shiners, and nasal congestion. Controlled challenges employed to demonstrate the association of foods with allergic tension fatigue have been observed by some clinicians to result in common symptoms (e.g., pain, diarrhea, and hyperactivity) appearing to be the physical expression of pathology. This tends to explain the emotional presentation observed. Whether tension fatigue is a symptom of underlying pathology or an isolated symptom complex remains uncertain.

Allergy and Organic Brain Syndromes

In patients demonstrating clear-cut evidence of atopic disease (asthma, rhinitis, and eczema), the most consistent common factor experienced is the ingestion of drugs for purposes of ameliorating disease. In many cases, drug administration is initiated early in life and exposure may become chronic through the formative years. These same drugs may continue to be experienced in adult life with subtle implications that are frequently not appreciated by patient, parent, teacher, or clinician. The potential toxic effects of methylxanthines and, as a corollary, caffeine, are debated in the medical literature. In contrast, the physiologic potential for stimulation to promote clarity of thought and inhibition of sleepiness and fatigue is not disputed. This stimulation of the respiratory center and the influence on vasomotor and vagal tone has been clearly identified. Effects on coronary artery and cerebral vascular flow, as well as pulmonary profusion, increase in heart rate, bronchodilatation, and diuresis, all speak to the broad effects of this drug. Nervousness, headaches, flushing, palpitations, nausea, gastric distress, diarrhea, tachypnea, hyperesthesia, tinnitus, scotomata, agitation, hyperexcitability, and heightened arousal patterns are all associated with the toxic effects of this single medication, which is often introduced to a child in the first few months of life (29). It is safe to say that a similar provenance can be ascribed to adrenalin, ephedrine compounds, corticosteroids, and antihistamines. The failure to recognize the pharmacologic dependency and the physiologic consequences of prolonged exposure to these substances complicates the necessary distinction between a direct drug effect and an alleged food allergy. The frequent use of alcohol and opiates in many pediatric compounds as naturally occurring toxicants, and contact with these materials in foods, could readily lead to misinterpretation as to the cause of behavioral and cognitive dysfunction. Little debate exists about the sedative effect of antihistamines, which has led to a pharmaceutical scramble in search of chemicals with nonsedating properties. One hopes that clinicians will keep in mind the potential effects of these new and useful drugs when interpreting social and cognitive aberrations in both children and adults who use them.

Specific Foods and Behavior

Thorough media attention, as well as the response of the consumer to books and articles containing sensational testimonies of patients and physicians regarding food and behavior, has incriminated some common foods in well-characterized psychiatric conditions (30). To date, none of these associations has been reliably confirmed. Concepts of cyclical and masked allergy leading to typical clinical presentations of addiction, characterized by withdrawal of food resulting in increased symptoms associated with depression and reintroduction of food resulting in cessation of symptoms and stimulation or euphoria, have been proposed (31). The interpretations permitted by this scheme provide an "explanation" for every conceivable observation associated with behavior, regardless of origin and, therefore, lend themselves to therapy schemes uninhibited by historical facts, physical observations, or laboratory findings. Insights into alcohol addiction and evidence for genetic predisposition to alcohol addiction (32) have no corollary that has been identified for foods such as wheat, corn, and yeast. Anecdotal reports and inadequate epidemiologic reviews of the psychiatric population have suggested that wheat and rye consumption affects the therapy outcome of hospitalized schizophrenics (33, 34). While these reports suggest a potential relationship for glutenin intolerance with schizophrenia, the analysis of the data originally presented contains a statistical error. Cumulative frequency of patient discharge at different time intervals over a one-year period was used, when actual frequency in each time interval is the correct dependent measure for Fisher's exact test. Our analysis of the same data found that the group of schizophrenics on a wheat-free diet did not differ from controls. Two large studies failed to find evidence for an association between celiac disease and schizophrenia (35, 36). Soft associations for correlations between glutenin intolerance and schizophrenia may be found in the observation that as many as 20% of schizophrenics have antibodies to wheat gliadin (37, 38), and that whole wheat and rye antibodies are observed more frequently in schizophrenic than in control subjects, while 50% of schizophrenics have lymphocyte reactivity to glutenin, a percentage similar to that found in celiac disease.

It is important to concede that, although absence of proof does not mean proof of absence in such relationships, clear-cut indications of such associations remain to be demonstrated. Comparisons of immunoglobulin E (IgE) titers in depressed patients with those in control populations have led to the observation that a greater percentage of the depressed patients demonstrated IgE specific for some foods, such as eggs. Yet no evidence has been forthcoming to demonstrate a causative relationship between any specific food and a psychological effect. The limited literature on this subject prohibits the drawing of any conclusions on this matter.

When patients who believed that foods are a cause of psychological disease were compared with a group of mentally ill patients without such a belief, highly significant concordance was noted. When the same parameters were compared in a group of patients with well-characterized food allergy but without such a belief, discordance was found. In addition,

patients with verified food allergy were not found to be significantly different from a control group of nonallergic, nonpsychologically impaired subjects (39). Lessof and associates studied 100 patients with food intolerance. No exclusively psychiatric symptoms were found in the patients with documented evidence for immediate food hypersensitivity (40). Patients with psychological problems are resistant to a designation of psychogenic or psychosomatic illness. Most of these patients will seek an alternative explanation onto which they project their problem. Therefore, food is an attractive alternative as an explanation for symptoms. With as many as 20% of the population estimated to experience some kind of emotional disorder, nutrophobia can be expected to persist as a major clinical obstacle to wellness.

Candida: *Yeast and Behavior*

A number of patients believe that yeast—specifically *Candida*—is responsible for all or part of their psychological and polysomatic complaints. This belief is an extension of the attention given the original observations of Truss (41) and has been presented by publications that have not been subjected to comprehensive scientific review. The yeast theory suggests a cascade of events in which candidal colonization, a normal homeostatic event, results in the release of various products (antigens, toxins, and metabolic factors), which leads to immune reactions including autoimmunity and food allergy. These events are suggested to have consequences for organ system dysfunction (potentially all organ systems), which in turn leads to systemic illness and polysomatic complaints. These vulnerabilities then enhance total food allergy, which contributes to a perpetuating phenomenon from which no escape appears possible. Predisposing factors leading to patient susceptibility include a litany of factors such as impaired immunity, nutritional and dietary deficiencies, disruptions to normal host-defense mechanical factors such as skin and mucosal barrier deficiencies, and even hormonal events associated with menses and pregnancy. Also, the use of medications such as antibiotics, steroids, and hormones (oral contraceptives), as well as the existence of endocrinopathies or malignancies, are all suggested to enhance patient susceptibility.

Careful reading of a review of this theory reveals little support in comprehensively reviewed scientific literature for the construct that underpins this theory. Furthermore, it is difficult to identify substantial authoritative evidence that suggests the existence of such a condition (42). Overapplication of this diagnosis may lead to problems.

CASE NO. 1

A mother of three children complained of headaches and vague polysomatic conditions referable to the neuromuscular system. A rotation diet and specific food elimination had been recommended following sublingual and subcutaneous provocation food testing. Short-term, immediate relief of symptoms and a weight loss of approximately 15 pounds (from 145 to 130 pounds) resulted over several months.

During our examination, results of prick testing for foods were negative and a comprehensive dietary history did not suggest the probability of food involvement in this patient's current complaints. A comprehensive medical history suggested the possibility of childhood trauma because of the patient's reticence to discuss her early childhood and a near-complete amnesia for events prior to the age of 10 years. Despite attempts to engage the patient further, she was lost to follow-up for approximately one year.

During this time the patient consulted a nutritionist, who initiated candidal treatment strategies and referred the patient to a kinesiologist who "confirmed" the presence of yeast in the patient's blood by utilizing a "special blood test." The condition of the patient continued to deteriorate, which was ascribed to chemical sensitivity as a consequence of mycotoxin produced by the *Candida*. She was then referred to an environmental ecology center. Her husband intervened at this point and she was again seen in our office. She weighed 89 pounds and was suffering from severe malnutrition.

Short-term psychotherapy revealed that this woman had been subjected to incestuous sexual abuse at 6 years of age, which continued until she literally fled her home at 17 years of age. Although she was married and a mother, her father continued his advances and she perceived him to be a significant threat. Although the prognosis in this case is guarded, long-term psychotherapy has reversed the progressive starvation and signs and symptoms of "food allergy."

Unproved Diagnostic Techniques

Provocation tests (sublingual and subcutaneous), accustress, and other controversial strategies have been employed with many patients, leading to the proposed identification of a cause-and-effect relationship between food and psychological impairment (43). In our opinion, no body of information exists in the competently reviewed scientific literature to support these contentions. In a study by King (44), 30 patients with symptoms including anxiety, confusion, difficulty in concentration, and depression were characterized by the Minnesota multiphasic personality inventory (MMPI). They showed elevated scores on scales of depression, schizophrenia, hysteria, and hypochondriasis. Using a sublingual provocation technique, King found cognitive–emotional symptom scores to be greater after allergen administration than after placebo in this population. In some patients, scores after placebo were greater than scores after allergen. The validity of the procedure has been questioned because of the likelihood that subjects were able to distinguish between placebo and active challenges. Similarly, in our experience, patients subject to such diagnostic strategies and subsequently identified as having food allergy often have been demonstrated in therapy to have severe psychological difficulties; when these difficulties are appropriately addressed, symptoms allegedly caused by food ingestion often resolve.

CASE NO. 2

A young interior designer complained of experiencing daily headaches and general malaise since early childhood. These headaches did not fit a typical migraine or cluster pattern and were associated with severe gastrointestinal symptoms. Single-blind, sublingual provocation testing had identified positive reactions to several foods. No repeat or control challenges had been performed. After attempts at avoidance and rotation of foods failed to alter her symptoms, she sought a second opinion. Standard skin testing for incriminated foods was negative.

Reactions to randomized, double-blind, placebo-controlled sublingual and subcutaneous tests for incriminated foods failed to distinguish active food challenges from control challenges. While reviewing these results with the patient, a nonconfrontational inquiry suggested that psychological factors could be of major importance. Psychotherapy revealed profound physical and sexual abuse beginning in infancy and continuing until puberty, involving incest and multiple offenders. As these events were uncovered and brought to the patient's conscious awareness, symptoms resolved, as did her alleged food allergy. A striking association was revealed in this case between specific foods and specific abuse. These associations offered a remarkable demonstration of the importance of the senses of sight, odor, and taste in the development of well-focalized psychotherapy.

Hyperventilation, Vocal Cord Dysfunction, and the Allergic Patient

It is tempting to dismiss symptoms as hyperventilation, the condition of patients with chronic recurrent respiratory disease, often to the exclusion of other clinical signs that may suggest psychological problems. Acute episodes of hyperventilation are generally well recognized by clinicians in association with panic syndromes. On the other hand, chronic hyperventilation as induced by organic toxins, including drugs, or as the result of emotional factors, most notably anxiety, is often confusing. The subsequent development of hyperventilation as a coping style is not well recognized by many clinicians. Our experience would suggest that anxiety and fear as a consequence of abandonment (physical and emotional), and fear as a consequence of abuse occurring in early childhood, can lay the foundation for hyperventilation as well as other increasingly well-characterized respiratory

syndromes such as paradoxical vocal cord dysfunction.

CASE NO. 3

A 29-year-old teacher came to our attention with a history of asthma from age 11. Her condition had been inadequately controlled despite prescription of multiple medications, including corticosteroids, which left her cushingoid. Recurrent episodes of "severe asthma" had been attributed to her exposure to the odor of corn. The smell of popcorn in a theater, for instance, would result in an emergency room visit and potential hospitalization with severe, protracted respiratory obstruction. Yet methacholine challenges, isocapnic hyperventilation, and exercise challenges failed to induce asthma under controlled conditions. A controlled challenge to the odor of corn resulted in marked obstruction that seemed to be focalized in the upper airway. Flexible fiber-optic examination revealed a chink deformity of the posterior commissure as described by Christopher (45). Skin testing and in vitro testing failed to identify evidence of immunoglobulin E specific to corn. A confrontation with the evidence that the patient did not have asthma, and that she, in fact, was experiencing an obstruction of the upper airway, which could have significant psychological overtones, was followed by intense psychotherapy. It revealed evidence of severe psychotrauma, which was brought into the patient's conscious awareness, resulting in the ability to challenge this patient with the odor of corn and, subsequently, to the patient's ingestion of corn without respiratory symptoms (46).

On the other hand, chronic hyperventilation is easily overlooked in some patients (47). Hypocapnia associated with hyperventilation leads to a fall in organic phosphorus disproportionate to respiratory alkalosis. This decline results in symptoms of dizziness and paresthesias with numbness and tingling of the extremities, mental changes leading to disorientation, and a generalized malaise. At the same time, alkalosis results in neuromuscular complaints, while cerebral hypoxia enhances lightheadedness and dizziness and compounds cerebral vasoconstriction. An intriguing scenario emerges here of a patient developing, as a result of chronic hypoxia, an altered perception of the ability to breathe. The respiratory center activity in response to partial pressure of carbon dioxide in arterial blood results in a sensation of dyspnea, yet partial pressures of oxygen and carbon dioxide are normal. This condition can lead to a vicious cycle that is commonly encountered and often not recognized in patients suffering from chronic hyperventilation. They will complain of the inability to breathe comfortably. Their condition is punctuated by intermittent, very deep breaths that serve to sustain the metabolic abnormalities.

In this physiologic mode, a minimal amount of stress results in changes in respiration, which can then lead to acute symptoms. These symptoms include general malaise and affect the central nervous, cardiovascular, respiratory, gastrointestinal, and neuromuscular systems. When a patient has been introduced to the idea that these symptoms are related to food allergy, suspicion of a particular food or eating in general with the potential for exposure to unrecognized suspect foods can lead to apprehension. This fear exacerbates the cycle of adrenergic activity leading to hyperventilation. At the same time, the psychiatric expressions of anxiety, depression, and what is often recognized as panic are obvious in the indiscriminate fast-food culture and must be distinguished from hyperventilation. Rapid ingestion of food and carbonated beverages can often lead to bloating and distention as well as aerophagia. Esophageal refluxing can lead to stimulation of distal esophageal reflexes, which may induce bronchospasm and chest pain.

Lymphocyte Subpopulations in Food Allergies

Patients with alleged adverse food reactions have been reported to have depressed absolute T- and B-lymphocyte counts, both chronically and as an apparent consequence of food challenge (48). These observations are uncontrolled, and their significance is questionable in view of other studies (49, 50) that have shown similar variations in lymphocyte populations in patients with depressive disorders and bereavement. At this writing, no convincing evidence has documented significant variations in lymphocyte population as a result of food allergy. On the other hand, in our experience, stress factors can often be identified in patients who maintain a belief that food allergy is responsible for psychosomatic complaints. This belief often has its origins with clinicians who rely on unproved and controversial techniques in suggesting to the patient a cause-and-effect relationship between food exposure and illness. Suggestion can be profound, and patient susceptibility is often associated with primary gain. Primary gain requires an alternative to the painful prospect of confronting severe psychotrauma, and the patient is grateful to the clinician who suggests a convenient alternative— i.e., food allergy. The clinician becomes an accomplice in the patient's need to circumvent unresolved conflicts that underlie his or her polysomatic complaints.

Conditioning

Laboratory animals can be conditioned to experience anaphylaxis with marked increase through measurable mediators such as histamine upon the perception of an odor. The classic conditioning experiment of Russell and associates demonstrated that with parenteral sensitization to bovine serum albumin, guinea pigs could experience anaphylaxis with the perception of an odor that was simultaneously associated with anaphylaxis induced by bovine serum albumin feedings (51). Histamine release resulted from the perception of this odor, triethylamine (fishy odor) and dimethylsulfide (sulfur odor), which is immunologically unrelated to bovine serum albumin and to which controlled guinea pigs did not demonstrate anaphylaxis.

Bronchi have been observed to constrict and dilate as a result of suggestion, and exercise-induced bronchospasm can be clearly demonstrated to be influenced by hypnosis. An atropine blockade of suggestion response seems to indicate a parasympathetic pathway is involved. The pioneering experiments of Wolff in the early 1950s, which demonstrated the effects of conditioning and food provocation on cutaneous eruption, nasal secretion, and even peripheral blood eosinophilia, are striking examples of the impact of suggestion and the importance of controlled observations in food allergy (52).

Double-Blind Challenge Procedures

Amazingly, many physicians are willing to ascribe depression, mania, and a host of other psychological symptoms to food on the basis of open food challenge. It has been clearly shown that such challenges can result in the production of any symptom. Blinded challenges have demonstrated repeatedly how unreliable the history can be for food allergy.

CASE NO. 4

Several years ago, we evaluated a 42-year-old teacher who complained of severe "asthma" and gastrointestinal symptoms that resulted in her inability to maintain employment (53). She professed a belief that she was "universally allergic" and mentioned allergic reactions to a large variety of foods. The patient was evaluated under controlled environmental conditions in a specially constructed diagnostic facility. Double-blind, placebo-controlled challenges with a variety of foods resulted in "total-body reactions" lasting for as long as two days, during which she felt totally incapacitated and was bedridden. The patient experienced fear prior to each challenge and characterized this feeling as "like walking into doom." After being confronted in a supportive fashion with the nature of her reactions and the false-positive symptoms that she had demonstrated to the placebo challenge, she described herself as feeling worthless and useless.

This experience served as an opportunity for the initiation of psychotherapy, which has continued to this date and during which she uncovered traumatic abuse in early childhood. At two years of age, she was hospitalized in a home for children with sexually transmitted diseases, with gonorrhea that she had contracted from her father. She recalled lying in her crib and hearing her father's threats of abandonment if he was discovered. These threats were realized and compounded by her mother's placing blame on her and punishing her by leaving her in this hospital for six months without visitation. This child was rejected further when she was reunited with the family. Coping with these abuses led to profound psychodynam-

ics. This patient has been restored to society, is able to maintain a productive job, and is financially self-sustaining.

Psychological problems continue, however. She recently arrived in an emergency room with total-body pruritus after eating a restaurant-prepared meal. An examination failed to reveal any obvious signs of food reaction, and careful assessment of this episode in psychotherapy led to the patient's recognition that the pruritus was associated with physical sensations she had experienced while hospitalized and under treatment for the gonorrhea.

This incident triggered psychological expressions of panic subsequently traced to issues of loss and fear of abandonment related to the transfer of a supervisor on whom she was very dependent. These revelations were uncovered in a psychotherapy session necessitated by a hysterical episode and during which all symptoms resolved. As demonstrated in this case, the importance of double-blind challenges cannot be overstated. Eliminating patient and observer bias is essential to objectifying food intolerance.

Learned Sensitivity and Psychological Symptoms: A Cascading Model

In food challenges, the symptoms observed are usually assumed to be directly caused by the food being tested. This need not always be the case, however. In an alternative model, physical symptoms, which may in fact be caused by the food, serve as triggers for additional psychological or psychophysiologic symptoms associated with fear and panic. This model may be viewed as a cascading sequence of responses, each serving as a trigger for further responses. In the case just presented, symptoms of pruritus served as triggers to sensory memories associated with gonorrhea, leading to images of parental abandonment that elicited the subjective and physiologic experiences of panic and fear.

Food Allergy and Learned Sensitivity

The September 1986 issue of *National Geographic* contains a remarkable review of what is referred to as "the intimate sense." The survival significance of the sense of smell is found in the evolutionary trail from sea life to humans. The author recounts the poignant experience of sniffing, on impulse, an old deerskin belonging to his grandfather and being transported: "Suddenly I was a boy again, and there in all but the flesh was my grandfather, methodically reloading his shotgun as the flushed quail sailed beyond the mesquite." This description goes on to include recall of exquisite detail involving sight, taste, and touch in a process that is no doubt unique to humans in its completeness.

Our experience suggests that the depth of our heritage may entail trauma that, at times, overwhelms the psychological host defense. As coping styles are exhausted, these events result in a patient with clinical symptoms that must be recognized by the clinician as major pathology. The frequency with which these patients are subjected to polypsychopharmaceutical therapy, without the professional investment required to elucidate underlying pathology, is very troubling. When the allergist is approached by such a patient, a unique opportunity presents itself for utilizing the history-taking talents and investigational skills of the physician. By not rejecting the patient out of hand as mentally ill, but rather recognizing the signs of possible learned sensitivity, the physician can help many of these patients. Using controlled challenge testing, it is possible either to identify a real intolerance and develop dietary avoidance strategies, or to reveal to the patient evidence of nonresponse and dispel inaccurate belief of food intolerance instilled by nonmedical suggestion. Salvaging such patients makes the physician investment most rewarding and adds a significant dimension to the traditional role of the allergist.

REFERENCES

1. Garfinkel PE, Coscina DV. The physiology and psychology of hunger and satiety. In: Zales MR, ed. Eating, sleeping and sexuality. New York: Brunner/Mazel, 1982, 5–42.
2. Benedict CR, Anderson GH, Sole MJ. The influence of oral tyrosine and tryptophan feeding on plasma catecholamines in man. Am J Clin Nutr 1983;38:429–435.
3. Youngman MW, Keisel SH. Diet and sleep patterns in newborn infants. N Engl J Med 1983;309:1147–1149.
4. Wurtman RM. Nutrients that modify brain function. Sci Am 1982;246:50–59.
5. Roth J, LaRoith D, Collier ES, *et al*. Evolutionary origins of neuropeptides, hormones and receptors: possible applications to immunology. J Immunol 1985;135:816–819.
6. Shavitt Y, Terman GW, Martin FC, Lewis JW, Liebeskind JC, Gale RP. Stress, opioid peptides, the immune system and cancer. J Immunol 1985;135:834–837.
7. Murphy RC, Pickett WC, Culp BR, Lands W. Tetraene and pentaene leukotrienes: selective production from murine mastocytoma cells after dietary manipulation. Prostaglandins 1981;22:613–622.
8. Sperling RI, Weinklatt M, Robbin JL. Effects of dietary fish oil on vitro leukocyte leukotriene generation and activity of disease in rheumatoid arthritis. Arthritis Rheum 1986; 29.S18(abstr 41).
9. Anderson JA. Food allergy: an overview. Immunol Allergy Pract 1984;6:13–20.
10. Feingold BF. Why your child is hyperactive. New York: Random House, 1975.
11. Consensus conference: defined diets and childhood hyperactivity. JAMA 1982;248:290–292.
12. Connors CK. Food additives and hyperactive children. New York: Plenum Press, 1980.
13. Weiss B. Color me hyperactive. Am Health 1982;1:1485.
14. Swanson JM, Kinsbourne M. Food dyes impair performance of hyperactive children on a laboratory learning test. Science 1980;207:1485–1487.
15. Shaywitz R, Goldenring JR, Wool RS. The effects of chronic administration of food colorings on activity levels and cognitive performance in normal and hyperactive developing rat pups. Ann Neurol 1978;4:196A.
16. Buchanan S. The most ubiquitous toxin. Am Psychologist 1984;39:1327–1328.
17. Milich R, Pelham WF. Effects of sugar ingestion on classroom and playground behavior of attention deficit disordered boys. J Consult Clin Psychol 1986;54:714–718.
18. Behar D, Rapaport JL, Adams AJ, Berg CJ, Cornblath M. Sugar challenge testing with children considered behaviorally "sugar reactive." J Nutr Behavior 1984;1:277.
19. Wolraich ML, Milich R, Stumbo P, Schultz F. Effects of sucrose ingestion on the behavior of hyperactive boys. J Pediatr 1985;106:675–682.
20. Mahan K, Furakawa CT, Chase M, Shapiro GG, Pierson WE, Bierman W. Sugar and children's behavior. Presented at the annual meeting of the American Academy of Pediatrics, Chicago, September 1984.
21. Ferguson B. The effects of sugar and aspartame on children's cognition and behavior: a challenge study. Presented at the American Medical Association Conference on Diet and Behavior, Arlington, Va., November 1984.
22. Merimee TJ, Tyson JE. Hypoglycemia in man: pathologic and physiologic variants. Diabetes 1977;26:161–165.
23. Hale F, Margen S, Rabak D. Postprandial hypoglycaemia and "psychological" symptoms. Biol Psychiatry 1982;17:125–130.
24. Wurtman RJ, Wurtman JJ. Carbohydrates and depression. Sci Am 1989;260:68–75.
25. Zioudrou C, Streaty TS, Klee WA. Opioid peptides derived from food proteins: the exorphins. J Biol Chem 1979;254:2446–2449.
26. Rowe AH. Allergic toxaemia and migraine due to food allergy. Calif Med 1930;33:785–793.
27. Randolph TG. Fatigue and weakness of allergic origin (allergic

toxaemia) to be differentiated from nervous fatigue and neurasthenia. Ann Allergy 1945;3:418–430.

28. Speer F. The allergic–tension–fatigue syndrome. Pediatr Clin North Am 1954;1:1029–1037.

29. Hendeles L, Massanari M, Weinberger M. Theophylline. In: Middleton E, Reed CE, Ellis EF, eds. Allergy, principles and practice, 3rd ed. St. Louis: CV Mosby, 1988, 673–714.

30. Philpott WH, Kalita D. Brain allergies. New Canaan, Conn.: Keats Publishing, 1980.

31. Randolph TG. Bulletin of the Human Ecology Research Foundation. Chicago, 1980.

32. Goodwin DW. Genetic aspects of alcoholism. Drug Therapy 1982;(October):57–66.

33. Dohan FC. The possible pathogenic effect of cereal grains in schizophrenia. Celiac disease as a model. Acta Neurol (Napoli) 1976;31:195–205.

34. Dohan FC, Grasberger JC. Relapsed schizophrenics: earlier discharge from the hospital after cereal-free, milk-free diet. Am J Psychiatry 1973;130:685–688.

35. Dean G, Hanniffy L, Stevens F, et al. Schizophrenia and coeliac disease. J Irish Med Assoc 1975;68:545–546.

36. Stevens FM, Lloyd RS, Gerachty SMJ, et al. Schizophrenia and coeliac disease—the nature of the relationship. Psychol Med 1977;7:259–263.

37. Dohan FC, Martin L, Grasberger JC, et al. Antibodies to wheat gliadin in blood of psychiatric patients: possible role of emotional factors. Biol Psychiatry 1972;5:127–137.

38. Hekkens WThJM, Schipperijn AJM, Freed DLJ. Antibodies to wheat proteins in schizophrenia: relationship or coincidence? In: Hemmings G, ed. Biochemistry of schizophrenia and addiction. Lancaster, U.K.: MTP Press, 1980, 125–133.

39. Rix KJB, Pearson DJ, Bentley SJ. A psychiatric study of patients with supposed food allergy. Br J Psychiatry 1984;145:121–126.

40. Lessof MH, Wraith DG, Merrett TG, Merrett J, Buisseret PD. Food allergy and intolerance in 100 patients—local and systemic effect. Qu J Med 1980;195:259–271.

41. Truss CO. The role of Candida albicans in human illness. Orthomol Psychiatry 1981;10:228.

42. Kroker G. Chronic candidiasis and allergy. In: Brostoff J, Challacombe SJ, eds. Food allergy and intolerance. East Sussex, UK: Baillières Tindall 1987, 850–872.

43. Selner JC, Condemi JJ. Unproven diagnostic and treatment methods. In: Middleton E, Reed CE, Ellis EF, eds. Allergy, principles and practice, 3rd ed. St. Louis: CV Mosby 1988, 1571–1597.

44. King DS. Can allergic exposure provoke psychological symptoms? A double-blind test. Biol Psychiatry 1981;16:3–19.

45. Christopher K. Vocal cord dysfunction presenting as asthma. N Engl J Med 1983;308:1566–1570.

46. Selner JC, Staudenmayer H, Koepke JW, Harvey R, Christopher K. Vocal cord dysfunction: the importance of psychological factors and provocation inhalation challenges. J Allergy Clin Immunol 1987;79:726–733.

47. Pearson DJ, Rix KJB. Psychological effects of food allergy. In: Brostoff J, Challacombe SJ, eds. Food allergy and intolerance. East Sussex, UK: Baillières Tindall, 1987, 688–708.

48. Rea WJ. Environmentally-triggered cardiac disease. Ann Allergy 1978;40:243–251.

49. Schleifer SJ, Keller SE, Meyerson AT, et al. Lymphocyte function in major depressive disorder. Arch Gen Psychiatry 1984;41:484–486.

50. Beauchemin JA. Allergic reactions in mental diseases. Am J Psychiatry 1935;92:1190.

51. Russel M, Dark KA, Cummins RW, Ellman G, Callaway E, Peeke HVS. Learned histamine release. Science 1984;225:733–734.

52. Wolff HG. Life stress and bodily disease—a formulation: the nature of stress in man. In: Proceedings of the Association for Research in Nervous and Mental Disease. Baltimore: Williams and Wilkins, 1950, 1059–1094.

53. Selner JC, Staudenmayer H. The relationship of environment and food to allergic and psychiatric illness. In: Young SH, Rubin JM, Daman H, eds. Psychobiological aspect of allergic disorders. New York: Praeger Press, 1986, 102–146.

37

CONNECTIVE TISSUE REACTIONS TO FOODS

Richard S. Panush
Sami L. Bahna

A variety of symptoms affecting virtually every organ system have been attributed to hypersensitivity reactions to foods (1–9). Many of these symptoms reflect the concept of "delayed" reactions, which presumes that certain clinical allergies to food develop over a period of hours or days (or longer) and are caused by immunologic mechanisms other than immediate-type hypersensitivity mediated by immunoglobulin E (IgE) (10, 11). Alleged delayed food allergies related to connective tissue remain controversial.

Historical Perspective

Considerable literature about food and rheumatic diseases appeared earlier in this century. Most observers remained unimpressed by the consistent relationship determined between diet or food and rheumatic diseases (10–12) (summarized in Table 37.1). In 1932, Weatherbee analyzed 350 cases of arthritis and concluded that "Dietary treatments of all types had been tried in many cases [but] . . . little definite improvement from dietary management alone was reported" (13). In 1933, Minot wrote: "There exist many peculiar facts concerning diets for arthritis" (14). Two years later, Bauer stated, "There exists no unanimity of opinion concerning the correct diet for an arthritic patient," although he believed that allergy to foods provoked arthritis in certain patients (15). An authoritative, comprehensive review of the English-language rheumatology literature in 1940 concluded, "The incidence of food allergy among rheumatic patients is not significant" (16). This same group also noted, "We cannot approve the emphasis laid on the factor of food allergy in cases of atrophic arthritis; it is neither common nor do we consider it important. Variations in articular systems are so common from day to day that it is easy to blame erroneously some food for the day's ill feeling. Cases of atrophic arthritis with undoubted and repeated articular exacerbations from foods are few and far between" (17).

Based on this literature, one of the last rheumatology textbooks to extensively consider the relationship between food and arthritis (published in 1954) included the statement, "It is almost universally acknowledged that rheumatoid arthritis cannot be overcome by any dietary manipulations which have thus far been proposed" (18). In its 1981 informational pamphlet for patients, "The Truth About Diet and Arthritis," the Arthritis Foundation summarized: "The possible relationship between diet and arthritis has been thoroughly and scientifically studied. The simple proven fact is: no food has anything to do with causing arthritis and no food is effective in treating or 'curing' it" (19).

On the other hand, provocative observations have supported the idea that specific dietary manipulation ameliorated arthritis. These treatments were predicated on the hypothesis that foods or food additives were injurious and caused or perpetuated arthritis. Most of these data may be inadequate because prospective, blinded, controlled, experimental studies

Table 37.1
Nutrition and Rheumatic/Vasculitic Diseases. Reproduced with permission from the publisher with slight modification from Panush RS. Foods, diets, nutrition, and other questionable remedies for arthritis. In: Koopman WJ, ed. Arthritis and allied conditions, 13th ed.

Reference	Observations	Comments
Pottenger 1928 (63)	Allergies frequent among arthritis patients.	Uncontrolled. Arthritis undifferentiated.
Weatherby 1932 (13)	Dietary management ineffective for arthritis.	Uncontrolled. Arthritis undifferentiated.
Minot 1933 (14)	"There is, of course, no standard diet for arthritis."	Review.
Lewin and Taub 1936 (66)	Allergic synovitis due to walnuts.	Uncontrolled, unblinded.
Berger 1939 (67)	Intermittent hydrarthrosis improved on elimination diet.	Unproven.
Hench et al. 1941 (16, 17)	Food allergy suspected but unproven in palindromic rheumatism.	Review.
Hench and Rosenberg 1941 (20)	Food allergy suspected in 16 patients with palindromic rheumatism.	Unproven.
Vaughn 1943 (68)	Palindromic rheumatism in 2% of allergic patients.	Unblinded, uncontrolled.
Miller 1949 (cited in ref. 32)	Allergic (palindromic) arthritis.	Three anecdotes.
Zeller 1949 (21)	Possible food allergy "as a factor" in RA.	Four anecdotes.
Kaufman 1953 (64)	"Food induced allergic musculoskeletal syndromes."	Anecdotal.
Zussman 1966 (22)	Foods suspected of causing inflammatory arthritis.	Four patients.
Epstein 1969 (70)	Sodium nitrate associated with palindromic rheumatism.	Blinded, controlled challenges.
Millman 1972 (65)	"An allergic concept of the etiology of RA."	Review.
Rowe 1972 (23)	Food allergy caused arthralgias/arthritis.	10 patients.
Marguardt et al. 1973 (71)	Behçet's syndrome associated with black walnuts.	Incompletely blinded, controlled.
Randoph 1976 (69)	RA and myalgias associated with foods.	Anecdotes.
Skoldstam et al. 1979 (cited in ref. 32)	Fasting ameliorated RA symptoms.	Controlled.
Mandell and Conte 1980 (29)	"Rheumatic joint" reactions in 88% of patients.	Abstracted and presented. Questionable controls, blinding.
Parke and Hughes 1981 (77)	RA exacerbated by milk.	Incompletely blinded, controlled.
Williams 1980 (cited in ref. 32)	Dairy products associated with arthritis.	Anecdote.
Sundqvist et al. 1982 (cited in ref. 32)	Fasting improved RA.	Controlled, unblinded.
Wraith 1982 (80)	RA-like arthritis associated with food (tartrazine).	Double-blind challenge.
Hanson et al. 1983 (cited in ref. 32)	No therapeutic benefit from evening primrose oil.	Prospective, open trial.
Panush et al. 1983 (28)	Restriction diet comparable to placebo diet for RA and OA.	Prospective, controlled, blinded.
Reidenberg et al. 1983 (75)	SLE associated with hydrazine.	Unblinded challenge.
Stroud 1983 (51)	Fasting antirheumatic; foods exacerbated arthritis.	Incompletely blinded, controlled.
Roberts and Hayashi (73)	SLE exacerbated by alfalfa (L-canavanine).	Anecdotal.
Uden et al. 1983 (18)	Fasting improved RA.	Controlled.
Burne et al. 1985 (cited in ref. 32)	Six patients with arthritis and coeliac disease.	Food-related?
Jantti et al. 1985 (cited in ref. 32)	No appreciable therapeutic benefit from sunflower oil (linoleic acid) for inflammatory arthritis.	Prospective, single-blind, placebo-controlled; 10 patients.
Kremer et al. (cited in ref. 32)	Eicosapentanoic acid (EPA) modestly improved some subjective symptoms of RA.	Double-blind, controlled prospective.
O'Driscoll et al. 1985 (cited in ref. 32)	Normal incidence of atopy in RA.	
Ratner et al. 1985 (83)	Milk associated with arthritis in lactase deficiency.	Incompletely blinded, controlled.
Darlington et al. 1986 (84)	Food elimination improved and challenge worsened some RA patients.	Unblinded, controlled.

Table 37.1
(Continued)

Reference	Observations	Comments
Panush et al. 1986 (29)	RA-like arthritis and immunologic hypersensitivity to milk.	Prospective, double-blind, controlled, repeated challenges on clinical research unit.
Kremer et al. 1987 (cited in ref. 32)	EPA modestly improved subjective symptoms of RA.	Double-blind, controlled, prospective.
Moore et al. 1987 (cited in ref. 32)	EPA did not benefit SLE.	Randomized, controlled.
Sperling et al. 1987 (cited in ref. 32)	EPA modestly improved some symptoms of RA.	Double-blind, controlled.
Tanner et al. 1987 (cited in ref. 32)	28% of RA patients noted association of food with clinical status: 11% unfavorable, 6% favorable, 10% both.	Prospective survey.
Belch et al. 1988 (cited in ref. 32)	Fish oil (EPA) reduced NSAID requirement in RA.	Controlled.
Beri et al. 1988 (cited in ref. 32)	Diet restrictions ameliorated RA.	Incompletely described.
Cleland et al. 1988 (cited in ref. 32)	Modest subjective, symptomatic benefit from fish oil for RA.	Double-blind, non-crossover study.
Hafstrom et al. 1988 (cited in ref. 32)	Antirheumatic effects of fasting, possibly mediated by neutrophils.	Prospective crossover study.
Malone and Metcalfe 1988 (86)	IgE-dependent, mast cell-mediated "arthritis" in rats.	Experimental model.
Kremer et al. 1990 (cited in ref. 32)	Fish oil (EPA) improved RA tenderness and swelling in dose-dependent fashion.	Prospective, randomized, controlled.
Panush 1990 (34)	Foods definitely but infrequently induced palindromic, RF(−) inflammatory arthritis.	Prospective, double-blind, controlled, repeated challenges on clinical research unit.
van der Tempel 1990 (cited in ref. 32)	Fish oil was modestly beneficial for RA.	Randomized, double-blind, placebo-controlled crossover.
Westberg and Tarkowski 1990 (cited in ref. 32)	Max EPA was not beneficial for SLE.	Randomized, double-blind, placebo-controlled, 9-month crossover trial.
Clark et al. 1990 (cited in ref. 32)	Max EPA therapy led to biochemical but not clinical change in lupus nephritis.	Open, unblinded, uncontrolled.
Lassus et al. 1990 (cited in ref. 32)	EPA/DHA provided subjective benefit for psoriatic arthritis.	Uncontrolled, unblinded.
Perez-Mareda et al. 1991 (cited in ref. 32)	Antibodies to milk proteins in RA cross-react with epitodes on Type I collagen, C1q, and vitamin D.	Intriguing.
Kjeldsen-Kragh et al. 1991 (60)	Notable benefit for RA patients from individually adjusted diet modifications.	Important methodological limitations.
Walton et al. 1991 (cited in ref. 32)	Max EPA was beneficial in SLE.	Prospective, double-blind, crossover.
Fahrer et al. 1991 (cited in ref. 32)	Fish (4–6 times weekly) produced lipid changes similar to fish oil.	Normal volunteers.
Panush 1991 (12)	A comprehensive review of nutrition and rheumatic disease.	21 contributions.
Kjeldsen-Kragh et al. 1992 (cited in ref. 32)	Mild benefit of EPA/DHA for RA.	Randomized, controlled comparison with naproxen.
Lunardi et al. 1992 (100)	4 of 5 patients with hypersensitivity vasculitis and personal or family history of allergy remitted and 1 of 5 benefited from elimination diets.	3-week elimination diets followed by open and double-blind food challenges.
Karjalainer et al. 1992 (cited in ref. 32)	Patients with insulin-dependent diabetes mellitus have antibodies cross-reacting with bovine albumin a beta cell surface protein.	Intriguing.
Stammers et al. 1992 (cited in ref. 32)	Cod liver oil was ineffective for OA.	Double-blind, placebo-controlled.
Epstein et al. 1992 (cited in ref. 32)	Urticarial vasculitis resolved in association with elimination diet.	Single patient, uncontrolled.

Table 37.1
(Continued)

Reference	Observations	Comments
Shigemasa *et al.* 1992 (cited in ref. 32)	SLE improved in association with vegetarian diet.	Single patient, uncontrolled.
Skoldstam *et al.* 1992 (cited in ref. 32)	Modest benefit of fish oil for RA.	Randomized, controlled, blinded.
Panush 1993 (25)	Questionable arthritis remedies	Review.
Leventhal *et al.* 1993 (cited in ref. 32)	Modest benefit from plant-seed–derived gammalinolenic acid for RA.	Randomized, double-blinded, placebo-controlled, 24-week trial.
Rossi and Costa 1993 (cited in ref. 32)	Fish oil prevented miscarriages in women with spontaneous abortions and antiphospholipid antibodies.	Uncontrolled, unblinded.
Lau *et al.* 1993 (cited in ref. 32)	Fish oil reduced NSAID requirement in RA.	Randomized, single-blind, placebo-controlled.
Wuthrich 1993 (99)	A case of bisulfite-induced urticarial vasculitis and a case of anaphylactoid purpura caused by tartrazine and benzoate.	Confirmed by placebo-controlled oral provocation.
Geusens *et al.* 1994 (cited in ref. 32)	Significant clinical benefit of fish oil for RA.	Randomized, double-blind, controlled, 12-month trial.
Appelboom and Durez 1994 (76)	Many spondyloarthropathy patients responded to milk elimination.	Incompletely controlled.
Haugen *et al.* 1994 (cited in ref. 32)	Some RA patients may respond to elimination of foods.	Small study (17 patients), small differences in groups.
Leventhal *et al.* 1994 (cited in ref. 32)	Black walnut seed oil suppressed disease activity in RA.	Randomized, double-blind, placebo-controlled, 24-week trial.

RA, rheumatoid arthritis; OA, osteoarthritis; SLE, systemic lupus erythematosus; NSAID, nonsteroidal anti-inflammatory drug.

were not carefully conducted. In addition, different types of arthritis were considered as a single entity, making conclusions about a specific disease difficult.

In 1941, Hench and associates concluded that food allergy occasionally caused "atrophic arthritis" (rheumatoid arthritis) (16, 17). In describing palindromic rheumatism, allergy was suggested to constitute an etiologic factor in certain cases (20). Several allergists wrote about the relationship of allergy and "rheumatism." Zeller related four case reports to support his thesis that ingested foods exacerbated rheumatoid arthritis and that dietary exclusions improved its course (21). Some patients failed to improve on exclusion diets, however. Zussman also presented patients whose histories suggested an exacerbation of their musculoskeletal problems following ingestion of certain foods (22). Twenty percent of 1000 consecutive adults with allergic complaints (e.g., asthma, hayfever, or urticaria) had rheumatic complaints. Most of these patients experienced allergic symptoms attributed to food, although 27 (of the original 1000) had rheumatic symptoms exacerbated by ingestion of specific foods. Rowe reviewed literature from 1917 to 1972 and concluded that "Food allergy as a cause of arthritis pain or arthralgia and swelling occurs not infrequently," citing literature and personal cases to support his conclusion (23).

Thus, both physicians and patients have long been intrigued by the possibility that some foods might provoke arthritis and others ameliorate it. If this hypothesis is true, then arthritis would be expected to respond to appropriate nutritional therapy (12, 24–32). Diet therapy for rheumatic disease has been generally considered quackery; indeed, more than 90% of arthritis patients annually spend billions of dollars on this and related questionable therapies (12, 25, 26). Despite the skepticism of rheumatologists and the fervor of its advocates, little objective information existed about nutritional therapy for rheumatic diseases until recently. This lack of knowledge is considered an important contemporary issue, and such therapy has been identified among major future clinical advances anticipated in rheumatology (33). Most conclusions have been based on improper study design or inadequate data, however (10–12, 24–32).

Possible Relationships Between Nutrition and Rheumatic Diseases

A relationship between nutrition and rheumatic diseases could occur through two possible mechanisms that are not mutually exclusive. First, nutritional factors might alter immune and inflammatory responses, thereby modifying manifestations of rheumatic diseases. Second, food-related antigens might provoke hypersensitivity responses—food allergies—leading to rheumatologic symptoms (10–12, 24–32).

This brief and necessarily selective review considers the evidence for the latter possibility—that certain patients with rheumatic diseases may experience food-sensitive symptoms. The published data are largely, but not exclusively, anecdotal, and several of the anecdotes (which may be a valid basis for generating scientific hypotheses) appear persuasive. Several reasons exist to give serious consideration to the hypothesis that food allergy might relate to rheumatic diseases:

1. Foods may evoke immune responses.
2. Foods may cause immunologically mediated symptoms.
3. Immunologic mechanisms of tissue injury play important roles in the pathogenesis of rheumatic diseases.
4. The antigens that might trigger abnormal immune events in rheumatic disease remain unknown.
5. Rheumatic diseases have been associated with foods in anecdotal reports (34).

The etiology of rheumatoid arthritis and most forms of inflammatory joint disease remains unknown. Much speculation has arisen about the putative role of microbial and other environmental agents in the pathogenesis of these disorders. It seems no less reasonable to consider food or related antigens as candidates for initiation of immunologically mediated inflammation in certain patients. Studies in this area may potentially identify antigens capable of inducing or perpetuating inflammatory arthritis and elucidate pathogenetic pathways for such patients. This information may, in turn, influence the study of patients with rheumatic diseases.

Food sensitivity as a cause of rheumatic disease has been controversial, in large part because of unsubstantiated claims in the lay press based on little or no solid data. Nutritional therapy for disease also has inspired controversy. Inappropriate advocacy of this notion prejudiced its consideration as a potentially useful approach for selected situations. Firm evidence now exists to prove nutritional modulation of experimental autoimmunity. Thus, food sensitivity in rheumatic disease constitutes an important issue in contemporary clinical immunology.

FOOD ALLERGY, RHEUMATIC DISEASE, AND THE GASTROINTESTINAL TRACT

If hypersensitivity to foods actually causes arthritis, then food antigens would have to cross the gastrointestinal barrier and circulate in antigenic form until they were recognized by effector or intermediary cells in the immune system. Experimental data indicate that food antigens can, indeed, cross this barrier and subsequently circulate as both food antigens and immune complexes (35–38).

In immunologically compromised individuals, intrinsic abnormalities of the gastrointestinal mucosa may permit the transport of larger quantities or different types of antigenic material. Selective IgA deficiency has been associated with both gastrointestinal disorders and immunologic disease. Increased titers of antibodies to cow's milk were found in IgA-deficient subjects and correlated with the presence of circulating immune complexes (39) and with serologically defined autoimmune disease (35). Patients with hypogammaglobulinemia demonstrated both increased absorption of bovine milk antigens and prolonged persistence of these antigens in the circulation (40).

Some studies have suggested that patients with rheumatic disease experience abnormal digestive and absorptive function. Abnormal fecal fat excretion and vitamin A and D-xylose absorption have been demonstrated in such individuals (41, 42). Furthermore, some investigations have noted that the gastrointestinal tracts of patients with rheumatoid arthritis may be more easily penetrated by food antigens than the tracts of normal individuals, although this finding has been inconsistent (43, 44). The abnormal intestinal permeability may also be due to effects produced by nonsteroidal anti-inflammatory drugs (45). Antigens of the intraluminal contents (other than food antigens) have been seen to stimulate lymphocyte transformation and production of leukocyte inhibitory factor in patients with spondyloarthropathies (46). Patients with jejunoileal bypass for obesity have developed an arthritis indistinguishable from rheumatoid. These patients also displayed immunologic abnormalities, including circulating immune complexes, of which the antigen was intraluminal (47).

FASTING, ELEMENTAL NUTRITION, AND DIETS

Fasting appeared to ameliorate disease in some patients with rheumatic disease (Tables 37.1 and 37.2) (48–50). Five of 15 patients with classic rheumatoid arthritis who fasted for 7 to 10 days benefited, while only 1 of 10 control subjects showed an improvement. Fasting patients experienced lessened pain, stiffness, and medication requirements, and demonstrated decreased Ritchie index score and finger size. Continuation of a lactovegetarian diet did not show a consistent benefit (48).

Another controlled study on the effects of fasting on patients with rheumatoid arthritis involved 14 patients who fasted for seven days; they were then crossed over to a control regimen. The majority experienced clinical improvement during fasting, while their condition remained unchanged or worsened during the control period. Improvement during the fasting period was accompanied by decreased erythrocyte sedimentation rate, Ritchie and Lansbury indices, morning stiffness, and joint counts. Serum cortisol levels did not change (50).

A prospective study investigated the effects of a complete fast on patients with rheumatoid arthritis. The investigation was carried out in a specialized, "environmentally controlled" unit. Forty-three patients underwent a water fast that lasted seven days. Tenderness, swelling, grip strength, dolorimeter scores, joint circumference, functional activity, and erythrocyte sedimentation rate improved significantly during the fast. It was suggested that short-term fasting may induce rapid clinical improvement in rheumatoid arthritis (51).

Our own studies also found that short-term fasts proved antirheumatic for some patients with rheumatoid arthritis (28, 29). Improvement might have been caused by reduced gastrointestinal permeability, decreased neutrophil function, depressed lymphocyte response to mitogens, or increased cortisol concentrations during fasting (52–55).

In other studies, we examined a specific prescription "arthritis" diet (no red meat, fruits, dairy products, herbs, spices, preservatives, additives, or alcohol). Outpatients who had long-standing, progressive, active rheumatoid arthritis fared no better than comparable patients receiving a placebo diet. Some patients did improve on the experimental diet, however, and experienced recurrence of symptoms when they deviated from this regimen (28).

Limited information is available about other specific diets for arthritis. Various types of elimination, vegetarian, or other diets have been utilized in some other studies—usually not entirely controlled—with some possible benefit (81–87). Elemental nutrition also provided benefits in some experiences (12, 29, 34, 57, 58, 60, 62) (Tables 37.1 and 37.2).

FOOD ALLERGY AND PALINDROMIC RHEUMATISM, SYSTEMIC LUPUS ERYTHEMATOSUS, AND OTHER SYSTEMIC RHEUMATIC DISEASES

Several clinical observations suggest relationships between food intake and systemic rheumatic disease (16, 17, 20–22, 63–69) (Table 37.1). Reports include

Table 37.2
Diets, Fasting, Elemental Nutrition, Vitamins, Minerals, and Foods and Rheumatic Diseases. Reproduced with permission from the publisher from Panush RS. Foods, diets, nutrition, and other questionable remedies for arthritis. In: Koopman WJ, ed. Arthritis and allied conditions, 13th ed.

- Fasting had short-term antirheumatic effects.
- Elemental nutrition was inconsistently antirheumatic.
- Specific diets have not proved consistently beneficial for patients with rheumatic diseases.
- Vitamins, minerals, or nutritional supplements have not proved consistently antirheumatic.
- Rare patients with rheumatic disease have had clinical symptoms convincingly documented to be associated with food or food-product sensitivity.

that of a dermatologist who documented his own palindromic rheumatism as being due to sodium nitrate hypersensitivity (70). Black walnut ingestion was linked to clinical exacerbations of Behçet's syndrome and to abnormal cellular hypersensitivity responses (71). Ingestion of alfalfa seed and sprout has been associated with systemic lupus erythematosus in both humans and monkeys (72, 73). The disease induced in primates was characterized by an autoimmune hemolytic anemia with low complement levels, positive antinuclear antibodies, anti-DNA, positive lupus erythematosus cell preparations, and deposition of immunoglobulin and complement in the skin. Induction of the disease was attributed to L-canavanine, a nonprotein amino acid component of alfalfa. Antibody to the alfalfa seed cross-reacted with DNA and may have activated B lymphocytes (74). Systemic lupus erythematosus in a young woman was linked to environmental exposure to hydrazine (75). Milk elimination might have proved beneficial to patients with spondyloarthropathy (76) (Tables 37.1 and 37.2).

FOOD ALLERGY AND INFLAMMATORY ARTHRITIS

Parke and Hughes reported a challenge test in a patient who had suffered from progressive rheumatoid arthritis for 11 years (77) (Table 37.1). She showed a poor response to NSAIDs and daily prednisolone, and could not tolerate penicillamine, gold, or azathioprine. The patient gave a history of eating cheese daily for the previous 18 years. A milk-free diet brought improvement within three weeks. Hospital-based challenge with dairy products produced marked exacerbation of her arthritis as measured by increased pain, Ritchie index score, morning stiffness, swelling, and decreased grip strength. Stroud reported a largely uncontrolled study that found an antirheumatic effect attributable to fasting; in addition, chemical or food challenges—particularly wheat, corn, and beef—caused deterioration of grip strength and dolorimeter and arthrocircameter scores in patients with rheumatoid arthritis (51).

A preliminary report of a prospective study of patients with definite or classic rheumatoid arthritis indicated that withdrawal of allergenic substances (as identified by an elimination diet) brought responses varying from "complete success with total abolition of all rheumatic symptoms to deterioration" (78). A double-blind provocation study, also reported on a preliminary basis, found that challenges "with food extracts and other incitants including alternaria, house dust, tobacco smoke and petrochemicals induced 'rheumatic' joint and muscle reactions, indistinguishable from presenting complaints . . . in . . . (87.5% of 40) . . . subjects" (79).

Other reports related food sensitivity in at least five patients with rheumatoid arthritis, including one in whom double-blind challenge studies implicated tartrazine as the culprit. Many of these patients had circulating immune complexes containing IgE and IgG anti-IgE; these complexes were speculated to be related to the pathogenesis of symptoms (80). Hill (81) and Brostoff and coworkers (82) have reported on patients with juvenile and adult rheumatoid-like arthritis with food sensitivities, respectively. Ratner and coworkers have suggested that lactose-intolerant individuals may be susceptible to milk-induced arthritis (83). Darlington and colleagues extended their earlier observations (78), reporting that some patients with rheumatoid arthritis benefited from food elimination and experienced symptomatic deterioration following reintroduction of offending foods (84). These studies were not rigorously controlled, however, and thus have not definitely proved that foods can exacerbate inflammatory joint disease (12, 24–26, 32).

Our own initial studies of effects of food on arthritis naively used a prescription diet (no red meat, fruit, dairy products, herbs, spices, preservatives, additives, or alcohol) and found that outpatients with long-standing, progressive, active rheumatoid arthritis fared no better than when receiving placebo diet (28). Some patients did improve on the experimental diet, however, and later experienced a recurrence of symptoms when deviating from it. A prospective, blinded, controlled trial in a clinical research center was then initiated to determine whether joint symptoms were associated with food sensitivities in selected patients. The first patient, who had rheumatoid arthritis, had previously noted an exacerbation of symptoms associated with dairy products and other foods. She exhibited marked, consistent improvement, as measured on both subjective and objective bases, during fasting, which was sustained with elemental nutrition. Four different, blinded challenges with milk reproducibly exacerbated symptoms, whereas placebo and other foods had no effect. Symptoms peaked 24 to 48 hours after challenge and resolved over a period of 1 to 3 days. Immunologic studies suggested both delayed and immediate cutaneous reactivity to milk, no elevation in anti-milk IgE, marked increases of anti-milk IgG and IgG4 levels, marginally increased IgG-milk circulating immune complexes, and in vitro cellular sensitivity to milk. Symptomatic exacerbation of arthritis and immunologic hypersensitivity to milk coexisted in this patient (29).

In further studies, 30% of our patients with rheumatoid arthritis alleged food-related ("allergic") arthritis. Sixteen patients completed 19 double-blind, placebo-controlled food challenge studies, and three demonstrated subjective and objective rheumatologic symptoms following double-blind, encapsulated food challenges; these subjects were virtually asymptomatic when placed on an elemental nutrition diet (30, 34). These seronegative patients exhibited palindromic symptoms and nonerosive disease. Fasting or elemental nutrition also benefited several of these patients (30, 34). Most patients alleging food-induced rheumatic symptoms did not show such reactions on blinded challenge, although some did. We tentatively concluded that immunologic sensitivity to food was an uncommon cause of symptom among rheumatic disease patients. Such patients have been identified only in controlled challenge studies. These observations suggest a possible role for food allergy in at least some patients with rheumatic disease. In related work, our group and other investigators have noted that the substitution of cow's milk for water led to inflammatory synovitis in certain rabbit strains (10, 31, 85). One study demonstrated that synovial membrane mast cells can be activated by IgE- and non–IgE-mediated stimuli (86). Golding (87) reported three patients who had recurrent joint pain—sometimes associated with swelling—that was precipitated by milk in two subjects and by cheese and egg in one individual. Milk challenge in one subject caused knee

swelling within a few hours; 30 mL of fluid was aspirated and indicated synovitis.

FOOD ALLERGY AND VASCULITIS

Allergic vasculitis constitutes a relatively small group of vasculitic syndromes. It affects the small blood vessels, mostly of the skin, to a lesser extent the mucous membranes, and occasionally the joints or other organs. The skin lesions, which usually take the form of palpable purpura, can be large. In some patients, the condition may mimic urticaria or erythema multiforme. Food hypersensitivity has been implicated as causing vasculitis in certain patients (mostly adults). The relationship was not widely accepted, probably because of its rarity and because of the anecdotal nature of most of the reports.

In 1914 Osler became the first to suggest a role for protein sensitivity in certain patients with purpura (88). In 1929, six cases of Henoch-Schonlein purpura were reported in which avoidance of certain foods resulted in improvement and reintroduction of those foods caused a recurrence of symptoms (89). In 1951, a patient was reported with recurrent purpura following ingestion of crab meat; his platelet count was normal and his serum transferred passive hypersensitivity (Prausnitz-Küstner reaction) to crab (90). In 1953, Ackroyd reported 23 patients with allergic purpura related to specific foods, most commonly egg, milk, chocolate, wheat, and beans (91). A few other patients were noted as having purpura related to fish (92, 93). Other authors also recognized that food hypersensitivity might cause vasculitis (94, 95). In a few patients, azo dyes—particularly tartrazine—were implicated (96–99). Lunardi *et al.* (100) described five patients who had allergy and vasculitis for 1 to 13 years in whom the offending agent was confirmed by double-blind challenge to the food (two patients), food additive (two patients), and both (one patient). While subjects followed an elimination diet, none experienced a recurrence of vasculitis during the two-year follow-up.

From the limited information available in the literature and from our own experience, it appears that vasculitis, if caused by food allergy, is rare, albeit perhaps underdiagnosed. The underlying immunologic mechanism may be predominantly a type III (immune complex or Arthus-type) reaction. In some cases, a type I (IgE-mediated) reaction may be involved as well, causing increased vascular permeability and enhanced deposition of immune complexes. Histologic examination of a biopsy specimen taken from the edge of a lesion will verify the presence of vessel wall necrosis, extravasation of red cells, perivascular polymorphonuclear cellular infiltrate, fibrin deposits, and often nuclear debris—hence leading to the name leukocytoclastic vasculitis (101, 102). Immunofluorescence studies may demonstrate immune complex deposits in vessel walls along the basement membrane. The nature of the antigen and antibody involved can sometimes be determined.

Studies are certainly needed to verify that food-induced vasculitis is possible, to delineate its pathogenesis, and to develop simple tests for its diagnosis.

Acknowledgments

The authors appreciate the excellent secretarial assistance of Nancy Rodriguez in the preparation of this chapter. Tables 37.1 and 37.2 were reproduced from reference 32 with permission.

REFERENCES

1. Bahna SL, Heiner DC. Allergies to milk. New York: Grune and Stratton, 1980.
2. Anderson JA, Sogn DD, eds. Adverse reactions to foods. American Academy of Allergy and Immunology Committee on Adverse Reactions to Foods, and National Institute of Allergy and Infectious Diseases. NIH publication 84-2442. Bethesda, MD: National Institutes of Health, 1984.
3. Brostoff J, ed. Food allergy. Clin Immunol Allergy 1982;2:1–260.
4. Panush RS, Webster EM. Food allergies and other adverse reactions to foods. Med Clin North Am 1985;69:533–546.
5. Metcalfe DD. Food hypersensitivity. J Allergy Clin Immunol 1984;73:749–766.
6. Metcalfe DD, Goldblatt MJ, Simopoulos AP, eds. Adverse reactions to foods and food additives. J Allergy Clin Immunol 1986;78:125–252.
7. Sampson HA, McCaskill CM. Food hypersensitivity and atopic dermatitis: evaluation of 113 patients. J Pediatr 1985;107:669–680.
8. Bahna SL. Pathogenesis of milk hypersensitivity. Immunol Today 1985;6:153–154.
9. Bahna SL. The dilemma of pathogenesis and diagnosis of food allergy. Immunol Allergy Clin North Am 1987;7:299–312.
10. Panush RS. Possible role of food sensitivity in arthritis. Ann Allergy 1988;61:31–35.
11. Panush RS. Delayed reactions to foods. Food allergy and rheumatic diseases. Ann Allergy 1986;56:500–503.
12. Panush RS, ed. Nutrition and rheumatic diseases. Rheum Dis Clinics 1991;17:xii–xiv, 197–456.
13. Weatherbee M. Chronic arthritis. The clinical analysis of three hundred and fifty cases. AMA Arch Intern Med 1932;50:926–994.
14. Minot GR. General aspects of the treatment of chronic arthritis. N Engl J Med 1933;208:1285–1290.
15. Bauer W. What should a patient with arthritis eat? JAMA 1935;104:1–6.
16. Hench BS, Bauer W, Dawson MH, et al. The problem of rheumatism and arthritis. Review of American and English literature (6th rheumatism review). Ann Intern Med 1940;13:1838–1990.
17. Hench BS, Bauer W, Boland E, et al. Rheumatism and arthritis. Review of the American and English literature, for 1940 (8th rheumatism review). Ann Intern Med 1941;15:1002–1008.
18. Rosenberg EF. Diet and vitamins in rheumatoid arthritis. In: Hollander JL, ed. Comroe's arthritis and allied conditions, 5th ed. Philadelphia: Lea and Febiger, 1954, 542–546.
19. Arthritis Foundation. Arthritis, the basic facts. Atlanta: Arthritis Foundation, 1981.
20. Hench PS, Rosenberg EF. Palindromic rheumatism. Proc Staff Meet Mayo Clin 1941;16:808–815.
21. Zeller M. Rheumatoid arthritis—food allergy as a factor. Ann Allergy 1949;7:200–239.
22. Zussman BM. Food hypersensitivity simulating rheumatoid arthritis. South Med J 1966;59:935–939.
23. Rowe AH. Food allergy and arthropathies. In: Food allergy: its manifestations and control. Springfield, IL: Charles C. Thomas, 1972, 435–443.
24. Panush RS. Nutrition and rheumatic diseases. Postgrad Adv Rheumatol 1985;1:1–16.
25. Panush RS. Is there a role for diet or other questionable therapies in managing rheumatic diseases? Bull Rheum Dis 1993;42:1–4.
26. Panush RS. Non-traditional remedies. In: Schumacher HR, ed. Primer on the Rheumatic Diseases, 10th ed. Atlanta: Arthritis Foundation, 1993, 323–327.
27. Corman LC, Panush RS. Nutrition and arthritis: a perspective. Rheumatol News 1985;6:3.
28. Panush RS, Carter RL, Katz P, Kowsari B, Longley S, Finnie S. Diet therapy for rheumatoid arthritis. Arthritis Rheum 1983;26:462–471.
29. Panush RS, Stroud RM, Webster E. Food-induced (allergic) arthritis. Inflammatory arthritis exacerbated by milk. Arthritis Rheum 1986;29:220–226.
30. Panush RS, Corman L, Webster E, et al. Food-induced ("allergic") arthritis. Clinical and serological studies. Arthritis Rheum 1986;29(suppl):S33 (abstract).
31. Panush RS, Webster E, Endo L, Searle M, Hammack S, Woodard JC. Food-induced ("allergic") arthritis. A unique new model of inflammatory synovitis in rabbits. Arthritis Rheum 1986;29(suppl):S33 (abstract).
32. Panush RS. Arthritis, food allergy, diets, and nutrition. In: Koopman WJ, ed. Arthritis and allied conditions—a textbook of rheumatology, 13th ed. Baltimore, MD: Williams & Wilkins, in press.

33. Klinenberg JR. ARA presidential address: 1984–2034: the next half-century for American rheumatology. Arthritis Rheum 1985;28:1–7.

34. Panush RS. Food-induced ("allergic") arthritis: clinical and serological studies. J Rheumatol 1990;17:291–294.

35. Walker WA, Isselbacher KJ. Uptake and transport of macro-molecules by the intestine. Possible role in clinical disorders. Gastroenterology 1974;67:531–550.

36. Paganelli R, Levinsky RJ, Brostoff J, Wraith DG. Immune complexes containing food proteins in normal and atopic subjects after oral challenges and effect of sodium cromoglycate on antigen absorption. Lancet 1979;1:1270–1272.

37. Cunningham-Rundles C, Brandeis WE, Pudifin DJ, Day NK. Auto-immunity in selective IgA deficiency: relationship to anti-bovine protein antibodies circulating immune complexes and clinical disease. Clin Exp Immunol 1981;45:299–304.

38. Paganelli R, Levinsky RJ, Atherton DJ. Detection of specific antigen within circulating immune complexes: validation of the assay and its application to food antigen–antibody complexes formed in healthy and food-allergic subjects. Clin Exp Immunol 1981;46:44–53.

39. Cunningham-Rundles C, Brandeis WE, Good RA, Day NK. Bovine antigens and the formation of circulating immune complexes in selective immunoglobulin deficiency. J Clin Invest 1979;64:272–279.

40. Cunningham-Rundles C, Carr RI, Good RA. Dietary protein antigenemia in humoral immunodeficiency. Correlation with splenomegaly. Am J Med 1984;76:181–185.

41. Siurala M, Julkuven H, Torvoneu S, Selkveu R, Saxen F, Pathaven F. Digestive tract in collagen disease. Acta Med Scand 1965;173:13.

42. Peterson R, Wegelius U, Skrifrans B. Gastrointestinal disturbances in patients with severe rheumatoid arthritis. Acta Med Scand 1970;188:139.

43. Rooney PJ, Jenkins RT, Goodacre RL, Sivakumaran T. Gut permeability of small molecules in rheumatoid disease. Clin Res 1983;31:106A (abstract).

44. Sundqvist T, Lindstrom F, Magnusson KE, Skoldstom L, Stjernstom I, Tagesson C. Influence of fasting on intestinal permeability and disease. Scand J Rheumatol 1982;11:33–38.

45. Bjarnason I, Williams P, So A, et al. Intestinal permeability and inflammation in rheumatoid arthritis: effects of nonsteroidal anti-inflammatory drugs. Lancet 1984;2:1171–1173.

46. Gross WL, Ludemann G, Ullman U, Schmidt KL. Klebsiella induced LIF response in Klebsiella infection and ankylosing spondylitis. Br J Rheumatol 1983;22(suppl):50–52.

47. Wands JR, Lamont JT, Mann E, Isselbacher KJ. Arthritis associated with intestinal bypass procedure for marked obesity: complement activation and characterization of circulating cryoproteins. N Engl J Med 1976;294:121–124.

48. Skoldstam L, Larsson L, Lindstrom FD. Effects of fasting and lactovegetarian diet on rheumatoid arthritis. Scand J Rheumatol 1979;8:249–255 (abstract).

49. Gershwin ME, Beach RS, Hurley LS. Nutrition and immunity. New York: Academic Press, 1985.

50. Uden AM, Trang L, Venizelos N, Palmbad J. Neutrophil functions and clinical performance after total fasting in patients with rheumatoid arthritis. Ann Rheum Dis 1983;42:45–51.

51. Stroud RM. The effect of fasting followed by specific food challenge on rheumatoid arthritis. In: Hahn BH, Arnett FC, Zizic TM, Hochberg MC. Current Topics in Rheumatology. Kalamazoo: Upjohn, 1983, 145–157.

52. Hafstrom I, Ringertz B, Gyllenhammar H, et al. Effects of fasting on disease activity, neutrophil function, fatty acid composition, and leukotriene biosynthesis in patients with rheumatoid arthritis. Arthritis Rheum 1988;31:585–591.

53. Palmblad J, Halfstrom I, Ringertz B. Antirheumatic effects of fasting. Rheum Dis Clin 1991;17:351–362.

54. Skoldstam L, Magnusson KE. Fasting, intestinal permeability, and rheumatoid arthritis. Rheum Dis Clin 1991;17:363–372.

55. Panush RS, Su M. Antirheumatic effects of fasting. Internal Medicine for the Specialist 1991;12:57–59.

56. Darlington LG, Mansfield JR. Food allergy and rheumatoid disease. Ann Rheum Dis 1983;42:319 (abstract).

57. Darlington LG, Ramsey NE, Mansfield JR. Placebo-controlled, blind study of dietary manipulation in rheumatoid arthritis. Lancet 1986;1:236–276.

58. Darlington LG. Dietary therapy for arthritis. Rheum Dis Clin 1991;17:273–286.

59. Henderson CJ, Lovell DJ. Nutritional aspects of juvenile rheumatoid arthritis. Rheum Dis Clin 1991;17:403–414.

60. Kjeldsen-Kragh J, Haugen M, Brochgrevink CF, Laerom E, Eck M, Mowinkel P, Hori K, Forre O. Controlled trial of fasting and one-year vegetarian diet in rheumatoid arthritis. Lancet 1991;338:899–902.

61. Van de Laar MAFJ, van der Korst JK. Food intolerance in rheumatoid arthritis. I. A double blind, controlled trial of the clinical effects of elimination of milk allergens and azo dyes. Ann Rheum Dis 1992;51:298–302.

62. Haugen MA, Kjeldsen-Kragh J, Forre O. A pilot study of the effect of an elemental diet in the management of rheumatoid arthritis. Clin Exp Rheum 1994;12:275–279.

63. Pottenger RT. Constitutional factors in arthritis with special reference to incidence and role of allergic disease. Ann Intern Med 1928;12:323–333.

64. Kaufman W. Food induced allergic musculoskeletal syndromes. Ann Allergy 1953;11:179–184.

65. Millman M. An allergic concept of the etiology of rheumatoid arthritis. Ann Allergy 1972;30:135–141.

66. Lewin P, Taub SJ. Allergic synovitis due to ingestion of English walnuts. JAMA 1936;106:2144.

67. Berger H. Intermittent hydroarthrosis with an allergic basis. JAMA 1939;112:2402–2405.

68. Vaughn WT. Palindromic rheumatism among allergic persons. J Allergy 1943;14:256–263.

69. Randolph TG. Ecologically oriented rheumatoid arthritis. In: Dickey LD, ed. Clinical ecology. Springfield, IL: Charles C. Thomas, 1976, 201–212.

70. Epstein S. Hypersensitivity to sodium nitrate: a major causative factor in cases of palindromic rheumatism. Ann Allergy 1969;27:343–349.

71. Marguardt JL, Snyderman R, Oppenheim JJ. Depression of lymphocyte transformation and exacerbation of Behçet's syndrome by ingestion of English walnuts. Cell Immunol 1973;9:263–272.

72. Malinow MR, Bardana EJ, Pirofsky B, Craig S, McLoughlin P. Systemic lupus erythematosus-like syndrome in monkeys fed alfalfa sprouts: role of a nonprotein amino acid. Science 1982;216:415–417.

73. Roberts JL, Hayashi JA. Exacerbation of SLE associated with alfalfa ingestion (letter). N Engl J Med 1983;308:1361.

74. Bardana EJ, Malinow MK, Craig S, McLoughlin P. Cross-reacting antibody to alfalfa seed and deoxyribonucleic acid

in systemic lupus erythematosus. J Allergy Clin Immunol 1983;71:102 (abstract).

75. Reidenberg MM, Durant PJ, Harris RA, Boccardo GP, Lahita R, Stenzel RH. Systemic lupus erythematosus-like disease due to hydrazine. Am J Med 1983;75:365–370.

76. Appelboom T, Durez P. Effect of milk product deprivation on spondyloarthropathy. Ann Rheum Dis 1994;53:481–482.

77. Parke AL, Hughes GRV. Rheumatoid arthritis and food: a case study. Br Med J 1981;282:2027–2029.

78. Darlington LE, Mansfield JR. Food allergy and rheumatoid disease. Ann Rheum Dis 1983;42:219 (abstract).

79. Mandell M, Conte A. The role of allergy in arthritis, rheumatism, and associated polysymptomatic cerebro-viscerosomatic disorders: a double blind provocation test study. Ann Allergy 1980;44:51 (abstract).

80. Wraith DG. Allergic joint symptoms. Presented at the 4th International Food Allergy Symposium of the American College of Allergy, Vancouver, Canada, July 25–29, 1982.

81. Hill DJ. Food antigens as a cause of chronic arthritis in children. Presented at the 5th International Food Allergy Symposium, Atlanta, October 1984.

82. Brostoff J, Scadding G, Monroe J. Immune complexes and platelet aggregation in food-induced disease. Presented at the 5th International Food Allergy Symposium, Atlanta, October 1984.

83. Ratner P, Schneeyour A, Eshel E, Teitler A. Does milk intolerance affect seronegative arthritis in lactose-deficient women? Isr J Med Sci 1985;21:532–534.

84. Darlington LG, Ramsey NW, Mansfield JR. Placebo-controlled, blind study of dietary manipulation therapy in rheumatoid arthritis. Lancet 1986;1:236–238.

85. Panush RS, Webster EM, Endo LP, Greer JM, Woodard JC. Food-induced ("allergic") arthritis: inflammatory synovitis in rabbits. J Rheumatol 1990;17:285–290.

86. Malone DG, Metcalfe DD. Mast cells and arthritis. Ann Allergy 1988;61:27–30.

87. Golding DN. Is there an allergic synovitis? J Royal Soc Med 1990;83:312–314.

88. Osler W. The visceral lesions of purpura and allied conditions. Br Med J 1914;1:517–525.

89. Alexander HL, Eyermann CH. Allergic purpura. JAMA 1929;92:2092–2094.

90. Ancona GR, Ellenhorn MJ, Falconer EH. Purpura due to food sensitivity: use of skin testing in etiological diagnosis. J Allergy 1951;22:487–493.

91. Ackroyd JF. Allergic purpura including purpura due to foods, drugs, and infections. Am J Med 1953;14:605–632.

92. Jensen B. Schonlein-Henoch's purpura. Acta Med Scand 1955;152:61–70.

93. Robinson BWS. Henoch-Schonlein purpura due to food sensitivity. Br Med J 1977;1:510–511.

94. Harkavy J. Vascular allergy and its systemic manifestations. Washington, DC: Butterworths, 1963.

95. Theorell H, Blomback M, Kockum C. Demonstration of reactivity to airborne and food allergens in cutaneous vasculitis by variations in fibronopeptide A and other blood coagulation, fibrinolysis and complement parameters. Thromb Haemost 1976;36:593–604.

96. Criep LH. Allergic vascular purpura. J Allergy Clin Immunol 1971;48:7–12.

97. Michaelsson G, Pettersson L, Juhlin L. Purpura caused by food and drug additives. Arch Dermatol 1974;109:49–52.

98. Kubba R, Champion RH. Anaphylactoid purpura caused by tartrazine and benzoates. Br J Dermatol 1975;93(suppl 11):61–62.

99. Wuthrich B. Adverse reactions to food additives. Ann Allergy 1993;71:379–384.

100. Lunardi C, Bambara LM, Biasi D, Zagvi P, Caramaschi P, Pecor ML. Elimination diet in the treatment of selected patients with hypersensitivity vasculitis. Clin Exp Rheumatol 1992;10:131–135.

101. Fauci AS. Vasculitis. J Allergy Clin Immunol 1983;72:211–223.

102. Elkestamm E, Kallen JP. Cutaneous leukocytoclastic vasculitis, clinical and laboratory features of 82 patients seen in private practice. Arch Dermatol 1984;120:484–489.

38

UNPROVED DIAGNOSTIC AND THERAPEUTIC TECHNIQUES

John J. Condemi

*I*t is obvious that the understanding of adverse reactions to foods has benefited from the application of scientific principles to both immunologic and non-immunologic causes. Currently, the accepted method for determining whether a patient is having an adverse reaction to foods involves avoidance of the suspected food. If clinical improvement appears, a double-blind, placebo-controlled food challenge is performed to determine if symptoms can be induced. This labor-intensive manipulation is unlikely to be performed by some physicians and may be feared by some patients. A reliable laboratory test to guide the physician regarding foods that might be reasonable to avoid and for which a double-blind food challenge should be performed would, therefore, be extremely desirable. Skin testing and the radioallergosorbent test (RAST), for example, have been validated to determine the potential for a subject to have an IgE-mediated or immediate reaction to foods (1, 2), but no such tests exist to guide physicians as to the potential for delayed or non–IgE-mediated reactions. These types of reactions present particular concerns for women, who typically act as major purchasers for their families. Two studies indicated that 16.2% to 27.5% of women interviewed felt that someone in their household was allergic to food products (3; Lomar International Corporation, private study). When diet manipulations were performed by this group, 70% acted without the advice of a physician and most of the reactions listed were found to be either delayed or non–IgE-mediated. In my own experience, many patients have read articles in the lay press indicating that a wide variety of reactions may be related to the ingestion of foods. Such individuals may seek physicians who will guide them in de-

termining if a relationship exists between their symptoms and foods (4–6). Some health care practitioners may utilize the unproved and controversial diagnostic and treatment methods described in such literature. These unproved diagnostic tests, if employed, may reinforce food avoidance and contribute to malnutrition and social isolation. As almost every physician will meet patients seeking information on food allergy after having read such literature, it is appropriate to have some understanding of these diagnostic and therapeutic techniques. The following example describes a case in which malnutrition and social isolation occurred.

A 19-year-old female was referred for allergy to intravenous plastic tubing, manifested by abdominal pain. Her illness began four years prior to our evaluation, following an exposure to formaldehyde in a biology class. The symptoms due to formaldehyde exposure were shortness of breath, vision problems, and blacking out. At that time, evaluation by an allergist revealed positive skin test results for inhalants, eggs, and milk. She avoided eggs and milk and experienced improvement, but after one year she developed increasing symptoms, which were believed to be due to bread. As a result, grains were eliminated from her diet.

She was next evaluated for persistent symptoms by another physician, who performed tests that indicated that she was allergic to all foods. He referred her to an out-of-state environmental control center. At that center the patient's nutritional status was so poor that a subclavian line was required for supplemental nutrition. When four lines were replaced over a five-month period of time, she was told that she was allergic to the plastic used in the subclavian line.

When she proved unable to keep a nasogastric tube down, she was told that she was also allergic to the nasogastric tube. She remained at the environmental center for a total of six months, during which time her weight fell from 120 to 69 pounds. She also had not been out of bed for five months.

She returned home with a central line for supplemental feeding and continued to experience the same symptoms, some of which were considered to be due to plastic tubing. Her symptoms at admission consisted of headaches, dizziness, foggy thinking, difficulty in breathing, nausea, palpitations, throat swelling, difficulty in swallowing, photophobia, and repeated dislocations of shoulder, hip, neck, back, knees, and ankle, which were treated by a chiropractor on a weekly basis. The patient was said to be allergic to 31 different medications that had been used for treating her symptoms. The home environment had been modified to remove as many plastics as possible. No hair spray, perfumes, or chemicals were allowed in the house. Heating was provided with electricity. Travel was difficult because of her sensitivity to automobile fumes. The patient also suspected that she would have symptoms when the environment included high-power electric lines. She had porcelain electric heaters at home and utilized membrane-distilled water. Her treatment was that of sublingual drops, which she used prior to eating any foods, and 6 L of oxygen by face mask.

Some of the following diagnostic and therapeutic techniques were utilized to evaluate this patient's symptoms. As almost every physician will encounter patients who have read the lay literature indicating that these unproved techniques may have value, it is appropriate to have some understanding of them to educate patients.

Cytotoxicity Testing (Bryan's Tests)

Leukocytotic testing is based on the belief that the addition of specific allergen in vitro to whole blood or to serum leukocyte suspensions will reduce white blood cells (7) or kill the leukocytes (8–12). It is claimed to be useful for the diagnosis of both food and inhalant allergy. No physiologic basis exists for the test, however, and controlled studies have not demonstrated its effectiveness in the diagnosis of inhalant or food allergy (13–21). Franklin and Lowell studied whole blood obtained from ragweed-sensitive patients and noted no difference in white blood cell counts with either saline or ragweed pollen extract (16). Chambers and associates studied a variety of allergens and noted no difference between leukocytes exposed to allergens to which patients were sensitive and those to which they were not sensitive (17). Liebermann and coworkers, in a controlled study of the cytotoxic effect of specific allergens on white cells, determined that the test did not correlate with IgE-mediated reactions to foods or with reactions such as headache, diarrhea, and fatigue (18). Benson and Arkins noted that positive cytotoxic effects are frequently obtained with foods that produce no clinical symptoms, while negative results are obtained with foods that do produce clinical symptoms (19). This test continues to be utilized by some investigators in the evaluation of patients claiming to have adverse reactions to foods.

Provocative Testing and Neutralization Treatment

Provocative testing and neutralization is a technique for both diagnosis and treatment of allergic disease. The provoking dose is the quantity of allergen or chemical substance sufficient to induce subjective symptoms or objective signs in the subject. A positive response may include the exact symptoms corresponding to the patient's complaints; alternatively, any sign or symptom may be accepted as evidence for allergy to the test substance. Neutralization of symptoms can be accomplished by injecting or placing sublingually a fivefold weaker or stronger dilution of the provoking material. The amount capable of neutralizing the allergic reaction is then utilized to relieve symptoms due to food and chemicals.

SUBLINGUAL TESTING

Sublingual provocative testing and neutralization for food-allergic reactions probably began with Hansel in 1944 (22). In addition to the diagnosis and treatment of food-related symptoms, it has been used to determine inhalant and chemical sensitivity (23, 24). In general, the method currently used for diagnosis consists of placing three drops of an aqueous extract (weight–volume ratio of 1 : 100) under the tongue of the patient and waiting 10 minutes for symptoms to appear. If symptoms occur, a neutralizing dose (usually three drops of a more dilute solution of the same extract) is placed under the tongue. These symptoms are expected to disappear in approximately the same temporal sequence in which they appear. If a patient experiences headache, blurring of vision, and foggy thinking, the headache resolves first, followed by the blurring of vision and then foggy thinking. This neutralizing dose can also be administered prior to challenge to prevent symptoms. Patients are then given this neutralizing solution and are told to utilize it before eating a meal containing the offending food. A number of anecdotal reports claim the accuracy of this treatment, although none is based on prospective, double-blind, well-controlled protocols (22–27). Control studies have been performed by several groups (28–31). These studies report that sublingual provocative food testing did not discriminate between placebo controls and food extracts. Kailin evaluated the effectiveness of sublingual provocative testing by five different physicians, all of whom had been using this method for at least seven years (30). The physicians were allowed to select patients previously tested and known to have positive reactions. On this occasion, however, the sublingual technique was performed according to a double-blind protocol. No distinction was observed between reactions to placebo and to active food extracts. Lehman also reported that the symptoms or signs occurred as frequently after provocation with placebo as with food extracts (31). Critical reviews on both provocation and neutralization have not supported the validity of this technique for diagnosis or treatment (13, 14, 33, 34). As a result of these double-blind, multicenter, controlled investigations, neither the American College of Allergy and Immunology nor the American Academy of Allergy and Immunology could recommend the sublingual provocation technique as a reliable indicator of food allergy or as a treatment (34).

SUBCUTANEOUS TESTING

Subcutaneous provocative testing and neutralization were first described by Lee and colleagues for the diagnosis and treatment of subjects with food allergy (35). Subsequently, this technique has been utilized to evaluate inhalants and chemicals in the environment (36, 37). Additional articles reporting a favorable response in evaluating the food-allergic patient have raised concerns about objectivity, observer bias, appropriateness of controls, and adequacy of statistical methods employed in reaching conclusions (38–40). Miller reported a favorable response in eight subjects to subcutaneous food injections in a double-blind, crossover study (40). The concern with this study centered on the wide variety of symptoms reportedly improved by food neutralization treatment. Concern also arises about the scoring of symptomatic improvement and the statistical analysis of the data.

A study by Monro and associates also deserves comment (41). This group reported improvement in 11 migraine sufferers selected from a group of 280 headache patients. These patients were identified as having mild symptoms with intradermal injections of fixed amounts of food extract and relief with a more dilute injection. This therapeutic dose, translated into a sublingual neutralization dose and given four times a day 20 minutes prior to meals, prevented migraine symptoms. Patients were subsequently supplied with sublingual solutions that contained an unspecified number of potential allergens selected from 50 foods, inhalants, and chemicals. They received two sublingual solutions: one containing the material to which they were sensitive and a placebo. Double-blind conditions were claimed because one independent nonallergic observer was asked to taste the solutions and proved unable to distinguish between them. This entire study hinged on the assertion of one person who was unable to distinguish active from placebo solutions.

Several studies have been unable to confirm the validity and reproducibility of provocation testing (31, 42–44). Crawford and colleagues, in a multigroup study performed on 61 atopic subjects studied with five common foods, could not confirm the validity and reproducibility of results from subcutaneous food testing using symptoms as the end point (42). In addition to studying symptoms, Bronsky and associates evaluated objective signs such as pulse, electrocardiogram, fluctuation in white blood cell count, peak expiratory flow rates, and results of a chest examination in 20 asthmatic children before and after provocation testing with foods (43). They found no correlation of symptom induction or of these measurements with food injection challenges. Draper performed intradermal provocative tests in 121 subjects, followed by deliberate feeding tests (44). He found 38% of the positive intradermal test results could not be confirmed by deliberate feeding and urged that verification of all results be obtained by deliberate feeding. Kailin and Collier studied the ability of the neutralizing dose to relieve symptoms by both subcutaneous and sublingual administration in a double-blind study using saline as the control (30). No difference appeared in the results between saline and aqueous food extracts in their ability to relieve symptoms.

The neutralization procedure based on end-point determination has been suggested to be a "phasic" phenomenon capable of influencing specific immune responses involving antigen processing, immune complex formation, and mediator release in non–IgE-mediated symptoms (45). One dose provokes an immune reaction, a weaker dose neutralizes this response, and an even weaker dose provokes a response again. Some suggest that anti-idiotype downregulation or cellular suppression occurs with the weaker concentrations. Presently, no scientific data support any of these statements. Both the American Academy of Allergy and Immunology and the American College of Allergy and Immunology have stated that subcutaneous and sublingual provocation and neutralization treatment should be reserved for use in only controlled experiments (46). A recent study concluded that "when the provocation of symptoms to identify food sensitivities is evaluated under double-blind conditions, this type of testing, as well as the treatments based on neutralizing such reactions, appears to lack scientific validity. The frequency of positive responses to the injected extracts appears to be the result of suggestion and chance" (47).

Autogenous Urine Immunization

Autogenous urine injection therapy for allergic diseases was introduced by Plesch (48). The data consist of brief case histories from 12 patients who had diverse illnesses, including jaundice, posthepatitis weakness, depression, abdominal pain, constipation, eczema, asthma, hayfever, urticaria, and food allergy. This form of therapy is used by certain physicians who advertise its efficacy to the public. No other articles have been published on this subject in scientific journals since the original article by Plesch. Concern has arisen that this form of treatment might initiate production of antibodies to the glomerular basement membrane capable of causing nephritis, as humans excrete antigens immunologically related to soluble antigens from normal human glomerular basement membrane (GBM) (49). The antigens in human urine appear identical in different normal adults, and they have proved capable of evoking anti-GBM antibodies in sheep (50). In humans, Goodpasture's syndrome is caused by anti-GBM antibodies. Eluting these antibodies from nephritic human kidney and then transferring the antibody to monkeys has produced glomerulonephritis in the monkeys (51). Circulation of anti-GBM antibodies in humans has also resulted in glomerulonephritis in allografted kidneys (52). The California Society of Allergy and Clinical Immunology and the California Blue Shield, aided by the Blue Shield advisory panels on allergy, internal medicine, and dermatology, have stated: "It is the unanimous opinion of members of the advisory panels on allergy, internal medicine, and dermatology that urine injections are not acceptable medical practice in the treatment of allergic diseases" (53). Advisory panel members of the American Academy of Allergy and Immunology agreed with the California Society of Allergy and Clinical Immunology's position paper on this subject. They also emphasized that this treatment modality must be considered experimental until controlled studies prove its benefit and, furthermore, that physicians using urine injection therapy should be encouraged strongly to do such studies (46).

IgG4 and Food Allergy

Considerable controversy exists concerning the role of the IgG4 subclass in allergic diseases. Several studies indicate a role for IgG4 in non–IgE-, mast-cell-mediated diseases, which can be used to support the thesis that this antibody might cause some symptoms of food allergy. Antibodies of the IgG4 subclass have been described as homocytotropic for human basophils and may be the short-term sensitizing antibodies described by Parrish (54). Vijay and Perelmutter reported that human basophils have receptors for IgG4 that can be passively sensitized with IgG4 and that subsequently release histamine on exposure to a specific antigen (55, 56). Fagan and coworkers reported that white cells of 14 nonallergic subjects released histamine when incubated with monoclonal mouse anti-IgG4 antibody, but not when incubated with monoclonal antibodies to the other IgG subclasses (57).

Nagakawa and colleagues were able to reproduce these results using flow cytometry (58). Other investigators, however, have not been able to confirm a role for IgG4 as a homocytotropic antibody capable of causing histamine release from basophils (59–61). The failure of IgG4 to trigger release of mediators from basophils is suspected to be due to the fact that IgG4 is monomeric and, therefore, not capable of cross-linking; it also has low affinity for its receptor (57, 61). Johansson claims that the IgG4 present on basophils is actually directed against IgE (62). Cross-linking may also be accomplished by an IgM rheumatoid factor directed against IgG4 (64). In addition, the ability of some investigators to demonstrate IgG4 receptors, while others cannot, raises the question of whether some IgG4 subtypes can sensitize basophils (65).

Another serious concern about implicating IgG4 in allergic disease is the fact that allergen-specific IgG4 often appears in sera of individuals with no apparent clinical sensitivity to that allergen (66–70). Its presence in both allergic and nonallergic subjects is explained by chronic immune stimulation's ability to synthesize IgG4 antibodies (71–73). Considering the amount of food eaten, it is not surprising that IgG4 antibodies have been demonstrated to foods. Several studies have suggested that IgG4 may play a

role in allergic disease. Clinically increased levels of IgG4 have been described in patients with atopic dermatitis (74) and allergic asthma (75, 76). Bronchial provocation studies have suggested that IgG4 antibodies could be involved in late-onset reactions in allergic patients who fail to show positive prick skin test reactions or RAST results to a specific allergen (77). Rafei and associates studied food-allergic patients by double-blind, oral challenge, skin tests, and determination of IgG4 levels. These preliminary studies suggested a slight correlation between early and late challenge responses and the presence of IgE and IgG (78). This finding, however, may not indicate a pathogenic role for IgG_4, but may indicate a greater antigen load or genetic predisposition to develop an immune response to a specific food. Its presence in the honeybee-allergic patients, as well as in beekeepers who were nonallergic but were frequently stung, and as a response to immunotherapy has stimulated interest in its role as a blocking antibody (72). After performing serial studies in children with a history of immediate allergic reactions to cow's milk, Schwartz and coworkers suggest that the presence of IgG4 alone reflects dietary intake of cow's milk, and the presence of both IgG4 and IgE reflects continuing sensitization in a sensitive individual (79). Additional milk challenges in these children must be performed to confirm this conclusion.

Thus, at present little evidence suggests that IgG4 is responsible for, or contributes to, immediate reactions to foods. Considerable evidence indicates that it is a normal response to ingested foods. Further studies, however, will be necessary to determine whether it is an indicator of those patients who are at risk to develop late reactions to foods and, prove its pathogenic role in these patients, and in those patients who have "outgrown" their food allergy. At present, no apparent clinical value exists in obtaining food-specific IgG4 in the evaluation of a patient suspected of having food-related symptoms.

Food Immune Complexes

Despite a number of nonspecific as well as antigen-specific mucosal barrier mechanisms that limit antigen uptake, experimental and clinical evidence suggests that intact antigens and antigen fragments are capable of traversing the epithelial barrier and stimulating the immune system (80–86). The quantities absorbed—although nutritionally irrelevant—are sufficient for immunization. Both antibody and cell-mediated responses to dietary antigens have been described (87). In most normal children and adults, low titers of serum antibody of different classes and subclasses against dietary proteins occur without evidence of adverse reactions to the ingested food (88, 89). Increased permeability of the gastrointestinal tract to macromolecules has been demonstrated with local antibody IgA deficiency (86, 90), inflammation of the gastrointestinal tract (91), and decreased gastric acidity (92). The predominant antibodies are members of the IgA and IgG classes. For a number of antigens, the dominant subclasses were IgG1 and IgG4. IgG2 and IgG3 antibodies usually existed at low or undetectable levels (93). In subjects with specific serum food antibodies, the subsequent reintroduction of the specific food might be capable of generating immune complexes with the food as the antigen (94–102). These food immune complexes contain IgE, IgG, and IgA antibodies. Paganelli *et al.* (101) and Brostoff *et al.* (103) have suggested that IgA complexes are predominantly formed in nonatopic persons and IgG or IgE complexes in atopic persons. IgG or IgE complexes are not necessarily responsible for symptoms, however (104). Immune complexes have also been found after ingestion of cow's milk by IgA-deficient patients (97). In IgA-deficient patients, a high correlation occurs between the presence of immune complexes and large amounts of circulating antibody. In these patients with large amounts of circulating immune complexes after drinking milk, bovine casein and bovine globulin can be identified within the complex (95, 105). The appearance of these circulating immune complexes in IgA-deficient individuals is not accompanied by any obvious clinical illness, and complement activation has not been demonstrated for a great majority of these patients. An unexplained correlation is noted between IgA deficiency and the appearance of an autoimmune disease. In patients with eczema, immune complexes also appear with higher titers of antibodies (100).

In addition to determining immune complexes after challenges, complement studies have been performed with no reduction of serum C3 or C4 level in children with intestinal cow's milk allergy (106, 107). This aspect, however, should be restudied to determine the presence of complement split products that result from complement activation. These products represent more sensitive indicators of complement activation than C3 or C4 levels.

In evaluating a pathogenic role for immune complexes, one should also consider that they may be formed in situ in the submucosa of the intestinal tract. Their presence in that location may not be associated with detection of circulating immune complexes, but may be responsible for local inflammation. In two infants with cow's milk sensitivity, C3 was demonstrated in jejunal biopsy material obtained 6 to 12 hours after challenge (108). Immune complexes and antigen have also been demonstrated in intestinal biopsy samples from food-allergic patients (109, 110).

In conclusion, immune complex formation is essentially a normal event that occurs in the course of an immune response and allows antigen elimination (111). As assays are now available to measure food immune complexes, it is reasonable to determine their relationship to late allergic reactions to food. The data indicate that further research must be done to determine the size and nature of antigens, duration in circulation, complement-fixing characteristics, location of formation (intravascular versus extravascular), and clearance before conclusions can be drawn concerning their role in food-related diseases and symptoms. Until these studies are performed, commercially available food immune complex tests are not indicated in clinical practice.

Electrodermal Testing

Electrodermal testing is performed with an electrical machine that utilizes a galvanometer to measure the electrical activity of the skin at designated acupuncture points (112, 113). The patient holds the negative electrode in one hand, while the positive electrode is pressed at selected acupuncture points on the skin. Points on the lower extremities are said to relate to food allergy. Food extracts in closed glass vials come in contact with an aluminum plate within the circuit. If touching of the skin by the probe yields a drop in electrical current, the diagnosis of allergy to the food being tested is made. Presently, no theory explains the procedure, nor have scientific or clinical studies documented its use in food allergy. The equipment is expensive and the manufacturer warns that its use in the United States is for investigational purposes only.

Applied Kinesiology

Applied kinesiology involves the testing for a specific food allergen by measuring the patient's muscle strength. Allergens for testing are placed in a sealed glass bottle that the patient holds in one hand while subjective estimates of muscle strength are performed in the opposite arm with and without the suspected food. Typically, the patient extends his or her arm and the investigator determines how far the arm can be pushed down with briefly applied pressure. A decrease in muscle power while the food is held indicates a positive test. For uncooperative infants, a parent is usually tested while holding the child's hand and when holding the food. One published report describes blinded testing to multiple foods in 20 subjects (114). Results were random and not reproducible. This procedure has no credible theory and is without scientific support.

Dietary Manipulation

The determination of food allergy depends on the improvement of symptoms when a food is withdrawn and the precipitation of symptoms when the food is reintroduced. Some writings, however, contain certain controversial terms and speculative phenomena with which physicians should be familiar.

MASKING AND ADDICTION

The controversial statement is sometimes made that allergies to foods consumed every day are more difficult for the patient to recognize because masking

involves the opposite of the expected result. Avoidance or removal of a food to which a patient is sensitive thus creates a transient worsening of the symptoms, whereas eating the food produces initial improvement. Eating a food to reduce or avoid symptoms was termed "food addiction" by Randolph, who explained obesity and alcoholism by this phenomenon (112–114). Although masking in response to aspirin and caffeine is recognized, this phenomenon has not been proved for foods (115).

ROTARY DIET

The rotary diet is based on the belief that the degree of sensitivity to a food relates to its incidence in the diet. Increased frequency of intake thus increases sensitization. The type of reaction is described as "nonfixed" because tolerance to ingestion will occur after prolonged omission (116). For patients with multiple allergies, a rotary diet is utilized in diagnosis and treatment (5). The diet is organized so that no individual food or closely related foods are eaten on consecutive days. It rotates exposure to each individual food family through a four- or five-day cycle. Once established on such a diet and asymptomatic, the patient can introduce foods to determine whether symptoms develop. For some patients, this dietary regimen may be used on a temporary basis to define foods that should be excluded, for other patients, it is a lifelong diet. Although the basis for initially using this diet has not been verified, it can be utilized as an elimination diet. Its disadvantage is its complexity.

FASTING

The complete removal of food for the diagnosis of food allergy was first described by Randolph (113). The fast includes treatments with epsom salts or milk of magnesia to evacuate the bowel. Bottled spring water from multiple sources is allowed, but even toothpaste is eliminated. In analyzing the subjective and objective results of fasting, the profound effects of starvation must be considered. The altered metabolic and endocrine effects of starvation may cause improvement in symptoms, rather than the withdrawal of an allergic food (117–120).

REFERENCES

1. Sampson HA. IgE mediated food intolerance. J Allergy Clin Immunol 1988;81:495–504.
2. Bock SA, Lee WY, Reinego LK, May CD. Studies of hypersensitivity reactions to foods in infants and children. J Allergy Clin Immunol 1987;62:327–334.
3. Women's opinions of food allergies. A Good Housekeeping Institute Report. Consumer Research Department, September 1984.
4. Mandell M, Waller S, Camlon L, Dr. Mandell's five day allergy relief system. New York: Thomas Y. Crowell, 1979.
5. Feingold BE. Why your child is hyperactive. New York: Random House, 1975.
6. Crook WG. The yeast connection. Jackson, TN: Professional Books, 1984.
7. Squier TL, Lee HJ. Lysis in vitro of sensitized leukocytes by ragweed antigen. J Allergy 1947;18:156–163.
8. Black AP. A new diagnostic method in allergic disease. Pediatrics 1956;17:716–724.
9. Bryan WTK, Bryan MP. The application of in vitro cytotoxic reactions to clinical diagnosis of food allergy. Laryngoscope 1960;70:810.
10. Bryan WTK, Bryan MP. Diagnosis of food allergy by cytotoxic reactions. Trans Am Soc Ophthal Otolaryngol Allergy 1967;8:14.
11. Bryan WTK, Bryan MP. Cytotoxic reactions in the diagnosis of food allergy. Otolaryngol Clin North Am 1971;4:523.
12. Bryan WTK, Bryan MP. Allergy in otolaryngology. In: Paparella MM, Shumrick DA, eds. Otolaryngology, vol. 3. Philadelphia: WB Saunders, 1973, 69–94.
13. Golbert TM. A review of controversial diagnostic and therapeutic techniques employed in allergy. J Allergy Clin Immunol 1975;56:170–190.
14. Lowell FC. Some untested diagnostic and therapeutic procedures in clinical allergy. J Allergy Clin Immunol 1975;56:168–169.
15. Van Metre TE. The advancement of the knowledge and practice of allergy. J Allergy Clin Immunol 1979;64:235–241.
16. Franklin W, Lowell FC. Failure of ragweed pollen extract to destroy white cells from ragweed-sensitive patients. J Allergy 1949;20:375–377.
17. Chambers W, Hudson BH, Glaser J. A study of the reactions of human polymorphonuclear leukocytes to various antigens. J Allergy 1958;29:93–102.
18. Lieberman P, Crawford L, Bjelland J, Connell B, Rice M. Controlled study of the cytotoxic food test. JAMA 1974;231:728–730.
19. Benson TE, Arkins JA. Cytotoxic testing for food allergy: evaluations of reproducibility and correlation. J Allergy Clin Immunol 1976;58:471–476.
20. Lehman CW. The leukocytic food allergy test: a study of its reliability and reproducibility. Effect of diet and sublingual food drops on this test. Ann Allergy 1980;45:150–158.
21. Lowell FC, Heiner DC. Food allergy cytotoxic diagnostic technique not proven. JAMA 1972;220:1624–1630.
22. Hansel FK. Allergy and immunity in otolaryngology, 2nd ed. Rochester, MN: American Academy of Ophthalmology and Otolaryngology, 1968, 134–135.
23. Galapeaux EA. Chemical testing and therapy. In: Dickey LD, ed. Clinical ecology. Springfield, IL: Charles C. Thomas, 1976.
24. Hosen H. The relationship of FD&C dyes and respiratory allergy. J Asthma Res 1972;10:131–134.
25. Morris DL. Use of sublingual antigen in diagnosis and treatment of food allergy. Ann Allergy 1971;27:289–294.
26. Dickey LD. Sublingual antigens. JAMA 1971;217:214.
27. Green M. Sublingual provocative testing for food and FD and C dyes. Ann Allergy 1974;33:274.
28. Breneman JC, Crock WC, Deamer W, et al. Report of the Food Allergy Committee on the sublingual method of provocative testing for food allergy. Ann Allergy 1973;31:382–383.
29. Breneman JC, Metzler C, Hurst A, et al. Final report of the Food Allergy Committee of the American College of Allergists on the clinical evaluation of sublingual provocation testing method for diagnosis of food allergy. Ann Allergy 1974;33:164–166.
30. Kailin EW, Collier R. "Relieving" therapy for antigen exposure. JAMA 1971;217:78.
31. Lehman CW. A double-blind study of sublingual provocative food testing: a study of its efficacy. Ann Allergy 1980;45:144–149.
32. Samter M. Sublingual desensitization for allergy not recommended. JAMA 1972;215:1210.
33. Golbert TM. Sublingual desensitization. JAMA 1971;217:1703–1704.
34. Position statements—controversial techniques. J Allergy Clin Immunol 1981;67:333–338.
35. Lee CH, Williams RT, Binkley EL. Provocative testing and treatment for foods. Arch Otolaryngol 1969;90:87.
36. Boris M, Weindorf S, Corriel RN, et al. Antigen induced asthma attenuated by neutralization therapy. Clin Ecology 1985;3:59.
37. Lee CH, Williams RI, Binkley EL. Provocative inhalant testing and treatment. Arch Otolaryngol 1969;90:173.
38. Rinkel HJ, Lee CH, Brown DW, Willoughby JW, Williams JM. The diagnosis of food allergy. Arch Otolaryngol 1964;75:71.
39. Willoughby JW. Provocative food test technique. Ann Allergy 1965;23:543–554.
40. Miller JB. A double-blind study of food extract injection therapy: a preliminary report. Ann Allergy 1977;38:185–191.
41. Monro J, Carini C, Brostoff J. Migraine: is it an allergic disease? Lancet 1984;2:719–721.
42. Crawford LV, Lieberman P, Harfi HA, et al. A double blind study of subcutaneous food testing sponsored by the Food Committee of the American Academy of Allergy. J Allergy Clin Immunol 1976;57:236 (abstract).
43. Bronsky EA, Burkley DP, Ellis EE. Evaluation of the provocative skin test technique. J Allergy 1971;47:104 (abstract).
44. Draper LW. Food testing in allergy: intradermal provocative vs. deliberate feeding. Arch Otolaryngol 1972;95:169.
45. American Academy of Environmental Medicine. Position paper—a new medical specialty designed to identify and treat environmental and ecologic illness, 1984–1985.
46. American Academy of Allergy. Position statements—controversial techniques. J Allergy Clin Immunol 1981;67:333–338.
47. Jewett DL, Fein G, Greenberg MH. A double-blind study of symptom provocation to determine food sensitivity. N Engl J Med 1990;323:429–433.
48. Plesch J. Urine therapy. Medical Press 1947;218:128.
49. McPhaul JJ, Dixon FJ. Basement membrane antigens in serum and urine. Transplant Proc 1969;1:964–967.
50. Lerner RA, Dixon FJ. The induction of acute glomerulonephri-

tis in rabbits with similar antigens isolated from normal homologous and autologous urine. J Immunol 1968;100:1277.

51. Hawkins D, Cochran CG. Glomerular basement membrane damage in immunological induced glomerulonephritis. Immunology 1968;14:665–681.

52. Glassock RJ, Edgington TJ, Watson JL, Dixon FJ. Autologous immune complex nephritis induced with renal tubular antigen. II. The pathogenetic mechanism. J Exp Med 1968;127:573–587.

53. California Medical Association Scientific Board Task Force on Clinical Ecology. Clinical ecology—a critical appraisal. West J Med 1986;144:239–245.

54. Parrish WE. The clinical relevance of heat stable, short term, sensitizing anaphylactic IgG antibodies and of related activities of IgG4 and IgG2. Br J Dermatol 1981;105:223–231.

55. Vijay HM, Perelmutter L. Inhibition of reagin-mediated PCA reactions in monkeys and histamine release from human leukocytes by human IgG4 subclass. Int Arch Allergy Appl Immunol 1977;53:78–87.

56. Vijay HM, Perelmutter L, Bernstein JL. Possible role of IgG4 in discordant correlation between intracutaneous skin tests and RAST. Int Arch Allergy Appl Immunol 1978;56:517–522.

57. Fagan DL, Slaughter CA, Capra JD, Sullivan TJ. Monoclonal antibodies to immunoglobulin G4 induced histamine release from human basophils in vitro. J Allergy Clin Immunol 1982;70:399–404.

58. Nakagawa T, Stadler BM, Heiner DC, Skvaril F, Week AL. Flow-cytometric analysis of human basophil degranulation. II. Degranulation induced by anti-IgE, anti-IgG4 and the calcium ionophore A23187. Clin Allergy 1981;2:21–30.

59. van Toorenenbergen AW, Aalberse RC. IgG4 and passive sensitisation of basophil leukocytes. Int Arch Allergy Appl Immunol 1981;65:432–440.

60. van Toorenenbergen AW, Aalberse RC. IgG4 and release of histamine from human peripheral blood leukocytes. Int Arch Allergy Appl Immunol 1982;67:117–122.

61. Devey ME, Bleasdale KM, French MAH, Harison G. The IgG4 subclass is associated with a low affinity antibody response to tetanus toxoid in man. Immunology 1985;55:565–567.

62. Johansson SGO. Anti-IgE antibodies in human serum. J Allergy Clin Immunol 1986;77:555–557.

63. Aalaberse RC, van der Gaag R, van Leeuwen J. Serologic aspects of IgG4 antibodies. I. Prolonged immunisation results in an IgG4-restricted response. J Immunol 1983;130:722–726.

64. Shakib E. The role of antiglobulins in IgG4 mediated allergic disease. N Engl Regional Allergy Proc 1988;9:35–42.

65. Walten MR, Bird P, Ulaeto DI, Godall DM, Jeffers R. Immunogenic and antigenic epitopes of immunoglobulins, antigenic variants of IgG4 proteins revealed with monoclonal antibodies. Immunology 1986;57:25–28.

66. Merrett J, Burr ML, Merrett TG. A community survey of IgG4 antibody levels. Clin Allergy 1983;13:397–407.

67. Layton GT, Stanworth DR. The quantitation of IgG4 antibodies to three common food allergens by ELISA with monoclonal anti-IgG4. J Immunol Methods 1984;73:347–356.

68. Shakib F, Brown HM, Stanworth DR. Relevance of milk- and egg-specific IgG4 in atopic eczema. Int Arch Allergy Appl Immunol 1984;75:107–112.

69. Nakagawa T. Egg white specific IgE and IgG subclass antibodies and their association with clinical egg sensitivity. N Engl Regional Allergy Proc 1988;9:67–73.

70. Halpern GM, Scott JR, Sun J, Rock HS, Xia ZL. IgG4 antibodies resume levels in normal healthy adults; a follow-up study. J Allergy Clin Immunol 1986;77:124.

71. Vander Giessen M, Homan WL, van Kernebeek G, et al. Subclass typing of IgG antibodies formed by grass pollen allergic patients during immunotherapy. Int Arch Allergy Appl Immunol 1976;50:625–640.

72. Halpern GM. IgG4 as a blocking antibody. Immunol Allergy Pract 1989;11:11–15.

73. Gentlesk MD, Halpern GM, Scott JR, Rock HS, Harris MS. Determination of IgG4 antibodies in treated hymenoptera sensitive patients. N Engl Regional Allergy Proc 1988;9:17–22.

74. Shakib F, McLaughlan P, Stanworth DR, Smith E, Fairburn E. Elevated serum IgE and IgG4 in patients with atopic dermatitis. Br J Dermatol 1977;97:59–63.

75. Gwynn CM, Morrison-Smith J, Leon G, Stanworth DR. Role of IgG4 subclass in childhood allergy. Lancet 1978;1:910–911.

76. Gwynn CM, Morriston-Smith J, Leon G, Stanworth DR. IgE and IgG4 subclass in atopic families. Clin Allergy 1979;9:119–123.

77. Gwynn CM, Ingram J. Bronchial provocation tests in atopic patients with allergen specific IgG4 antibodies. Lancet 1982;1:254–256.

78. Rafei AE, Peters SM, Harris N, Bellanti JA. Diagnostic value of IgG4 measurements in patients with food allergy. Ann Allergy 1989;62:91–93.

79. Schwartz RH, Keefe MW, Harris N. Specific IgG4 and IgE in children with a history of immediate allergic reaction to cow's milk. J Allergy Clin Immunol 1989;83:240.

80. Udall JN, Walker WA. The physiologic and pathologic basis for the transport of macromolecules across the intestinal tract. J Pediatr Gastroenterol Clin Nutr 1982;1:295.

81. Walker WA. Allergen absorption in the intestine: importance for food allergy in infants. J Allergy Clin Immunol 1986;78:1003–1009.

82. Walker WA. Gastrointestinal host defense: importance of gut closure in control of macromolecular transport. CIBA Found Symp 1976;70:201.

83. Walker WA. Pathophysiology of intestinal uptake and absorption of antigens in food allergy. Ann Allergy 1987;59:716.

84. Walker WA, Bloch KJ. Gastrointestinal transport of macromolecules in the pathogenesis of food allergy. Ann Allergy 1983;51:240–245.

85. Walker WA, Isselbacher KJ. Uptake and transport of macromolecules by the intestine: possible role in clinical disorders. Gastroenterology 1974;67:531–550.

86. Cunningham-Rundles C. Selective IgA deficiency and the gastrointestinal tract. Immunol Allergy Clin North Am 1988;8:435–449.

87. Strober W, Brown WR. The mucosal immune system. In: Samter M, Talmage DW, Frank MM, Austen FK, Claman HN, eds. Immunologic disease. Boston: Little, Brown, 1988.

88. Korenblatt RE, Rothberg RM, Minden P, Farr RS. Immune response of human adults after oral and parenteral exposure to bovine serum albumin. J Allergy 1968;41:226–236.

89. Rothberg RM, Farr RS. Anti-bovine serum albumin and anti-alpha lactalbumin in the serum of children and adults. Pediatrics 1965;35:571–588.

90. Buckley RH, Dees SC. Correlation of milk precipitins with IgA deficiency. N Engl J Med 1969;281:465–469.

91. Taylor KB, Truelove SC. Circulating antibodies to milk proteins in ulcerative colitis. Br Med J 1961;2:924–929.

92. Kraft SC, Rothberg RM, Knauer CM, et al. Gastric acid output and circulating anti-bovine serum albumin in adults. Clin Exp Immunol 1967;2:321–330.

93. Urbanek R, Kemeny MD. IgG and IgG subclasses response to dietary antigens in patients with immediate and non-immediate food allergy. Food Allergy 1988;17:71.

94. Delire M, Cambiaso CL, Masson PL. Circulating immune complexes in infants fed on cow's milk. Nature 1978;272:632.

95. Paganelli R, Levinski RJ, Brostoff J, Wrath DK. Immune complexes containing food proteins in normal and atopic subjects after oral challenge and effect of sodium cromoglycate on antigen absorption. Lancet 1979;1:1270–1272.

96. Brostoff J, Carini C, Wrath DG, Paganelli R, Levinsky RJ. Immune complexes in atopy. In: Pepys J, Edwards AM, eds. The mast cells. London: Putnam, 1979.

97. Cunningham-Rundles C, Brandeis WE, Good RA, Day NK. Milk precipitins, circulating immune complexes and IgA deficiency. Proc Natl Acad Sci USA 1978;75:3387–3389.

98. Cunningham-Rundles C, Brandeis WE, Good RA, Day NK. Bovine proteins and the formation of circulating immune complexes in selective IgA deficiency. J Clin Invest 1979;64:272–279.

99. Inganas M, Johansson SGO, Dannaeus A. A method for estimation of circulating immune complexes after oral challenge with ovalbumin. Clin Allergy 1980;10:293–302.

100. Paganelli R, Atherton DJ. Detection of specific antigen within circulating immune complexes: validation of the assay and its application to food antigen–antibody complexes formed in healthy and food-allergic subjects. Clin Exp Immunol 1981;46:44–53.

101. Paganelli R, Atherton DJ, Levinsky R. The differences between normal and milk-allergic subjects in their immune response after milk ingestion. Arch Dis Child 1983;58:201.

102. Leary HL, Halsey JE. An assay to measure antigen specific immune complexes in food-allergy patients. J Allergy Clin Immunol 1984;74:190–195.

103. Brostoff J, Carini C, Wraith DG, Johns P. Production of IgE complexes by allergen challenge in atopic patients and the effect of sodium cromoglycate. Lancet 1979;1:1268–1270.

104. Practice Standards Council. Measurement of circulating IgG and IgE food-immune complexes. J Allergy Clin Immunol 1988;81:758–760.

105. Frick OL. Beta-lactoglobulin in immune complexes in milk-sensitive children. J Allergy Clin Immunol 1982;69:157.

106. Matthews TS, Soothill JF. Complement activation after milk feeding in children with cow's milk allergy. Lancet 1970;2:893–895.

107. Savilohti E. Cow's milk allergy. Allergy 1981;36:73–88.

108. Shiner M, Ballard J, Smith ME. The small intestinal mucosa in cow's milk allergy. Lancet 1975;1:136–140.

109. Shiner M. Ultrastructural features of allergic manifestations in the small intestine of children. Scand J Gastroenterol 1981;70(suppl):49.

110. Bock SA, Remigio LK, Gordon B. Immunochemical localization of proteins in the intestinal mucosa of children with diarrhea. J Allergy Clin Immunol 1983;72:262–268.

111. WHO report of a scientific group. The role of immune complexes in disease. Technical Report Series No. 606. Geneva: WHO, 1977.

112. Tsuei JJ, Lehman CW, Lam FMK, Zhu DAH. A food allergy study utilizing the EAV acupuncture technique. Am J Acupuncture 1984;12:105.

113. Voll R. The phenomenon of medicine testing in electroacupuncture according to Voll. Am J Acupuncture 1980;8:87.

114. Garrow JS. Kinesiology and food allergy. Br Med J 1988;296:1573.

115. Randolph TG. Descriptive features of food addictions, addictive eating and drinking. QJ Studies Alcohol 1956;17:198.

116. Randolph TG. An ecologic orientation in medicine—comprehensive environment control in diagnosis and therapy. Ann Allergy 1965;23:7–22.

117. Randolph TG. The role of specific sugars. The role of specific alcoholic beverages. In: Dickey LD, ed. Clinical ecology. Springfield, IL: Charles C. Thomas, 1976, 310–333.

118. Stevenson DD, Pleskow WW, Simon RA, et al. Aspirin-sensitive rhinosinusitis asthma: a double-blind crossover study of treatment with aspirin. J Allergy Clin Immunol 1984;73:500–507.

119. Rinkel HJ, Randolph TG, Zeller M. Food allergy. Springfield, IL: Charles C. Thomas, 1951.

120. Palmblad J, Levi L, Burger A, et al. Effects of total energy withdrawal (fasting) on the levels of growth hormone, thyrotropin, cortisol, adrenalin, noradrenalin, T4, T3, and rT3 in healthy males. Acta Med Scand 210:15.

121. Landsberg L, Young JB. Fasting, feeding, and regulation of the sympathetic nervous system. N Engl J Med 1978;298:1295–1301.

122. Cahill GF, Sherwood LM, Parris EE. Starvation in man. N Engl J Med 1970;282:668.

123. Cahill GF. Starvation in man. Clin Endocrinol Metab 1976;5:397.

INDEX